Sudden Death in Infancy, Childhood and Adolescence

This unique, comprehensive survey of virtually all aspects of sudden death in infancy and childhood will be an essential reference source for pathologists, clinicians, and lawyers who deal with such cases. Individual sections deal in detail with deaths due to inflicted and non-inflicted injuries and due to natural diseases. This new edition includes 1200 new references, 300 new illustrations, and an extensively revised chapter on sudden infant death syndrome. The intentional injury chapter has additional material on head trauma, the biomechanics of injury, neonaticide, suicide, and subtle and unusual trauma. The chapter on non-intentional injury has also been expanded to reflect more accurately its importance as a cause of death. Deaths in the first week of life are also covered. In addition, this new edition addresses the full range of natural causes of death and their pathological investigation undertaken in light of advances in our understanding of genetic susceptibility and pathophysiology.

Roger W. Byard qualified in medicine in Australia in 1978 and obtained an LMCC in Canada in 1982. He holds fellowships in anatomical pathology in Canada (FRCPC), the UK (FRCPath), and the USA (FCAP), and in family medicine with the Canadian College of Family Physicians (CCFP). He has a specific interest in sudden infant and childhood death. He has written over 270 papers in peer-reviewed journals, and 35 chapters, many of which deal with this subject. He has also presented or co-authored over 200 papers at national and international meetings. In addition to *Sudden Death in Infancy, Childhood and Adolescence* he has co-edited *Sudden Infant Death Syndrome: Problems, Progress and Possibilities* (2001), and is also currently co-editing an encyclopedia of forensic and legal medicine. He has an interest in preventive pathology and coordinates childhood accident prevention through the "Keeping Your Baby and Child Safe Program" in South Australia. Professor Byard has presented workshops on pediatric forensic pathology and medicine in a number of countries in Europe, North America, Africa, and Asia.

From reviews of the first edition

"This is an outstanding book for practitioners, pathologists, and researchers . . . Each chapter reads like a conference in which the pathologist holds the clues and answers questions from the clinician and other investigators from the autopsy table."
R. L. Ariagno, *New England Journal of Medicine*

" . . . the overall impression is of a volume based on sound scholarship and experience."
W. R. Roche, *Lancet*

" . . . a valuable new addition to the literature."
S. Gould, *Archives of Disease in Childhood*

"I highly recommend this book as a unique and indispensable reference for all forensic pathologists."
S. Dana, *American Journal of Forensic Medicine and Pathology*

" . . . it is the book to turn to when faced with the investigation of a sudden death in infancy or childhood, or the interpretation of findings in these cases."
J. Keeling, *Paediatric and Perinatal Epidemiology*

"The authors have produced a single, comprehensive source of information on virtually all aspects of sudden death in infants and children."
From the foreword to the 1st edition by V. DiMaio, Editor in Chief, *American Journal of Forensic Medicine and Pathology*

Sudden Death in Infancy, Childhood and Adolescence

Second Edition

Roger W. Byard

Specialist Forensic Pathologist, Forensic Science
Centre, Adelaide; Clinical Professor, Departments
of Pathology and Paediatrics, University of
Adelaide; Consultant Paediatric Forensic
Pathologist, Child Protection Unit, Women's &
Children's Hospital, Adelaide, Australia

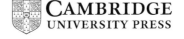
CAMBRIDGE
UNIVERSITY PRESS

PUBLISHED BY THE PRESS SYNDICATE OF THE UNIVERSITY OF CAMBRIDGE
The Pitt Building, Trumpington Street, Cambridge, United Kingdom

CAMBRIDGE UNIVERSITY PRESS
The Edinburgh Building, Cambridge CB2 2RU, UK
40 West 20th Street, New York, NY 10011–4211, USA
477 Williamstown Road, Port Melbourne, VIC 3207, Australia
Ruiz de Alarcón 13, 28014 Madrid, Spain
Dock House, The Waterfront, Cape Town 8001, South Africa

http://www.cambridge.org

First published 2004

Printed in the United Kingdom at the University Press, Cambridge

Typefaces Utopia 8.5/12 pt. and Dax   *System* LATEX 2$_\varepsilon$ [TB]

A catalog record for this book is available from the British Library

Library of Congress Cataloging in Publication data
Byard, Roger W.
Sudden death in infancy, childhood, and adolescence / Roger W. Byard. – 2nd edn
    p.   cm.
Includes bibliographical references and index.
ISBN 0 521 82582 2
1. Sudden death in children.   2. Sudden death in adolescence.   3. Sudden infant death
syndrome.
I. Title.
RJ520.S83B98   2004
618.92′0078 – dc21   2003055126

ISBN 0 521 82582 2 hardback

What greater pain can mortals bear than this;
to see their children die before their eyes?

Attributed to Euripides 480–406 BC

(Russell-Jones, D. L. (1985). Sudden infant death in
history and literature. *Archives of Disease in
Childhood*, **60**, 278–81.)

To Renée, Alice, and Sophie

Contents

Foreword

It is a somewhat daunting task to provide a foreword to such an impressive work of scholarship, which now encompasses a wide spectrum of deaths from birth to early adulthood. I have watched Professor Byard's *magnum opus* develop over a number of years, as I was an examiner for his doctoral thesis from which the first edition of his textbook evolved, and I now see the second edition to be a more extensive expansion of the original work. He can reasonably be considered as the most internationally respected specialist in the realm of sudden childhood death, and this new edition will consolidate his position further.

The area of medicine in which he has chosen to work must be one of the most difficult of all, not only for its scientific and technical problems but also because it contains the interface between the highly emotive issue of death in childhood and the extremely controversial issue of child abuse. Recent years have thrown up trial after trial where fiercely fought legal battles in both criminal and civil courts have raged over allegations of child abuse and child killing. In some of these, the standard of medical evidence has left a great deal to be desired, and ignorance and prejudice have in a few instances undoubtedly led to scandalous miscarriages of justice. Although this book addresses an enormous range of medical conditions, there is no doubt that a substantial part of its utilization will be to clarify the controversies and disputes that exist over the relationship between sudden infant death syndrome (SIDS) and alleged suffocation and other forms of deliberate harm to children. Indeed, Professor Byard has been involved so often in such issues that his original career as a mainstream pediatric pathologist has veered towards forensic pathology, and he is one of the few who have managed to successfully bestride both specialties.

The content of this second edition is even more ambitious and comprehensive than the first. The author has extended his age range down to the moment of birth, deaths in the first week of life formerly being excluded. Young adult deaths are also considered, as there is no true temporal cut-off between some childhood conditions and those of early adulthood.

Together with Stephen Cohle, another well-known expert in the field, the first part of the book deals with trauma. The tricky problem of the nomenclature and semantics of the various categories of injury is addressed at length.

A major part of the work is then devoted to natural disease, generally dealt with in the conventional way by organ systems, though there are caveats about keeping in mind the frequency with which multisystem disorders occur.

SIDS is then considered in great detail, with further warnings about distinguishing sudden death in infancy from SIDS, which too often are confused in the minds of many people. A marked feature of the volume is the increase in both illustrations and references, the latter now virtually providing a total capture of all relevant papers on the subject matter of the book. At the end, there are a series of appendices relating to autopsy practice, with protocols and guidelines for a variety of situations, including SIDS, non-accidental injury, metabolic disorders, infective conditions, and possible poisoning.

A foreword should not be repetitive of either the table of contents or the author's preface, but should attempt to summarize the worth of the book to the medical and also, in this case, the legal communities. There can be no doubt that this second edition, even more than the previous one, is the current international benchmark in the subject – and it is likely to remain so against any potential competitors until the next edition.

Some textbooks, like Gray's *Anatomy* and Greenfield's *Neuropathology*, sit monolithic and enduring in the annals of medicine – and in the turbulent and controversial waters of childhood deaths, Byard's book remains a similar beacon for those who seek guidance.

Professor Bernard Knight, CBE
Cardiff, UK

Preface

The second edition of this text comes at a time when there has been considerable focus by the legal and medical professions and the public on inflicted and non-inflicted injuries in infants and young children. At the same time, there have been substantial developments in the field of pediatric natural diseases, with the discovery of genetic mutations associated with a wide array of disorders. As many of these diseases and injuries may be identified for the first time at autopsy, there is a great need for accuracy in postmortem diagnosis, with appropriate tissue sampling and investigation.

In an attempt to deal with this new information, sections of the text have been defined more clearly, with, for example, separation of sudden infant death syndrome (SIDS) from other conditions that have been grouped under the headings of unintentional trauma, intentional trauma, and natural disease. Much has occurred in the SIDS field over the past decade, with identification of many risk factors resulting in a marked reduction in incidence. However, despite continued research, it still represents a "diagnosis" in search of causal diseases due to its lack of specific pathological features and its heterogeneous etiology. New developments in the areas of non-intentional injury and homicide have also necessitated substantial revision and expansion of this chapter. Several high-profile trials have drawn attention to the complexities of inflicted pediatric trauma and the problems that may arise in attempting to clearly establish causes of death. Thus, the intentional injury chapter has added, or expanded, sections on head trauma, the biomechanics of injury, neonaticide, subtle and unusual trauma, death by starvation, and irresponsible testimony by medical experts. Additional new sections also deal with murder–suicides and suicide.

Extensive referencing has been a deliberate feature of the text in an attempt to provide readers with access to substantial background information to allow them to find out more about individual conditions, many of which are seen rarely in everyday practice. This second edition has over 1200 new references and 300 additional figures.

Despite the somewhat tarnished reputation of the "case report," observational studies remain extremely useful in providing examples of unusual features of a disorder and in illustrating pathophysiological principles. Thus, wherever possible, case descriptions of particular conditions and diseases have been given.

Debate has occurred in recent years concerning the use of terminology such as "accidental" compared with "non-intentional." While there is no doubt that many injuries in children are both non-intentional and preventable, the term "accident" has not been dispensed with completely as it is one that is familiar to readers and is distinct from inflicted injury. The chapter on non-intentional injury has also been expanded to reflect more accurately the importance of non-inflicted trauma as a cause of death in childhood and adolescence, and to demonstrate again the significant role that pathology may play in injury prevention in the community.

Deaths in the first week of life have been included in this edition, and the age range of cases has also been extended into the early twenties in several of the rarer entities, as there is often no difference in the susceptibility to, and manifestations of, disease in this age range compared with adolescence.

On a more theoretical level, we are still no closer to understanding the pathophysiological basis of many conditions, as it is now apparent that mechanisms and mutations causing disease may be as complex and varied as phenotype. Multiple mutations or diverse injuries may have similar manifestations, and the features that we use to diagnose a condition may be coincidental to lethal processes. Unfortunately, tissues and organs have only a relatively limited range of responses to a variety of environmental insults and mutations.

Where does that leave us? On a positive note, it would seem that we are on the threshold of discovering mechanisms for many childhood conditions that will lead us to improve diagnoses and to develop screening tests and treatment regimes. Given the rarity of many of these conditions, thorough postmortems may be essential in identifying cases and enabling further studies to be undertaken.

Pediatric forensic pathology represents a developing discipline that is attempting to apply established forensic techniques to pediatric cases. The step from pediatric hospital to forensic mortuary is not, however, an easy one – conditions are rare and often quite complex, autopsy findings are subtle, and diagnoses may have considerable ramifications beyond the confines of pathology departments. Although the significance of certain findings remains uncertain, this will not stop the need for opinions to be formulated, substantiated, and defended in that most public of forums, the courtroom. Despite these problems, it is hoped that this text may provide some background information and guidance to assist pathologists, clinicians, and lawyers who find themselves dealing with the sometimes uneasy and changing interface of law, pathology, and pediatrics.

Roger W. Byard
Adelaide, Australia
2003

Preface to the first edition

Although there is a considerable body of literature on sudden adult death, there has been less interest in comprehensively classifying rare and diverse causes of sudden death in children. For example, publications dealing with sudden infant death tend to concentrate on sudden infant death syndrome (SIDS), and older children and adolescents are often included in the same series as adults. As well, some series have specifically excluded children who were hospitalized or under one year of age.

This book represents an attempt to redress the perceived deficit in the literature by gathering together in a single text the range of diseases, malformations, and conditions that can cause sudden, and often unexpected, death in both infants and children. Due to the unique nature of the neonatal period, perinatal deaths have not been included, and the age range of cases is generally between one week and 19 years of age.

It is our goal to provide a comprehensive, system-by-system review of a wide range of entities, including both "common" and more arcane disorders, along with illustrations of the conditions and back-up references for further reading. More attention has been paid to some of the rarer conditions that are unique to childhood than to some of the more common conditions found at all ages, as these are described well in general texts. For example, idiopathic arterial calcinosis has deliberately been dealt with in much greater depth than bacterial pneumonia, although the latter is far more common.

While the book has been divided into chapters based loosely on organ systems, a number of conditions may involve multiple systems. In these cases, the most detailed descriptions are to be found in the chapters that seem to deal best with the underlying pathological process that leads to sudden death.

As well as a general text, this book is also intended for use as an autopsy manual for pathologists confronted with an infant or child who has died unexpectedly, by providing protocols and checklists to serve as reminders of more obscure disorders that may otherwise be overlooked in a busy autopsy room.

Unfortunately, the number of disorders that may cause sudden death in childhood is quite vast, ranging from congenital abnormalities of early life to the acquired disorders of early adulthood. While we have attempted to cover as many conditions as possible within the limitations of this short text, some will not have been included, due either to deliberate exclusion or to oversight on the authors' part. As well, due to the professional background and experience of the authors, the text tends to be ethnocentric, with a concentration on diseases and conditions that are found predominantly in Western countries rather than in other areas of the world. We apologize for any omissions. Given these imperfections, we hope that the text will be of practical and theoretical use to physicians and students who are engaged in the practice and study of pediatric medicine and pathology.

RWB, Adelaide, Australia
SDC, Grand Rapids, USA
March 1994

Acknowledgments

I would like to acknowledge and thank pathologists and colleagues at the Forensic Science Centre and the Women's and Children's Hospital, Adelaide, specifically Dr Terry Donald, Dr Ross James, Dr John Gilbert, Dr Hilton Kobus, and Mr David Eitzen, for their continued and much appreciated support. Professor Peter Blumbergs, Dr Tony Bourne, Dr Terry Donald, Det. S/C Rick Fielder, Professor Yee Khong, Dr Jill Lipsett, Dr Lynette Moore, Dr Lloyd Morris, Dr Rebecca Scroop (Adelaide, Australia), Dr Joyce deJong (Grand Rapids, USA), and Professor Cenk Büyükünal (Istanbul, Turkey) are also thanked for contributing photographs and artwork. The permission of Mr Wayne Chivell, South Australian State Coroner, to publish details of cases is also acknowledged gratefully, as is the help of his staff. Dr John Gilbert, Roland Hermanis and the South Australian Police (SAPOL) Physical Evidence and Photographic Sections are also thanked for photographic work.

The extensive update in references was only possible due to the excellent work of Ms Bet Witton, Librarian, Department of Administrative and Information Services, Adelaide. Finally, this text would not have been possible without the continued support and untiring editorial and indexing work of Ms Renée Amyot.

Copyright owners are thanked for permission to use the following previously published photographs and materials: Figures 2.3 and 2.4 – *Am. J. Forensic Med. Pathol.* 2002;23:45–7 ©2002, Lippincott Williams & Wilkins; Figures 2.5 and 2.51 – *J. Clin. Forensic Med.* 2001;8:214–7 ©2001, Churchill Livingstone; Table 2.2, Figures 2.6, 2.7, 2.9, 2.23, 2.44, 2.58, 2.63, 2.69, and 2.74 – *Perspect. Pediatr. Pathol.* 2000;3:405–18 ©2000, Springer-Verlag GmbH & Co. KG; Figures 2.11 and 2.12 – *Arch. Pathol. Lab. Med.* 1992;116:654–6 ©1992, American Medical Association; Figure 2.24 – *Am. J. Forensic Med. Pathol.* 2002;23:45–7 ©2002, Lippincott Williams & Wilkins; Figures 2.26, 2.31, 2.32, 2.35, 2.36, 2.37 and 2.42 – *J. Clin. Forensic Med.* 2001;8:214-17 ©2001, Churchill Livingstone; Figure 2.29 – *Am. J. Forensic Med. Pathol.* 1993;14:296–302 ©1993, Lippincott Williams & Wilkins; Figure 2.30 – *J. Paediatr. Child Health* 2000;36:66–8 ©2000, Blackwell Science Asia; Figure 2.38 – *J. Paediatr. Child Health* 2001;37:201–2 ©2001, Blackwell Science Asia; Figure 2.39 – *J. Paediatr. Child Health* 1997;33:171–3 ©1997, Blackwell Science Asia; Figure 2.41 – *Am. J. Forensic Med. Pathol.* 1995;16:177–80 ©1995, Lippincott Williams & Wilkins; Figure 2.42 – *Forensic Sci. Int.* 1996;83:105–9 ©1996, Elsevier Science; Figures 2.48, 2.55, and 2.57 – *J. Forensic Sci.* 1996;41:438–41 Copyright ASTM International, reprinted with permission; Figure 2.54 – *Pediatr. Pathol.* 1990;10:837–41 – with permission; Figure 2.60 – *Am. J. Forensic Med. Pathol.* 1988;9:252–4 ©1988, Lippincott Williams & Wilkins; Figure 2–68 – *J. Paediatr. Child Health* 2003;39:46–8 ©Blackwell Science Asia; Figures 2.70–2.73 – *Am. J. Forensic Med. Pathol.* 1999;20:73–7 ©1999, Lippincott Williams & Wilkins; frontispiece, Chapter 3 – *Pediatr. Surg. Int.* 1991;6:401–6 – with permission; Figure 3.51 – *J. Forensic Sci.* 1995;40:212–18 Copyright ASTM International, reprinted with permission; Figure 3.65 – *J. Clin. Forensic Med.* 2000;7:6–9 ©2000, Churchill Livingstone; Figure 3.70 – *Am. J. Forensic Med. Pathol.* 2001;22:391–4 ©2001, Lippincott Williams & Wilkins; Figure 4.12 – *Int. J. Pediatr. Otorhinolaryngol.* 1993;28;77–81 ©1993, Elsevier Science; Figure 4.17 – *J. Forensic Sci.* 2002;47:202–4 Copyright ASTM International, reprinted with permission; Figure 4.31 – *Arch. Dis. Child* 1991;66:155–6, with permission; Figure 4.36 – *Surg. Pathol.* 1993;5:55–62 ©1993, Westminster publications; Figure 5.5 – *Am. J. Cardiovasc. Pathol.* 1990;3:333–6, with permission; Color Plate 12 – *Med. Sci. Law* 1997;37;84–7 ©1997, British Academy of Forensic Sciences; Color Plate 12 – *Pediatr. Surg. Int.* 1992;7:464–7, with permission; Figures

6.7, 6.9, and 6.55 – *Cardiovasc. Pathol.* 1996;5:243–57 ©1996, Elsevier Science; Figures 6.13 and 6.15 – *Arch. Pathol. Lab. Med.* 1991;115:770–73 ©1991, American Medical Association; Figures 6.19 and 6.20 – *Pediatr. Pathol.* 1992;12:231–6, with permission; Figure 6.22 – *J. Forens. Sci.* 1991;36:1234–9 – Copyright ASTM International, reprinted with permission; Figure 6.26 – *Pathology* 2001;33:235–8 ©2001, Taylor & Francis, *http://www.tandf.co.uk/journals;* Figures 6.31 and 9.2, and Color Plate 28 – *Med. Sci. Law* 1991;31:157–61 ©1991, British Academy of Forensic Sciences; Figure 6.34 – *Forens Sci. Int.* 1991;51:197–202 ©1991, Elsevier Science; Figures 6.38 and 7.12 – *Eur. J. Pediatr.* 1991;150:224–7 ©1991, Springer-Verlag GmbH & Co. KG; Figure 6.40 – *J. Forensic Sci.* 2001;46:274–7 Copyright ASTM International, reprinted with permission; Figure 6.52 – *Arch. Pathol. Lab. Med.* 1990;114:142–4 ©1990, American Medical Association; Figure 6.49 – *Pediatr. Pathol. Lab. Med.* 1995;15:333–40 ©1995, Taylor and Francis, *http://www.tandf.co.uk/journals;* Figure 6.56 – *J. Forens. Sci.* 1995;40:599–601 Copyright ASTM International, reprinted with permission; Figure 6.57 – *Cardiovasc. Pathol.* 2002;11:296–9 ©Elsevier Science; Figure 7.3 – *Forensic Sci. Int.* 1994;66:117–27 ©1994, Elsevier Science; Figure 7.4a – *Pediatr. Surg. Int.* 1992;7:464–7 with permission; Figures 7.4b and 7.5 – *J. Paediatr. Child Health* 1990;26:12–6 ©1990, Blackwell Science Asia; Figures 7.6 and 7.7 – *Int. J. Pediatr. Otorhinolaryngol.* 1990;20:107–12 ©1990 Elsevier Science; Figures 7.8 and 7.10 – *Am. J. Forensic Med. Pathol.* 1996;17:255–9 ©1996, Lippincott Williams & Wilkins; Figures 8.6, 8.9–8.13, and 8.15 – *Pediatr. Neurosci.* 1991–92;17:88–94 with permission; Figure 8.16 – *J. Forens. Sci.* 1993;38:210–303 Copyright ASTM International, reprinted with permission; Figures 8.20 and 8.21 – *Am. J. Forensic Med. Pathol.* 1996;17:260–63 ©1996, Lippincott Williams & Wilkins; Figure 2.24 – *Am. J. Forensic Med. Pathol.* 2001;22:207–10 ©2001, Lippincott Williams & Wilkins; Figure 8.23 and 8.24 *J. Forens. Sci.* 1991;36:1229–33 Copyright ASTM International, reprinted with permission; Figures 8.26–8.28 – *J. Forens. Sci.* 2001;46:913–15 Copyright ASTM International, reprinted with permission;

Figures 9.10–9.12 – *J. Clin. Forensic Med.* 2001;8:160–62 ©2001, Churchill Livingstone; Figures 10.8–10.10 –*J. Clin. Forensic Med.* 2001;8:81–5 ©2001, Churchill Livingstone; Figure 10–17 – *Can. J. Gastroenterol.* 1989;3:58–60 with permission; Figure 10.21 – *Pathology* 1992;24:170–71 ©1992, Taylor and Francis, *http://www.tandf.co.uk/journals;* Figure 10.26 – *Am. J. Forensic Med. Pathol.* 2000;21:90–92 ©2000, Lippincott Williams & Wilkins; Figure 12.2 – *Am. J. Clin. Pathol.*1990;93:579–82 with permission of the *American Journal of Clinical Pathology*; Figure 13.5 – *J. Clin. Pathol.* 1993;46;108–12 ©1993 BMJ Publishing Group; Figure 13.8 – *Am. J. Clin. Nutr.* 1994;60:189–94 Reproduced with permission by the *American Journal of Clinical Nutrition.* ©*Am. J. Clin. Nutr.*; American Society for Clinical Nutrition. Figure 13.11 – *Am. J. Forensic Med. Pathol.* 2000;21:311–14 ©2000, Lippincott Williams & Wilkins; Figure 13.26 – *Pediatr. Pathol.* 1993;13:53–7 ©1993, Taylor & Francis, *http://www.tandf.co.uk/journals.*

Part I

Introduction

Sudden pediatric death: an overview

Introduction

There have been considerable developments in our understanding of pediatric natural diseases, with many complex genetic links being discovered. More than 900 disease genes have been documented, each of which has from one to many hundreds of mutations. This now places considerable responsibility on pediatric and forensic pathologists to correctly identify diseases that may present as sudden and unexpected childhood deaths, as family screening and genetic counseling may be required (Dietz & Pyeritz, 1994; Goodwin, 1997; Gregersen, Andresen & Bross, 2000).

The pathologist also has to continually evaluate non-inflicted and inflicted trauma, liaising with coroners, product safety experts, and community groups dealing with childhood injury prevention. Preventive pathology refers to this type of activity, with information being taken from the morgue back to the community for use in educational and intervention programs (Byard, 1999; Byard, 2000; Rivara, Grossman & Cummings, 1997a; Rivara, Grossman & Cummings, 1997b). Pathological evaluation of cases of sudden childhood death involves, therefore, considerably more than simple dissection and slide examination.

A question that sometimes arises concerns the definition of terms such as "sudden" and "unexpected," but as long as it is stated clearly how the words are being used then there really should not be any problems in terminology.

How sudden is "sudden?"

The definition of sudden death is quite variable, with different authors setting limits of zero, one, six and 24 hours from the time of onset of symptoms and signs to the time of death. There has again been considerable flexibility in the inclusion of cases in this edition, both from the literature and from personal files, as too rigid an adherence to definitions is impractical and may result in the exclusion of important disease entities. However, generally victims have either been completely well or have been suffering from only an apparently minor illness. If they did have a major illness, then they had been thought to be stable. The common theme uniting all of these cases is that rapid deterioration occurred, culminating in death, although the unavoidable reliance on the presenting history to make this assessment does leave scope for inaccuracy. Quite often the children described in the text were found dead in bed, or suffered a cardiorespiratory arrest while they were engaged in usual activities.

How unexpected is "unexpected?"

It can be argued that the term "unexpected" might not be appropriate to describe death in children who have diseases that are known to be lethal. If this philosophy is applied too rigidly, however, it would be impossible to call a death unexpected in any child suffering from a number of conditions such as Marfan syndrome, tetralogy of Fallot, sickle cell disease, aortic stenosis, myocarditis, and bronchopulmonary dysplasia, to name but a few. The only way to avoid the problems associated with this form of semantic tangle was to avoid the term "unexpected" and to concentrate instead on deaths that occurred suddenly. In this way, cases of sudden death due to fungal thromboemboli in immunocompromised leukemic patients, or due to massive intracranial hemorrhage in patients with brain tumors, could be discussed without having to go into an excessive analysis of whether the case was truly "unexpected." The common feature of these cases is that death occurred before it was anticipated.

What constitutes being "well?"

A child has been accepted as being well, or only mildly unwell, if neither the parents nor the attending physician felt that there was any evidence of serious disease of a type that would require immediate hospitalization or emergency treatment. This will not always be accurate, particularly in cases of parental neglect and in cases of inflicted injury.

Should conditions be described if sudden death has been reported only in adults, or if sudden death in childhood is only a theoretical possibility?

If the clinicopathological features are otherwise similar in all age groups, then it appears reasonable to accept that these entities may be potential, albeit rare, causes of sudden pediatric death.

Overview

Cases fall into three broad groups:

1 Apparently completely well infants and children who suffered an unexpected cardiac arrest/collapse and died within hours, or who were found dead in bed. Examples include certain types of congenital cardiac defects, cerebral hemorrhage, trauma, and sudden infant death syndrome (SIDS).

2 Infants and children who were considered to be mildly unwell and who presented in a similar manner to the first group. Examples include a variety of diverse infectious diseases, such as viral myocarditis, bacterial meningitis, and epiglottitis. A number of infants who succumb to SIDS would also be included in this group, as a history of low-grade fever, upper respiratory tract infection, and non-specific malaise is often elicited. This group also includes (a) children who had minor illnesses completely coincidental to the underlying lethal process, (b) infants who exhibited only relatively minor symptoms and signs of a serious disease, and (c) those in whom major symptoms and signs were either missed or deliberately ignored, as in cases of inflicted injury and neglect. On occasion there may be an additive effect of an acquired disease to a previously established abnormality with lethal consequences, for example an infant with an anomalous coronary artery circulation who decompensates when the added stress of anemia exacerbates myocardial hypoxia.

3 Children with a known serious but stable condition who suddenly die. Examples include children with asthma and epilepsy.

Detailed tables in the following chapters list conditions that are associated with sudden death in the pediatric age group. Some of these conditions are unique to early childhood, usually causing death before the second decade is reached, while others are found more often in later adolescence. Examples of this age-related variability in mortality include certain congenital cardiovascular anomalies, which may manifest within the first few months of life, compared with sudden death in asthma, which tends to occur in later childhood.

Frequency

The incidence of pediatric sudden death is difficult to determine precisely, since there is variability from community to community, and from year to year in the same population (Denfield & Garson, 1990). In addition, death certificate diagnoses are known to be inaccurate, particularly in cases that do not come to autopsy. It has been estimated that sudden natural death in the age range of 1–20 years ranges from 1.1 to 13.8 per 100,000 of the pediatric population per year (Denfield & Garson, 1990; Morentin *et al.*, 2000), accounting for 2–5% of deaths in that group (Berger, Dhala & Friedberg, 1999; Driscoll & Edwards, 1985; Molander, 1982). As for trauma, a study from Melbourne, Australia, reported an overall mortality rate from injury in children aged from 0 to 14 years of 10.6 per 100,000 per year (Nolan & Penny, 1992). This compares with a lethal injury rate of 30.3 per 100,000 per year that has been quoted in the USA for the age range 0–19 years (Guyer & Gallagher, 1985). The sudden death rate is higher in boys than in girls (Gillette & Garson, 1992).

Causes of sudden death

SIDS remains the most common cause of sudden and unexpected death in infancy (one week to one year of age) despite dramatic falls in rates over the past decade (Byard, 1991; Côté, Russo & Michaud, 1999). Over one year of age, the major causes of sudden natural death are malignancies, congenital anomalies, and infections (Corey Handy & Buchino, 1998; Denfield & Garson, 1990; Vetter, 1985).

Infectious disorders that are most commonly associated with sudden pediatric death include myocarditis, meningitis, epiglottitis, bronchopneumonia, bronchiolitis, tracheobronchitis, septic shock, gastroenteritis, and peritonitis. Acute infections were responsible for the greatest number of deaths in a study of 207 sudden deaths in the age range 1–21 years, the median age of death being 4.3 years (Neuspiel & Kuller, 1985).

Cardiovascular anomalies or diseases rank along with infections as major causes of sudden death in childhood, although the age of death tends to be older than for infections, the median age being 16.2 years in the study of Neuspiel & Kuller (1985). The usual cardiovascular disorders are hypertrophic cardiomyopathy, dilated cardiomyopathy, aortic stenosis, congenital coronary artery anomalies, tetralogy of Fallot, Ebstein anomaly, pulmonary

hypertension, mitral valve prolapse, conduction disturbances, and Eisenmenger syndrome (Klitzner, 1990). The relative percentages of these entities depend on the particular series. For example, while Topaz & Edwards (1985) found mitral valve prolapse to be equal in frequency to myocarditis (24%), with only 4% of cases having aortic stenosis, Lambert and colleagues (1974) found an incidence of 18% for aortic stenosis with only one case of "myxomatous" mitral valve disease. Sudden death following surgery in children with congenital heart defects, particularly tetralogy of Fallot and transposition of the great vessels, also accounts for a significant number of cases (Vetter, 1985).

The most likely etiology for sudden death in young athletes or children engaged in strenuous physical activity is cardiovascular. For example, Maron and colleagues (1980) found a structural cardiovascular anomaly in 28 of 29 competitive athletes aged between 13 and 30 years who died suddenly. The most common abnormality in that series was hypertrophic cardiomyopathy (48%), contrasting with a similar study by Corrado and colleagues (1990), in which the most common abnormality found was right ventricular dysplasia (27%). Whether this variability in results reflects a difference in the populations studied, a difference in diagnostic practice, or a difference in the pattern of referral of autopsy cases for review is difficult to ascertain.

Other "common" causes of sudden pediatric death include epilepsy, intracranial hemorrhage, and asthma (Kitada, Nakagawa & Yamaguchi, 1990; Neuspiel & Kuller, 1985; Norman, Taylor & Clarke, 1990). Less usual causes involve hematologic, gastrointestinal, genitourinary, metabolic, endocrine, genetic, and immunologic disorders.

Use of the term "accident" has been discouraged in recent years by some clinicians as it is argued that most injuries are predictable and preventable (Davis & Pless, 2001). Certainly there is merit in this view, but not all injuries are preventable and most people have a clear concept of what is meant when the term "accident" is used. Additionally, standard categories for the manner of unnatural death in forensic terminology are homicide, suicide, accident, and undetermined. For these reasons, the term "accidental death" has continued to be used in this edition until a comparable and generally accepted term has been devised.

Deaths due to accidents (i.e. traumatic episodes arising from non-inflicted injury) in children are most often caused by traffic accidents and drowning; other causes of injury in the pediatric age range include burns, scalds, falls, poisoning, choking, and non-accidental trauma (Nolan & Penny, 1992; Norton, 1983).

The percentage of cases of sudden death in childhood that remain unexplained even after an autopsy has been conducted will vary greatly depending on the rigor with which the postmortem examination has been conducted and the significance that is subsequently attached to the findings. The cases that are left serve to highlight the inadequacy of investigations into childhood death and the insensitivity of standard pathological techniques in ascertaining the cause of certain pediatric fatalities.

REFERENCES

Berger, S., Dhala, A. & Friedberg, D. Z. (1999). Sudden cardiac death in infants, children, and adolescents. *Pediatric Clinics of North America*, **46**, 221–34.

Byard, R. W. (1991). Possible mechanisms responsible for the sudden infant death syndrome. *Journal of Paediatrics and Child Health*, **27**, 147–57.

Byard, R. W. (1999). Preventative pathology and childhood injury. *Injury Prevention*, **5**, 292–3.

Byard, R. W. (2000). Accidental childhood death and the role of the pathologist. *Pediatric and Developmental Pathology*, **3**, 405–18.

Corey Handy, T. & Buchino, J. J. (1998). Sudden natural death in infants and young children. *Clinics in Laboratory Medicine*, **18**, 323–38.

Corrado, D., Thiene, G., Nava, A., Rossi, L. & Pennelli, N. (1990). Sudden death in young competitive athletes: clinicopathologic correlations in 22 cases. *American Journal of Medicine*, **89**, 588–96.

Côté, A., Russo, P. & Michaud, J. (1999). Sudden unexpected deaths in infancy: what are the causes? *Journal of Pediatrics*, **135**, 437–43.

Davis, R. M. & Pless, B. (2001). BMJ bans "accidents". *British Medical Journal*, **322**, 1320–21.

Denfield, S. W. & Garson, A., Jr (1990). Sudden death in children and young adults. *Pediatric Clinics of North America*, **37**, 215–31.

Dietz, H. C. & Pyeritz, R. E. (1994). Molecular biology – to the heart of the matter. *New England Journal of Medicine*, **330**, 930–32.

Driscoll, D. J. & Edwards, W. D. (1985). Sudden unexpected death in children and adolescents. *Journal of the American College of Cardiology*, **5**, 118–21B.

Gillette, P. C. & Garson, A., Jr. (1992). Sudden cardiac death in the pediatric population. *Circulation*, **85**, I64–9.

Goodwin, J. F. (1997). Sudden cardiac death in the young. A family history of sudden death needs investigation. *British Medical Journal*, **314**, 843.

Gregersen, N., Andresen, B. S. & Bross, P. (2000). Prevalent mutations in fatty acid oxidation disorders: diagnostic considerations. *European Journal of Pediatrics*, **159** (Suppl 3), S213–18.

Guyer, B. & Gallagher, S. S. (1985). An approach to the epidemiology of childhood injuries. *Pediatric Clinics of North America*, **32**, 5–15.

Kitada, M., Nakagawa, T. & Yamaguchi, Y. (1990). A survey of sudden death among school children in Osaka prefecture. *Japanese Circulation Journal*, **54**, 401–11.

Klitzner, T. S. (1990). Sudden cardiac death in children. *Circulation*, **82**, 629–32.

Lambert, E. C., Menon, V. A., Wagner, H. R. & Vlad, P. (1974). Sudden unexpected death from cardiovascular disease in children. A cooperative international study. *American Journal of Cardiology*, **34**, 89–96.

Maron, B. J., Roberts, W. C., McAllister, H. A., Rosing, D. R. & Epstein, S. E. (1980). Sudden death in young athletes. *Circulation*, **62**, 218–29.

Molander, N. (1982). Sudden natural death in later childhood and adolescence. *Archives of Disease in Childhood*, **57**, 572–6.

Morentin, B., Aguilera, B., Garamendi, P. M. & Suarez-Mier, M. P. (2000). Sudden unexpected non-violent death between 1 and 19 years in north Spain. *Archives of Disease in Childhood*, **82**, 456–61.

Neuspiel, D. R. & Kuller, L. H. (1985). Sudden and unexpected natural death in childhood and adolescence. *Journal of the American Medical Association*, **254**, 1321–5.

Nolan, T. & Penny, M. (1992). Epidemiology of non-intentional injuries in an Australian urban region: results from injury surveillance. *Journal of Paediatrics and Child Health*, **28**, 27–35.

Norman, M. G., Taylor, G. P. & Clarke, L. A. (1990). Sudden, unexpected, natural death in childhood, *Pediatric Pathology*, **10**, 769–84.

Norton, L. E. (1983). Child abuse. *Clinics in Laboratory Medicine*, **3**, 321–42.

Rivara, F. P., Grossman, D. C. & Cummings, P. (1997a). Injury prevention. First of two parts. *New England Journal of Medicine*, **337**, 543–8.

Rivara, F. P., Grossman, D. C. & Cummings, P. (1997b). Injury prevention. Second of two parts. *New England Journal of Medicine*, **337**, 613–18.

Topaz, O. & Edwards, J. E. (1985). Pathologic features of sudden death in children, adolescents, and young adults. *Chest*, **87**, 476–82.

Vetter, V. L. (1985). Sudden death in infants, children, and adolescents. *Cardiovascular Clinics*, **75**, 301–13.

Part II

Unintentional trauma

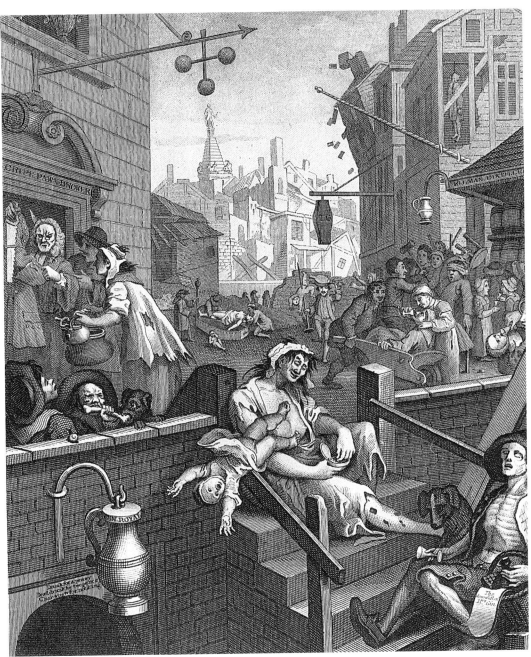

Gin Alley, a nineteenth-century etching by Hogarth, which demonstrates vividly the dangers to infants from trauma associated with poverty and poor living conditions.

Accidents

with Stephen D. Cohle

Forensic Pathologist, Spectrum Health, Grand Rapids, Michigan, USA

Introduction

Accidents account for nearly half of all deaths of individuals aged from one to 24 years old in the USA – 25,814 of 54,239 in 1987 (*Accident Facts*, 1990). Accidents cause only 3% of deaths in infants less than one year of age, but cause 71% of deaths in those aged 15–19 years. At all ages motor vehicle crashes account for a significant percentage of non-intentional deaths (Johnston, Rivara & Soderberg, 1994), from 23% in infants under one year to 80% of deaths in the 15–19-year group. These results are summarized in Table 2.1. Generally, the term "adolescence" refers to the 13–19-year-old age group and "young adulthood" after this.

In the *Accident Facts* survey, suffocation was the second leading cause of death in infants under one year of age. In older age groups, drowning was next to motor vehicle accidents (MVAs). Firearm deaths were the third major cause of accidental deaths in 15–19-year-olds in the USA. About half of drownings and motor vehicle-related deaths involve alcohol (Rosenberg, Rodriguez & Chorba, 1990).

Injury mortality for those aged between one and 19 years from 1984 to 1986 in the USA exceeded that of other countries, with an overall mortality rate of 30.5/100,000 of the population, compared with 26.1/100,000 for Canada, 22.3 for Norway, 21.5 for France, 15.6 for England and Wales, and 13.1 for the Netherlands (Williams & Kotch, 1990). In Australia more recent data on accidental death show a mortality rate of 10.8/100,000 for children under four years, 5.3/100,000 in five- to nine-year-olds, 6.4/100,000 in 10–14-year-olds, and 29.2 in 15–24-year-olds (National Injury Surveillance Unit, 1995). Again, drowning and motor vehicle deaths account for the majority (65%) of cases (Pitt, Balanda & Nixon, 1994).

In North Carolina Runyan and colleagues (1985) found fires and burns to be the leading cause of death due to non-inflicted injuries in the under four years age group, followed by motor vehicle accidents, pedestrian injuries, suffocation, and drowning. In the 15–19 years age group, motor vehicle fatalities and drowning were the major causes of death, with suicides and homicides also accounting for many deaths in that age group. Of 267 children with life-threatening injuries treated at a regional trauma center, 55% were injured in motor vehicle accidents, 27% were hurt in falls, 10% were due to sports and other injuries, and 8% were assault victims. In 75% of the motor vehicle accidents, the child was a pedestrian. Fifty one percent of those injured had involvement of one organ system, 29% two organ systems, and 20% three or more organ systems. Fourteen of the 17 deaths resulted from head injury, primarily accounting for the mortality of 6.7% (Colombani *et al.*, 1985).

In Peclet and colleagues' study (1990) of 3472 children up to 14 years of age admitted to an urban trauma center, traffic-related injuries accounted for 29% of all patients. School-age children (5–10 years) tended to have falls and traffic-related injuries. Child abuse, drowning, and penetrating injuries accounted for 5% of all injuries but 40% of all deaths. Seventy five percent of the deaths in this study involved head injury.

Table 2.1. Types of accidental deaths by age (percentages) (derived from *Accident Facts*, 1990)

	Age (years)				
	<1	1–4	5–9	10–14	15–19
Percentage of deaths due to accidents	3	39	48	48	55
Motor vehicle accidents	23	34	55	59	80
Drownings	13	23	15	13	6
Fires, burns	11	24	13	5	1
Firearms	<1	1	3	7	3
Poisoning	2	1	1	<1	1
Falls	4	2	1	1	1
Mechanical suffocation	19	2	2	3	1
Other accidents	28	13	9	11	7

There is marked variability between communities in the rates of childhood gunshot deaths. For example, in 1992 firearms were responsible for 72% of homicides in the 10–14-years age group in the USA (O'Donnell, 1995), but in Australia such deaths are rare. A significant, although small, number of childhood firearm homicides in a study from South Australia were perpetrated by parents in murder/suicide situations (Byard *et al.*, 1999b).

Accidental deaths occurring during the first year of life have been described by Corey and colleagues (1992) and also in a study produced by the New York State Department of Health (1991). Corey and colleagues reported 36 unintentional deaths in this age group over an 11-year period. Nineteen (53%) died from asphyxia: eight were in mechanically unsafe sleeping environments, six were overlaid, three suffocated in plastic bags, and two asphyxiated on foreign objects. Four (11%) drowned, three (8%) each died in house fires, of scald burns, and in motor vehicle accidents, two (6%) died of hypothermia, one (3%) fell from a height, and one (3%) died of alcohol toxicity. The New York study found that injuries were the third leading cause of death after perinatal conditions and congenital anomalies. Between 1984 and 1988 there were 343 deaths due to injury in this series. Homicide accounted for 116 (34%) deaths. Of the remaining 227 deaths, the intention was unknown in

71, and these were not described further. Of the remaining 156 deaths, 39 (25%) were caused by fires and 60 (38%) were caused by asphyxia: 27 by suffocation, 22 by choking on food, and 11 by choking on a foreign object. Nineteen (12%) died in motor vehicle accidents, 15 (10%) drowned, and 23 (15%) died of miscellaneous causes. Infants and young children are particularly vulnerable to injury or death due to their high dependency, and may be at particular risk if a carer dies or becomes incapacitated. For example, three deaths occurred in South Australia in children aged one, two and a half, and three years, respectively, due to dehydration when children became trapped in houses with carers who had died (Byard, 2002) (Figure 2.1).

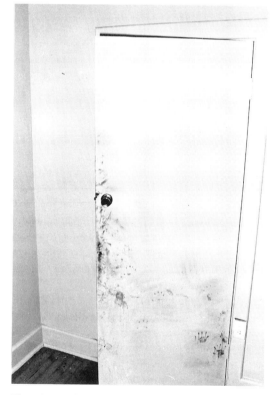

Figure 2.1 Handprints left on a closed bedroom door by a 2.5-year-old boy who was unable to reach the handle. Both the boy and his one-year-old brother died of dehydration in the room after their mother had died in bed of epilepsy.

Table 2.2. Details of 369 cases of accidental death of children aged from 0 to 16 years in South Australia from 1963 to 1996

Category	n	Male	Female	Age range	Mean
Motor vehicle accident					
Unspecified	66	35	31	1–14 years	6 years 5 months
Passenger	27	13	14	1 month–13 years	4 years 9 months
Pedestrian	69	47	22	6 months–15 years 11 months	7 years 5 months
Cyclist	24	17	7	5 years 7 months–15 years 8 months	10 years 2 months
Motorcyclist	3	2	1	6 years 6 months–13 years	9 years 10 months
Drowning	63	46	17	3 months–12 years 8 months	3 years 6 months
Cot/bed asphyxia	40	25	15	1 month–4 years	10 months
Fire/flame/scald	24	11	13	1 year 1 month–14 years 2 months	5 years 1 month
Foreign body aspiration	14	12	2	3 months–8 years	2 years 2 months
Poisoning	10	5	5	1 year 1 month–6 years	2 years 9 months
Farm-related*	10	6	4	2 years 6 months–11 years 6 months	4 years 10 months
Electrocution	6	4	2	2 years–12 years	5 years 8 months
Other asphyxia	5	5	0	3–9 years	5 years 5 months
Sporting	4	4	0	3 years 9 months–14 years 10 months	9 years 3 months
Falls	2	1	1	3 years 2 months–14 years	8 years 7 months
Industrial	1	0	1	9 years 6 months	9 years 6 months
Train	1	1	0	12 years 4 months	12 years 4 months
Total	369	234	135	1 month–15 years 11 months	5 years 2 months

*In addition, there were five other deaths on farms included in other categories: two asphyxias, one drowning, one incineration, and one motorcycle accident.

As a background to this chapter, two studies were undertaken. In the first, pediatric autopsies (age 16 years and younger) performed in Grand Rapids, Michigan, USA, from 1983 to September 1991 were reviewed. A total of 568 children were autopsied, including 330 natural deaths, 168 accidents, 42 homicides, and 15 suicides. The manner of death in 13 cases was indeterminable. The 168 accidental deaths serve as the focus for this chapter. Under the Michigan Medical Examiner Law, all sudden and unexpected deaths and all unnatural deaths (accidents, suicides, and homicides) must be investigated by a physician medical examiner, who, as part of his or her investigation, may order an autopsy. These 168 autopsies were thus ordered by the investigating medical examiner. There were 44 cases of craniocerebral trauma (defined as fatal injury to the head or neck), 38 cases of multiple injuries (defined as serious or fatal injuries involving at least two different areas, e.g. head and chest), 30 cases of asphyxia, 26 drownings, 22 fire deaths, and eight miscellaneous causes of death.

In the second study, a review of 369 cases of non-intentional childhood deaths occurring in South Australia over a 34-year period from 1963 to 1996 was undertaken (Byard, 2000; Byard, 2001). In South Australia, which has a population of approximately 1.5 million people, all violent or unusual deaths are reported to the State Coroner. Children's autopsies were performed at the Forensic Science Centre or the Adelaide Children's Hospital. Of the 369 cases, there were 189 motor vehicle accidents, 63 drownings, 40 sleeping accidents, 24 fire/flame/scalds, 14 foreign body aspirations, 10 poisonings, six electrocutions, five miscellaneous asphyxias, four sports-related deaths, two falls, one industrial death, and one train death. Fifteen of the deaths occurred on farms. The details are summarized in Table 2.2.

Multiple injuries

Road accidents

Motor vehicle drivers and passengers

Thirty-seven children in the Michigan study died of multiple injuries. The types of injuries found were determined largely by the circumstances and speed of impact, with characteristic head, chest, and abdominal trauma. Three of the deceased, all 16-year-old boys, were the drivers of motor vehicles, of whom two were at fault. It is unknown whether seatbelts were worn in two cases, and seatbelts were not used in one case. One driver ran a stop sign and was hit by a truck, one was hit head-on by another automobile, and the third failed to negotiate a curve and was ejected as his car rolled. The speed was unknown in each case.

Eleven children were passengers in a motor vehicle. They ranged in age from three weeks to 16 years, with a mean age of 10.5 years. There were five males and six females. Two were wearing seatbelts, eight were not, and in one case seatbelt use is unknown. In five cases the driver was at fault, in one case the driver was not at fault, and in five cases fault is unknown. In one case the speed at the time of the crash was at or just under 72 kph (45 mph), three accidents were "high speed" (greater than the highway speed limit of 105 kph (65 mph)), and in seven cases the speed was unknown.

Of the 37 children with multiple injuries, 33 had head injuries, 33 had chest injuries, and 31 had abdominal injuries. Twenty-nine had head injuries that would have been fatal in isolation. Included in this number were nine children with atlanto-occipital fracture-dislocations and associated pontomedullary lacerations or transections; six of these were motor vehicle passengers, two were pedestrians hit by motor vehicles, and one was a cyclist hit by an automobile. Fifteen had rib fractures, seven had aortic lacerations or transections, six had cardiac lacerations (Figure 2.2), and 28 had pulmonary contusions or lacerations. Twenty-two children had liver lacerations and 21 had splenic lacerations. Of the 11 drivers and passengers on whom

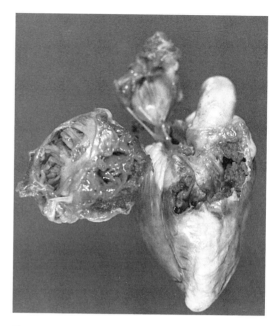

Figure 2.2 Multiple cardiac lacerations with avulsion of the infundibulum from a crush injury of the chest sustained when a 14-year-old cyclist was dragged for half a mile beneath a dump truck.

information was available, two wore seatbelts and nine did not.

Several recent cases from South Australia have demonstrated additional unusual mechanisms of death that may occur in vehicle accidents, including two children who suffered lethal aortic and carotid artery injuries from seat belts (Figures 2.3 and 2.4), a 16-year-old boy who was trapped in a vehicle and exposed to significant amounts of gasoline vapor, and a 12-year-old boy who asphyxiated when the truck that he was traveling in overturned, filling the cabin with soil (Figure 2.5) (Byard *et al.*, 2002a; Hanson *et al.*, 2002; Riches *et al.*, 2002). A breakdown of childhood motor vehicle passenger fatalities per age group is provided in Figure 2.6.

Pedestrians

Sixteen pedestrians were killed during the period of the Michigan study. Their ages ranged from two to 16 years, with a mean age of six years. There were

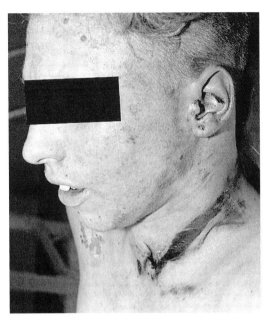

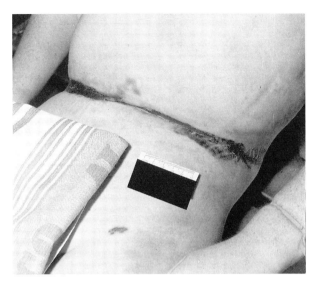

Figure 2.4 Deeply indented and parchmented abrasion across the abdomen of a 10-year-old boy corresponding to the position of a lap seatbelt, which transected his aorta.

Figure 2.3 Oblique parchmented abrasion on the left side of the neck of a 15-year-old boy corresponding to the position of a lap-shoulder seatbelt, which transected his underlying common carotid artery.

10 boys and six girls. Ten children (with a mean age of four years) ran into the path of a vehicle, two were run over in a driveway, two were killed by the same out-of-control automobile while they were on the sidewalk, one was struck from behind by an at-fault vehicle, and one jumped off a snowmobile and was hit by a car.

The most common lethal injury in childhood pedestrians in a South Australian study involved the head in 91.2% of cases, followed by the abdomen in 50%, the chest in 47.1%, and the neck in 38.2% (Byard *et al.*, 2000a). The injuries were often severe, resulting in rapid death, with the most significant injury combinations involving the head, chest, and abdomen in 14.7% of children, the head and chest in 11.8%, and the head, neck, and abdomen in 11.8%. Significant chest injuries may occur in children without related rib fractures due to the elasticity of the chest wall in the young (Pollak & Stellwag-Carion, 1991; Nakayama, Ramenofsky & Rowe, 1989). Limb injuries tended to not be life-threatening and occurred in

88% of cases (Byard *et al.*, 2000a). As in the Michigan study, a distinct subgroup was also identified of younger children who were backed over by vehicles, often driven by a parent, in the home driveway (Byard *et al.*, 2000a; Roberts, Kolbe & White, 1993; Winn, Agran & Castillo, 1991). A breakdown of childhood pedestrian fatalities per age group is provided in Figure 2.7.

Bicyclists/motorcyclists

Seven children in the Michigan study riding bicycles or motorcycles died of multiple injuries, including soft tissue damage (Figure 2.8 and Color Plate 1). They ranged from five to 16 years, with a mean age of 11 years. There were six boys and one girl. Six rode their bicycle into the path of a motor vehicle and thus were at fault. One was hit by a truck; fault could not be determined. A breakdown of cyclist fatalities per age group is provided in Figure 2.9.

Mechanisms of blunt force injury

The mechanisms of blunt force injury to the chest and abdomen have been summarized by Cooper &

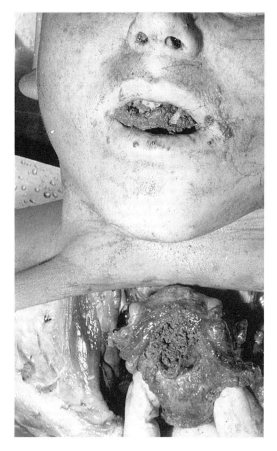

Figure 2.5 Filling of the upper aerodigestive tract with soil in a 12-year-old boy following a vehicle rollover.

Taylor (1989). When blunt force is applied to the body wall, there is inward displacement, which is the primary mechanism of energy transfer and thus of injury. Experiments in which the torsos of swine were struck with blunt objects have shown that there is very little rebound velocity, indicating that the body is very viscous. This viscoelasticity means that displacement upon impact loading is rate-dependent. The rate and magnitude of body wall distortion determine the type and severity of internal injury.

A slow velocity of compression (>20–50 ms) usually causes little or no injury even in the face of severe inward displacement, while rapid compression

(<5 ms) may produce serious internal injury with compression of only 3–4 cm. The likelihood of sustaining injury depends upon mechanical failure of tissues and the propagation of different types of waves (stress waves, shock waves, and shear waves) into the body cavities, as well as on crush injury (Cooper & Taylor, 1989).

Stress (compression) waves can produce small but rapid distortions of tissue (strain). In organs such as lung and bowel, in which there are large differences in material properties (e.g. air and tissue), the pressure differentials cause capillary hemorrhage, hence intestinal and pulmonary contusions result from stress waves. There are two actions of stress waves that tend to cause indirect injuries: (1) reflection from surfaces such as a bronchus or the mediastinum causing at least a doubling of pressure at the surface, and (2) synergistic action after reflection producing focally high pressures within the body away from the body surface and the site of impact. For example, a blow to the lateral chest wall may cause maximum injury to the hilar portion of the lung. Stress waves are the most common mechanism of injury in high-speed (>106 kph or 66 mph) accidents (Cooper & Taylor, 1989). The inward movement of the body wall generates the stress wave, but the peak velocity of the body wall determines the severity of injury (Cooper & Taylor, 1989).

Shock waves are high-pressure, high-velocity waves traveling faster than the speed of sound in the tissue. This type of wave tends to occur with explosions (Cooper & Taylor, 1989).

Shear waves are transverse waves of long duration and low velocity. Internal injury from a body wall impact may result from collision of viscera with stiff structures, asynchronous motion of adjacent connected structures, or stretching (strain) at sites of attachment. Shearing can result in contusion or laceration, including laceration of the mesentery, the splenic pedicle, the liver at the falciform ligament, and the aorta at the ligamentum arteriosum. Shear injuries are characterized by marked displacement of the body wall over a relatively long period of time. These injuries require significant momentum (mass × velocity) and are the most common type of

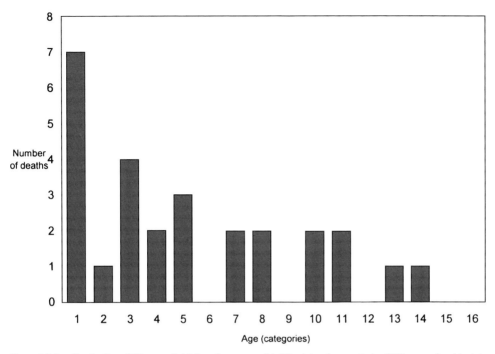

Figure 2.6 Age distribution of 27 cases of childhood passenger fatalities taken from a study of 369 cases of accidental childhood death in South Australia, showing reduced vulnerability with increasing age (1 = first year).

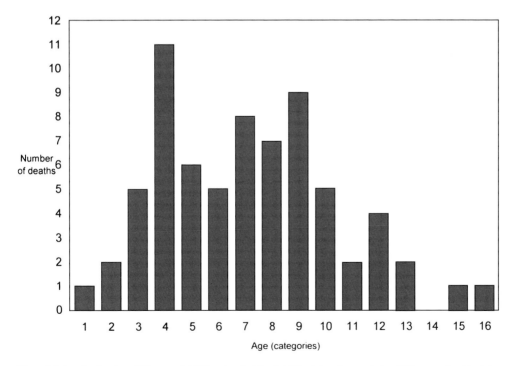

Figure 2.7 Age distribution of 69 cases of childhood pedestrian fatalities taken from a study of 369 cases of accidental childhood death in South Australia, showing increased risk between the fourth and ninth years of life (1 = first year).

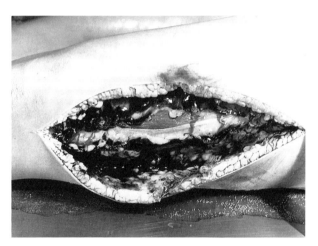

Figure 2.8 Crush injury of the lateral aspect of the thigh in a nine-year-old cyclist hit by a car.

impact injury associated with low-velocity (<53 kph or 33 mph) motor vehicle accidents (Cooper & Taylor, 1989).

Crush injuries result from the application of large, relatively static loads to the body, as might cause compression of the anterior abdominal wall to the retroperitoneum (Cooper & Taylor, 1989).

Aortic injuries

Aortic lacerations from blunt force injuries range in incidence from 2.1% of all children aged 16 years or younger dying of accidental injuries (Eddy *et al.*, 1990) to 26% of people of all ages (average age 39 years) dying in accidents (Allgood, Scholten & Cohle, 1990). Most aortic lacerations are received in motor vehicle crashes. In the series of Eddy and colleagues (1990), child pedestrians most frequently suffered aortic lacerations, followed by motor vehicle occupants, as shown in Table 2.3. In all series, the ligamentum arteriosum (isthmus) of the aorta was the most common site of laceration (Figure 2.10), followed by the ascending aorta. None of the motor vehicle occupants in Eddy and colleagues' series (1990) were restrained, and 58% of the patients in Allgood and colleagues' series (1990) were unrestrained. Of the three children in the Michigan study about whom

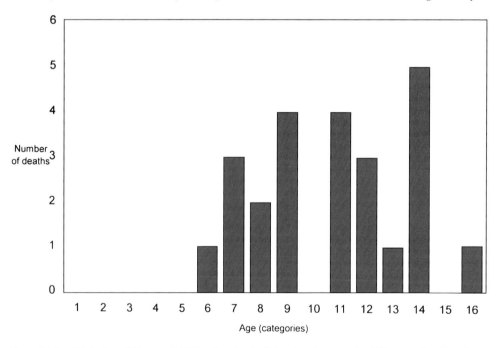

Figure 2.9 Age distribution of 24 cases of childhood cycling fatalities taken from a study of 369 cases of accidental childhood death in South Australia, showing an increased risk in early adolescence (1 = first year).

Table 2.3. Characteristics of fatal aortic injuries

	Reference		
	Eddy *et al.* (1990)	Parmley *et al.* (1958)	Allgood *et al.* (1990)
Age (years)	≤16	18–85	39 (mean)
Incidence	12/551 (2.2%)	275/1174 (23%)	113/443 (26%)
Motor vehicle occupant (%)	38	58	72
Pedestrian (%)	46	6	11
Other (%)	15	36	17
Ligamentum arteriosum (%)	75	45	50
Ascending aorta (%)	17	23	9
Aortic arch (%)	8	8	0
Other site (%)	0	24	31

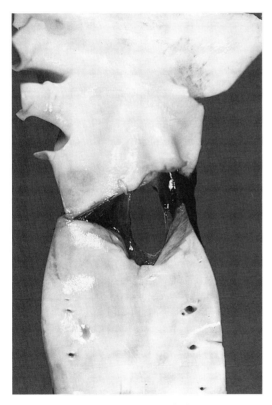

Figure 2.10 Transection of the aorta at the ligamentum arteriosum in a motor vehicle driver. The left subclavian and left internal carotid arteries are above, with paired intercostal arteries below.

information is available, two were not wearing seatbelts. Aortic laceration may also rarely be caused by seatbelt webbing (Riches *et al.*, 2002).

The speed in four of the five cases in which it could be estimated was greater than 86 kph (55 mph) in Eddy and colleagues' series (1990), the average speed in 19 of Allgood and colleagues' (1990) cases was 87 kph (56 mph), and the mean velocity in eight of the cases reported by Newman & Rastogi (1984) was 61 kph (38 mph).

Aortic ruptures extend horizontally, usually at the isthmus. If the adventitia, the strongest layer of the aortic wall, is not lacerated, rupture may be delayed. Failure to rupture may result in pseudoaneurysm formation. There are four different types of force that may tear the aorta: horizontal deceleration, vertical deceleration, severe chest compression, and massive crush injury (Culliford, 1989). Horizontal deceleration, as occurs in a motor vehicle crash, causes shearing of the aorta at the ligamentum arteriosum, which is located at the junction of the fixed descending aorta and the relatively mobile heart and aortic arch. Bending stress, caused by angulation of the aortic arch upon the descending aorta held fast by the intercostal arteries, adds to the tendency of the aorta to rupture at this point. The ascending aorta may be torn by torsion stress, brought about by anterior-posterior compression of the chest, displacing the heart into the left pleural cavity. Experimental subjection of dogs to horizontal linear trauma to the

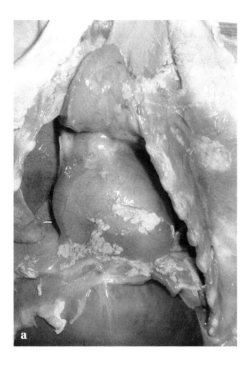
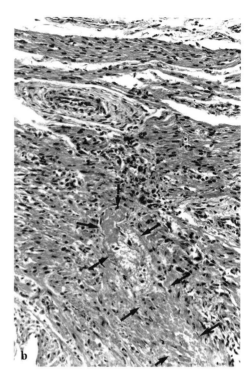

Figure 2.11 Sudden death in an infant due to a hydropericardium (a) associated with penetration of the right ventricular wall by an intravascular catheter. Microscopic section of the wall of the right ventricle showed partial-thickness necrosis along the catheter tract (arrows) (b). E = epicardium. (Hematoxylin and eosin, ×250.)

sternum caused a sharp increase in intra-aortic pressure (the "water hammer" effect), which is greatest in the ascending aorta (Sevitt, 1977a; Symbas, 1989). A study of the breaking strength of strips of aorta from different locations showed the ascending aorta to be the strongest area, followed by the descending aorta, with the isthmus being the weakest point (Sevitt, 1977a). This is probably due to the disarray of the elastic and smooth muscle fibers at the attachment point of the ligamentum arteriosum. The pressure necessary to rupture the aorta is equal to an intravascular pressure of 2500 torr (333.3 kPa) (Parmley *et al.*, 1958).

Cardiac tamponade

The diagnosis of acute tamponade immediately following an accident or medical procedure may be obvious, but situations may also arise when there is delay between the injury and the development of symptomatic fluid accumulation (Byard *et al.*, 1992; Nadroo *et al.*, 2001). If fluid other than blood has caused the tamponade, then this may be derived from intravascular lines that have been removed. In these circumstances it may be difficult at autopsy to determine the precise site of injury. Taking samples for biochemical analysis may be the only way to confirm the cause and source of the intrapericardial fluid accumulation (Figures 2.11 and 2.12).

Commotio cordis

Non-penetrating chest injuries may cause cardiac lacerations, valvular damage, papillary muscle rupture, transmural necrosis, and compromise of coronary artery patency (Curfman, 1998; Jones, 1970).

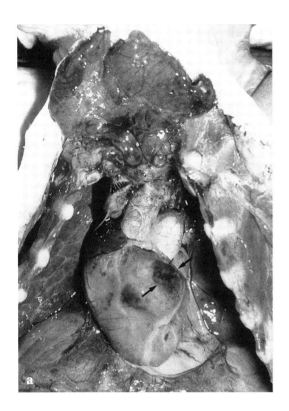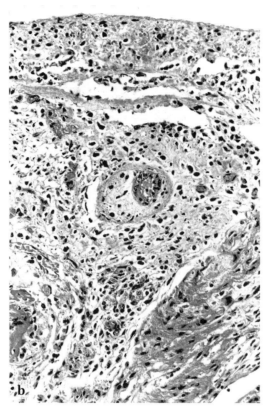

Figure 2.12 Sudden death due to acute cardiac tamponade following delayed rupture of the heart after catheter insertion.
(a) Thinning and discoloration of the conus at the point of perforation (arrows). (b) Corresponding full-thickness necrosis.
E = epicardium. (Hematoxylin and eosin, ×250.)

Rarely, sudden death in childhood or adolescence may result from a blow to the chest, with no apparent significant acute damage to the heart or vessels being discernable (Frazer & Mirchandani, 1984; Kohl *et al.*, 2001), although on occasion there may be epicardial hemorrhage at the site of impact (Froede, Lindsey & Steinbronn, 1979). A typical scenario involves sudden impact to a small area of the precordium from a hard object such as a baseball or hockey puck (Maron *et al.*, 1995; Nesbitt, Cooper & Kohl, 2001).

Known as commotio cordis, the etiology of death in this form of cardiac concussion is uncertain; however, both ventricular fibrillation and acute bradyarrhythmias have been documented (Abrunzo, 1991; Estes, 1995; Link *et al.*, 1998). Postulated

mechanisms include reflex vasoconstriction with redirection of coronary blood flow, or an abnormal autonomic response with resultant fatal ventricular arrhythmia (Frazer & Mirchandani, 1984). Support for a vascular etiology in some cases derives from a 10-year-old boy who died suddenly after a boxing match and was found to have an occlusive thrombus of the left anterior descending coronary artery, but these cases are rare (Bor, 1969). In possible cases, the diagnosis is suggested when there is a classical history of closed chest trauma followed immediately, or very soon after, by collapse with no abnormal findings at autopsy to adequately explain death. Homicide due to commotio cordis following blows to the chest in children has also been reported (Denton & Kalelkar, 2000).

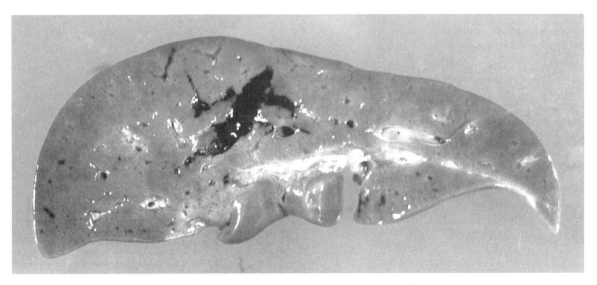

Figure 2.13 Liver laceration in a two-month-old infant passenger in a motor vehicle accident.

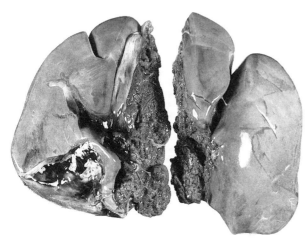

Figure 2.14 Transection of the liver in an older child with extensive intraperitoneal hemorrhage following a motor vehicle accident.

Abdominal injuries

Saladino, Lund & Fleischer (1991) studied 77 children with liver or spleen injuries. The mean age was nine years and three months, with nearly 80%

aged between four and 15 years. Nearly half suffered a direct blow to the abdomen, with the most frequent mechanism in this category being a blow from bicycle handlebars. In contrast, Galat, Grisoni & Gauderer (1990) found motor vehicle–pedestrian accidents to be the most common cause of injury. Rivkind, Siegel & Dunham, (1989) also found motor vehicle accidents to be the most common cause of hepatic injury in their series of adults with abdominal trauma.

Saladino, Lund & Fleischer (1991) found that 70% of children had injury to the spleen only, 23% had hepatic injury only, and in 7% of cases both the liver and the spleen were injured. Vital signs were not accurate predictors of intra-abdominal injury, as they were normal in the majority of patients. Abdominal examination was the most sensitive diagnostic maneuver, with abdominal tenderness present in 94% of patients. Although the two patients who died also had severe head injuries, two-thirds of all patients had liver or spleen trauma as their only severe injury (Figures 2.13 and 2.14).

In general, solid abdominal organs are more susceptible than hollow organs to blunt force injury. Experiments using impactors into the abdomens of animals have revealed that organs such as the spleen and liver require smaller impact forces to produce injury than do hollow lower abdominal organs. In a survey of mostly unrestrained motor vehicle occupants involved in frontal impacts, the liver sustained 38.2% of the injuries, the spleen 24.2%, and the kidneys 13.7%, while the intestines and urinary bladder received only 18.5% of the injuries (Miller, 1991).

The maximum viscous criterion (VC_{max}), defined as the product of maximum velocity of deformation and compression, was the most important predictor of injury in experiments using pigs struck in the abdomen with an impactor. Miller (1991) reported a tolerance level of 1.29 m/s for the lower abdomen, 1.20 m/s for the upper abdomen, and 1.00 m/s for the thorax. The chest, being surrounded by the ribs, has the greatest viscoelastic potential, followed by the upper abdomen, partly covered by ribs and containing the liver. The lower abdomen has the least viscoelastic potential, and thus requires a greater velocity of deformation to cause injury.

Blunt force to the lower abdomen may cause injury when the hollow organs therein are distended with fluid or gas and trapped between the intruding structure and the vertebral column (Huelke & Melvin, 1980). At the same force and velocity, there is more damage caused by a localized force than by a diffusely applied force. However, the injury caused by application of force over a prolonged time is greater than that produced by the same velocity over a shorter duration (Stalnaker, McElhaney & Roberts, 1973).

Craniocerebral trauma

Approximately 30% of all childhood deaths result from head injury, accounting for 7000 deaths in children in 1986 in the USA. About 5% of head injuries in children result in death (Division of Injury Control, 1990).

In 1986 the most frequent causes of head injury by age group were as follows: under four years, falls (55%); five to nine years, falls, motor vehicle accidents, and sports/recreational injuries (each about 30%); 10–14 years, sports/recreational injuries (43%); 15–19 years, motor vehicle accidents (55%). There were twice as many boys as girls (Kraus, Rock & Hemyari, 1990). Motor vehicle accidents accounted for 37% of all head injuries, fatal and non-fatal. Of these, 19% were occupants, 8% were motorcycle riders, 6% were pedestrians, and 4% were cyclists colliding with motor vehicles. Falls accounted for 24% (15% from a height and 9% from a level surface). Sports and recreational injuries accounted for 21% of the head injuries: bicycle accidents not involving motor vehicles (11%), sports injuries (7%), and playground accidents (3%). Other accidents accounted for 8% of head injuries in the study. Of serious head injuries, motor vehicle accidents were the cause in 29%, assaults in 34%, falls in 7%, sports/recreational injuries in 6%, and other trauma in 20% (Kraus, Rock & Hemyari, 1990).

In the Michigan series, 45 children (27% of accidental deaths) died of craniocerebral trauma, defined as fatal injury to the head or neck with no fatal injuries elsewhere. Twenty (11 males, nine females) were passengers in motor vehicles. They ranged in age from two weeks to 16 years, with a mean age of six years. Seven were restrained and 12 were not (in one child this was not known). Four children were thrown from a car, six sustained an impact on their side of the car, there was a head-on collision against either another vehicle or a fixed object in eight cases, one was in a vehicle hit from behind by another car, and in a final case the circumstances of the crash were unknown.

There were four motor vehicle drivers who died of craniocerebral trauma alone, three males (all aged 16) and one female (aged 14). Three victims were unrestrained and one was burned too badly to tell. Three motor vehicles collided with trees, and one left the roadway and rolled multiple times.

There were 16 pedestrians in the Michigan study who died of craniocerebral trauma alone, eight boys and eight girls. Their ages ranged from one month to 14 years, with a mean age of four years. The speeds of the cars were available in three cases and were estimated at 40–48 kph (25–30 mph), 56–64 kph (35–40 mph), and 64 kph (40 mph).

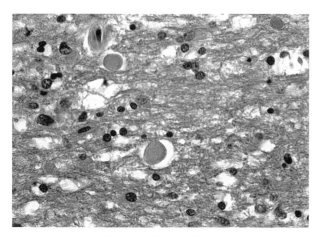

Figure 2.15 Diffuse axonal injury following head trauma 11 days previously. Swollen "retraction balls" can be readily identified. (Hematoxylin and eosin, ×400.)

Five cyclists (four boys, one girl), all of whom collided with motor vehicles, ranged in age from seven to 13 years, with a mean age of 10 years. The motor vehicle was at fault in two cases, and the child was at fault in three. In the one case where speed was known, the automobile was travelling at 64 kph (40 mph) when it collided with the victim.

Six children (four boys, two girls) with an age range of 3–16 years and a mean age of 10 years, died in a variety of ways. Two fell off horses, one fell from a tree, one hit a telephone pole while snow sledding, one hit her head against a door jamb, and one motorcyclist hit a tree.

Mechanisms of craniocerebral injury

Brain injury is related to acceleration and deceleration of the head. If the duration of the acceleration/deceleration is short, as happens in falls, then the primary results are subdural hematoma and cerebral contusion. Accidents, such as motor vehicle crashes, that cause a longer duration of acceleration/deceleration tend to cause diffuse axonal injury (DAI) in addition to hematomas and contusions. Experiments with primates have shown that acceleration of the head in the lateral (coronal) plane causes the most severe DAI, with less severe injury

associated with acceleration in the sagittal or oblique planes (Gennarelli *et al.*, 1982).

Grossly, DAI appears as hemorrhage in the corpus callosum, the parasagittal white matter, the superior cerebellar peduncles, and the dorsolateral quadrants of the brainstem (Gennarelli *et al.*, 1982). In some cases it may present grossly as diffuse white matter petechial hemorrhage, with no apparent fatal injury. Microscopically, DAI appears as eosinophilic or argyrophilic swellings in the white matter (Figure 2.15). These lesions, or "retraction balls", are located adjacent to areas of perivascular hemorrhage. Although they are not microscopically detectable on routine staining until 6–24 hours postinjury, they are described here as they may be found in individuals who have been kept alive by artificial means for some time following lethal trauma. They may also be detected much earlier using immunohistochemical staining for amyloid precursor protein (APP). The healed lesion is non-specific, consisting of attenuation of the neuropil with subsequent astrocytosis and hemosiderin-laden macrophage accumulation. The mechanism of DAI involves shearing of axons from rapid back-and-forth movement of the brain parenchyma at the time of injury. The brain is predisposed to shearing, as its consistency varies due to the tracts and nuclei arranged throughout (Leestma, 1988). Those who suffer severe DAI are usually unconscious from the moment of injury and remain unconscious, or at least severely impaired, until death.

Contusions occur at the crests of the gyri and have a hemorrhagic, streak-like appearance on cut section. In young infants, blunt force head injury causes tears or separations at the gray–white junction, and sometimes within the cortex, rather than contusions (Adams, 1984). These "contusional tears" result from a variation in the elasticity of the cortex and subjacent white matter in the less myelinated brain of infants (Leestma, 1988). In older children, *coup* contusions occur at the site of impact of a blunt object with the head, in the absence of a fracture. *Contrecoup* contusions are located opposite the point of impact, and occur because of sudden deceleration, such as occurs with a fall (Figure 2.16). Classically,

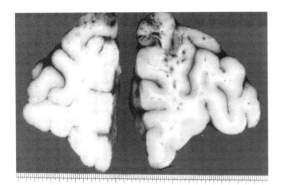

Figure 2.16 Contrecoup lesions of the frontal lobes of the brain in a 14-year-old equestrian who was thrown from a horse, landing on the occiput.

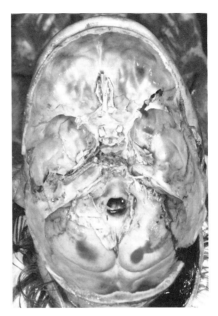

Figure 2.17 Crushed skull of a four-year-old who was run over by a truck. The base of the skull reveals multiple fractures. The brain, however, was not contused.

contrecoup contusions are seen on the orbital surface of the frontal lobes and tips of the temporal lobes in a fall on the occipital part of the skull.

Intermediary *coup* contusions occur in the deep structures of the brain and are caused by shearing of blood vessels and axons in severe closed head injury. The shearing forces are generated by oscillations of the brain following impact and by lateral stretching of the brain caused by deformation of the skull in the anterior-posterior direction. Intermediary *coup* contusions occur most frequently in the white matter, the basal ganglia, the corpus callosum, the hypothalamus, and the brainstem. Contusions, caused by shearing of blood vessels, are much more likely to occur when the head is freely movable rather than when the head is fixed. In fact, with severe crush injury of a non-movable skull, such as might occur when the head is run over by a truck (Figure 2.17), the skull may have numerous comminuted fractures with few or no cerebral contusions (Leestma, 1988).

Subdural hemorrhage is caused by tearing of the bridging veins (Figure 2.18), and epidural hemorrhage is due most often to laceration of the middle meningeal artery as it courses along the inner table of the skull external to the dura mater. Epidural hemorrhage is almost always caused by skull fracture. However, in children less than 10 years of age, in whom the skull is deformed but not fractured, the dura mater may be torn from the inner table of the

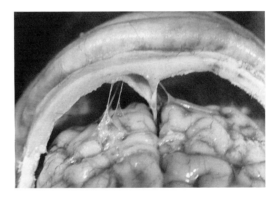

Figure 2.18 Bridging veins, which lead to subdural hematomas when torn.

skull with laceration of a nearby branch of the middle meningeal artery without skull fracture (Leestma, 1988). Epidural (extradural) hematomas are a cause of expanding intracranial injuries with clinical deterioration in those who have had a lucid interval after injury followed by death (Adams, 1984) (Figure 2.19).

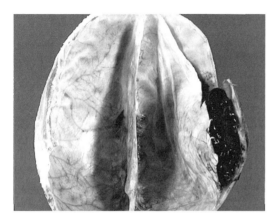

Figure 2.19 Epidural hematoma in an eight-year-old whose head hit a fixed pole while sledding.

Severe posterior or lateral hyperextension of the neck, found in pedestrians who are struck from behind by a motor vehicle, and in passengers or drivers who receive a forceful blow to the underside of the chin or forehead, may result in pontomedullary laceration, cervicomedullary laceration, or avulsion of these structures (Leestma, 1988). These injuries are usually accompanied by atlanto-occipital fracture-dislocation or a "ring fracture" of the skull around the foramen magnum (Figure 2.20). Skin and soft tissue injuries associated with certain types of craniocerebral trauma may be characteristic and may assist in determining the mechanism of injury (Figure 2.21).

Drowning

The diagnosis of drowning is one of exclusion once the autopsy reveals no other cause of death. It requires a history of the child being recovered from water with no potentially fatal diseases present, unless these have precipitated the fatal episode. If death occurs in shallow water or in a bath, the possibility of an underlying natural disease, such as epilepsy or a cardiac problem, or inflicted injury, must be considered (Saxena & Ang, 1993; Stumpp, Schneider & Bär, 1997). The peak age ranges for drowning are under

four and between 15 and 19 years (Division of Injury Control, 1990).

The 26 drowning victims in the Michigan series had a mean age of four years, with a range of two months to 13 years. There were 20 males and six females. Three infants, aged eight to nine months, were left alone in the bathtub for times ranging from five minutes to an hour. The common denominator in these cases was that all were relatively helpless. Two infants, both aged 11 months, were found with their heads submerged, one in a toilet and the other in a bucket of water. Both of these infants were mobile but lacked coordination. One was unobserved for two to three minutes and the other for five minutes.

Thirteen children fell into a body of water or were caught in an undertow while swimming. There were 10 boys and three girls, with a mean age of six and a half years and a range of 1–13 years. In the four cases in which information was available, the time out of the carer's sight ranged from 10 to 20 minutes. These children were old enough to play on their own without immediate supervision.

Seven children drowned in swimming pools. Five children were two years old, one was seven, and one was only one year. The six younger individuals were missing from five minutes to an hour. Except for the seven-year-old, these children were at a stage in which they were mobile and curious but too young to be able to swim. One two-month-old infant was recovered from a river; how he entered the water is unknown.

In their review of 58 deaths certified as drowning, Smith, Byard & Bourne (1991) found that six had pre-existing medical conditions that could have precipitated the drowning or caused death. Four patients had epilepsy, one had subarachnoid hemorrhage from a ruptured arteriovenous malformation, and one had a hypoplastic right coronary artery (see Figure 6.21). Figure 2.22 illustrates a case of drowning in a two-year-old girl who was subsequently found on retrospective examination of autopsy tissues to have a previously unsuspected mucopolysaccharidosis, Sanfilippo syndrome.

While findings at autopsy in typical drowning cases may include marked pulmonary edema,

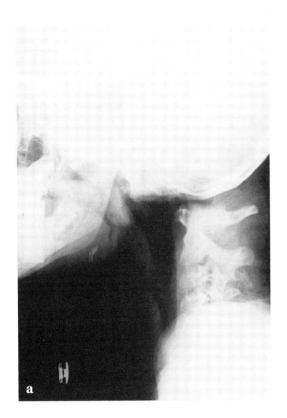

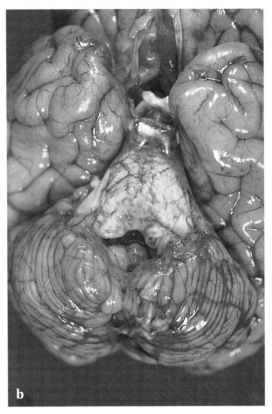

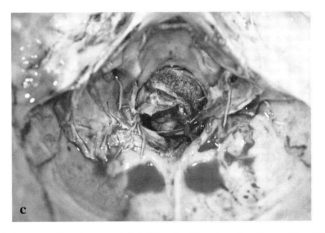

Figure 2.20 Skull radiograph demonstrating atlanto-occipital dislocation (a) and resultant transection of the brainstem (b) in a five-year-old who was a belted rear-seat passenger in a motor vehicle that hit another. (c) Skull with atlanto-occipital dislocation from an eight-year-old cyclist who was hit by a motor vehicle. The fragmented atlas can be seen in the spinal canal.

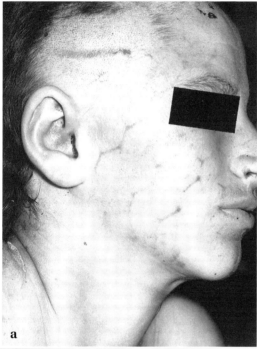

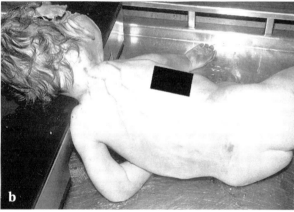

Figure 2.21 Impressions left by motor vehicle tire tread on the face of a 14-year-old boy (a) and on the back of a 13-month-old boy (b), both of whom died of cerebral trauma following vehicle accidents.

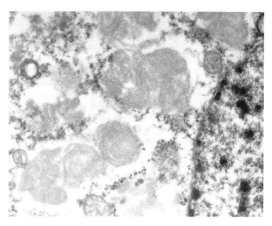

Figure 2.22 Electron micrograph of intraneuronal inclusions from a two-year-old girl who had drowned, revealing membrane-bound bodies containing loose lamellar structures in keeping with Sanfilippo syndrome (×21,000). Review of the case was undertaken after a subsequent sibling was found to have the syndrome.

Hemodilution, which occurs more in freshwater drowning, may result in intimal staining of major vessels (Lawler, 1992). Demonstration of diatoms in the lungs and comparison of blood chloride levels in the right and left ventricles have not proven to be reliable tests for drowning (DiMaio & DiMaio, 2001).

The risk of drowning varies with age, with nearly 90% of drowning in young children occurring in residential pools, compared with adolescents who drown in a variety of other environments (Cass, Ross & Lam, 1996; Edmond et al., 2001; Kibel et al., 1990; Pearn, 1992; Pitt & Cass, 2001; Warneke & Cooper, 1994; Wintemute 1990). As noted above, half (13) of the Michigan drowning cases were less than three years of age: six drowned in swimming pools, three in the bathtub, two in bodies of water, one in a toilet, and one in a bucket. The preponderance of victims in every age group are males, with 12 times the number of males compared with females in the 15–19 years age group. Alcohol may be detected in 40–50% of adolescent drownings.

Pearn et al. (1979) drew attention to bathtub drownings. These occur in toddlers with a median age of nine months, who can sit alone and pull themselves up to stand (Byard & Lipsett, 1999). These

so-called "emphysema aquosum," this is not specific for drowning, and it may occur in such diverse conditions as epilepsy, congestive heart failure, and drug overdose, or following prolonged resuscitation.

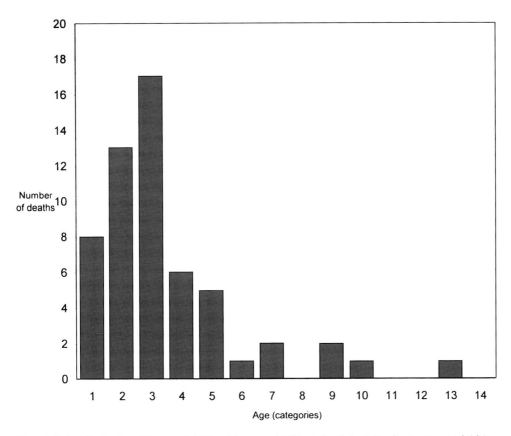

Figure 2.23 Age distribution of 56 cases of childhood drowning fatalities in South Australia, showing increased risk in the young (1 = first year).

children typically come from large families of lower socioeconomic class (O'Shea, 1991) and tend to be left unsupervised in the tub. Concerns have also been raised that the presence of an older sibling in the bath may increase the risk of drowning (Byard *et al.*, 2001b). Also at risk are epileptic infants and those with febrile convulsions, especially when such a child with a fever is put into a hot bath. A breakdown of childhood drowning deaths per age group is provided in Figure 2.23, with an analysis of the location of drowning for children under the age of two years in Figure 2.24.

Jumbelic and Chambliss (1990), Hyma (1990), and Kibel and colleagues (1990) all warn of the dangers of large (five-gallon) buckets. The infants and toddlers in Jumbelic & Chambliss' series of 12 cases

averaged 11.6 months of age (range 9–16 months), and all buckets were heavy, plastic, and rigid. The large size and heavy construction of the buckets coupled with the toddlers' high center of gravity and poor motor coordination kept them from extricating themselves after leaning over the edge (Mann, Weller & Rauchschwalbe, 1992). All had been left unattended from one minute to several hours prior to death, and all were found with their heads submerged and their feet in the air. Most buckets contained soapy water and were filled from 10% to 90% of capacity. As in other drownings, the bulk of victims were male (75%) (Jumbelic & Chambliss, 1990).

The mechanism of death in drowning is complex, involving not only asphyxia but also hydrostatic and osmotic effects of inhaled fluid within the alveoli

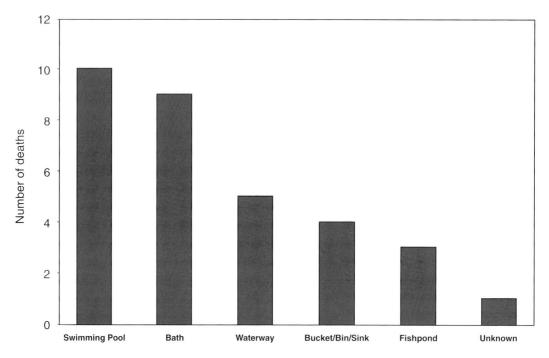

Figure 2.24 Numbers of drowning deaths according to site of death taken from a study of 32 infants and young children under the age of two years who drowned in South Australia.

(Lawler, 1992). In approximately 7–10% of cases, the victim suffers laryngeal spasm (Modell, 1971). At autopsy in these cases, the lungs are pink and spongy and contain no edema fluid. Some children may survive immersion episodes for considerable lengths of time, particularly if the water is cold (<21 °C (70 °F)) (Spyker, 1985). The physiological sequence that has been proposed to explain this phenomenon involves reflex inhibition of breathing when cold water contacts the face. This prevents water from entering the lungs, and is followed by bradycardia and selective vasoconstriction of the periphery. This forms part of the diving response that diverts blood to the brain, which is protected further by a marked reduction in metabolic rate (Gooden, 1992).

Asphyxia

Asphyxia occurring during sleep

Infants and young children may die by hanging or wedging (Clark *et al.*, 1993; Collins, 2001; Cooke,

Cadden & Hilton, 1989), the latter representing a well-recognized cause of asphyxial death in infants (Altmann & Nolan, 1995; Byard, 1996a; Byard, Beal & Bourne, 1994; Gilbert-Barness *et al.*, 1991; Nixon *et al.*, 1995; Smialek, Smialek & Spitz, 1977; Sturner, 1980). Typically the infant is caught between the edge of a mattress and side rails or between the slats of a crib (Figures 2.25 and 2.26). Infants put to sleep on adult beds or mattresses on the floor may become wedged between the mattress and bed or an adjacent dresser. Sofas may also have gaps that may entrap an infant (Figure 2.27). Cribs that are broken or in poor repair may have large gaps that increase the risk of accidental asphyxia (Corey *et al.*, 1992; Variend & Usher, 1984). Careful examination of the head in such cases may reveal bruising or abrasions resulting from wedging (Figures 2.28 and 2.29).

Of 11 infants in the Michigan review who were asphyxiated after they had been put down to sleep, seven were wedged and four were asphyxiated in other ways. The wedged infants ranged from four to 11 months of age, with a mean age of seven months.

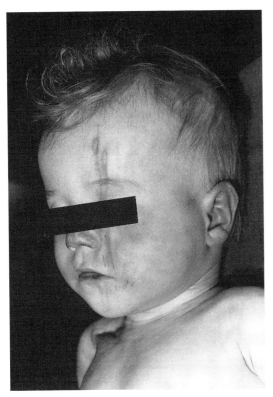

Figure 2.25 Linear marks on the face of a 10-month-old girl who was wedged between the side of an adult bed mattress and a wall.

One infant was wedged between the end and side rails of a crib, and another was wedged between the mattress and broken side rails of a poorly maintained crib. Three infants were wedged between mattresses on the floor on which they had been placed to sleep, and an adult bed, dresser, and wall, respectively. Of two infants sleeping on an adult bed, one was wedged between the bed and the wall, and the other between the bed and a footboard. The remaining four infants ranged in age from three months to one year, with a mean age of seven months. There were two girls and two boys. One infant suffocated from a blanket that wrapped around his head, one wrapped a plastic sheet around his face, one was asphyxiated beneath the arm and chest of a sleeping carer ("overlaying"), and one, with periventricular leukomalacia and a history of choking when face down, was found dead face down in bed.

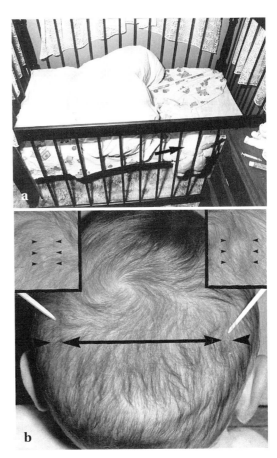

Figure 2.26 A teddy bear (arrow) shows where an 8.5-month-old girl was found wedged between the sliding side of her crib and the mattress and frame (a). The back of her head demonstrates two linear indentations (see insets with arrowheads) that correspond to the bars of the crib (b). The distance between the indentations and the bars was the same (60 mm).

Severely disabled children are known to be at increased risk of accidental asphyxia, sometimes with involvement of devices that were designed to prevent them from falling out of bed (Figures 2.30 and 2.31) (Amanuel & Byard, 2000). In the Michigan series a severely retarded 11-year-old who had encephalitis as an infant caught her neck in the side rails of her crib.

In most cases of infantile asphyxia, the autopsy findings are non-specific (Beal & Byard, 1995; Byard & Krous, 1999), although facial petechiae may be

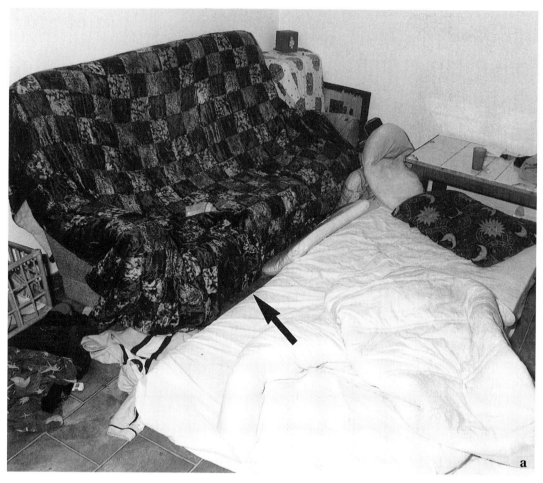

Figure 2.27 A gap between a mattress and a couch into which a 10-month-old infant had rolled and suffocated (arrow) (a). His head was wrapped in a heavy blanket, with his face pressed into an area that was sodden with vomit (white line = position of head) (b).

detected in hanging deaths in infants (Moore & Byard, 1993) (Figure 2.32). Impressions of clothing around the neck may also be found in cases where young children have become suspended by their clothes from the side of cribs (Figure 2.33). Toddlers placed in cribs within reach of curtain cords or electric flexes may be in danger of hanging or strangulation if they wrap the cords or flexes around their necks (Figure 2.34) (Byard, 1996a; Rauchschwalbe & Mann,1997; Shepherd, 1990). Figure 2.35 demonstrates a situation where the death scene findings were changed by a mother who had found her

18-month-old son hanging from a looped cord attached to a cupboard door knob. She had removed the boy from the ligature and repositioned the cord to where it should have been, above his reach. Although investigating police officers were initially suspicious about the death scene findings, the explanation was soon elicited, and the reasons for the "cover-up" were considered understandable. Accidental hanging while playing or experimenting with ligatures may also occur in older children, with death resulting from suspension around the neck or trunk (Busuttil & Obafunwa, 1993; Wyatt *et al.*, 1998).

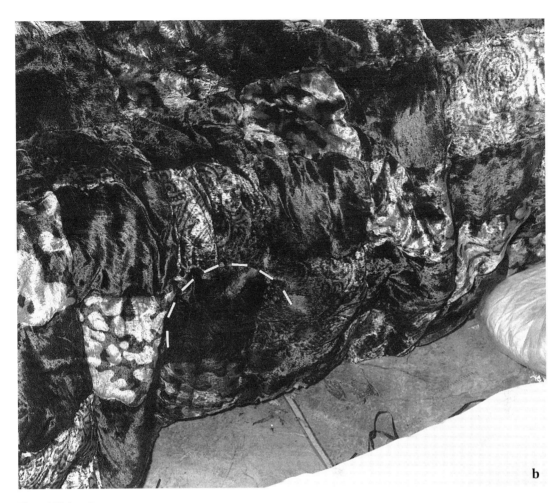

Figure 2.27 (cont.)

Infants and young children may also slip down in restraining seats and hang themselves (Figures 2.36 and 2.37). In these situations the lethal outcome may be due not to the product as such but to the manner in which it was used. For example, in the case shown in Figure 2.36, the product label warned specifically against leaving a child in the harness unattended; in the case shown in Figure 2.37, the infant had been left unsupervised for two hours. Car windows may also entrap children's heads, either by creating a space for potential hanging if partially open (Figure 2.38), or if power windows are operated while a child is looking out (Byard & James, 2001; Simmons, 1992).

To identify an asphyxial death properly, there must be a scene investigation. If, as is usually the case, the infant or child has been removed from the scene or at least from the position initially found, placing a similarly sized doll in the location in which the infant was found may be invaluable.

Asphyxial deaths have been reported in infants sleeping on polystyrene-filled cushions (Kemp & Thach, 1991; Gilbert-Barness & Emery, 1996). Kemp & Thach (1991) used rabbits under conditions similar to those in infants sleeping face down on cushions, and showed that the animals asphyxiated from rebreathing carbon dioxide after three hours. They

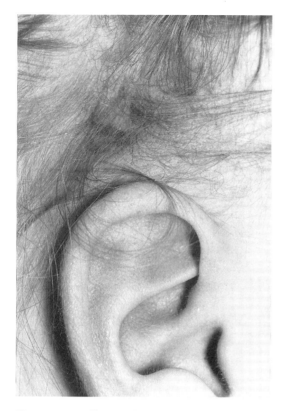

Figure 2.28 Area of bruising above the ear in a nine-month-old boy who was found wedged in a gap between a mattress and crib side.

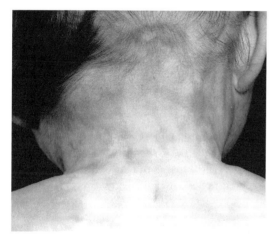

Figure 2.29 Livid area over the occiput in a 10-month-old infant wedged between a crib side and mattress.

also reviewed the deaths of 25 infants (mean age 57 days) that had occurred on infant cushions. Although the cause of death had been certified as SIDS in 19 of 23 autopsied cases, they concluded that the deaths were probably due to rebreathing of carbon dioxide. Other recently reported unsafe sleeping arrangements have involved V-shaped pillows, waterbeds, mesh-sided cots, stroller prams, and overhead-suspended rocking cradles (Figures 2.39–2.41) (Ackerman & Gilbert-Barness, 1997; Beal *et al.*, 1995; Byard & Beal, 1997; Byard, Bourne & Beal, 1996; Byard *et al.*, 1996a; Moore *et al.*, 1995; Morrison *et al.*, 2002). Infants may also become trapped between a thick mattress and the side of a mesh cot, hang from the mesh if it is torn, or become caught in the "V" of the side bars if they collapse (Figures 2.42 and 2.43). The age distribution of a series of deaths due to accidental asphyxia related to dangerous sleeping environments is shown in Figure 2.44.

Traumatic asphyxia

In the Michigan series, nine children (seven boys, two girls) died of traumatic asphyxia, defined as external compression of the chest preventing respiratory motion. The age range was 2–16 years, with a mean age of eight years. Four died from having caught their head or chest in a window or dresser drawer, and one child's chest and abdomen were compressed beneath an electric garage door. Three others were pinned beneath cars: one was an unbelted passenger in a rollover accident, one became pinned beneath a car that she had been pushing, and one was a moped driver who became pinned beneath a car during the course of an accident. The final victim was pinned under an all-terrain vehicle (ATV) that flipped and landed on him. Autopsy findings in such cases usually include facial petechiae (Figure 2.45) (Byard, Hanson & James, 2003).

Miscellaneous causes of asphyxia

Nine children (four boys, five girls) died of asphyxia due to a variety of other causes. Three siblings aged four, five, and six years suffocated in an abandoned freezer. One 19-month-old died of anoxic encephalopathy from choking on a pill at eight months of age. A 13-year-old motorcyclist hit his neck on a steel cable and had severe soft tissue injuries, resulting in airway occlusion from surrounding interstitial edema and hemorrhage. Two 15-year-old runaway girls died of carbon monoxide intoxication from a charcoal grill on which they were cooking in an abandoned house.

Foreign body impaction/migration

The peak age range for choking on foreign bodies is two to three years (Friedman, 1988), with 90% of cases occurring in children under five years (Harris *et al.*, 1984). Round foods (hot dogs, carrots, candy, nuts, and grapes) are the most frequently aspirated foreign objects causing death, although a variety of objects, including toy parts, metal screws, and plastic pen components, may impact in the upper airway (Figures 2.46–2.50) (Al-Hilou, 1991; Baker & Fisher, 1980; Banerjee *et al.*, 1988; Bhana, Gunaselvam & Dada, 2000; Kenna & Bluestone, 1988; Laks & Barzilay, 1988; Lima, 1989; Linegar *et al.*, 1992; Mantel & Butenandt, 1986; Mittleman, 1984; Wiseman, 1984). Balloons have been found to be the most common cause of childhood airway obstruction due to toys (Lifschultz & Donoghue, 1996; Meel, 1998). Foreign bodies causing acute upper airway obstruction in children usually lodge in the pharynx or within the tracheobronchial tree (Byard *et al.*, 2001c). The problem has been recognized for many centruries with Bradwell, a London doctor, commenting in 1633: "Of Things that endanger stopping of the breath in swallowing, some are Sharp, and some Blunt . . . I have heard of a Child in Woodstreet strangled with a grape" (Harris *et al.*, 1984).

Symptoms, which include choking, gagging, coughing, and wheezing, may subside when a foreign body moves into a bronchus. Toddlers are at particular risk of inhaling food, as incisor teeth erupt at 10 months to two years, before the second molars at 20–30 months. This means that they are able to bite off portions of hard food before they can effectively chew (Byard *et al.*, 1996b). Problems may arise in childcare centers when young children are

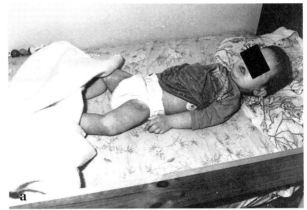

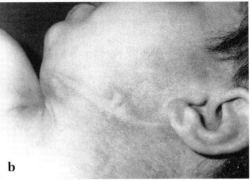

Figure 2.30 A four-year-old boy with severe congenital hydrocephalus was found dead in bed with his head over the side of the bed and his neck resting on a plank of wood that had been attached to the bed to prevent him from falling out (a). An area of irregular linear blanching was present on the left side of his neck, corresponding to the position of the plank under his neck (b).

exposed to food that they may not have encountered before and are not able to properly masticate (Byard, 1994a).

The diagnosis of foreign body aspiration may be delayed in 30% of cases, and only 80% will have a positive history. The chest X-ray may be normal, and foreign material aspirated into the trachea may cause delayed death (Humphries, Wagener & Morgan, 1988). If there has been medical attention, the foreign object may have been removed and thus the autopsy may not reveal the cause of death. In such cases, the medical record should provide an

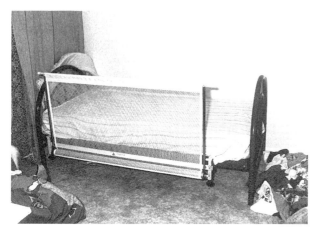

Figure 2.31 A four-year-old severely developmentally delayed boy was found wrapped in a thick quilt wedged between the side of a bed and a retractable mesh barrier that had been attached to the bed to prevent him from falling out.

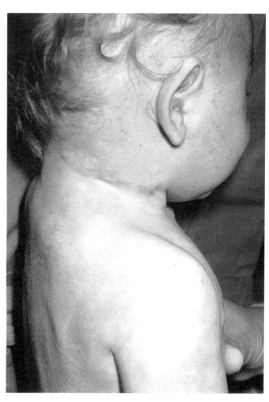

Figure 2.33 Linear mark around the neck of a 16-month-old boy who was found suspended by clothing from the side of his crib.

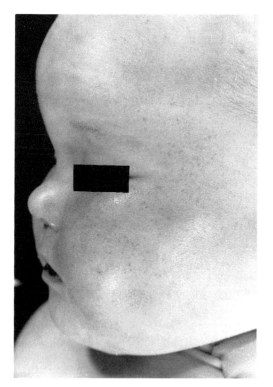

Figure 2.32 Facial petechiae in a girl aged eight and a half months who slipped down in her car seat and was found hanging.

appropriate description of events. Optimally, the foreign body can be retrieved by the pathologist for examination and photographic documentation (Figures 2.51 and 2.52).

Upper airway occlusion may also be caused by inhalation of soil in trench or tunnel cave-ins (Figure 2.53).

Foreign material that has passed into the esophagus may also compromise the upper airway, although again symptoms may not be immediate. Over time, compression of the trachea combined with local inflammation may cause acute airway blockage. Such was the case in a four-month-old infant who presented as a probable SIDS death. The only prior history was of a mild upper respiratory tract infection, which had appeared to be responding to decongestants (Byard, Moore & Bourne, 1990). At autopsy, a one-cent coin was found within the esophagus, which had caused compression of the adjacent trachea (Figure 2.54). Acute airway obstruction resulted from the combined effects of anteroposterior flattening of the trachea, chronic inflammatory infiltrate, and mucus plugging. If the coin had not resulted in death from airway compromise, death may have resulted from hemorrhage, as the edges of the coin had opened a tract that extended towards the common carotid artery. Inflicted injury from the feeding of inappropriate material should also be considered when intra-esophageal foreign bodies are found (Nolte, 1993).

Sudden death due to exsanguination from vessel perforation or cardiac tamponade is a well-recognized complication of migrating or perforating intra-esophageal foreign bodies in children (Figure 2.55) and may be extremely rapid if an aorto-esophageal fistula develops (Atkins, 1895; Byard, 1996b; Dahiya & Denton, 1999; Grey *et al.*, 1988; Jiraki, 1996; Norman & Cass, 1971). In addition to coins and sharp objects, button batteries may be particularly hazardous, as leakage of contents may hasten perforation.

Although most foreign bodies that pass through the esophagus are not associated with a serious outcome, occasional cases may occur in which there is perforation of a viscus (Amyand, 1736); there may even be unexpected death due to either associated vessel perforation or sepsis. Perforation of the wall of the bowel by a sharp foreign body in the case of a seven-year-old mentally retarded boy who died unexpectedly following a brief illness was due to a wood screw that had initiated bacterial septicemia (Figure 2.56). Mechanisms of possible childhood death following foreign body ingestion/inhalation are summarized in Figure 2.57. The age distribution of a series of deaths due to accidental foreign body aspiration is shown in Figure 2.58.

Overlaying

Overlaying refers to the accidental suffocation of an infant by a sleeping adult. It is an uncommon

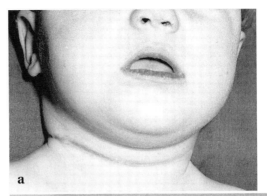
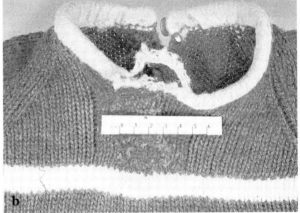

Figure 2.34 Linear abrasion around the neck of an infant who was found hanging from a curtain cord (a). A sweater worn by a toddler who was found hanging from a wing nut that projected into her crib. The torn area was caught by the nut (b).

occurrence but is most likely to occur when an infant is placed to sleep under covers on a soft mattress between two adults (Byard, 1994b). Parental fatigue, intoxication, and sedation increase the risk of suffocation, and cases have been reported (including among hospital in-patients) where infants have died when their breastfeeding mother has fallen asleep. As some infants are extremely susceptible to even transient airway occlusion (Byard, 1998; Byard & Burnell, 1995), it is not surprising that there are no specific autopsy findings (Byard, 1994c; Byard, 1995; Byard & Hilton, 1997; Mitchell, Krous & Byard, 2002). An increased risk of infant death while cosleeping has been documented in mothers who smoke, for

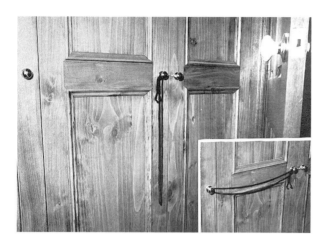

Figure 2.35 A looped cord attached to a cupboard door knob from which an 18-month-old boy was found hanging. The inset shows where the cord should have been positioned, out of the boy's reach.

reasons that remain unclear (Scragg *et al.*, 1993), and also in situations where an adult is sleeping with an infant on a sofa (Byard *et al.*, 2001a). Scene findings are usually unhelpful, although staining of parental clothing with serosanguinous oronasal secretions from the dead infant may confirm that contact was made and show the relative positions of the infant and parent at some stage during the night (Figure 2.59).

An unusual variant of non-lethal asphyxia while cosleeping involved a 27-month-old boy who became entangled in his mother's waist-length hair. The child was found to have a ligature mark around his neck, with facial petechiae (Kindley & Todd, 1978).

Autoerotic asphxia

Rarely, fatal asphyxia may occur during autoerotic activity, often involving adolescent boys who are using hypoxia to augment solitary sexual activities (Byard & Bramwell, 1991; Sabo *et al.*, 1996). Death is accidental and results from failure or unexpected effect of a device, material, or substance that was integral to the activity. Cases occur at all ages but

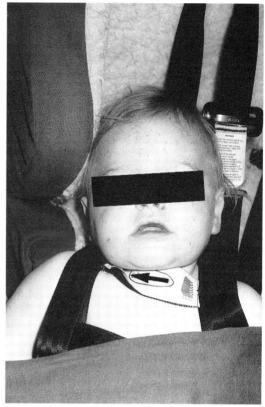

Figure 2.36 A 16-month-old boy was left sleeping in a car in a child restraint harness. He was found hanging when his parents returned. The arrow indicates safety instructions that warned against leaving a child in the harness unattended.

classically involve males aged between 15 and 25 years who are found hanging in secluded or secure places. There is usually evidence of antemortem sexual activity, with exposure of the genitals and adjacent pornographic pictures. There may be evidence that the activity has previously taken place, with multiple rope marks on the suspension point. A finding characteristic of male cases is the presence of female underclothing, which is either worn or placed nearby, sometimes in association with sado-masochistic and bondage equipment. Ropes around the neck may be padded to prevent abrasions and bruising, and there is usually no history of suicidal ideation (Byard, 1994d). Occasionally, inhalation of volatile substances may be used to enhance the effects of hypoxia. The youngest victim so far reported was nine years of age (Byard, Hucker & Hazelwood, 1990).

While bizarre props and pornographic literature at the death scene are clues to this type of activity in young males, cases in young women often lack this paraphernalia. Such was the case in a 19-year-old female who was found deceased, face down in her bed, with a rope looped around her neck and tied to her ankles. Extending her legs would have increased the pressure on her neck, which unfortunately was maintained once she had lost consciousness, resulting in death (Figure 2.60). A hairbrush handle within her vagina indicated antemortem sexual activity associated with self-induced hypoxia. There was no evidence of anyone else being involved in the death (Byard & Bramwell, 1988).

Embolism

Air embolism

Air embolism causing sudden death has been reported as a complication of many different procedures, including phlebotomy, central venous catheter placement, angiography, cesarian section, cervical surgery during pregnancy, and criminal abortion (Knight, 1997; Mitterschiffthaler *et al.*, 1989). Rouse & Hargrove (1992) reported the death of an 11-month-old infant due to gas embolism caused by attachment of tubing from an oxygen cylinder to an intravenous line. Gas embolism may also follow trauma if laceration or incision of any large superficial vein results in air gaining access to the circulation.

Sudden death has been documented in pregnant adolescents following oral sex or vaginal manipulation (Fatteh, Leach & Wilkinson, 1973), when air forced into the vagina causes tearing of distended submucosal veins. Histories of these types of activities are not often forthcoming at the time of autopsy, and so this possibility should be considered in cases

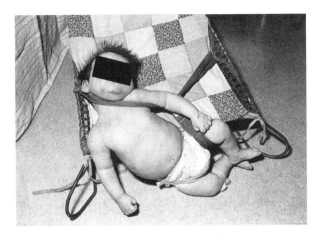

Figure 2.37 A three-month-old girl found hanging in a baby bouncer. She had been left unattended for two hours.

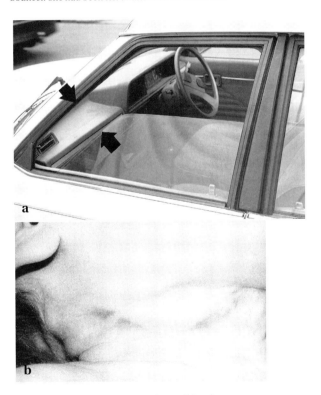

Figure 2.38 A gap between the window and doorframe (arrows) of a standard car providing a space that could entrap the head of a young child (a). V-shaped linear abrasion on the neck of a three-year-old boy found hanging from a similar, partly opened car window (b).

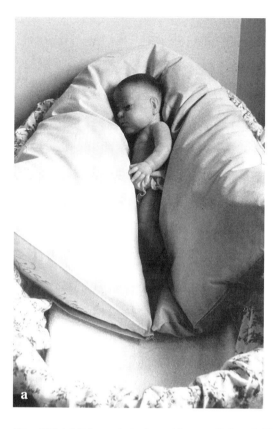 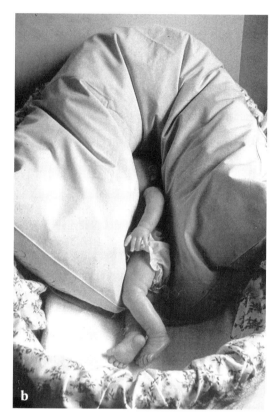

Figure 2.39 A doll demonstrates the positions on a V-shaped pillow on which an infant was (a) placed to sleep, and (b) subsequently found. Death was due to suffocation.

of sudden collapse and death of a pregnant female of any age.

A rare cause of possible air embolism associated with air travel and possible tension pneumothorax occurred in a young woman who collapsed shortly after take-off. At autopsy, the major abnormality found was a single large bulla occupying most of the right lung (Neidhart & Suter, 1985).

Air embolism may also occur during scuba diving if there has been an uncontrolled ascent from considerable depth. In cases of diving accidents, it is important to have detailed information of the circumstances of death and not to commence the autopsy until clinicians with experience in barotrauma are present. Preliminary chest radiographs should also be taken, looking for air within the heart and major

vessels. Detailed examination of the equipment used is required. The specialized techniques that are required for such autopsies have been described elsewhere (Knight, 1997; Bajanowski, West & Brinkmann, 1998).

Foreign body embolism

Embolization of catheter tips may occur after cardiac catherization. This occurred in a three-month-old boy with transposition of the great vessels, and was followed by paradoxical embolization of the fragment of catheter into his circumflex coronary artery, with myocardial infarction (Klys, Salmon & De Giovanni, 1991). Cerebral ischemia from embolization of an intracardiac shotgun pellet to the middle cerebral artery in a 12-year-old boy following a shooting accident has been reported (Vascik & Tew, 1982).

Other embolism

Bone marrow and fat embolism (Figure 2.61) are relatively common findings within the small vessels of the lungs following trauma that includes both cardiopulmonary resuscitation and intraosseous infusion. Emboli are merely markers for the underlying process and are usually not considered to be of significance clinically, except possibly in cases where there may be right-to-left cardiac shunting (Orlowski, *et al.*, 1989). If there is significant fat embolism, however, there may rarely be a rapid onset of tachycardia, fever, and a characteristic petechial rash, followed by coma and death (Sevitt, 1977b).

Fire deaths

In the Michigan series, 22 (13%) children died as a result of fire. The mean age was five years, with a range of two months to 16 years. There were 14 males and eight females. In the seven patients who had attempted resuscitation, blood carbon monoxide (CO) levels ranged from 7% to 47%, with a mean of 29%. CO saturation ranged from 20% to 95% (mean 71%) in the 14 children who died without resuscitation. In healthy adults, blood carboxyhemoglobin levels have to be at least 50–60% to be considered lethal; however, it may be lower in infants, possibly because their higher respiratory rate causes more rapid absorption (Knight, 1997).

Of the four children who died without resuscitation, and in whom the CO saturation was less than 50%, there were other factors contributing to death. A four-year-old (37% CO saturation) suffered 70% body surface area (BSA) burns from a fire that arose when adults were cleaning car parts with a volatile solvent. A 16-year-old who died in a house fire of unknown origin had 45% BSA burns and a blood cyanide level of 5.4 μmol/l (140 ng/ml) (normal levels: 0–0.6 μmol/l; 0–16 ng/ml). Cyanide, known to be generated by the combustion of plastic objects, is

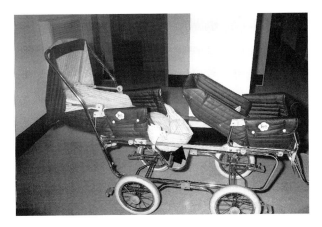

Figure 2.40 A stroller pram in which a three-month-old boy was found hanging with his head over the side bar (arrow), after the foot plate that he had been sleeping on had collapsed.

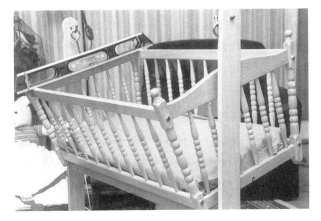

Figure 2.41 An overhead-suspended rocking cradle in which an 11-month-old girl was found dead, lying face down in the angle between the base and one side. The locking pin had been removed, resulting in tilting of the cradle.

assayed in cases in which there is insufficient CO or other causes to explain death from a fire. A six-year-old who had a CO level of 28% had a cyanide level of 54.8 μmol/l (1425 ng/ml) and 95% BSA burns. The CO saturation was 20% in a 15-year-old who also had 100% BSA burns.

Multiple children died in fires in five cases. Four fires each killed two children, while three children died in one fire. Thus, five fires accounted for half

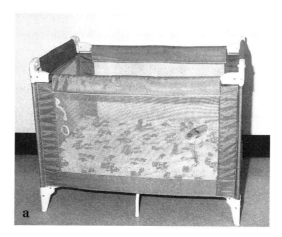

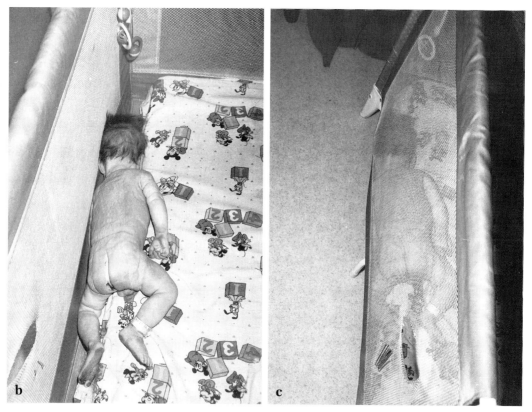

Figure 2.42 A mesh-sided portable crib (a) in which a 3.5-month-old boy was found lying face down between the side of the mattress and the stretched mesh wall (b). The elastic recoil of the mesh held the body firmly in position (c). The tear in the mesh side represented another potentially dangerous situation.

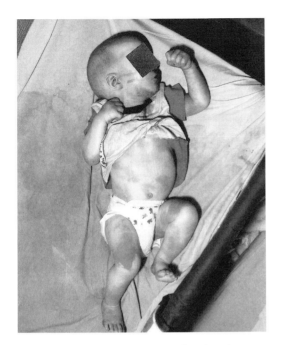

Figure 2.43 Unusual facial blanching with a triangular pattern due to wedging of the head between a mattress and the side of a portable mesh cot in a seven-month-old boy who had asphyxiated. A thicker mattress had been added to the cot.

the deaths in this group. The origin of the fire was unknown in nine cases, was caused by improper use of volatile liquids in four cases, was caused by children playing with matches in three instances, was the result of a defective fireplace chimney in two cases (this fire killed two children), and arose from a cigarette, a cigarette lighter, and a faulty heater in one case each. Cyanide was assayed in four cases, in three of these because the CO saturation was too low to explain the death by itself. The cyanide levels ranged from 5.4 to 54.8 μmol/l (140–1425 ng/ml).

Twenty of the 22 children were burned, with mean BSA burns of 67% (range 19–100%). Both of the un-burned children died in house fires and had under-gone attempted resuscitation; one had a CO satura-tion of 36% and the other a CO saturation of 40%. Of the 14 children found dead at the scene, the mean BSA burned was 82% (range 45–100%). Those surviv-ing to reach the hospital had a range of BSA burns of 0–90% (mean 41%).

In the investigation of a fire death, the presence of soot in the airway (Figure 2.62) and a blood CO of greater than 5% (greater than 10% in a smoker) indicates that the individual was alive for at least some time during the fire. If the CO is not elevated, and if the victim has not had attempted resuscita-tion (which hastens the elimination of CO), then contributing factors such as cyanide, thermal burns, young age, or associated medical conditions should be sought. The absence of soot in the airway and low levels of CO and/or cyanide indicate that the victim was dead before the fire, raising the possibility of an attempt to conceal a homicide.

In another study of childhood fire deaths (Byard, Lipsett & Gilbert 2000), a number of cases involved children who had been left for variable periods of time in motor vehicles. Unfortunately, vehicles pro-vide a confined and highly flammable space, with lockable doors and non-childproof lighters. Once a fire has started, young children are not good at self-escape but tend to practice avoidance by moving into the back seat area.

Burns from scalding in the bath have a char-acteristic distribution (Color Plate 2) that corre-sponds to the position of the infant. This enables differentiation from deliberately inflicted scalds (see Chapter 3). The age distribution of a series of deaths due to burns/scalds is shown in Figure 2.63.

Electrocution

There was only one case of electrocution in the Michigan review, in which a portable electric heater fell into a bathtub containing water, resulting in the death of its occupant, a three-year-old boy. South Australian data also confirm that fatal electrocu-tion in childhood and adolescence is uncommon, and usually occurs at home when children are play-ing around electrical wiring or with faulty electrical equipment (Byard *et al.*, 2003). Workplace deaths, suicides, and high-voltage electrocutions in chil-dren are rare. The pathological presentations are the same as similar events in adults. Skin injuries, which may be lacking in low-voltage electrocutions, may,

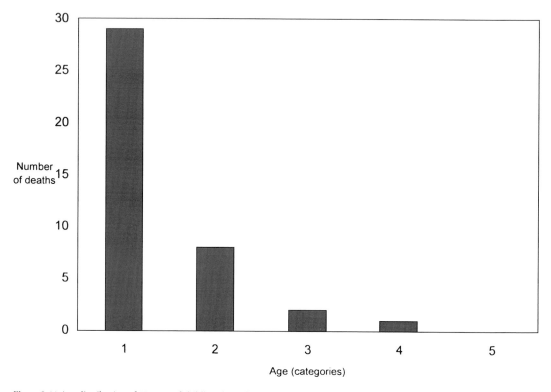

Figure 2.44 Age distribution of 40 cases of childhood accidental asphyxia taken from a study of 369 cases of accidental childhood death in South Australia, showing an increased risk in infancy (1 = first year).

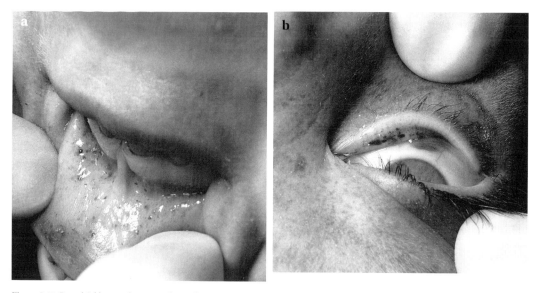

Figure 2.45 Petechial hemorrhages on the oral mucosa (a) and inner aspect of the eyelid (b) in a three-year-old-boy who was crushed in a conveyor belt accident at a chemical works.

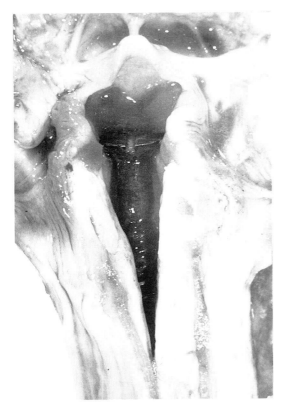

Figure 2.46 Wood screw found wedged firmly in the larynx and upper trachea in a case of childhood asphyxiation.

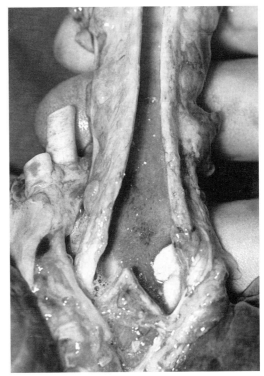

Figure 2.47 Aspirated tablets filling the right main bronchus associated with collapse of the right lung in a two-year-old boy who suffered cardiopulmonary arrest soon after ingesting them.

however, be quite variable in appearance. Typical lesions are shown in Figures 2.64–2.68 and Color Plate 3.

Poisoning

Children in the toddler age group usually ingest adult medicines, while adolescents most commonly poison themselves in suicide attempts or in the course of recreational drug abuse (DiMaio & Garriott, 1974; Yamamoto, Wiebe & Matthews, 1991). Poisoning should be suspected when no other cause of death can be found, especially in the one–five years age group and in teenagers. As younger children are more likely to be poisoned at home (Yamamoto,

Wiebe & Matthews 1991), a thorough inventory of the medicines available in the house should be taken. A case in which a two-year-old child was given a bath by the father, who had been out drinking before coming home, was considered to be homicide when the child was discovered dead in bed the next morning as several loud thuds had been heard during the bathing. Autopsy revealed no injuries, however, but disclosed 15 partially digested potassium chloride tablets in the stomach that the child had apparently obtained from the grandmother's medication bottle.

Sibert & Routledge (1991) divided the most common toxic substances into medicines, household products, and plants. The former included antiepileptics, benzodiazepines, digoxin, tricyclic antidepressants, salicylates, theophylline, opiates,

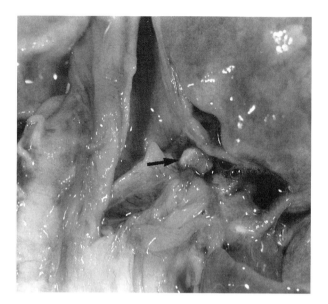

Figure 2.48 Occlusion of the right main bronchus by an aspirin tablet (arrow). The three-month-old victim had collapsed at home soon after ingesting the tablet.

iron, lithium, mefenamic acid, metoclopromide, mianserin, quinine, and hyoscine. Very toxic household products included alcoholic beverages, acids and alkalis, ethylene glycol, essential oils, petroleum distillates, methanol, methylene chloride, organochloride and organophosphate insecticides, paradichlorobenzene moth balls, weedkillers, phenolic compounds, and metaldehyde. Very toxic plants included arum lily, deadly nightshade, oleander, laburnum, and yew. Yamamoto, Wiebe & Matthews (1991) in Hawaii found that the most common agents precipitating treatment at an emergency department included prescription drugs, household items, natural items, liquor, street drugs, and multiple substances. In Rfidah and colleagues' study (1991) of poisoning in Dublin in children under 10 years of age admitted to an emergency department, 93% were under five; the most common agents were medicines (65%), household or garden products (34%), and plants (1%). Drugs most frequently ingested included paracetamol, benzodiazepines, cough suppressants and expectorants,

antidepressants, oral contraceptives, and bronchodilators. Ingested household products included bleach, cosmetics, white spirits, turpentine, caustic cleaners, and detergents.

In their study of poisoned children admitted to a Montreal pediatric intensive care unit, Lacroix, Gaudreault & Gauthier (1989) found that most children were under three years of age or older than 12 years. The most commonly ingested agents included tricyclic antidepressants (22%), benzodiazepines (15%), theophylline (10%), ethanol (10%), hallucinogens (8%), salicylates (8%), narcotics (8%), antihistamines (7%), and carbamazepine (5%). One-fifth of the children had multiple drug ingestions, particularly in suicide attempts. The death rate of 1% in poisonings reported by Lacroix, Gaudreault and Gauthier (1989) is in accord with the relatively low lethality of poisoning reported in other series.

There has been a dramatic fall in fatal childhood poisoning in Australia, from 3.5 deaths per 100,000 in 1921 to 0.3/100,000 in 1978 (O'Connor, 1983), with only three deaths registered nationally between 1990 and 1994 in children under 14 years. This compares with 48 fatal poisonings in the 15–24 years age group. The marked fall in cases, particularly in young children, has been due to the success of safety campaigns, with changing patterns of drug prescribing, safer packaging for medication, and colouring toxic fluids such as kerosene blue (Pearn *et al.*, 1984; Reith, Pitt & Hockey, 2001; Sibert, Craft & Jackson, 1977). The reason for the age difference lies in the increased tendency for adolescents to deliberately use drugs and toxins for recreational activities or for suicide (Byard *et al.*, 2000b). The age distribution of a series of deaths due to poisoning from South Australia is shown in Figure 2.69.

Farm deaths

Agriculture ranks second only to mining in terms of occupational danger, with proportionately more children than adults dying. Although only 2% of children in the USA live on farms, there are almost

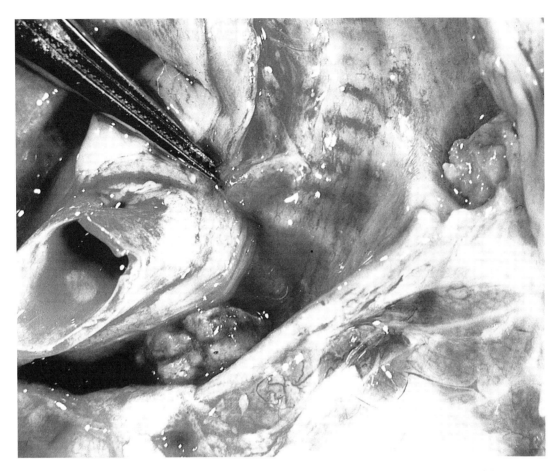

Figure 2.49 Fragments of meat plugging both main bronchi in an eight-month-old boy who collapsed while being fed.

as many deaths from farm machines as there are deaths due to falls or poisoning in the home (Byard *et al.*, 1999a; Dunn & Runyan, 1993; Fragar 1996; Wolfenden & Sanson-Fisher, 1993).

Farms provide a unique blend of home and industrial environments in which there are many hazards for children. Studies of farm deaths have shown that children are at risk of death and serious injury from tractor run-overs, drowning in dammed areas of water, suffocation in wheat silos, and unsupervised access to machinery (Byard *et al.*, 1998b; Mandryk & Harrison, 1995; Salmi *et al.*, 1989). Long working hours during peak seasons, working during all weather conditions, use of old machinery, and

involvement of all family members in farm activities have all been cited as contributing factors to the high rates of morbidity and mortality (Swanson *et al.*, 1987). Injuries are severe, characterized by amputations, evisceration, and crushing (Figures 2.70–2.73) (Byard *et al.*, 1999a). Younger children tend to be injured from animal kicks, vehicle run-overs, and falls, while older children are injured while riding horses or using equipment without proper supervision (Cameron, Bishop & Sibert, 1992; Holland *et al.*, 2001). Fatal falls are uncommon, as children generally survive falls from heights of three stories or less (Barlow *et al.*, 1983). The age distribution of a series of farm-related fatalities is shown in Figure 2.74.

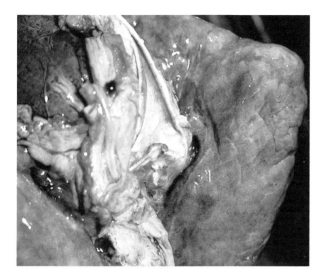

Figure 2.50 Filling of the airways with wheat pellets in a boy who asphyxiated in a grain storage silo.

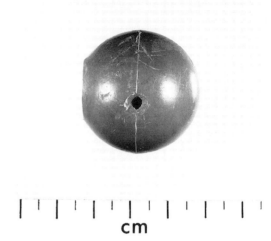

Figure 2.52 A 33-mm plastic ball that was attached loosely to the handle of a toy was found impacted in the oropharynx of an 18-month-old girl.

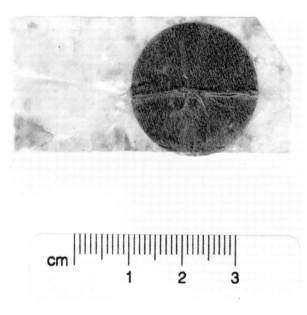

Figure 2.51 A piece of tape with a circular sticker, most likely from a rented videotape, that was wedged in the glottis of a seven-year-old boy who choked. The autopsy findings were non-specific.

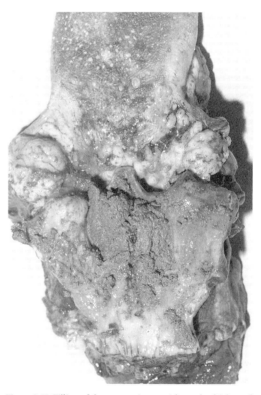

Figure 2.53 Filling of the upper airway with sand, which can be seen spilling out of the glottis in a 12-year-old boy who was buried while digging a hole.

Deaths due to animal activity

Deaths attributed to animal actions are quite varied, and include anaphylaxis from insects, toxic effects from snake or spider envenomation, trauma from falling off horses, shark attacks, and kicks from large farm animals (Lee, 2000). While injuries from large predators are reasonably obvious, snake, spider, and insect bites or stings may be extremely difficult to identify at autopsy. Infants and young children may also be more susceptible to envenomation than adults due to their smaller size. Domestically, the most common form of lethal episode is from dog attack. In 1995–96, 25 people in the USA died from dog attacks, 80% of whom were children aged from neonates to 11 years (Centers for Disease Control, 1997).

Children are particularly vulnerable to attacks by dogs as they are small and are often incapable of either self-defense or escape. Provocation of the attacking animal is also a possibility, and toxicological assessment of victims has been recommended (Lauridson & Myers, 1993). Injuries from dog attacks consist of puncture/stab wounds and lacerations/incised wounds of the face and extremities, with fatalities resulting from crushing head or neck injuries or exsanguination from multiple injuries (Wiseman, Chochinov & Fraser, 1983). The combination of considerable canine biting strength, with forces measured at 200–400 pounds per square inch, and the relative softness of the infant skull predisposes to cerebral trauma (Pinckney & Kennedy, 1980; Wilberger & Pang, 1983).

At autopsy there may be bites to all parts of the body, consisting of linear punctate abrasions or puncture wounds, with avulsion of the nose, skin, lips, and ears. There may be abrasions and lacerations from claws, with crushing injuries to the cranium (Figures 2.75 and 2.76). Rarely, a perpetrator may attempt to disguise a homicide by feeding the dismembered remains of a corpse to a dog (Boglioli et al., 2000).

Odontological examination of the bite marks may be useful, as the shape of the wounds will depend on the facial characteristics of the attacking dog, which

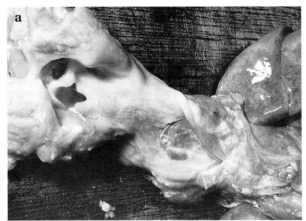

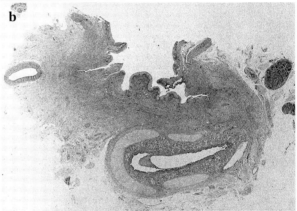

Figure 2.54 A one-cent coin wedged firmly in the upper esophagus in a four-month-old boy who was initially considered to have died of SIDS (a). Histologic cross-section after removal of the coin revealed ulceration on either side of the esophagus, with compression of the adjacent trachea, which contained mucopurulent debris (b). (Hematoxylin and eosin, ×6.)

are breed- and dog-specific, enabling confirmation of the identification of the particular animal (Clark et al., 1991). As many attacks occur in a domestic setting and involve a dog known to the child, identification may not be an issue.

Pit bull breeds and German shepherds have been the most common breeds involved in attacks (Sacks, Sattin & Bonzo, 1989), although dingos (wild dogs) in Australia have also been known to attack infants and children.

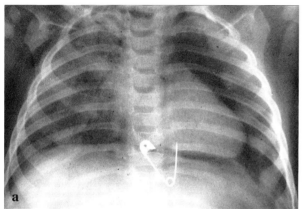

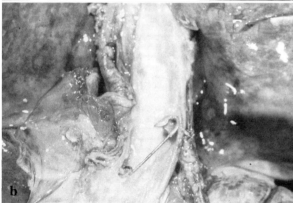

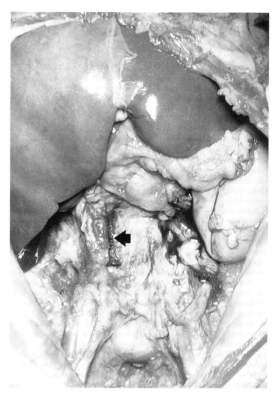

Figure 2.56 A swallowed wood screw (arrow) found in the retroperitoneum of a mentally retarded boy associated with bacterial septicemia.

Figure 2.55 A chest X-ray of an eight-month-old boy who collapsed in a doctor's office, showing an opened safety pin piercing the heart (a). At autopsy, the safety pin was found to have penetrated the anterior wall of the esophagus (b) and the posterior wall of the left ventricle, causing death from cardiac tamponade.

Drug and substance abuse

Cocaine

Cocaine, used by 30 million Americans (Barnes, 1988), many of whom are teenagers, may cause death by a variety of different mechanisms. The underlying pathogenesis of cocaine toxicity is prevention of reuptake of norepinephrine at adrenergic nerve endings and inhibition of reuptake and subsequent metabolism of circulating epinephrine (Hueter, 1987). Cocaine can cause lethal re-entrant arrhythmias and ischemic heart disease by inducing coronary artery spasm, accelerating the development of fixed atherosclerotic lesions (Karch & Billingham, 1988), causing intimal hyperplasia (Simpson & Edwards, 1986) and initiating coronary thrombosis (Stenberg *et al.*, 1989). Contraction band necrosis frequently occurs; less commonly, hypersensitivity myocarditis, chronic heart failure, and valvular heart disease may be observed (Karch & Billingham, 1988).

Volatiles

Inhaled volatile substances have included antiperspirants, flyspray, air fresheners, cigarette lighters, coronary artery dilators, shoe polish, typewriter correction fluid, degreasers, solvents, paint remover,

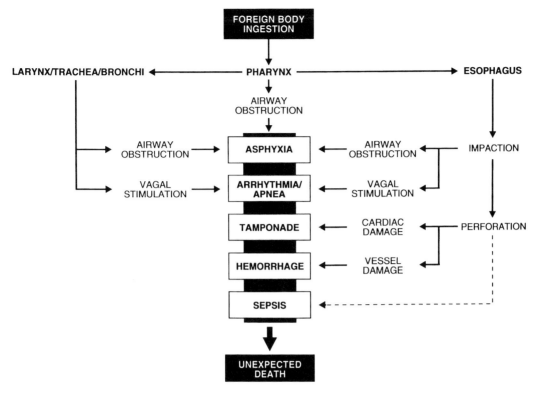

Figure 2.57 A summary of possible causes and mechanisms of sudden and unexpected death in infancy and childhood following foreign body ingestion.

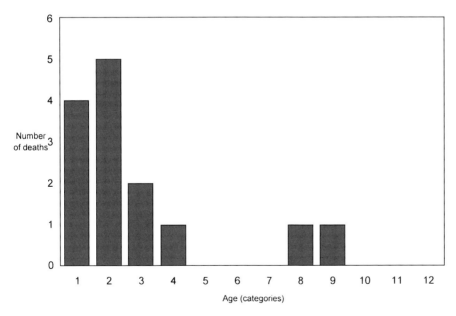

Figure 2.58 Age distribution of 14 cases of accidental asphyxia in childhood from foreign body asphyxia taken from a study of 369 cases of accidental childhood death in South Australia, showing a preponderance of cases in infancy and early childhood (1 = first year).

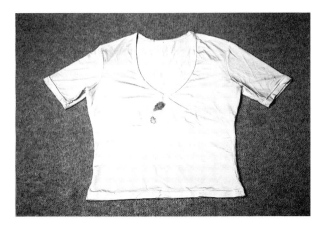

Figure 2.59 Staining of a mother's shirt with serosanguinous fluid from the nose and mouth of her two-month old infant who was found dead beside her in bed. Death was attributed to overlaying. The staining of the shirt confirmed that the infant had been in contact with his mother at some stage during the night.

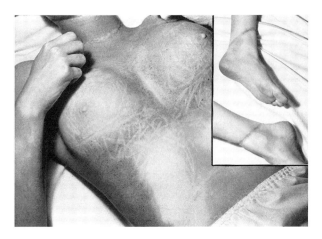

Figure 2.60 Rope marks around the neck and ankles of a 19-year-old woman who died during an autoerotic asphyxial episode.

adhesives, cleaning fluid for textiles, and felt tip marking pens (Bowen, Daniel & Balster, 1999; Fosseus, 1991; King, Smialek & Troutman, 1985; McHugh, 1987). Deaths occur mainly in adolescents (King, Smialek & Troutman, 1985), although older individuals may be involved (McBride & Busuttil,

1990). In their evaluation of 34 cases of death from inhalant abuse, Garriott & Petty (1980) found that 16 children died from inhaling freon (halogenated methane), five from nitrous oxide, three from 1,1,1 trichloroethane or trichloroethylene, three from alkane gas (natural gas), and the remainder from paint, carbon tetrachloride, toluene, and miscellaneous substances. They noted that freon deaths decreased dramatically after the local media publicized the danger of sniffing freon-containing products. Deaths may be due to accidents such as drowning or falling while the victim is intoxicated, or from direct inhalant toxicity (Chao *et al.*, 1993). While deaths are usually accidental, suicides using inhalants occasionally occur (Klitte *et al.*, 2001).

Inhalants produce a dose-related, rapid-onset, short-duration effect ranging from mild euphoria and disorientation to sedation requiring deep pain for arousal (Troutman, 1988). The main mechanism of death is sensitization of the myocardium to endogenous catecholamines, leading to arrhythmias that may be precipitated by exercise or fright (Adgey, Johnston & McMechan, 1995; Rohrig, 1997). Other mechanisms include asthma, aspiration of gastric contents, asphyxia from the plastic bag into which the volatile substance was sprayed prior to sniffing, central respiratory depression, and cerebral edema with herniation (D'Costa & Gunasekera, 1990; Esmail *et al.*, 1993; Troutman, 1988). Chronic abuse may lead to cerebellar degeneration and liver cirrhosis (Al-Alousi, 1989; Garriott & Petty, 1980). Parker, Tarlow & Milne Anderson (1984) reported a case of cerebral infarct that followed an episode of sniffing trichloroethylene and that was thought to be due to spasm of the left middle cerebral artery. Since 1982, mustard oil has been added to some batches of typewriter correction fluid to prevent abuse, but nonetheless in one of the three sniffing deaths reported by Troutman (1988) addition of this substance had not prevented abuse. Steadman *et al.* (1984) reported sudden death (unmonitored) and non-fatal ventricular fibrillation in two adolescent boys, respectively, who inhaled bromochlorodifluoromethane sprayed from a fire extinguisher into a plastic bag.

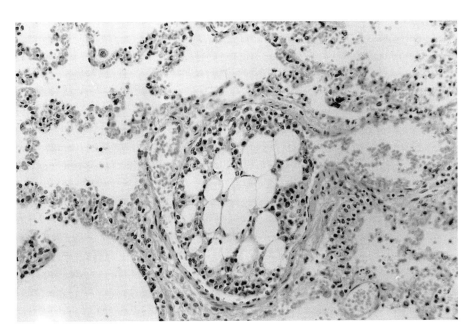

Figure 2.61 Bone marrow embolus within a small pulmonary vessel in a case of failed cardiopulmonary resuscitation.

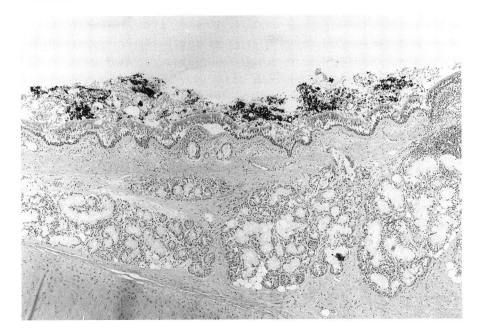

Figure 2.62 Carbon staining of the mucosal surfaces of the upper airway of a five-year-old boy who died in a house fire. His blood carboxyhemoglobin level was 65%, with an elevated cyanide level.

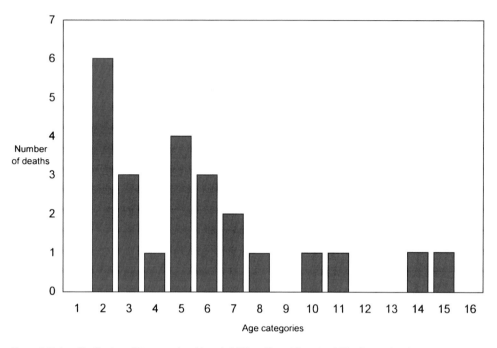

Figure 2.63 Age distribution of 24 cases of accidental childhood burn/flame/scald fatalities taken from a study of 369 cases of accidental childhood death in South Australia, showing a preponderance of cases in infancy and early childhood (1 = first year).

Glue or correction fluid may be found on the hands or around the nose and mouth at autopsy (Figure 2.77), and a "glue sniffer's rash" has been described around the nose in habitual users (Watson, 1978). However, given the generally non-specific findings at autopsy in such cases, death scene examination may play a vital role in the investigation of possible inhalant deaths with confirmatory head space analysis for volatiles during toxicological evaluation of blood and tissues.

Gasoline

Gasoline (petrol) inhalation forms a distinct subset of inhalant abuse that is found particularly in disadvantaged rural communities associated with sudden death. There is a high level of use among young indigenous people in Australia, Canada, the USA, Mexico, and South Africa (Steffee, Davis & Nicol, 1996). Prolonged gasoline sniffing leads to neurological impairment, with encephalopathy manifest by motor impairment and ataxia with seizures. The toxic effects arise from both volatile aromatic hydrocarbons and also tetraethyl lead. Deaths may arise from burns if the gasoline ignites (Flanagan & Ives, 1994). The latter may occur if the gasoline has been heated over a flame to enhance the amount of vapor present.

The autopsy assessment of such cases requires careful examination of the face for impressions of containers used to hold gasoline to the nose. Typical containers that may be with the body at the scene consist of tin cans molded to fit the shape of the face or cut-away plastic containers (Figure 2.78). The body may smell of gasoline, and there may be epistaxis with gasoline burns around the mouth and nose. Abnormalities may be present within the cerebellum, brainstem, or basal ganglia with chronic abuse, with loss of Purkinje cells and neuronal chromatolysis. There may also be gliosis and neuronal

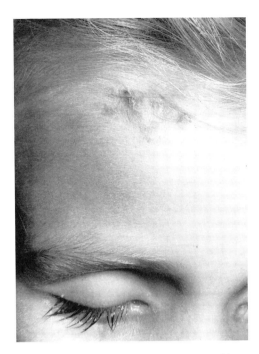

Figure 2.64 Burn on the forehead of a seven-year-old boy who bumped into a defective air conditioner and was electrocuted.

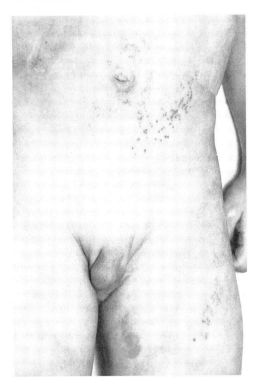

Figure 2.65 Electrical arc burns on the abdomen of a four-year-old boy who touched power lines while playing on a garage roof.

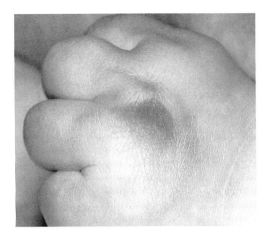

Figure 2.66 Classical electrical burns in a case of childhood electrocution, showing targetoid appearances with peripheral blanching and hyperemic borders.

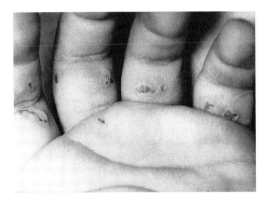

Figure 2.67 Finger burns in a child who grasped a live wire.

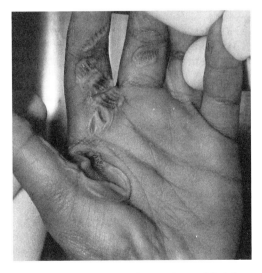

Figure 2.68 Patterned electrical contact burns of the left hand of a four-year-old girl who was electrocuted while playing with a faulty hairdryer.

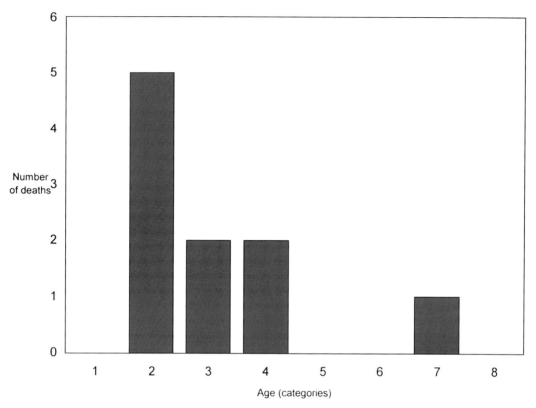

Figure 2.69 Age distribution of 10 cases of accidental childhood poisoning taken from a study of 369 cases of accidental childhood death in South Australia, showing a preponderance of cases between the second and fourth years (1 = first year).

depopulation of the cerebral cortex and hippocampus (Maruff *et al.*, 1998).

Confirmation of exposure requires toxicological assessment of head space vapor for gasoline constituents, such as aromatic hydrocarbons (benzene, xylene, and toluene), alkenes, paraffins, and naphthalene. Blood lead levels may also be elevated (Goodheart & Dunne, 1994).

Opiates

Intravenous narcotism, although unusual in children, should be suspected when the death scene includes characteristic drug paraphernalia such as syringes, tourniquets, powder, pills, razor blades, and straws. If death occurs sufficiently rapidly, then the needle may still be in the decedent's vein when the body is discovered. Gross autopsy findings may include fresh needle punctures, needle track scars, and frothy pulmonary edema emitting from the nose or mouth. Microscopic findings include infection (abscesses and/or infective endocarditis) and foreign body granulomas containing starch, talc, cotton, or other material, chiefly in the lungs but occasionally in the liver, lymph nodes, and spleen (Gross, 1978).

Amphetamines

In recent years there has been increasing use of "designer drugs" in the form of ring-derivative amphetamines. These drugs, the most widely known of which is 3,4-methylenedioxymethamphetamine (MDMA, or ecstasy), exert their effects through the

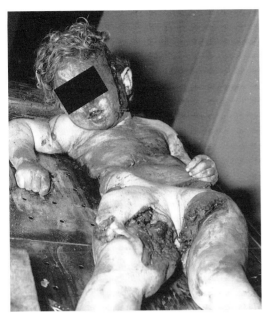

Figure 2.70 A four-year-old girl who fell from a tractor on a farm and was run over by a rotary hoe sustained multiple deep lacerations of the limbs and trunk, with extensive soft tissue, internal organ, and bone damage.

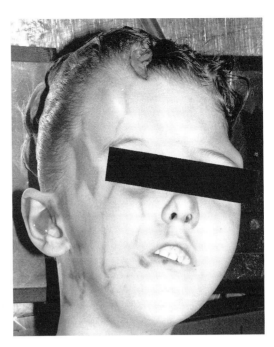

Figure 2.72 A three-year-old girl sustained a severe crush injury of the head after being run over by a tractor and trailer loaded with hay on a farm. The tread marks of the vehicle tires can be seen on her face.

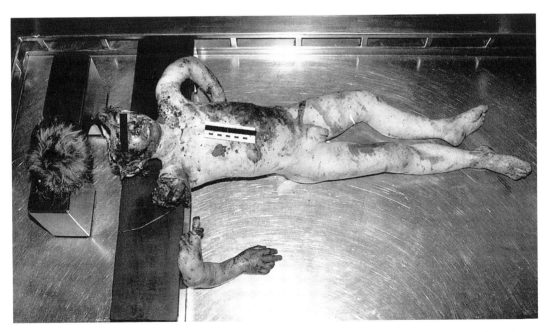

Figure 2.71 A five-year-old boy who fell from a tractor on a farm and was run over by a mower suffered amputation of his right arm and a severe head injury.

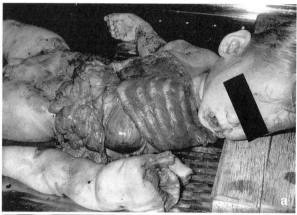

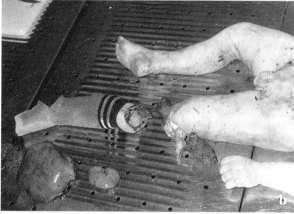

Figure 2.73 A three-year-old boy who became entangled in a tractor power take-off on a farm sustained amputation of his left arm and leg, with avulsion of his left kidney and liver and extensive degloving injuries of the chest and abdomen.

serotonergic, noradrenergic, and dopaminergic neurotransmitter pathways, and are popular in the "rave" dance scene. Although initially enhanced alertness and confidence is reported by users, toxic effects include hyperthermia with rhabdomyolysis (Figure 2.79), convulsions, disseminated intravascular coagulation, multiorgan failure, and death (Byard *et al.*, 1998a). Toxicity varies among the drugs in this group, with increasing numbers of fatalities being reported due to paramethoxyamphetamine (PMA) ingestion. This ring-derivative amphetamine is appropriately named "death" or "killer" on the streets (Byard *et al.*, 2002b).

Alcohol

Intoxication with alcohol is found in a large number of cases of motor vehicle accidents involving adolescents and young adults, in addition to being a significant contributor to drowning deaths (Rogers, Harris & Jarmuskewicz, 1987; Rosenberg, Rodriguez & Chorba, 1990). Aspiration of gastric contents, respiratory depression and postural asphyxia are other potentially lethal problems.

Hyperthermia and hypothermia

As there are often no characteristic autopsy findings in children, and as the autopsy may reveal only normal organs and tissues, a detailed history with clinical findings if available must be sought in cases of suspected hyper- or hypothermia. The duration of exposure to harmful environmental conditions is an important factor.

Hyperthermia

In hyperthermic deaths, the temperature, humidity, and ventilation (wind conditions) of the death scene should be documented. The body temperature should be noted, as should the degree of physical activity at the time of collapse (Benz, 1980). Medical conditions such as cystic fibrosis and congenital adrenal hyperplasia may predispose infants and children to unexpected death in hot weather. Environmental hazards include closed automobiles on hot days and overwrapping infants in front of heaters in the wintertime.

Hyperthermia (heat stroke) occurs when the environmental temperature is high and the rectal temperature exceeds 40.6 °C (105 °F) (Hiss *et al.*, 1994). There may have been signs of central nervous system malfunction, such as coma and muscle spasm, prior to death. Infants are particularly prone to heat stroke because of their higher metabolic rates, their incompletely developed hypothalamic thermoregulatory centers, and their inability to extricate themselves from unsafe environments (Ohshima

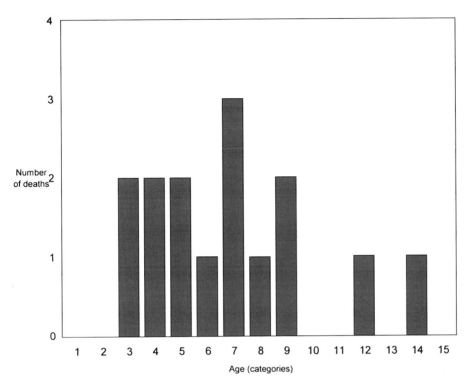

Figure 2.74 Age distribution of 15 cases of accidental childhood farm-related fatalities taken from a study of 369 cases of accidental childhood death in South Australia, showing a clustering of cases between the third and ninth years
(1 = first year).

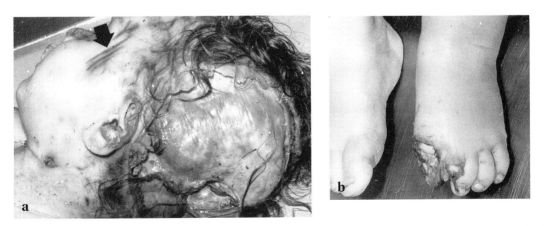

Figure 2.75 Exposure of the dura and brain of a 17-month-old boy who was attacked by two bull terrier dogs. Large amounts of scalp and skull were missing from the left side of the head. Parallel abrasions on the left side of the forehead were in keeping with scratches from paws (arrow) (a). There was also avulsion of toes from the left foot (b).

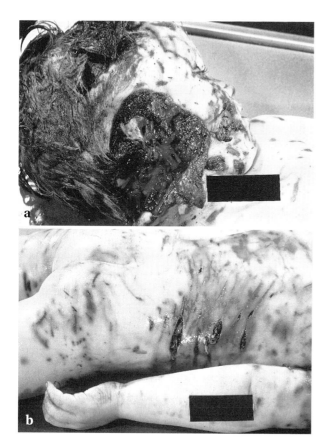
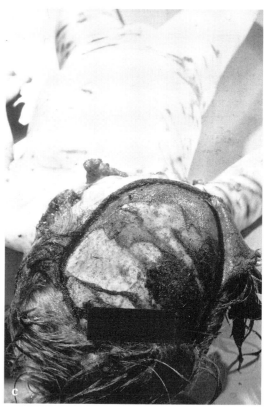

Figure 2.76 Head of a 17-month-old girl who was the victim of a dog attack, showing avulsion of the ear and surrounding skin, with numerous bite marks to the face and chest (a). The torso and buttocks also showed numerous bruises, abrasions, incisions, and stab wounds from dog teeth (b). A large part of the scalp had been removed, as in the previous case (Figure 2.75), with exposure of the skull. Crushing injuries from the dog's jaws included multiple skull fractures (c).

et al., 1992). Two groups of children tend to be at risk of hyperthermic death: febrile infants who are over-wrapped in a warm room, and children who are left, or become trapped, in a motor vehicle and are rapidly exposed to quite high environmental temperatures (Bacon, Scott & Jones, 1979; Krous *et al.*, 2001). In some cases, modification of the interior of a car, such as by inserting a cargo barrier (Figure 2.80), may create a trap for exploring children, as may automatic locking devices (Byard, Bourne & James, 1999; Byard, Noblett & Fotheringham, 2000).

Children and infants in hot environments may be dehydrated as well as hyperthermic, with sunken fontanelles and eyes, reduced skin turgor, and dry mucus membranes and internal organs, but this is not invariable (Whitehead *et al.*, 1996). Postmortem vitreous humor levels of sodium >155 mmol/l, chloride >135 mmol/l, and urea >40 mmol/l have been cited as reliable indicators of antemortem dehydration (Knight, 1997).

Hypothermia

In the investigation of hypothermic deaths, the degree of wetness of the body should be assessed, since a wet body loses heat much faster than a dry one.

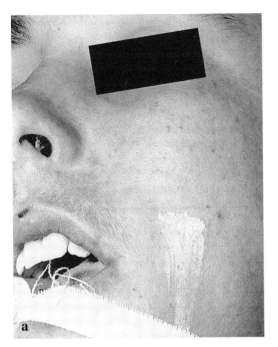

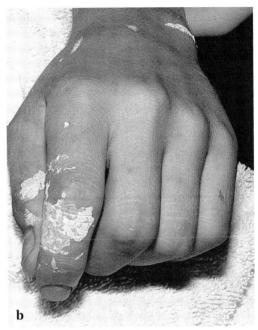

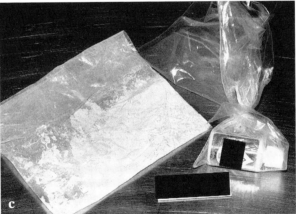

Figure 2.77 Typewriter correction fluid was found on the face (a) and hands (b) of this 15-year-old male who was found dead beside a plastic bag and correction fluid container (c).

The presence of frostbite indicates survival for some time following exposure to cold. Additional important information in the investigation of hypothermia deaths includes the environmental temperature, humidity, and windchill, the duration of exposure, the amount and type of clothing, the body temperature when found, evidence of alcohol or drug use, and the medical history.

Hypothermia occurs when the core temperature is less than 35 °C (95 °F), and may be due to exposure to low environmental temperatures or to an underlying disorder that interferes with thermoregulation

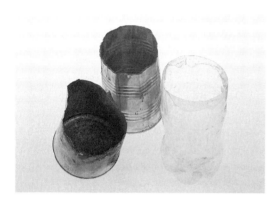

Figure 2.78 Metal and plastic containers used for gasoline sniffing by children in an isolated Aboriginal community in central Australia. The metal container on the left has been molded to better fit around the nose.

(Reuler, 1978; Ward & Cowley, 1999). Potentially lethal core temperatures range from 26 to 29 °C (79 to 85 °F), although children have been known to recover after enduring much lower temperatures (DiMaio & DiMaio 2001; Knight 1997; Spyker, 1985). The mechanism of death in hypothermia involves cardiac arrhythmias. For example, ventricular fibrillation occurs in patients externally cooled for cardiac surgery at 23 °C (73 °F), and asystole occurs at 20 °C (68 °F) (Southwick & Daglish, 1980). As with hyperthermia there are no characteristic autopsy findings (Benz, 1980), although the skin may show areas of pink discoloration, and gastric erosions (Figure 2.81), acute pancreatitis, and pulmonary edema have been noted in hypothermic adults (Knight, 1997). Coe (1984) found elevated levels of vitreous glucose in many

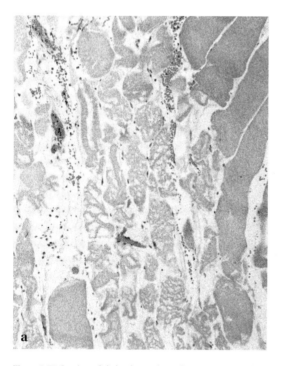
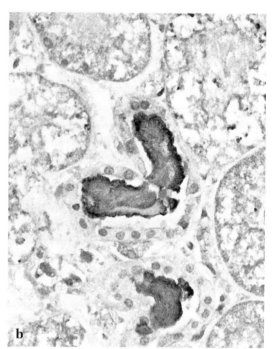

Figure 2.79 Section of skeletal muscle (a) from a 19-year-old male with lethal paramethoxyamphetamine toxicity, demonstrating edema and necrosis in keeping with rhabdomyolysis. Section of kidney demonstrating renal tubular necrosis with abundant granular casts shown on immunoperoxidase staining to be myoglobin (b). (Hematoxylin and eosin, ×100; immunoperoxidase staining, ×250.)

hypothermic deaths that were attributed to the effects of stress.

Sporting deaths

Collapse during exercise or sport is an unusual event in childhood. Deaths may be due to the direct consequences of severe trauma, such as a head or neck injury during a football match, or may be due to a simple blow to the chest from a projectile, such as a baseball or a hockey puck, so-called "commotio cordis" (*vide supra*) (Maron *et al.*, 1995). Death may be immediate or may be delayed from intracranial or abdominal complications such as hemorrhage or sepsis (Figure 2.82). Collapse may also be due to exacerbation of an underlying medical condition, which may be congenital, such as aortic stenosis, or may be acquired, such as myocarditis. There may be a complex interplay of a variety of factors producing the fatal episode, and toxicological assessment should always be performed for both prescription and non-prescription drugs (Byard, James & Gilbert, 2002).

Therapeutic misadventure

Murphy (1986) divided deaths occurring during medical procedures into anesthesia-related (30%), surgical (36%), those following therapeutic (18%) or diagnostic procedures (14%), and drug reactions (2%). The lone therapeutic misadventure in the Michigan series occurred when a two-year-old girl was overhydrated with 1000 ml of intravenous fluid following a tonsillectomy and adenoidectomy.

It is recognized that infants are at higher risk of dying during anesthesia (Graff *et al.*, 1964; Mancer, 1989). Twenty percent of the patients in Graff and colleagues' (1964) study of pediatric anesthetic deaths were infants less than one week of age. Anesthesia-related deaths may occur in the operating room, recovery room, or intensive care unit, or upon return to the patient's hospital room (Mancer, 1989). Graff *et al.* (1964) found that the primary factors leading

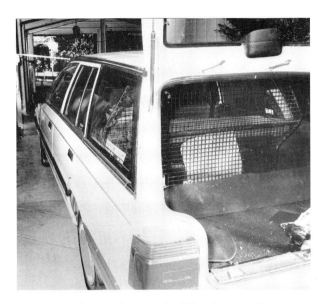

Figure 2.80 Back of a station wagon in which a nine-year-old boy and his three-year-old sister had become trapped while playing. Once the hatch had closed, they were unable to escape because of a mesh cargo barrier. The internal temperature of the car was estimated to have been 50 °C (122 °F). Both died of hyperthermia.

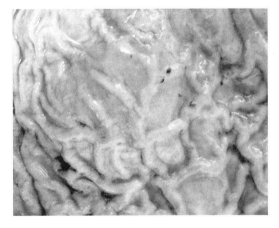

Figure 2.81 Scattered gastic erosions in a 19-year-old male who died of hypothermia (blood alcohol level 0.28%). Erosions may sometimes be quite subtle in appearance.

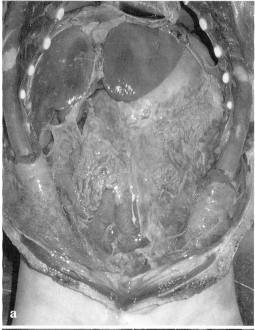

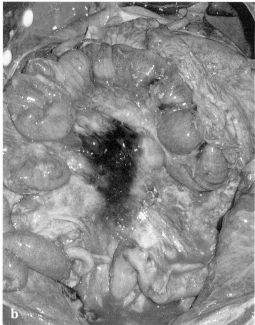

Figure 2.82 Peritonitis causing death in a four-year-old girl following a kick from a horse (a). Bruising of the mesentery was associated with rupture of the jejunum (b).

to anesthetic-related death in children were respiratory (83%) (including hypoventilation or aspiration of vomitus or blood), cardiovascular (16%) (primarily inadequate replacement of blood and fluid, and electrolyte imbalance), and neurologic (2%) (due to hyperpyrexia).

Hypoxia may arise from a slow respiratory rate, an inadequate tidal volume, or inadequate oxygenation of arterial blood. The latter may be caused by insufficient oxygen in the inspired gas caused by equipment failure (Mancer, 1989). Obstructive apnea may result from aspiration of gastric contents, pharyngeal obstruction, bronchospasm, or laryngospasm. Upper airway obstruction may render intubation difficult. Causes of obstruction include laryngotracheobronchitis, epiglottitis, foreign bodies, papillomas, airway burns, tumors, tracheomalacia, vascular abnormalities, and tonsillar hypertrophy (see Chapter 7). Airway obstruction may be worsened by anesthetic relaxation of the pharyngeal musculature (Berry, 1981).

The viscerocardiac reflex, manifest by bradycardia, hypotension, and ultimately asystole, is especially common at induction and termination of anesthesia. It can be brought about by intubation, extubation, tracheal suction, bronchoscopy, or manipulation of the viscera (Mancer, 1989). One percent of the population is predisposed to malignant hyperthermia, characterized by elevated body temperature, acidosis, hypoxia, and hyperkalemia. There are no characteristic autopsy findings.

Anesthetic agents may cause cardiac arrest and electrolyte imbalances, including hypo- and hyperkalemia, and hypercalcemia, and may be fatal. Anesthetic equipment malfunction from causes such as incorrect flowmeter settings, leaks, and misconnected gas lines may occur. Surgical complications include air embolism, intraoperative hemorrhage from inadvertant incision of the heart or great vessels, and visceral trauma (Murphy, 1986).

Anaphylactic reactions may occur during anesthesia, most often related to neuromuscular blocking agents. The estimated incidence is one in 6000 operations. The investigation of such cases involves assessing serum levels of tryptase, histamine, and specific immunoglobulin E (IgE) (Laroche *et al.*, 1992).

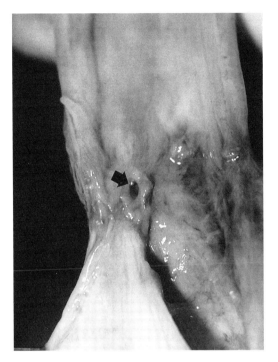

Figure 2.83 Perforation of the esophagus during a routine dilation procedure resulted in the death of a young child. The perforation (arrow) can be seen adjacent to a stricture that had resulted from previous successful surgical repair of a tracheo-esophageal fistula.

Sudden death may also occur during diagnostic procedures or treatment, such as from cardiac perforation during an endomyocardial biopsy or central hyperalimentation, or from rupture of viscera or vessels during dilation procedures for strictures (Figure 2.83) (Balaji, Oommen & Rees, 1991; Franciosi *et al.*, 1982; Karnak *et al.*, 1998). Embolization of catheter tips following cardiac catheterization may occur (Klys, Salmon & De Giovanni, 1991).

The investigation of a death occurring while a child is undergoing an operative procedure should include review of the operative record and previous medical history, interview of the surgeon and anesthesiologist, and consultation with an anesthesiologist and surgeon not associated with the case (Reay *et al.*, 1985).

Children may also be more sensitive than adults to certain drugs (Biederman, 1991). For example, the mechanism of sudden death in children treated with indomethacin for rheumatoid arthritis is unclear, although it may involve hepatotoxicity (Balduck *et al.*, 1987; Jacobs, 1967). Unfortunately, assessment of cases is sometimes complicated by uncertainty as to the significance of standard therapeutic and toxic ranges for medications in the very young.

Other deaths in hospitals

Accidents in hospital wards may occur, but fortunately they are seldom fatal. In a study of 781 in-hospital accidents, Levene & Bonfield (1991) found injuries in only 443 children. Falls accounted for 42% of cases, with 27% of accidents involving beds or cribs. One potentially lethal entrapment between a mattress and crib side occurred, and two fractured skulls were documented. Buchino, Corey & Montgomery (2002), in their review of sudden unexpected deaths in hospitalized children, separated causes of death into six categories: natural, failure to monitor, therapeutic misadventures, suicide, homicide, and unexplained.

REFERENCES

Abrunzo, T. J. (1991). Commotio cordis. The single, most common cause of traumatic death in youth baseball. *American Journal of Diseases of Children*, **145**, 1279–82.

Accident Facts. (1990). Chicago: National Safety Council.

Ackerman, J. & Gilbert-Barness, E. (1997). Suspended rocking cradles, positional asphyxia, and sudden infant death. *Archives of Pediatric and Adolescent Medicine*, **151**, 573–5.

Adams J. H. (1984). Head injury. In *Greenfield's Neuropathology*, 4th edn, ed. J. H. Adams, J. A. N. Corsellis & L. W. Duchan. New York: John Wiley & Sons, pp. 85–124.

Adgey, A. A. J., Johnston, P. W. & McMechan S. (1995). Sudden cardiac death and substance abuse. *Resuscitation*, **29**, 219–21.

Al-Alousi, L. M. (1989). Pathology of volatile substance abuse: a case report and literature review. *Medicine, Science and the Law*, **29**, 189–208.

Al-Hilou, R. (1991). Inhalation of foreign bodies by children: review of experience with 74 cases from Dubai. *Journal of Laryngology and Otology*, **105**, 466–70.

Allgood, S. C., Scholten, D. J. & Cohle, S. D. (1990). Epidemiology and management of traumatic rupture of the thoracic aorta: a clinical series and autopsy review. Presented at Grand Rapids Area Medical Education Council Research Day, April 1990.

Altmann, A. & Nolan, T. (1995). Non-intentional asphyxiation deaths due to upper airway interference in children 0 to 14 years. *Injury Prevention*, **1**, 76–80.

Amanuel, B. & Byard, R. W. (2000). Accidental asphyxia in bed in severely disabled children. *Journal of Paediatrics and Child Health*, **36**, 66–8.

Amyand, C. (1736). Of an inguinal rupture, with a pin in the appendix caeci encrusted with stone: some observations on wounds in the guts. *Philosophical Transactions*, **39**, 329–36.

Atkins, C. (1895). Case of swallowing a halfpenny, without symptoms: death two months afterwards from opening into the innominate artery. *British Medical Journal*, 4 May, 978.

Bacon, C., Scott, D. & Jones, P. (1979). Heatstroke in well-wrapped infants. *Lancet*, **i**, 422–5.

Bajanowski, T., West, A. & Brinkmann, B. (1998). Proof of fatal air embolism. *International Journal of Legal Medicine*, **111**, 208–11.

Baker, S. P. & Fisher, R. S. (1980). Childhood asphyxiation by choking or suffocation. *Journal of the American Medical Association*, **244**, 1343–6.

Balaji, S., Oommen, R. & Rees, P. G. (1991). Fatal aortic rupture during balloon dilatation of recoarctation. *British Heart Journal*, **65**, 100–101.

Balduck, N., Otten, J., Verbruggen, L., *et al.* (1987). Sudden death of a child with juvenile chronic arthritis, probably due to indomethacin. *European Journal of Pediatrics*, **146**, 620.

Banerjee, A., Rao, K. S. V. K. S., Khanna, S. K., *et al.* (1988). Laryngo-tracheo-bronchial foreign bodies in children. *Journal of Laryngology and Otology*, **102**, 1029–32.

Barlow, B., Niemirska, M., Gandhi, R. P. & Leblanc, W. (1983). Ten years of experience with falls from a height in children. *Journal of Pediatric Surgery*, **18**, 509–11.

Barnes D. M. (1988). Drugs: running the numbers. *Science*, **240**, 1729–31.

Beal, S. M. & Byard, R. W. (1995). Accidental death or sudden infant death syndrome? *Journal of Paediatrics and Child Health*, **31**, 269–71.

Beal, S. M., Moore, L., Collett, M., *et al.* (1995). The danger of freely rocking cradles. *Journal of Paediatrics and Child Health*, **31**, 38–40.

Benz, J. A. (1980). Thermal deaths. In *Modern Legal Medicine, Psychiatry, and Forensic Science*, ed. W. J. Curran, A. L. McGarry & C. S. Petty. Philadelphia: F. A. Davis, pp. 268–304.

Berry, F. A. (1981). Pediatric anesthesia. *Otolaryngology Clinics of North America*, **14**, 533–56.

Bhana, B. D., Gunaselvam, J. G. & Dada, M. A. (2000). Mechanical airway obstruction caused by accidental aspiration of part of a ballpoint pen. *American Journal of Forensic Medicine and Pathology*, **21**, 362–5.

Biederman, J. (1991). Sudden death in children treated with a tricyclic antidepressant. *Journal of the American Academy of Child and Adolescent Psychiatry*, **30**, 495–8.

Boglioli, L. R., Taff, M. L., Turkel, S. J., Taylor, J. V. & Peterson, C. D. (2000). Unusual infant death. Dog attack or postmortem mutilation after child abuse? *American Journal of Forensic Medicine and Pathology*, **21**, 389–94.

Bor, I. (1969). Myocardial infarction and ischaemic heart disease in infants and children. Analysis of 29 cases and review of the literature. *Archives of Disease in Childhood*, **44**, 268–81.

Bowen, S. E., Daniel, J. & Balster, R. L. (1999). Deaths associated with inhalant abuse in Virginia from 1987 to 1996. *Drug and Alcohol Dependence*, **53**, 239–45.

Buchino, J. J., Corey, T. S. & Montgomery, V. (2002). Sudden unexpected death in hospitalized children. *Journal of Pediatrics*, **140**, 461–5.

Busuttil, A. & Obafunwa, J. O. (1993). Recreational abdominal suspension: a fatal practice. *American Journal of Forensic Medicine and Pathology*, **12**, 141–4.

Byard, R. W. (1994a). Unexpected death due to acute airway obstruction in daycare centers. *Pediatrics*, **94**, 113–14.

Byard, R. W. (1994b). Is co-sleeping in infancy a desirable or dangerous practice? *Journal of Paediatrics and Child Health*, **30**, 198–9.

Byard, R. W. (1994c). Sudden infant death syndrome: historical background, possible mechanisms and diagnostic problems. *Journal of Law and Medicine*, **2**, 18–26.

Byard, R. W. (1994d). Autoerotic death – characteristic features and diagnostic difficulties. *Journal of Clinical Forensic Medicine*, **1**, 71–8.

Byard, R. W. (1995). Sudden infant death syndrome – a 'diagnosis' in search of a disease. *Journal of Clinical Forensic Medicine*, **2**, 121–8.

Byard, R. W. (1996a). Hazardous infant and early childhood sleeping environments and death scene examination. *Journal of Clinical Forensic Medicine*, **3**, 115–22.

Byard, R. W. (1996b). Mechanisms of unexpected death in infants and young children following foreign body ingestion. *Journal of Forensic Sciences*, **41**, 438–41.

Byard, R. W. (1998). Is breast feeding in bed always a safe practice? *Journal of Paediatrics and Child Health*, **34**, 418–19.

Byard, R. W. (2000). Accidental childhood death and the role of the pathologist. *Pediatric and Developmental Pathology*, **3**, 405–18.

Byard, R. W. (2001). Accidental childhood death and the role of the pathologist. In *Perspectives in Pediatric Pathology*, vol. 23, ed. J. E. Dimmick & D. B. Singer. New York: Springer, pp. 77–90.

Byard, R. W. (2002). Incapacitation or death of a socially isolated parent or carer may result in the death of dependent children. *Journal of Paediatrics and Child Health*, **23**, 417–18.

Byard, R. W. & Beal, S. M. (1997). V-shaped pillows and unsafe infant sleeping. *Journal of Paediatrics and Child Health*, **33**, 171–3.

Byard, R. W. & Bramwell, N. H. (1988). Autoerotic death in females – an underdiagnosed syndrome? *American Journal of Forensic Medicine and Pathology*, **9**, 252–4.

Byard, R. W. & Bramwell, N. H. (1991). Autoerotic death – a definition. *American Journal Of Forensic Medicine and Pathology*, **12**, 74–6.

Byard, R. W. & Burnell, R. H. (1995). Apparent life threatening events and infant holding practices. *Archives of Disease in Childhood*, **73**, 502–4.

Byard, R. W. & Hilton, J. (1997). Overlaying, accidental suffocation and sudden infant death. *Journal of Sudden Infant Death Syndrome and Infant Mortality*, **2**, 161–5.

Byard, R. W. & James, R. A. (2001). Car window entrapment and accidental childhood asphyxia. *Journal of Paediatrics and Child Health*, **37**, 201–2.

Byard, R. W. & Krous, H. F. (1999). Suffocation, shaking and sudden infant death syndrome: can we tell the difference? *Journal of Paediatrics and Child Health*, **35**, 432–3.

Byard, R. W. & Lipsett, J. (1999). Drowning deaths in toddlers and preambulatory children in South Australia. *American Journal of Forensic Medicine and Pathology*, **20**, 328–32.

Byard, R. W, Beal, S., Blackbourne, B., Nadeau, J. M. & Krous, H. F. (2001a). Specific dangers associated with infants sleeping on sofas. *Journal of Paediatrics and Child Health*, **37**, 476–8.

Byard, R. W., Beal, S. & Bourne, A. J. (1994). Potentially dangerous sleeping environments and accidental asphyxia in infancy and early childhood. *Archives of Disease in Childhood*, **71**, 497–500.

Byard, R. W., Beal, S. M., Simpson, A., Carter, R. F. & Khong, T. Y. (1996a). Accidental infant death and stroller-prams. *Medical Journal of Australia*, **165**, 140–41.

Byard, R. W., Bourne, A. J. & Beal, S. M. (1996). Mesh-sided cots – yet another potentially dangerous infant sleeping environment. *Forensic Science International*, **83**, 105–9.

Byard, R. W., Bourne, A. J. & James, R. (1999). Childhood deaths and cargo barriers in cars. *Journal of Paediatrics and Child Health*, **35**, 409–10.

Byard, R. W., Bourne, A. J., Moore, L., & Little, K. E. T. (1992). Sudden death in infancy due to delayed cardiac tamponade complicating central venous line insertion and cardiac catheterisation. *Archives of Pathology and Laboratory Medicine*, **116**, 654–6.

Byard, R. W., de Koning, C., Blackbourne, B., Nadeau, J. M. & Krous, H. F. (2001b). Shared bathing and drowning in infants and young children. *Journal of Paediatrics and Child Health*, **37**, 542–4.

Byard, R. W., Gallard, V., Johnson, A., *et al.* (1996b). Safe feeding practices for infants and young children. *Journal of Paediatrics and Child Health*, **32**, 327–9.

Byard, R. W., Gilbert, J., James, R. & Lipsett, J. (1999a). Pathological features of farm and tractor-related fatalities in children. *American Journal of Forensic Medicine and Pathology*, **20**, 73–7.

Byard, R. W., Gilbert, J., James, R. & Lokan, R. J. (1998a). Amphetamine derivative fatalities in South Australia – is "Ecstacy" the culprit? *American Journal of Forensic Medicine and Pathology*, **19**, 261–5.

Byard, R. W., Gilbert, J. D., Klitte, Å. & Felgate, P. (2002a). Gasoline exposure in motor vehicle accident fatalities. *American Journal of Forensic Medicine and Pathology*, **23**, 42–4.

Byard, R. W., Gilbert, J., Lipsett, J. & James, R. (1998b). Farm and tractor-related fatalities in children in South Australia. *Journal of Paediatrics and Child Health*, **34**, 139–41.

Byard, R. W., Green, H., James, R. A. & Gilbert, J. D. (2000a). Pathological features of childhood pedestrian fatalities. *American Journal of Forensic Medicine and Pathology*, **21**, 101–6.

Byard, R. W., Hanson, K. A., Gilbert, J. D., *et al.* (2003). Death due to electrocution in childhood and early adolescence. *Journal of Paediatrics and Child Health*, **39**, 46–8.

Byard, R. W., Hanson, K. A. & James, R. A. (2003). Fatal unintentional traumatic asphyxia in childhood. *Journal of Paediatrics and Child Health*, **39**, 31–2.

Byard, R. W., Hucker, S. J. & Hazelwood, R. R. (1990). A comparison of typical death scene features in cases of fatal male and female autoerotic asphyxia with a review of the literature. *Forensic Science International*, **48**, 113–21.

Byard, R. W., James, R. A. & Gilbert, J. D. (2002). Childhood sporting deaths. *American Journal of Forensic Medicine and Pathology*, **23**, 364–7.

Byard, R. W., Knight, D., James, R. A. & Gilbert, J. (1999b). Murder–suicides involving children – a 29 year study. *American Journal of Forensic Medicine and Pathology*, **20**, 323–7.

Byard, R. W., Lipsett, J. & Gilbert, J. (2000). Fire deaths in children in South Australia from 1989 to 1998. *Journal of Paediatrics and Child Health*, **36**, 176–8.

Byard, R. W., Markopoulos, D., Prasad, D., *et al.* (2000b). Early adolescent suicide: a comparative study. *Journal of Clinical Forensic Medicine*, **7**, 6–9.

Byard, R. W., Moore, L., & Bourne, A. J. (1990). Sudden and unexpected death: a late effect of occult intraesophageal foreign body. *Pediatric Pathology*, **10**, 837–41.

Byard, R. W., Noblett, H. & Fotheringham, B. (2000). Automatic car locking and toddler entrapment. *Journal of Paediatrics and Child Health*, **36**, 521.

Byard, R. W., Rodgers, N., James, R. A., Kostakis, C. & Camilleri, A. (2002b). Death and paramethoxyamphetamine – an evolving problem? *Medical Journal of Australia*, **176**, 496.

Byard, R. W., Williams, D., James, R. A. & Gilbert, J. D. (2001c). Diagnostic issues in unusual asphyxial deaths. *Journal of Clinical Forensic Medicine*, **8**, 214–17.

Cameron, D., Bishop, C. & Sibert, J. R. (1992). Farm accidents in children. *British Medical Journal*, **305**, 23–5.

Cass, D. T., Ross, F. & Lam, L. T. (1996). Childhood drowning in New South Wales 1990–1995: a population-based study. *Medical Journal of Australia*, **165**, 610–12.

Centers for Disease Control. (1997). Dog bite-related fatalities – United States, 1995–1996. *Morbidity and Mortality Weekly Reports*, **46**, 463–7.

Chao, T. C., Lo, D. S. T., Koh, J., *et al.* (1993). Glue sniffing deaths in Singapore – volatile aromatic hydrocarbons in post-mortem blood by headspace gas chromatography. *Medicine, Science and the Law*, **33**, 253–60.

Clark, M. A., Feczko, J. D., Hawley, D. A., *et al.* (1993). Asphyxial deaths due to hanging in children. *Journal of Forensic Sciences*, **38**, 344–52.

Clark, M. A., Sandusky, G. E., Hawley, D. A., *et al.* (1991). Fatal and near-fatal animal bite injuries. *Journal of Forensic Sciences*, **36**, 1256–61.

Coe, J. J. (1984). Hypothermia: autopsy findings and vitreous glucose. *Journal of Forensic Sciences*, **29**, 389–95.

Collins, K. A. (2001). Death by overlaying and wedging. A 15-year retrospective study. *American Journal of Forensic Medicine and Pathology*, **22**, 155–9.

Colombani, P. M., Buck, J. R., Dudgeon, D. L., Miller, D. & Haller, M. A. (1985). One-year experience in a regional pediatric trauma center. *Journal of Pediatric Surgery*, **20**, 8–13.

Cooke, C. T., Cadden, G. A. & Hilton, J. M. N. (1989). Hanging deaths in children. *American Journal of Forensic Medicine and Pathology*, **10**, 98–104.

Cooper, G. J. & Taylor, D. E. M. (1989). Biophysics of impact injury to the chest and abdomen. *Journal of the Royal Army Medical Corps*, **135**, 58–67.

Corey, T. S., McCloud, L. C., Nichols, G. R. & Buchino, J. J. (1992). Infant deaths due to unintentional injury. An 11 year autopsy review. *American Journal of Diseases of Children*, **146**, 968–71.

Culliford, A. (1989). Traumatic aortic rupture. In *Thoracic Trauma*, ed. R. Hood, A. Boyd & A. Culliford. Philadelphia: W. B. Saunders, pp. 224–44.

Curfman, G. D. (1998). Fatal impact – concussion of the heart. *New England Journal of Medicine*, **338**, 1841–3.

Dahiya, M. & Denton, J. S. (1999). Esophagoaortic perforation by foreign body (coin) causing sudden death in a 3-year-old child. *American Journal of Forensic Medicine and Pathology*, **20**, 184–8.

D'Costa, D. F. & Gunasekera, N. P. R. (1990). Fatal cerebral oedema following trichloroethylene abuse. *Journal of the Royal Society of Medicine*, **83**, 533–4.

Denton, J. S. & Kalelkar, M. B. (2000). Homicidal commotio cordis in two children. *Journal of Forensic Sciences*, **45**, 734–5.

DiMaio, D. J. & DiMaio, V. J. M. (2001). *Forensic Pathology*, 2nd edn. New York: Elsevier.

DiMaio, V. J. M. & Garriott, J. C. (1974). Lethal caffeine poisoning in a child. *Forensic Science*, **3**, 275–8.

Division of Injury Control. Centers for Disease Control. (1990). Childhood injuries in the United States. *American Journal of Diseases of Children*, **144**, 627–46.

Dunn, K. A. & Runyan, C. W. (1993). Deaths at work among children and adolescents. *American Journal of Diseases of Children*, **147**, 1044–7.

Eddy, A. C., Rusch, V. W., Fligner, C. L., Reay, D. T. & Rice, C. L. (1990). The epidemiology of traumatic rupture of the thoracic aorta in children: a 13 year review. *Journal of Trauma*, **30**, 989–92.

Edmond, K. M., Attia, J. R., D'Este, C. A. & Condon, J. T. (2001). Drowning and near-drowning in Northern Territory children. *Medical Journal of Australia*, **175**, 605–8.

Esmail, A., Meyer, L., Pottier, A. & Wright, S. (1993). Deaths from volatile substance abuse in those under 18 years: results from a national epidemiological study. *Archives of Disease in Childhood*, **69**, 356–60.

Estes, N. A. M. (1995). Sudden death in young athletes. *New England Journal of Medicine*, **333**, 380–81.

Fatteh, A., Leach, W. B. & Wilkinson, C. A. (1973). Fatal air embolism in pregnancy resulting from orogenital sex play. *Forensic Science*, **2**, 247–50.

Flanagan, R. J. & Ives, R. J. (1994). Volatile substance abuse. *Bulletin on Narcotics*, **46**, 49–78.

Fosseus, C. G. (1991). Danger of inhaling trichloroethane. *South African Medical Journal*, **80**, 629–30.

Fragar, L. J. (1996). Down on the farm: health and safety in Australian agriculture. *Medical Journal of Australia*, **165**, 69–70.

Franciosi, R. A., Ellefson, R. D., Uden D. & Drake R. M. (1982). Sudden unexpected death during central hyperalimentation. *Pediatrics*, **69**, 305–7.

Frazer, M. & Mirchandani, H. (1984). Commotio cordis revisited. *American Journal of Forensic Medicine and Pathology*, **5**, 249–51.

Friedman, E. M. (1988). Foreign bodies in the pediatric aerodigestive tract. *Pediatric Annals*, **17**, 640–47.

Froede, R. C., Lindsey, D. & Steinbronn, K. (1979). Sudden unexpected death from cardiac concussion (commotio cordis) with unusual legal complications. *Journal of Forensic Sciences*, **24**, 752–6.

Galat, J. A., Grisoni, E. R. & Gauderer, M. W. L. (1990). Pediatric blunt liver injury: establishment of criteria for appropriate management. *Journal of Pediatric Surgery*, **25**, 1162–5.

Garriott, J. & Petty, C. S. (1980). Death from inhalant abuse. *Clinical Toxicology*, **16**, 305–15.

Gennarelli, T. A., Thibault, L. E., Adams, J. H., *et al.* (1982). Diffuse axonal injury and traumatic coma in the primate. *Annals of Neurology*, **12**, 564–74.

Gilbert-Barness, E. & Emery, J. L. (1996). Deaths of infants on polystyrene-filled beanbags. *American Journal of Forensic Medicine and Pathology*, **17**, 202–6.

Gilbert-Barness, E., Hegstrand, L., Chandra, S., *et al.* (1991). Hazards of mattresses, beds and bedding in deaths of infants. *American Journal of Forensic Medicine and Pathology*, **12**, 27–32.

Gooden, B. A. (1992). Why some people do not drown. Hypothermia versus the diving response. *Medical Journal of Australia*, **157**, 629–32.

Goodheart, R. S. & Dunne, J. W. (1994). Petrol sniffer's encephalopathy. A study of 25 patients. *Medical Journal of Australia*, **160**, 178–81.

Graff, T. D., Phillips, O. C., Benson, D. W. & Kelly, E. (1964). Baltimore anesthesia study committee: factors in pediatric anesthesia mortality. *Anesthesia and Analgesia*, **43**, 407–14.

Grey, T. C., Mittleman, R. E., Wetli, C. V. & Horowitz, S. (1988). Aortoesophageal fistula and sudden death. A report of two cases and review of the literature. *American Journal of Forensic Medicine and Pathology*, **9**, 19–22.

Gross, E. M. (1978). Autopsy findings in drug addicts. *Pathology Annual*, **13**, part 2, 33–67.

Hanson, K. A., Gilbert, J. D., James, R. A. & Byard, R. W. (2002). Upper airway occlusion by soil – an unusual cause of death in vehicle accidents. *Journal of Clinical Forensic Medicine*, **9**, 96–9.

Harris, C. S., Baker, S. P., Smith, G. A. & Harris, R. M. (1984). Childhood asphyxiation by food. *Journal of the American Medical Association*, **251**, 2231–5.

Hiss, J., Kahana, T., Kugel, C. & Epstein, Y. (1994). Fatal classic and exertional heat stroke – report of four cases. *Medicine, Science and the Law*, **34**, 339–43.

Huelke, D. F. & Melvin, J. W. (1980). Anatomy, injury frequency, biomechanics and human tolerances. SAE Technical Paper Series 800098. Paper presented to Society of Automotive Engineers Congress, Detroit, February 25–29.

Hueter, D. C. (1987). Cardiovascular effects of cocaine. *Journal of the American Medical Association*, **257**, 979–80.

Holland, A. J. A., Roy, G. T., Goh, V., *et al.* (2001). Horse-related injuries in children. *Medical Journal of Australia*, **175**, 609–12.

Humphries, C. T., Wagener, J. S. & Morgan, W. J. (1988). Fatal prolonged foreign body aspiration following an asymptomatic interval. *American Journal of Emergency Medicine*, **6**, 611–13.

Hyma, B. A. (1990). Accidental drowning of toddlers in buckets. *Journal of the American Medical Association*, **264**, 1407.

Jacobs, J. C. (1967). Sudden death in arthritic children receiving large doses of indomethacin. *Journal of the American Medical Association*, **199**, 182–4.

Jiraki, K. (1996). Aortoesophageal conduit due to a foreign body. *American Journal of Forensic Medicine and Pathology*, **17**, 347–8.

Johnston, C., Rivara, F. P. & Soderberg, R. (1994). Children in car crashes: analysis of data for injury and use of restraints. *Pediatrics*, **93**, 960–65.

Jones, F. L. (1970). Transmural myocardial necrosis after nonpenetrating cardiac trauma. *American Journal of Cardiology*, **26**, 419–22.

Jumbelic, M. I. & Chambliss, M. (1990). Accidental toddler drowning in 5 gallon buckets. *Journal of the American Medical Association*, **263**, 1952–3.

Karch, S. B. & Billingham, M. E. (1988). The pathology and etiology of cocaine induced heart disease. *Archives of Pathology and Laboratory Medicine*, **112**, 225–30.

Karnak, I., Tanyel, F. C., Büyükpamukçu, N. & Hiçsönmez, A. (1998). Esophageal perforations encountered during the dilation of caustic esophageal strictures. *Journal of Cardiovascular Surgery*, **39**, 373–7.

Kemp, J. S. & Thach, B. T. (1991). Sudden death in infants sleeping on polystyrene filled cushions. *New England Journal of Medicine*, **324**, 1858–64.

Kenna, M. A. & Bluestone, C. D. (1988). Foreign bodies in the air and food passages. *Pediatrics in Review*, **10**, 25–31.

Kibel, S. M., Nagel, F. O., Myers, J. & Cywes, S. (1990). Childhood near-drowning – a 12 year retrospective review. *South African Medical Journal*, **78**, 418–21.

Kindley, A. D. & Todd, R. McL. (1978). Accidental strangulation by mother's hair. *Lancet*, **i**, 565.

King, G. S., Smialek, J. E. & Troutman, W. G. (1985). Sudden death in adolescents resulting from the inhalation of typewriter correction fluid. *Journal of the American Medical Association*, **253**, 1604–6.

Klitte, Å., Gilbert, J. D., Lokan, R. & Byard, R. W. (2001). Adolescent suicide due to inhalation of insect spray. *Journal of Clinical Forensic Medicine*, **8**, 1–3.

Klys, H. S., Salmon, A. P. & De Giovanni, J. V. (1991). Paradoxical embolisation of a catheter fragment to a coronary artery in an infant with congenital heart disease. *British Heart Journal*, **66**, 320–21.

Knight, B. H. (1997). *Forensic Pathology*, 2nd edn. London: Arnold.

Kohl, P., Nesbitt, A. D., Cooper, P. J. & Lei, M. (2001). Sudden cardiac death by *commotio cordis*: role of mechano-electric feedback. *Cardiovascular Research*, **50**, 280–89.

Kraus, J. F., Rock, R. & Hemyari, P. (1990). Brain injuries among infants, children, adolescents and young adults. *American Journal of Diseases of Children*, **144**, 684–91.

Krous, H. F., Nadeau, J. M., Fukumoto, R. I., Blackbourne, B. D. & Byard, R. W. (2001). Environmental hyperthermic infant and early childhood death. Circumstances, pathologic changes and manner of death. *American Journal of Forensic Medicine and Pathology*, **22**, 374–82.

Lacroix, J., Gaudreault, P. & Gauthier, M. (1989). Admission to a pediatric intensive care unit for poisoning: a review of 105 cases. *Critical Care Medicine*, **17**, 748–50.

Laks, Y. & Barzilay, Z. (1988). Foreign body aspiration in childhood. *Pediatric Emergency Care*, **4**, 102–6.

Laroche, D., Lefrançois, C., Gérard, J-L., *et al.* (1992). Early diagnosis of anaphylactic reactions to neuromuscular blocking drugs. *British Journal of Anaesthesia*, **69**, 611–14.

Lauridson, J. R. & Myers, L. (1993). Evaluation of fatal dog bites: the view of the medical examiner and animal behaviorist. *Journal of Forensic Sciences*, **38**, 726–31.

Lawler, W. (1992). Bodies recovered from water: a personal approach and consideration of difficulties. *Journal of Clinical Pathology*, **45**, 654–9.

Lee, K. A. P. (2000). Injuries caused by animals. In *The Pathology of Trauma*, 3rd edn, ed. J. K. Mason & B. N. Purdue. London: Arnold, pp. 265–82.

Leestma, J. (1988). *Forensic Neuropathology*. New York: Raven Press.

Levene, S. & Bonfield, G. (1991). Accidents on hospital wards. *Archives of Disease in Childhood*, **66**, 1047–9.

Lifschultz, B. D. & Donoghue, E. R. (1996). Deaths due to foreign body aspiration in children: the continuing hazard of toy balloons. *Journal of Forensic Sciences*, **41**, 247–51.

Lima, J. A. (1989). Laryngeal foreign bodies in children: a persistent, life-threatening problem. *Laryngoscope*, **99**, 415–20.

Linegar, A. G., Von Oppell, U. O., Hegemann, S., De Groot, M. & Odell, J. A. (1992). Tracheobronchial foreign bodies. Experience at Red Cross Children's Hospital, 1985–1990. *South African Medical Journal*, **82**, 164–7.

Link, M. S., Wang, P. J., Pandian, N. G., *et al.* (1998). An experimental model of sudden death due to low-energy chest-wall impact (commotio cordis). *New England Journal of Medicine*, **338**, 1805–11.

Mancer, K. (1989). Death resulting from paediatric surgery and anesthesia. In *Paediatric Forensic Medicine and Pathology*, ed. J. K. Mason. London: Chapman & Hall, pp. 319–37.

Mandryk, J. & Harrison, J. (1995). Work-related deaths of children and adolescents in Australia, 1982 to 1984. *Australian Journal of Public Health*, **19**, 46–9.

Mann, N. C., Weller, S. C. & Rauchschwalbe, R. (1992). Bucket-related drownings in the United States, 1984 through 1990. *Pediatrics*, **89**, 1068–71.

Mantel, K. & Butenandt, I. (1986). Tracheobronchial foreign body aspiration in childhood. A report on 224 cases. *European Journal of Pediatrics*, **145**, 211–16.

Maron, B. J., Poliac, L. C., Kaplan, J. A. & Mueller, F. O. (1995). Blunt impact to the chest leading to sudden death from cardiac arrest during sports activities. *New England Journal of Medicine*, **333**, 337–42.

Maruff, P., Burns, C. B., Tyler, P., Currie, B. J. & Currie, J. (1998). Neurological and cognitive abnormalities associated with chronic petrol sniffing. *Brain*, **121**, 1903–17.

McBride, P. & Busuttil, A. (1990). A new trend in solvent abuse deaths? *Medicine, Science and the Law*, **30**, 207–13.

McHugh, M. J. (1987). The abuse of volatile substances. *Pediatric Clinics of North America*, **34**, 333–40.

Meel, B. L. (1998). An accidental suffocation by a rubber balloon. *Medicine, Science and the Law*, **38**, 81–2.

Miller, M. A. (1991). Tolerance to steering wheel induced lower abdominal injury. *Journal of Trauma*, **31**, 1332–9.

Mitchell, E., Krous, H. F. & Byard, R. W. (2002). Pathological findings in overlaying. *Journal of Clinical Forensic Medicine*, **9**, 133–5.

Mitterschiffthaler, G., Berchtold, J. P., Anderl, P. & Unterdorfer, H. (1989). Total paradoxical air embolism during a routine obstetric procedure (cervical cerclage). *Anaesthesist*, **38**, 29–31.

Mittleman, R. E. (1984). Fatal choking in infants and children. *American Journal of Forensic Medicine and Pathology*, **5**, 201–10.

Modell, J. H. (1971). *Pathophysiology of Drowning and Near Drowning*. Springfield, Ill.: Charles C. Thomas.

Moore, L. & Byard, R. W. (1993). A comparison of hanging and wedging deaths in infants and young children. *American Journal of Forensic Medicine and Pathology*, **14**, 296–302.

Moore, L., Bourne, A. J., Beal, S., Collett, M. & Byard, R. W. (1995). Unexpected infant death in association with suspended rocking cradles. *American Journal of Forensic Medicine and Pathology*, **16**, 177–80.

Morrison, L., Chalmers, D. J., Parry, M. L. & Wright, C. S. (2002). Infant-furniture-related injuries among preschool children in New Zealand, 1987–1996. *Journal of Paediatrics and Child Health*, **38**, 587–92.

Murphy, G. K. (1986). Therapeutic misadventure. An 11 year study from a metropolitan coroner's office. *American Journal of Forensic Medicine and Pathology*, **7**, 115–19.

Nadroo, A. M., Lin, J., Green, R. S., Magid, M. S. & Holzman, I. R. (2001). Death as a complication of peripherally inserted central catheters in neonates. *Journal of Pediatrics*, **138**, 599–601.

Nakayama, D. K., Ramenofsky, M. L. & Rowe, M. I., (1989). Chest injuries in childhood. *Annals of Surgery*, **210**, 770–75.

National Injury Surveillance Unit (1995). Injury deaths Australia 1990–1994. www. nisu. flinders. edu. au (accessed 17 September 1996 and 12 December 1996).

Neidhart, P. & Suter, P. M. (1985). Pulmonary bulla and sudden death in a young aeroplane passenger. *Intensive Care Medicine*, **11**, 45–7.

Nesbitt, A. D., Cooper, P. J. & Kohl, P. (2001). Rediscovering commotio cordis. *Lancet*, **357**, 1195–7.

New York State Department of Health. (1991). Epidemiology notes. *New York State Medical Journal*, **91**, 118–19.

Newman, R. J. & Rastogi, S. (1984). Rupture of the thoracic aorta and its relationship to road traffic accident characteristics. *Injury*, **15**, 296–9.

Nixon, J. W., Kemp, A. M., Levene, S. & Sibert, J. R. (1995). Suffocation, choking, and strangulation in childhood in England and Wales: epidemiology and prevention. *Archives of Disease in Childhood*, **72**, 6–10.

Nolte, K. B. (1993). Esophageal foreign bodies as child abuse. Potential fatal mechanisms. *American Journal of Forensic Medicine and Pathology*, **14**, 323–6.

Norman, M. G. & Cass, E. (1971). Cardiac tamponade resulting from a swallowed safety pin. *Pediatrics*, **48**, 832–3.

O'Connor, P. J. (1983). Epidemiology of accidental poisoning in children. *Medical Journal of Australia*, **2**, 181–3.

O'Donnell, C. R. (1995). Firearm deaths among children and youth. *American Psychologist*, **50**, 771–6.

Ohshima, T., Maeda, H., Takayasu, T., Fujioka, Y. & Nakaya, T. (1992). An autopsy case of infant death due to heat stroke. *American Journal of Forensic Medicine and Pathology*, **13**, 217–21.

Orlowski, J. P., Julius, C. J., Petras, R. E., Porembka, D. T. & Gallagher, J. M. (1989). The safety of intraosseous infusions: risks of fat and bone marrow emboli to the lungs. *Annals of Emergency Medicine*, **18**, 1062–7.

O'Shea, J. S. (1991). House-fire and drowning deaths among children and young adults. *American Journal of Forensic Medicine and Pathology*, **12**, 33–5.

Parker, M. J., Tarlow, M. J. & Milne Anderson, J. (1984). Glue sniffing and cerebral infarction. *Archives of Disease in Childhood*, 59, 675–7.

Parmley, L. F., Mattingly, T. W., Manion, W. C. & Jahnke, E. J. (1958). Nonpenetrating traumatic injury of the aorta. *Circulation*, **18**, 1086–101.

Pearn, J. (1992). The urgency of immersions. *Archives of Disease in Childhood*, **67**, 257–61.

Pearn, J. H., Brown, J., Wong, U. & Bart, R. (1979). Bathtub drownings: report of seven cases. *Pediatrics*, **64**, 68–70.

Pearn, J., Nixon, J., Ansford, A. & Corcoran, A. (1984). Accidental poisoning in childhood: five year urban population study with 15 year analysis of fatality. *British Medical Journal*, **288**, 44–6.

Peclet, M. H., Newman, K. D., Eichelberger, M. R., *et al.* (1990). Patterns of injury in children. *Journal Of Pediatric Surgery*, **25**, 85–91.

Pinckney, L. E. & Kennedy, L. A. (1980). Fractures of the infant skull caused by animal bites. *American Journal of Roentgenology*, **135**, 179–80.

Pitt, W. R., Balanda, K. P. & Nixon, J. (1994). Child injury in Brisbane South 1985–91: implications for future injury surveillance. *Journal of Paediatrics and Child Health*, **30**, 114–22.

Pitt, W. R. & Cass, D. T. (2001). Preventing children drowning in Australia. *Medical Journal of Australia*, **175**, 603–4.

Pollak, R. & Stellwag-Carion, C. (1991). Delayed cardiac rupture due to blunt chest trauma. *American Journal of Forensic Medicine and Pathology*, **12**, 153–6.

Rauchschwalbe, R. & Mann, N. C. (1997). Pediatric window-cord strangulations in the United States, 1981–1995. *Journal of the American Medical Association*, **277**, 1696–8.

Reay, D. T., Eisele, J. W., Ward, R., Horton, W. & Bonnell, H. J. (1985). Investigation of anesthetic deaths. *Journal of Forensic Sciences*, **30**, 822–7.

Reith, D. M., Pitt, W. R. & Hockey, R. (2001). Childhood poisoning in Queensland: an analysis of presentation and admission rates. *Journal of Paediatrics and Child Health*, **37**, 446–50.

Reuler, J. B. (1978). Hypothermia: pathophysiology, clinical settings and management. *Annals of Internal Medicine*, **89**, 519–57.

Rfidah, E. I., Casey, P. B., Tracey, J. A. & Gill, D. (1991). Childhood poisoning in Dublin. *Irish Medical Journal*, **84**, 87–9.

Riches, K. J., James, R. A., Gilbert, J. D. & Byard, R. W. (2002). Fatal childhood vascular injuries associated with seat belt use. *American Journal of Forensic Medicine and Pathology*, **23**, 45–7.

Rivkind, A. I., Siegel, J. H. & Dunham, C. M. (1989). Patterns of organ injury in blunt hepatic trauma and their significance for management and outcome. *Journal of Trauma*, **29**, 1398–415.

Roberts, I., Kolbe, A. & White, J. (1993). Non-traffic child pedestrian injuries. *Journal of Paediatrics and Child Health*, **29**, 233–4.

Rogers, B. B., Berns, S. D., Maynard, E. C. & Hansen, T. W. R. (1990). Pericardial tamponade secondary to central venous catheterization and hyperalimentation in a very low birthweight infant. *Pediatric Pathology*, **10**, 819–23.

Rogers, P. D., Harris, J. & Jarmuskewicz, J. (1987). Alcohol and adolescence. *Pediatric Clinics of North America*, **34**, 289–303.

Rohrig, T. P. (1997). Sudden death due to butane inhalation. *American Journal of Forensic Medicine and Pathology*, **18**, 299–302.

Rosenberg, M. L., Rodriguez, J. G. & Chorba, T. L. (1990). Childhood injuries: where we are. *Pediatrics*, **86**, 1084–91.

Rouse, D. A. & Hargrove, R. (1992). An unusual case of gas embolism. *American Journal of Forensic Medicine and Pathology*, **13**, 268–70.

Runyan, C. W., Kotch, J. B., Margolis, L. H. & Buescher, P. A. (1985). Childhood injuries in North Carolina: a statewide analysis of hospitalizations and deaths. *American Journal of Public Health*, **75**, 1429–32.

Sabo, R. A., Hanigan, W. C., Flessner, K., Rose, J. & Aaland, M. (1996). Strangulation injuries in children. Part 1. Clinical analysis. *Journal of Trauma: Injury, Infection and Critical Care*, **40**, 68–72.

Sacks, J. J., Sattin, R. W. & Bonzo, S. E. (1989). Dog bite-related fatalities from 1979 through 1988. *Journal of the American Medical Association*, **262**, 1489–92.

Saladino, R., Lund, D. & Fleischer, G. (1991). The spectrum of liver and spleen injuries in children: failure of the pediatric

trauma score and clinical signs to predict isolated injuries. *Annals of Emergency Medicine*, **20**, 636–40.

Salmi, L. R., Weiss, H. B., Peterson, P. L., *et al.* (1989). Fatal farm injuries among young children. *Pediatrics*, **83**, 267–71.

Saxena, A. & Ang, L. C. (1993). Epilepsy and bathtub drowning. Important neuropathological observations. *American Journal of Forensic Medicine and Pathology*, **14**, 125–9.

Scragg, R., Mitchell, E. A., Taylor, B. J., *et al.* (1993). Bedsharing, smoking, and alcohol in the sudden infant death syndrome. *British Medical Journal*, **307**, 1312–18.

Sevitt, S. (1977a). The mechanisms of traumatic rupture of the thoracic aorta. *British Journal of Surgery*, **64**, 166–73.

Sevitt, S. (1977b). The significance and pathology of fat embolism. *Annals of Clinical Research*, **9**, 173–80.

Shepherd, R. T. (1990). Accidental self-strangulation in a young child – a case report and review. *Medicine, Science and the Law*, **30**, 119–23.

Sibert, J. R. & Routledge, P. A. (1991). Accidental poisoning in children: can we admit fewer children with safety? *Archives of Disease in Childhood*, **66**, 263–6.

Sibert, J. R., Craft, A. W. & Jackson, R. H. (1977). Child-resistant packaging and accidental child poisoning. *Lancet*, **ii**, 289–90.

Simmons, G. T. (1992). Death by power car window. An unrecognized hazard. *American Journal of Forensic Medicine and Pathology*, **13**, 112–14.

Simpson, R. W. & Edwards, W. D. (1986). Pathogenesis of cocaine induced ischemic heart disease. *Archives of Pathology and Laboratory Medicine*, **110**, 479–84.

Smialek, J. E., Smialek, P. Z. & Spitz, W. U. (1977). Accidental bed deaths in infants due to unsafe sleeping situations. *Clinical Pediatrics*, **16**, 1031–6.

Smith, N. M., Byard, R. W. & Bourne, A. J. (1991). Death during immersion in water in childhood. *American Journal of Forensic Medicine and Pathology*, **12**, 219–21.

Southwick, F. S. & Daglish, P. H. (1980). Recovery after prolonged asystolic cardiac arrest in profound hypothermia. A case report and literature review. *Journal of the American Medical Association*, **243**, 1250–53.

Spyker, D. A. (1985). Submersion injury. Epidemiology, prevention and management. *Pediatric Clinics of North America*, **32**, 113–25.

Stalnaker, R. L., McElhaney J. H. & Roberts, V. L. (1973). Human torso response to blunt trauma. In *Human Impact Response: Measurement and Simulation*, ed. W. F. King & H. J. Mertz. New York: Plenum Press, pp. 182–99.

Steadman, C., Dorrington, L. C., Kay, P. & Stephens, H. (1984). Abuse of a fire extinguishing agent and sudden death in adolescents. *Medical Journal of Australia*, **141**, 115–17.

Steffee, C. H., Davis, G. J. & Nicol, K. K. (1996). A whiff of death: fatal volatile solvent inhalation abuse. *Southern Medical Journal*, **89**, 879–84.

Stenberg, R. G., Winniford, M. D., Hillis, L. D., Dowling, G. P. & Buja L. M. (1989). Simultaneous acute thrombosis of two major coronary arteries following intravenous cocaine use. *Archives of Pathology and Laboratory Medicine*, **113**, 521–4.

Stumpp, J. W. H., Schneider, J. & Bär, W. (1997). Drowning of a girl with anomaly of the bundle of His and the right bundle branch. *American Journal of Forensic Medicine and Pathology*, **18**, 208–10.

Sturner, W. Q. (1980). Pediatric deaths. In *Modern Medicine, Psychiatry, and Forensic Science*, ed. W. J. Curran, A. L. McGarry & C. S. Petty. Philadelphia: F. A. Davis, pp. 219–47.

Swanson, J. A., Sachs, M. I., Dahlgren, K. A. & Tinguely, S. J. (1987). Accidental farm injuries in children. *American Journal of Diseases of Children*, **141**, 1276–9.

Symbas, P. (1989). Rupture of the aorta. In *Cardiothoracic Trauma*, ed. P. Symbas. Philadelphia: W. B. Saunders, pp. 190–212.

Troutman, W. G. (1988). Additional deaths associated with the intentional inhalation of typewriter correction fluid. *Veterinary and Human Toxicology*, **30**, 130–32.

Variend, S. & Usher, A. (1984). Broken cots and infant fatality. *Medicine, Science and the Law*, **24**, 111–12.

Vascik, J. M. & Tew, J. M., Jr (1982). Foreign body embolization of the middle cerebral artery: review of the literature and guidelines for management. *Neurosurgery*, **11**, 532–6.

Ward, M. E. & Cowley, A. R. (1999). Hypothermia: a natural cause of death. *American Journal of Forensic Medicine and Pathology*, **20**, 383–6.

Warneke, C. L. & Cooper, S. P. (1994). Child and adolescent drownings in Harris County, Texas, 1983 through 1990. *American Journal of Public Health*, **84**, 593–8.

Watson, J. M. (1978). Clinical and laboratory investigations in 132 cases of solvent abuse. *Medicine, Science and the Law*, **18**, 40–43.

Whitehead, F. J., Couper, R. T. L., Moore, L., Bourne, A. J. & Byard, R. W. (1996). Dehydration deaths in infants and young children. *American Journal of Forensic Medicine and Pathology*, **17**, 73–8.

Wilberger, J. E. & Pang, D. (1983). Craniocerebral injuries from dog bites. *Journal of the American Medical Association*, **249**, 2685–8.

Williams, B. C. & Kotch, J. B. (1990). Excess injury mortality among children in the United States: comparison of recent international statistics. *Pediatrics*, **86**, 1067–73.

Winn, D. G., Agran, P. F. & Castillo, D. N. (1991). Pedestrian injuries to children younger than 5 years of age. *Pediatrics*, **88**, 776–82.

Wintemute, G. J. (1990). Childhood drowning and near-drowning in the United States. *American Journal of Diseases of Children*, **144**, 663–9.

Wiseman, N. E. (1984). The diagnosis of foreign body aspiration in childhood. *Journal of Pediatric Surgery*, **19**, 531–5.

Wiseman, N. E., Chochinov, H. & Fraser, V. (1983). Major dog attack injuries in children. *Journal of Pediatric Surgery*, **18**, 533–6

Wolfenden, K. & Sanson-Fisher, R. (1993). Patterns of non-fatal farm injury in New England, NSW. *Australian Journal of Rural Health*, **1**, 3–10.

Wyatt, J. P., Wyatt, P. W., Squires, T. J. & Busutill, A. (1998). Hanging deaths in children. *American Journal of Forensic Medicine and Pathology*, **19**, 343–6.

Yamamoto, L. G., Wiebe, R. A. & Matthews, W. J. (1991). Toxic exposures and ingestions in Honolulu: I. A prospective pediatric ED cohort. *Pediatric Emergency Care*, **7**, 141–8.

Part III

Intentional trauma

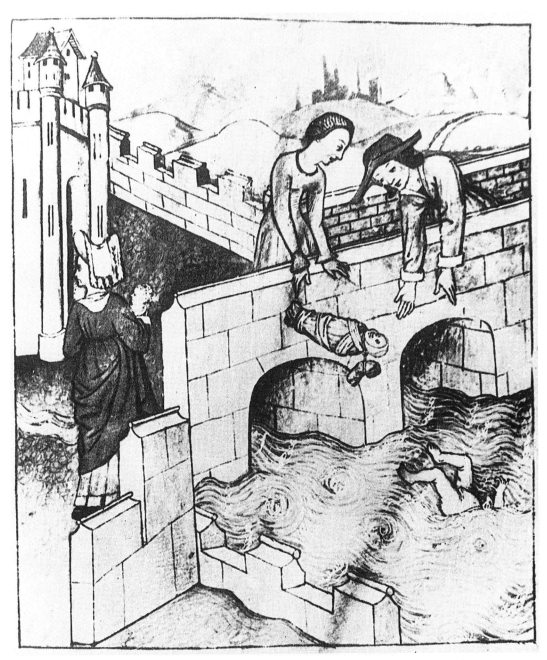

A sixteenth-century etching depicting infanticide, with mothers throwing their children into the Tiber river to drown.

Homicide and suicide

with Stephen D. Cohle

Forensic Pathologist, Spectrum Health, Grand Rapids, Michigan, USA

The child will not be quiet, the child will not be quiet:
Take it by the leg and hit it against the wall,
The child will not be quiet.

[Barn vil ikka teea, barn vil ikka teea:
Tak an leggen, slog an veggen,
Barn vil ikka teea.]

> Children's rhyme – Shetland Islands (translated from Old Norse) (Knight, 1986)

Introduction

This chapter deals with deaths of children due to intentional injury, the majority of which are homicides. In general, homicides can be divided into those occurring in very young children who are powerless to defend themselves against larger assailants, the typical "battered child" (Kempe *et al.*, 1962), and those occurring in older children who die of the same causes as adults. Examples of the former include blunt injuries, shaken infant syndrome, suffocation, and deaths caused by starvation and neglect (Figures 3.1 and 3.2) (Byard, Donald & Chivell, 1999). Young infants may also be drowned, a popular method of infanticide in previous centuries. Older children are more likely to be murdered by other means, such as gunshot and stab wounds, although this may occur at all ages (Figures 3.3–3.5). The findings at autopsy in lethally abused infants and children range from minimal to the extremely obvious, with evidence of severe and long-standing neglect and injury.

There are many factors to consider when trying to distinguish accidental from non-accidental injury. Clinical findings and radiologic imaging studies not in keeping with the history, and injuries of different ages, are key indicators of inflicted trauma, especially in infants (Barnes & Robson, 2000). An independent witness to the traumatic event is important for corroborating or negating a carer's version of the history. The age and stage of development of the child (e.g. could he/she move enough to become injured?), the timeliness of seeking treatment, other injuries (especially injuries of different ages), and the child's state of nutrition and cleanliness should all be taken into consideration when separating inflicted from non-inflicted injuries. If the diagnosis is difficult, then consultation with an expert in child abuse should occur. Abusive injuries tend to occur at odd hours, are allegedly unwitnessed by carers, and are often attributed to the actions of siblings (Rivara, Kamitsuka & Quan, 1988).

Homicide rates are greatest during infancy and the later teen years, with two defined patterns of "infantile" and "adolescent" (Christoffel, 1990; McClain *et al.*, 1993). In the infantile pattern, the child is young, the assailant is a parent or carer, death is caused by blunt force, intentional burns, or neglect, and the precipitating event often involves disciplinary action (see introductory verse). The adolescent type of homicide occurs in older children, is committed by peers, acquaintances, or gangs, and in the USA the cause of death is most commonly gunshot wound, followed by stabbing, strangulation, or motor vehicle hit-and-run incidents. The inciting event is usually

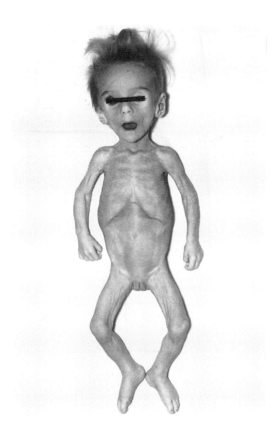

Figure 3.1 Marked cachexia in a one-year-old girl who was considered by her parents to be "all right" on the night of her death. Her condition indicates gross neglect.

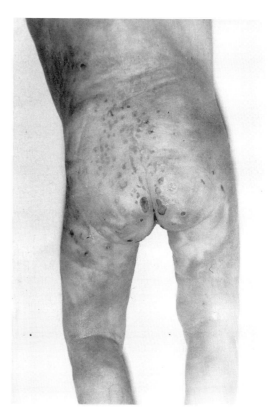

Figure 3.2 Wasted buttocks and impetigo in a grossly neglected and abused child.

an argument, or the victim dies during the commission of a crime such as robbery.

Of all traumatic deaths in children under the age of 19 years in the USA in 1985, homicide accounted for 12.8%, motor vehicle accidents for 47%, suicide for 9.6%, and drowning for 9.2%. In that year, there were 2877 homicides in the USA, a rate of 4.1 deaths per 100,000 individuals under 19 years of age (Division of Injury Control, 1990). The USA led all nations in homicide deaths in males aged between 13 and 19 years, with a rate of 13 per 100,000 of the population. Australia and Canada each had a rate of about 2.5 per 100,000, followed by France, the Netherlands, England and Wales, Sweden, and Japan, each with fewer than 0.5 deaths per 100,000. An identical rank,

although with a lower incidence, pertained to females within this age range. In a 10-year study of deaths of children in South Carolina, 60 cases (12%) were homicides. Head injuries accounted for 45% of the homicides, asphyxia and drowning for 25%, abdominal or body trauma for 12%, carbon monoxide poisoning or thermal injury for 10%, and neglect, stabbing, and poisoning for 8% (Collins & Nichols, 1999). At the Children's Hospital of Eastern Ontario (Ottawa, Canada), more recent data demonstrate that motor vehicle accidents and falls accounted for 63% of admissions for severe trauma, with child abuse making up 8% (Osmond, Brennan-Barnes & Shephard, 2002). Injury patterns and mechanisms in cases of fatal child abuse are detailed in Table 3.1.

Table 3.2, adapted from a Division of Injury Control (1990) report, shows that the most common

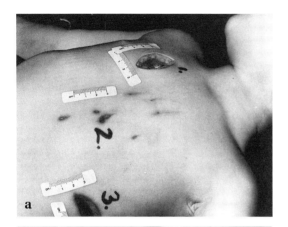

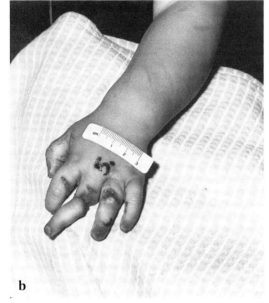

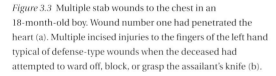

Figure 3.3 Multiple stab wounds to the chest in an 18-month-old boy. Wound number one had penetrated the heart (a). Multiple incised injuries to the fingers of the left hand typical of defense-type wounds when the deceased had attempted to ward off, block, or grasp the assailant's knife (b).

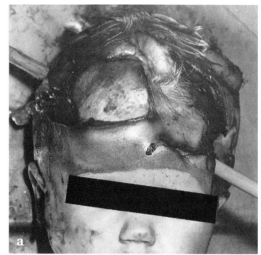

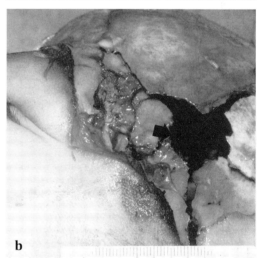

Figure 3.4 Shattering of the skull in a 10-month-old girl who was shot in the head by a .303 rifle. The rod demonstrates the projectile trajectory (a). Entrance wound in left temple (arrow) (b).

assaultive weapons in younger children in the USA are hands and fists, while firearms are used most frequently against older children and teenagers. In a study of 273 children with life-threatening injuries at a Baltimore trauma center, assaults accounted for 8% of admissions. Of these cases, 40% of the children had been shot, 27% had been stabbed, and 33% had received blunt force injuries (Colombani *et al.*, 1985). However, considerable geographic variability exists in methods of child homicide (Ellis, 1997; Fornes, Druilhe & Lecomte, 1995; Hargrave & Warner, 1992; Hutson, Anglin & Pratts, 1994). For example, the most

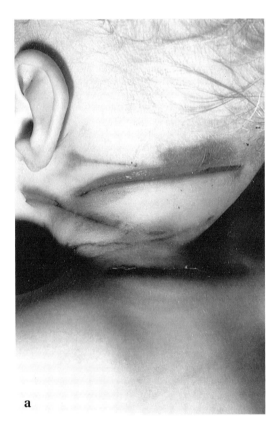 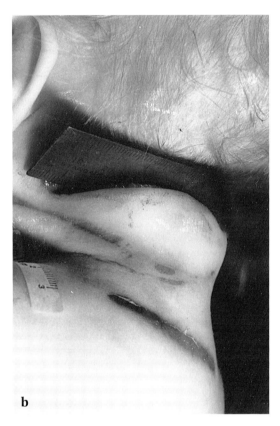

a   **b**

Figure 3.5 The back of the neck of a nine-month-old boy showing several incised wounds from an axe (a). Insertion of a metal ruler demonstrates the direction of the blow that transected his upper cervical spine and cord (b).

common cause of childhood death in cases of fatal inflicted injury in an Australian study was closed head injury, followed by asphyxia and strangulation (de Silva & Oates, 1993).

A review of child homicides autopsied in Grand Rapids, Michigan, USA, from 1983 to 2001, undertaken by one of the authors (SDC), revealed 72 cases, with a mean age of 24 months and a range of four weeks to seven years. Six infants killed within the first 24 hours of life were not included in this series. The sex of 51 children was known for the years 1991–2001 and was approximately equal (26 girls, 25 boys). The most common cause of death was blunt craniocerebral trauma (*n* = 40), including 11 cases of shaken infant syndrome. Eleven children were suffocated or asphyxiated. There were four cases each of gunshot

wounds and dehydration, three cases each of multiple stab wounds and blunt abdominal injuries, two cases of craniocerebral trauma with chest or abdominal injuries, two cases of scalds, one case each of blunt chest injuries and fat embolization from fractures, and one undetermined cause of death (Table 3.3). The most common initial history was of a child being found dead or unresponsive (43%), suffering a short fall (14%), falling down stairs (8%), striking his or her head against an object (4%), or suffering a collapse (4%) (Table 3.4).

In 51 (71%) cases the final history given was the same as the initial history. In five (7%) cases a carer admitted hitting a child, after initially denying the act, in four (6%) cases a carer admitted suffocating a child, and three (4%) caretakers admitted shaking

Table 3.1. Characteristic features of fatally abused children

General	<3 percentile for weight and > 3 percentile for height with absent subcutaneous fat, thymic atrophy, fatty liver, ascites, and no food in the gastrointestinal tract (in the absence of other lethal disease) – starvation
Skin and subcutis	Palm, sole, buttock: circular erosion – cigarette burn
	Perineum, buttocks, hands, feet: scald – immersion
	Wrists, ankles: contusions and abrasions – binding
	Corner of mouth: contusions and abrasions – gagging
	Lower back: contusions and abrasions – corporal punishment
	General: patterned hematomas – looped cord, shoe heel, household appliance, belt buckle, flyswatter, bite mark, finger or thumb impressions
Face	Lip: contusion – direct blow, forced feeding
	Frenulum of lip or tongue: laceration – direct blow, forced feeding
	Ear: hematoma – direct blow
	Nasal septum: hematoma, deviation – direct blow
	Eye: hematoma, hyphema, subconjunctival hemorrhage – direct blow
Head	Scalp: hematoma – direct blow or hair pulling (especially braids)
	Brain: subdural hematoma – shaking or direct blow
Genitalia	Hymen, fourchette: laceration – recent sexual assault
	Vulva: hematoma – recent sexual assault
	Scrotum, penis: hematoma, edema – twisting injury
	General: 1. venereal warts, gonorrhea – remote sexual assault
	2. bite marks, anal lacerations, poor sphincter tone – sexual assault
Chest	Thoracic cavity: hemopneumothorax – direct blow
Abdomen	Peritoneal cavity: mesenteric tears, ruptured hollow or solid viscera – direct blow
Skeleton	Rib, skull: fracture – direct blow
	Long bones: spiral fracture – twisting injury
	General: 1. callus – remote injury
	2. metaphyseal avulsion – jerking injury

Adapted from Caffey (1974), McNeese & Hebeler (1977), Curran, McGarry & Petty (1980), Spitz & Fisher (1980), and Zumwalt & Hirsch (1980).

Table 3.2. Weapons used in cases of homicide in children aged from 0 to 19 years (USA)

	Age (years, %)			
Weapon	0–4	5–9	10–14	15–19
Hands and fists	50	19	7.5	4
Firearms	8	39	51	67
Sharp objects	5	14	16	20
Blunt objects	7	2	7.5	4
Other	30	26	18	5

Adapted from Division of Injury Control report (1990).

Table 3.3. Causes of 72 childhood homicides in a study from Michigan, USA

Craniocerebral trauma	40
Suffocation and asphyxia	11
Gunshot wound	4
Dehydration	4
Multiple stab injuries	3
Blunt abdominal injuries	3
Craniocerebral trauma with chest or abdominal injuries	2
Scalding	2
Blunt chest injuries	1
Fat embolization from fractures	1
Undetermined	1

Table 3.4. Initial histories given by perpetrators to explain injuries in 72 childhood homicides in a study from Michigan, USA

History	Total
Found dead or unresponsive	31
Short fall	10
Fell down stairs	6
Hit own head against hard object	3
Witnessed collapse	3
Deterioration from prior assault	2
Shot	2
Shaken	2
Beaten	2
Accidental scald	2
Confession of suffocation	1
Choked on food	1
Wrestling with adult	1
Found wedged	1
Drowned in swimming pool	1
Hit head on padded furniture	1
Seizure	1
Shook few grains of pepper on to tongue	1
Thrown into water	1

Table 3.5. Final histories given by perpetrators to explain injuries in 72 childhood homicides in a study from Michigan, USA

History	Total
Unchanged	51
Caretaker hit baby	5
Baby suffocated	4
Baby shaken	3
Slammed against hard object	2
Pushed down stairs	1
Head hit doorway while being carried	1
Child stood up and hit head	1
Father squeezed baby's head	1
Shoved into wall	1
Found with garbage bag over head	1
Hit in abdomen	1

an infant (Table 3.5). Collins & Nichols (1999) and Feldman *et al.*, (2001) similarly found that falls or no suggested mechanism were the most common histories in their series of abused children.

Accidental injuries were compared with inflicted injuries in infants under one year of age who presented to the emergency departments of two Seattle hospitals and to the King County Medical Examiner's Office. Non-intentional injuries were 15 times more common than inflicted injuries. However, inflicted injuries were usually multiple and severe, and more commonly resulted in long-term disability. The mean injury severity score for non-intentionally injured infants was 1.6 (range 0–16), and for intentionally injured infants was 8.7 (range 0–33). In the accident group, falls were the most common cause of injury, accounting for 47% of cases; in the abuse group, the most common cause for the injury alleged by the carer was also a fall, most often from a bed or couch. These authors found that

accidents, except for those related to motor vehicles, rarely resulted in serious injury or death. In contrast, severe closed head injury, rib fractures, lower extremity fractures, abdominal injuries, and retinal hemorrhages were highly characteristic of inflicted injury.

Marshall, Puls & Davidson (1988) found that 51% of 382 children evaluated for abuse or neglect in their county hospital clinic were sexually abused, 34% were physically abused, and 15% had evidence of neglect. In nearly two-thirds of cases, perpetrators of physical abuse are males, such as the father, step-father, or mother's partner. Female babysitters have accounted for over one-sixth of assailants in some series (Starling, Holden & Jenny, 1995).

Falls from heights

One of the key factors in determining whether a fatal injury is unintentional or intentional is how well the injuries observed at autopsy correlate with the history given by the carer. Frequently a history of minor trauma is given to explain severe injuries, or the assailant may change the history in an attempt to adapt it to the autopsy findings. A useful comparison can be drawn from those accounts in the literature describing relatively short falls at home, in hospital, or on a

Table 3.6. Details of cases of short falls without fatalities

Reference	Cases (n)	Age (range or mean)	Site	Distance	Skull fractures (n)	Documented permanent sequelae	Death
Chadwick & Salerno (1993)	338	≤6 years	Home, daycare centers, buildings	–	0	0	0
Lyons & Oates (1993)	207	≤6 years	Hospital bed or crib	25–54 inches	1	0	0
Macgregor (2000)	85	<14 years	Beds or bunkbeds	–	0	0	0
Mayr *et al.* (1999)	103	7–30 months	Highchairs	–	16	0	0
Selbst, Baker & Shames (1990)	68	5.12 years	Bunkbeds	–	1	0	0
Smith *et al.* (1996)	36	≤10 years	Shopping carts	–	5	0	0
Tarantino, Dowd & Murdock (1999)	167	≤10 months	Bed, sofa, dropped	≤4 feet	12	0	0
Warrington & Wright (2001)	2554	≤6 months	Bed, sofa, dropped	–	<1%	0	0

playground, and those reports that describe the consequences of longer falls from buildings. Chadwick and colleagues (1991) have demonstrated clearly the unreliability of carers' histories in a study that showed that if the initial history of an injury is accepted, then the chance of dying from a fall of less than four feet was far greater (eight times) than from a fall of 10–45 feet. The obvious conclusion is that more than just a simple fall was involved in children in the first group and that their histories must have been falsified. Attributing death to such short falls has led to the designation "killer couches." One of the major problems in assessing this area of the literature is often the lack of adequate assessment of cases without formal forensic reviews based on substantiated and full histories. For this reason, there is sometimes considerable contradiction among reports.

Many authors have reported series of children who had short falls with no fatalities. These included falls at home from short distances, from hospital beds, highchairs, bunkbeds, shopping carts, and playground apparatus. Skull fractures were uncommon and fatalities were not reported (Table 3.6) (Ball & King, 1991; Chadwick & Salerno, 1993; Helfer, Slovis & Black, 1977; Levene & Bonfield, 1991; Lyons & Oates, 1993; Macgregor, 2000; Mayr *et al.*, 1999; Nimityongskul & Anderson, 1987; Selbst, Baker & Shames, 1990; Smith *et al.*, 1996; Tarantino, Dowd & Murdock, 1999; Warrington & Wright, 2001).

Chiaviello, Christoph & Bond (1994) and Joffe & Ludwig (1988) reported on children falling down stairs and found no deaths (Table 3.7). Skull fractures constituted 7% of Chiaviello, Christoph & Bond's series and 1.7% of Joffe & Ludwig's series, with no patients suffering permanent deficits. The most severe injuries, including most of the skull fractures, occurred in children who were being carried down stairs. Joffe & Ludwig found no correlation between the severity of injury and the number of steps fallen. They concluded that stairway injuries were much less severe than free falls of the same total vertical distance, as most stairway falls consisted of an initial mild to moderate impact followed by a series of low-energy non-injurious falls. Their closing comment is useful in assessing cases of childhood trauma attributed to falls down stairs: "When multiple, severe, truncal, or proximal extremity injuries are noted in a patient who reportedly fell down stairs, a different mechanism of injury should be suspected."

Table 3.7. Details of childhood falls down stairways

Reference	Cases (n)	Age (range or mean)	Intracranial hemorrhage/ cerebral contusion	Skull fractures (n)	Documented permanent sequelae	Death
Chiaviello, Christoph & Bond (1994)	69	<5 years (mean 2 years)	3 (4%)	5 (7%)	0	0
Joffe & Ludwig (1988)	363	<19 years	0	6 (1.7%)	0	0

Table 3.8. Details of cases of falls from heights

Reference	Cases (n)	Age (range or average)	Distance	Sites of falls (when documented)	Minimum lethal height	Deaths (n)
Barlow (1983)	61	<16 years	1–6 stories	Buildings	No deaths ≤3 floors	14
Keogh *et al.* (1996)	91	<16 years	6–100 feet	Buildings, trees, playgrounds	No deaths <15 feet	5
Musemeche *et al.* (1991)	70	≤15 years (mean 5 years)	≥10 feet (1–17 stories)	Buildings, fences	No deaths to 17 stories	0
Roshkow *et al.* (1990)	45	≤12 years	1–6 stories	Buildings	No deaths <3 floors	2
Williams (1991)	106	<3 years	≤ 70feet	Buildings	No deaths ≤40 feet	1

Reports of children who have fallen from buildings are instructive in allowing correlation between the distance fallen and the possibility of death (Table 3.8). In Barlow and colleagues' (1983) series of 61 children falling from one to six stories, all children falling three or fewer stories survived, while the mortality rate was 50% between the fifth and sixth floors (20% at four stories, 30% at five stories, and 83% at six stories). Roshkow and colleagues (1990) also studied falls from one to six stories in 45 children under 12 years of age. The two children who died had fallen three and five stories, respectively, and succumbed to medical complications of aspiration pneumonia and pulmonary embolism. Williams (1991) reviewed 106 cases of independently witnessed falls in children less than three years old who fell from heights of up to 70 feet. The single death was in a child who fell 70 feet. In Musemeche and colleagues' (1991) study of children with a mean age of five years falling at least 10 feet out of buildings, there were no deaths.

Distances fallen ranged from one to 17 stories, with a mean of two stories. Three children required rehabilitation, and three had residual defects. The preponderance of head and arm injuries in these series indicates that children are likely to fall headfirst and try to protect themselves by extending their arms. Of Smith, Burrington & Woolf's (1975) series of 66 children who fell from less than one storey to eight stories, only two (each falling four stories) died. Two other children falling four stories survived, as did a child who fell eight stories. The 64 survivors were returned to normal activities. Thus, despite Keogh and colleagues' (1996) report of five deaths in children under 16 years of age who fell from 15 to 100 feet, children are generally able to survive falls from considerable heights.

It is well recognized that skull fractures in children do not necessarily correlate with severe central nervous system injury (Root, 1992) (see also Table 3.6). For example, a 16-year-old girl from Grand Rapids,

Table 3.9. Details of cases of short falls with fatalities

Reference	Cases (n)	Age (range or mean)	Distance	Deaths (n)	Comment
Adesunkanmi et al. (1999)	305	–	≤10 feet	2	Distance fallen, surface struck, presence of witnesses not mentioned
Chadwick et al. (1991)	100	–	≤4 feet	7	All 7 fatalities thought to be homicidal. Only witness was caretaker. Five children had other injuries, including old fractures and genital trauma
Murray et al. (2000)	92	4.9 years	<15 feet	3	11/164 patients (including 72 with falls >15 feet) had multiple old fractures, acute and chronic subdural hemorrhages, and retinal hemorrhages. Presence of witnesses not indicated
Reiber (1993)	19	≤5 years	≤5–6 feet	2	No documented corroboration of histories
Wang et al. (2001)	393	<15 years	<15 feet	4	Surface struck not described; no documented corroboration of histories.

USA, fell 30 feet and landed on her head on concrete. Although she had multiple skull fractures, she subsequently returned to school with only a mild short-term memory loss.

Several authors have reported children dying after a carer has given a history of a short fall (Table 3.9). However, as the circumstances of these deaths are often not well documented, and significant information is often lacking, conclusions must be treated with caution. Adesunkanmi, Oseni & Bodru (1999) described two (0.7%) deaths out of their series of 305 children who had fallen 10 feet or less. The distances fallen, the surfaces upon which the children landed, and whether there were independent witnesses were not mentioned. Hall and colleagues (1989) reported deaths from head injuries in 18 children (average age 2.4 years) who either fell while running or fell less than three feet. In nine cases there was a delay of more than four hours in seeking medical treatment, which raises concerns about inflicted injury. In addition, pre-hospital and hospital records were not reviewed, and specific details of individual cases were not provided. Wang and colleagues (2001) described 729 cases of children under 15 years who had fallen. Although there were four deaths in falls of less than 15 feet (1% mortality), the authors do not describe

the specific height from which the four fatal falls occurred or the surfaces on to which the children fell.

Murray and colleagues (2000) identified three deaths out of 92 children with a mean age of 4.9 years who fell less than 15 feet. Eleven of the children had evidence of abuse, but whether those who died were abused was not indicated. Again, the surfaces on to which the fatally injured children landed were not described; neither was the presence of independent witnesses mentioned. Reiber (1993) reported 19 deaths in children with histories of falls of 1.5–1.8 m or less. Fourteen cases were homicides, in three the manner of death was ruled undetermined, and two were deemed accidental. The two children who died accidentally were aged 17 and 21 months, respectively. The 21-month-old fell 1.5–1.8 m off a bunkbed, and the 17-month-old fell backward from a rocking chair. Neither case had detailed descriptions of the falls or the neuropathology evaluations.

Plunkett (2001) reported 18 children who died following falls from platforms, from ladders, and in playgrounds. The victims, identified from Consumer Product Safety Commission databases, ranged in age from one to 13 years, and the distances fallen ranged from 0.6 to 3 m. Of these fatal cases, 10 were aged between one and five years, the most common age range for abusive head injuries. Only five of the 10 were autopsied. They showed significant injuries: two had large subdural hematomas, one had an epidural hematoma, one had thin bilateral subdural hemorrhages, and one had complex fractures of the left frontal and both temporal bones, small epidural and subdural hemorrhages, and *contrecoup* contusions. Five of the 10 falls in children aged five years or younger were unwitnessed, as were all of the falls in the group of four children younger than 23 months. Unfortunately, accurate assessments of heights of falls were not available in all cases. Furthermore, Plunkett (2001) defined the height of the fall as "the distance of the closest body part from the ground at the beginning of the fall." Schaber and colleagues (2002) have pointed out that the heights of the falls should have been taken as the distances of the victims' heads from the ground at the start of the falls. Given these omissions, it is difficult to derive any meaningful conclusions from these data, which certainly cannot be used to substantiate assertions that fatal childhood falls may be from low heights and may not be associated with immediate symptoms.

Head injuries from blunt force

Head injuries are the most common types of injuries seen in cases of fatal child abuse (Willging, Bower & Cotton, 1992). Billmire & Myers (1985) studied head injuries in 84 infants under one year of age. Eighteen of the 19 children with intracranial hemorrhage or other serious intracranial injuries had been abused, with the one accidentally injured child in this group being an unrestrained occupant in a motor vehicle accident. Fifty-six percent of the abused children suffered shaking injuries, and 89% of these had retinal hemorrhages. None of the accidentally injured children had retinal hemorrhages.

In a series of 100 head-injured children under two years of age, 24 had suffered inflicted trauma. Eight of these were said to have fallen, two caretakers admitted the assault, and in 14 cases no explanation of the injury could be given (Duhaime *et al.*, 1992). A clinical presentation of unexplained neurological deficit, seizures, apneic episodes, poor feeding, lethargy, rapidly developing unconsciousness, hydrocephalus, or increased intracranial pressure may occur in such cases (Hobbs, 1989a).

Clinical evaluation of the abused children in Duhaime and colleagues' (1992) series showed craniofacial soft tissue injuries in two children, linear or depressed skull fractures without dural hemorrhage in seven children, multiple, basilar, or stellate fractures in two children, intracranial hemorrhage in 13 children, and recent or healing long bone fractures in nine children. All depressed skull fractures in the accidentally injured children occurred in falls greater than four feet, or down stairs, or from an impact with a moving object. The clinical course was uncomplicated in falls that resulted in only focal cerebral contusions or focal subarachnoid hemorrhage (Duhaime *et al.*, 1992).

Skull fractures in accidentally injured children tend to be linear and involve the parietal bone (Hiss & Kahana, 1995). If depressed, fractures are usually localized, with a history of a fall on to a sharp object such as a table edge or a small, hard toy (Wheeler & Shope, 1997). In contrast, fractures resulting from assault are extensive, complex or branched, depressed, and wide (greater than 3 mm), and tend to involve several bones (Figures 3.6 and 3.7). Occipital or basilar fractures are especially likely to be non-accidental in origin (Hobbs, 1984; Hobbs, 1989a). Meservy and colleagues (1987) found that multiple fractures, bilateral fractures, and fractures that crossed suture lines were predictive of inflicted injury.

Mirror-image bilateral skull fractures may occur when a child's head is compressed between two hard, unyielding surfaces (Hiss & Kahana, 1995). These fractures can occur from mechanisms such as falling while holding a child, crushing the skull between the body of a carer and a floor, slamming a car door on a child's head, or stomping on an infant's head. Symmetric biparietal linear skull fractures may also occur accidentally, as in the case of a six-week-old infant who was witnessed independently to fall backwards two to three feet on to a concrete surface, with impact to the midline posteriorly; there were no associated intracranial injuries (Arnholz *et al.*, 1998).

The softness of infants' skulls means that calvarial bones may bend rather than fracture, and also that they may be more vulnerable to penetration by projectiles or sharp objects (Campbell-Hewson, D'Amore & Busuttil, 1998).

Subdural hemorrhage in children is usually always traumatic (Figure 3.8), except in cases of bleeding diatheses or vascular malformations (see Chapters 8 and 9), where hemorrhage may be spontaneous. It is unclear whether hemorrhage in such cases may also occur with lesser degrees of force. If diagnosed during the first three to four weeks of life, birth trauma may have been responsible (Newton, 1989). However, without adequate explanation, inflicted injury should always be considered (Hobbs, 1989a; Reece & Sege, 2000). Thirteen of the 24 abused children in Duhaime and colleagues' (1992) series had subdural hemorrhages, compared with only three of 76 accidentally injured children, each of whom was involved in a motor vehicle accident. The outcome for survivors when inflicted head injury is serious is generally poor (Gilles & Nelson, 1998; Holloway, Bye & Moran, 1994).

It is vital to check coagulation status as soon as possible in infants who present to hospital with suspected inflicted head injury, since coagulopathy may develop if there is intraparenchymal brain damage. Specifically, activated coagulation and mild prolongation of prothrombin times may be found (Hymel *et al.*, 1997a). It may not be possible at autopsy to refute suggestions of possible vitamin K deficiency if antemortem testing has not been performed. Those at highest risk of vitamin K deficiency are breastfed infants under six months of age who have had perinatal complications and are receiving antibiotics. Assessment of previous and family medical history for hemorrhagic disease is also important (Hymel *et al.*, 1997a). It should be emphasized, however, that children with bleeding disorders are not immune from inflicted injury (O'Hare & Eden, 1984).

Mechanisms of injury

Anatomic considerations

A number of anatomic factors predispose the brain of the young infant and child to injury. The skull of infants and young children is thin and pliable,

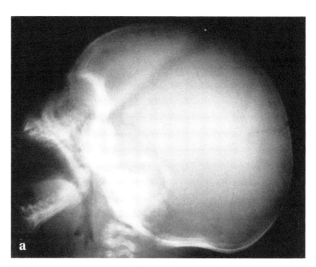

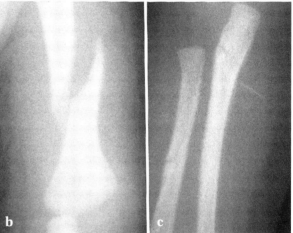

Figure 3.6 Fracture of the skull (a), spiral fracture of the left humerus (b), and fractures of the radius and ulna (c) in a six-week-old boy.

and its base is smooth and flat, lacking ridges that characterize the adult skull, and offering little resistance to a rapidly moving brain (Case *et al.*, 2001). Lack of myelination causes the brain to be soft, and many neurons lack dendritic connections. The head is disproportionately heavy and the neck muscles relatively weak, allowing extensive movement of the head and brain when accelerative and decelerative forces are applied to the infant's or child's head. Relatively more cerebrospinal

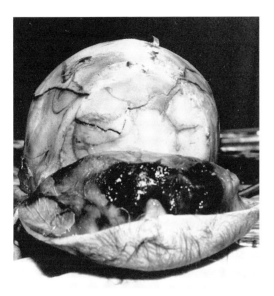

Figure 3.7 Shattering of the skull in a 3.5-month-old boy from severe blunt trauma. No adequate explanation for the injury was offered.

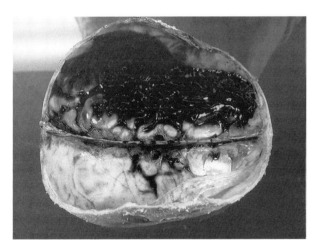

Figure 3.8 Typical fresh subdural hematoma formation following a blow to the head.

fluid is present, and the brain has a higher water content. These characteristics predispose the brains of infants and young children to shear injuries from shaking or impact (Case *et al.*, 2001; Finnie, 2001).

Biomechanics

Cranial trauma may result from impact or non-impact injuries. Impact causes focal injuries such as scalp lacerations, skull fractures, epidural hemorrhage, focal subdural or subarachnoid hemorrhage, and brain parenchymal contusions or lacerations, usually directly beneath the site of contact. Brain contusions resulting from impact injuries are referred to as *coup* contusions, while contusions opposite the site of impact (non-impact contusions) are referred to as *contrecoup* contusions. Non-impact injuries result from cranial acceleration or deceleration regardless of whether there is a direct blow to the cranium. These type of injuries derive from two direct mechanisms: (i) the brain may move relative to the skull and dura, tearing bridging veins; or (ii) there may be differential movement of various parts of the brain itself. Severe or fatal cranial injuries result most often from acceleration/deceleration rather than impact forces.

Following trauma, secondary hypoxia with alteration of cerebral blood flow, edema, and ischemia may subsequently exacerbate damage to brain tissues, from whatever cause or mechanism, as may the generation of free radicals and calcium influx into traumatized cells (Hymel *et al.*, 1998).

The forces causing head injury are mainly translational and rotational. Translational forces, as occur in a fall from a bed or changing table, are relatively benign and produce linear movement of the brain's center of gravity (Case *et al.*, 2001; Hymel *et al.*, 1998). Rotational or angular acceleration causes the brain to turn on its central axis or at its attachments at the junction of the brain and brainstem (Case *et al.*, 2001; Hymel *et al.*, 1998; Ommaya, Goldsmith, & Thibault, 2002). This results in shearing injuries, including diffuse axonal injury (DAI) and blood vessel laceration, by causing differential movements of brain structures (nuclei, white matter tracts) that have different densities depending upon the relative concentrations of myelin, neurons, and glial cells (Case *et al.*, 2001; Ommaya, Goldsmith & Thibault, 2002). At greatest risk for angular acceleration-induced strain are the junction of the cortex and white matter, the white matter and deep gray matter, and structures spanning the midline, including the corpus callosum and the superior and middle cerebellar peduncles (Case *et al.*, 2001). Severe angular acceleration, inducing differential motion between the brain and skull, causes subdural hematomas by tearing bridging veins (Hymel *et al.*, 1998; Ommaya, Goldsmith & Thibault, 2002). The difference between the initial rates of acceleration between the skull and brain is termed "deceleration lag" (Cory *et al.*, 2001).

Two types of force application, static and dynamic loading, cause different types of head injury. Static loading occurs slowly, compressing the skull (e.g. closing an elevator door on the head) (Hymel *et al.*, 1998); unless the force applied to the head is great, this may cause little or no injury. In contrast, dynamic loading, characterized by a rapid (usually <200 ms) application of force, causes abrupt deformation of the brain and is much more likely to cause strain injury, such as shearing (Finnie, 2001; Hymel *et al.*, 1998). Dynamic loading can be from either impulsive or impact loading. Impulsive loading results from a whiplash type of acceleration/deceleration without contact, with the forces transmitted through the neck. Impact loading occurs with contact, e.g. cranial collision (Hymel *et al.*, 1998).

Important variables in injury causation include the surface upon which a child lands, i.e. whether it is solid, such as concrete, or deformable, such as grass (Garrettson & Gallagher, 1985). A deformable surface absorbs some of the energy of the fall, reducing the force per unit area (stress) and therefore the severity of the injury. Strain refers to deformation of tissues in response to stress. Strain can be compressive when length is decreased, tensile when length is increased, or shearing when angular distortion occurs (Hymel *et al.*, 1998).

The deceleration of a body on impact can be expressed as the ratio of the height fallen to the deformation or stopping distance. Other factors determining severity of injury from a fall include the impact duration (the shorter the impact duration, the greater the force of the injury) and orientation of the body on impact. For example, a fall on to the feet with subsequent impact of the shoulders and head will result in the lower portions of the body absorbing the bulk of the impact energy. In most falls, however, a young child will land head down, as the head constitutes a large proportion of the body weight (Cory *et al.*, 2001).

Estimates have been made of the threshold for acceleration for fatal head injury using animal models and anthropomorphic dummies. However, flaws exist with such estimates, as anthropomorphic dummies cannot duplicate the complex biologic characteristics of the living human body, and animal and human skulls and brains differ in size, shape, and mechanical properties, such as density, pressure tolerance, and elasticity (Finnie, 2001). Head injury models may, however, be useful in predicting the likelihood that an injury could be caused by the event as described (Cory *et al.*, 2001).

Intracranial findings

Frequently, fatally abused children have little or no external injuries, despite having devastating injuries to the central nervous system. Children, unlike adults, tend to sustain contusional tears rather than more diffuse cerebral contusions (Shannon & Becker, 2001). Contusional tears are slit-like defects located in the subcortical white matter of the frontal and occipital lobes caused by shearing forces when a pliable skull is deformed by a blow to the head. When recent, they are lined by red blood cells and later become hemosiderin-stained (Lindenberg & Freytag, 1969; Calder, Hill & Scholtz, 1984). Characteristic injuries also observed on gross examination include epidural, subdural, subarachnoid, and retinal hemorrhages (Case *et al.*, 2001). Epidural hemorrhage, with or without fractures, results from brief, linear contact forces of the type associated with accidental falls or direct blows (Shugerman *et al.*, 1996).

Subdural hemorrhage results from shearing strains to bridging veins caused by differential acceleration of the skull and brain resulting from anterior-posterior rotational acceleration of relatively short duration and high magnitude. Specialized postmortem techniques have been described for demonstrating the site of bridging vein rupture

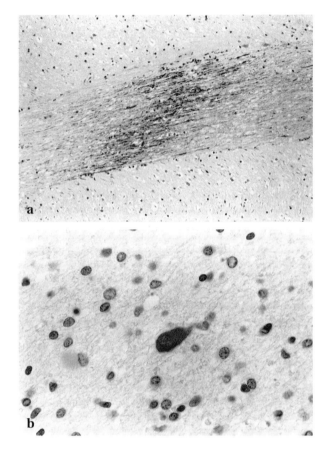

Figure 3.9 Immunohistochemical staining for beta-amyloid precursor protein (β-APP) in a victim of shaken infant syndrome, revealing injuries to the corpus callosum (a) (×100). Higher power reveals a typical axonal "bomb" (b) (×400).

using contrast material (Maxeiner, 1997; Maxeiner, 2001).

Cerebral swelling may occur quite rapidly after trauma, resulting in flattening of the gyri and cerebral herniation. This has been observed on computerized tomographic (CT) scan as early as one hour and 17 minutes after childhood trauma (Willman *et al.*, 1997). Swelling is due to a combination of increased cerebral blood flow from direct disturbance of vasomotor control, and leakage of fluid from damaged blood vessels. Vasodilation and hyperemia may begin within 30 minutes of trauma (Bruce *et al.*, 1981; Yoshino *et al.*, 1985).

Many authors believe that shearing injuries are responsible for severe neurological damage with DAI characterized by diffuse damage to axons in the cerebral hemispheres, corpus callosum, the brainstem, and occasionally the cerebellum (Adams *et al.*, 1989; Duhaime *et al.*, 1992; Case *et al.*, 2001). DAI has traditionally been identified when "retraction balls" or "bulbs" have been detected with silver or hematoxylin and eosin (H&E) staining of sections (Niess *et al.*, 2002). However, the most specific test for DAI is immunohistochemical detection of beta-amyloid precursor protein (β-APP). β-APP is a neuronal transmembrane glycoprotein transported by fast anterograde axoplasmic flow. Damage to the cytoskeleton of the axon interrupts transport of proteins including β-APP, causing accumulation at or near sites of injury, with resultant swelling and lobulation of the axon. Although other proteins are present at a site of injury, antibodies to β-APP are the most sensitive for detecting this type of damage (Figure 3.9) (Dolinak, Smith & Graham, 2000; Gleckman *et al.*, 1999; Medana & Esiri, 2003; Niess *et al.*, 2002). In the most severe forms of DAI, small hemorrhages may be seen in the corpus callosum and rostral brainstem (Niess *et al.*, 2002; Adams *et al.*, 1989). β-APP staining is not, however, specific for physical trauma, and it may result from other insults such as hypoxia and ischemia associated with parenchymal edema, fat embolization, or increased intracranial pressure (Dolinak, Smith & Graham, 2000; Geddes, Whitwell & Graham, 2000). This may create considerable difficulties in attempting to interpret injury patterns and mechanisms when there has been survival for several days following head trauma with diffuse hypoxic ischemic encephalopathy. In some cases, determining the relative contributions of trauma, hypoxia, and ischemia to β-APP staining may simply not be possible. β-APP immunoreactivity may remain positive for 30–99 days after head trauma (Medana & Isiri, 2003).

Several studies have assessed β-APP staining in head injury and hypoxic ischemic encephalopathy. In Gleckman and colleagues' (1999) study of rotational shaken and blunt impact head-injured infants, the most marked staining occurred in the internal capsule, midbrain, pons, and medulla, with less pronounced staining in the subcortical white matter. Non-traumatic controls (sudden infant death syndrome (SIDS), pneumonia, drowning, and suffocation) lacked β-APP positivity. Dolinak, Smith & Graham (2000) studied patients who had suffered cardiopulmonary arrest, status epilepticus, or carbon monoxide toxicity to evaluate the distribution of β-APP-positive axons. With the exception of carbon monoxide poisoning, they concluded that hypoxia per se did not cause axonal damage in the majority of cases and that most axonal injury in hypoxic patients could be attributed to vascular complications of raised intracranial pressure and herniation. Furthermore, non-traumatic axonal injury tended to have a vascular pattern. There was, however, some overlap with traumatic DAI, as a few cases had β-APP positivity in the corpus callosum, thalami, and brainstem. They also emphasized the need for specific and wide sampling of the brain to include the corpus callosum, parasagittal white matter bilaterally, both thalami, the posterior limb of the internal capsule, and the upper brainstem, including the cerebellar peduncles, if DAI is to be confirmed histologically.

While investigators have stressed the non-specificity of axonal injury, more work needs to be done. Niess and colleagues (2002) found that only 34% of their β-APP-positive cases were traumatic in origin, while approximately 61% had a non-traumatic etiology. However, many of their trauma patients died immediately, without sufficient time to manifest axonal changes. They also evaluated only parasagittal white matter and rostral pons for axonal injury. Oehmichen and colleagues (1999) examined the pons for DAI and compared traumatically injured brains in patients with focal cortical hemorrhage without dural involvement (caused by direct impact) with those with subdural hemorrhage without cortical involvement (caused by acceleration/deceleration). They found no significant difference between the two groups, concluding that β-APP positivity in the pons does not discriminate between traumatic brain injury and secondary damage caused by hypoxia/ischemia or edema. Geddes and colleagues (2001a), in a study of 53

non-accidentally head-injured children and infants, found a vascular pattern of axonal injury in 21 of 53 cases, while β-APP positivity in axons or bulbs scattered or in groups in the centrum semiovale, parasagittal white matter, corpus callosum, internal capsule, and cerebellar peduncles in the rostral brainstem was found in only three. In a subset of 37 infants nine months of age or younger, they observed vascular axonal injury in 13 cases and traumatic DAI in two children, both of whom had severe head injuries with multiple skull fractures. Eleven cases had epidural cervical hemorrhage and focal axonal injury to the brainstem and spinal nerve roots, suggesting to the authors that the craniocervical junction is vulnerable to stretch injury from cervical hyperextension and hyperflexion. They postulated that the main histologic abnormality in inflicted head injury in infants was diffuse vascular axonal damage, not DAI, and that brainstem-injury-induced apnea accounted for the hypoxic injury. They explained the lack of DAI by hypothesizing that either unmyelinated axons of infant cerebral hemispheres were resistant to trauma, or that shaking did not generate sufficient force to cause DAI (Geddes et al., 2001b).

Despite these proposals, however, it is generally believed that the finding of β-APP-positive axons in the brainstem, the corticospinal tracts of the cervical spinal cord, and spinal nerve roots in infants alleged to have suffered inflicted cerebral trauma suggests that the pathogenesis includes shaking with severe flexion/extension injuries of the brainstem and spinal cord. Certainly this could lead to hypoventilation or apnea, further exacerbating hypoxic/ischemic encephalopathy (Shannon & Becker, 2001; Shannon et al., 1998), but it does not explain diffuse β-APP staining in infants who do not have brainstem or upper cervical cord injuries.

There are several other limitations in assessing the brain for DAI. Although immunohistochemical evidence of DAI may be detected as early as one to three hours after injury (Dolinak, Smith & Graham, 2000; Gleckman et al., 1999), it may not be evident in victims who survive for shorter periods (Niess et al., 2002). Furthermore, adequate sampling of areas known to have DAI must be carried out, since different brain centers may demonstrate variable responses to injury. Such extensive sampling, accompanied by labor-intensive, expensive immunohistochemistry, may not be feasible for the average forensic laboratory and will require the expertise of a specialist neuropathology facility.

Retinal hemorrhage and eye injury

Massive retinal hemorrhage at all layers of the retina, in the absence of an independently verified or plausible history of accidental trauma, strongly suggests inflicted head injury, either from shaking or blunt head trauma, or a combination of both (Figures 3.10 and 3.11) (Bruce & Zimmerman, 1989; Levin, 2000; Munger *et al.*, 1993). Gilliland, Luckenbach & Chenier (1994) found that the cause of death in 62 of 70 children with retinal hemorrhage was craniocerebral trauma, which in 53 cases was inflicted. In Green and colleagues' (1996) study of 23 fatally abused children, 12 of 16 (75%) children dying from head injuries had retinal hemorrhages, compared with only one of 7 (14%) dying of non-central nervous system causes, a significant difference between the two groups ($P < 0.02$). Retinal hemorrhages are not, however, specific to shaking or other forms of inflicted head injury, and accurate dating is difficult (Duhaime *et al.*, 1998).

Non-inflicted retinal hemorrhage is rare and requires high-energy impact (Ophthalmology Child Abuse Working Party, 1999). For example, Elder, Taylor & Klug (1991) found no retinal hemorrhage in their series of 25 head-injured children, and in Schloff and colleagues' (2002) prospective study only one of 57 children had multiple retinal hemorrhages; this followed a motor vehicle accident. Three children reported by Christian and colleagues (1999) had injuries occurring at home: a 13-month-old boy in a walker fell down a flight of concrete stairs, a nine-month-old swung by his father struck his head on concrete, and a seven-month-old girl fell through a railing on to a concrete floor. In each case the retinal hemorrhage was ipsilateral to the intracranial hemorrhage and was confined to the posterior pole of the retina. Johnson, Braun & Friendly (1993) identified retinal hemorrhage in only two of 140 head-injured

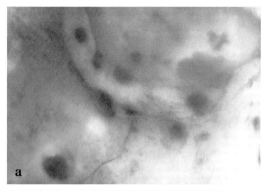

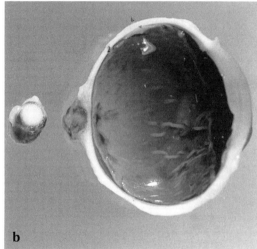

Figure 3.10 Retinal hemorrhages in a case of shaken infant syndrome, viewed through a dissecting microscope (a). Examination of the optic nerve and globe revealed hemorrhage around the nerve as well as confirming retinal hemorrhages (b).

children examined by an ophthalmologist. Both were restrained in the back seat of automobiles, sustaining impacts on the child's side. In another report, three of 18 infants and children under 24 months with head injuries from traffic accidents had retinal hemorrhages. These hemorrhages were located at the posterior pole and were flame-shaped (Vinchon *et al.*, 2002).

Retinal hemorrhages resulting from inflicted trauma are usually more severe, involving all layers of the retina, including the peripheral retina at the ora

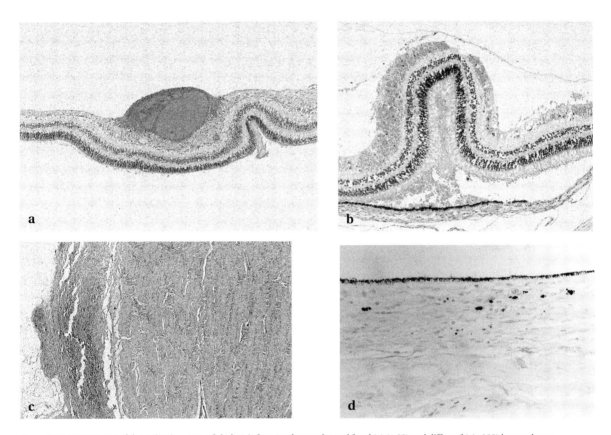

Figure 3.11 Microscopy of the retina in a case of shaken infant syndrome showed focal (a) ($\times 60$) and diffuse (b) ($\times 120$) hemorrhages at various levels within the retina, in addition to hemorrhage within the optic nerve sheath (c) ($\times 60$) (hematoxylin and eosin). Staining of the retina for iron in another case showed evidence of previous hemorrhage (d) (Perl's stain, $\times 180$).

serrata, and are often bilateral (Betz *et al.*, 1996). The authors have, however, seen a case with extensive bilateral retinal hemorrhages caused by rapidly increasing intracranial pressure due to a ruptured cerebral arteriovenous malformation. Thus, Levin (2000) has emphasized the need for accurate descriptions of the extent of the hemorrhages and the layers of the retina involved. With the most severe trauma, vitreous hemorrhage, traumatic retinoschisis, perimacular retinal folds, and retinal detachment may occur (Case *et al.*, 2001; Christian *et al.*, 1999; Duhaime *et al.*, 1998; Wilkinson *et al.*, 1989).

The most likely mechanism for traumatic retinal hemorrhage is traction on the retina from the vitreous caused by angular acceleration. Other postulated causes include increased pressure transmitted to the central retinal vein from increased thoracic pressure (Purtscher retinopathy) or from increased intracranial pressure, direct trauma to the retina from being struck by the vitreous moving within the eye, shearing between the vitreous and retina, intracranial hemorrhage (Terson syndrome), and acceleration/deceleration forces (Case *et al.*, 2001; Duhaime *et al.*, 1998; Elder, Taylor & Klug, 1991; Green *et al*, 1996; Levin, 2000; Ludwig & Warman, 1984; Riffenburgh & Sathyavagiswaran, 1991; Tomasi & Rosman, 1975).

Ipsilateral cerebral edema with ipsilateral subdural, subarachnoid and retinal hemorrhages, and bruising of the pinna may be caused by a blow to the head with angular acceleration. This has been termed "tin ear" syndrome (Feldman, 1992; Hanigan, Peterson & Njus, 1987).

Other causes of retinal hemorrhage include coagulopathies, sepsis, meningitis, intracranial neoplasms, leukemia, endocarditis, rupture of intracranial aneurysms, hypertension, increased intracranial pressure, galactosemia, spontaneous subarachnoid hemorrhage, scurvy, epilepsy, asphyxia, and rarely, if ever, cardiopulmonary resuscitation (CPR) (Case *et al.*, 2001; Duhaime *et al.*, 1998; Gilliland & Luckenbach, 1993; Green *et al.*, 1996; Kanter, 1986; McLellan, Prasad & Punt, 1986; Taylor, 2000). Retinal hemorrhages may be present in up to 40% of vaginally delivered newborns but resolve by approximately four weeks of age (Duhaime *et al.*, 1998; Spaide *et al.*, 1990).

Additional eye injuries from inflicted injury can include periorbital edema and contusion, subconjunctival hemorrhage, retinal detachment, retinal tears, lens subluxation, vitreous hemorrhage, subhyaloid hemorrhage, choroidal hemorrhage, and perineural hemorrhage (Case *et al.*, 2001; Green *et al.*, 1996; Rao *et al.*, 1988; Taylor, 2000). Optic atrophy, corneal opacity, macular scarring, and cataracts may be manifestations of previous injury (Harcourt & Hopkins, 1971; Harley, 1980). Although hemorrhage into the soft tissues behind the eyeball has been proposed as a marker for suffocation, this has not been the experience of the authors. In fact, manually disrupting small vessels in connective tissue at the back of the orbit at the time of enucleation will produce such a lesion, i.e. it may be created by postmortem dissection.

Shaken infant syndrome

Shaken infant syndrome (SIS), described in Caffey's landmark paper in 1974, is defined as intracranial injury in the absence of external signs of head trauma (Caffey, 1974; Wilkinson *et al.*, 1989). Gilliland & Folberg (1996) refined this definition by requiring two of the following three criteria: (i) finger marks and/or rib fractures, (ii) subdural and/or subarachnoid hemorrhage, and (iii) a history of vigorous

shaking. Thus, in many cases of fatal shaken infant syndrome there may be minimal or no external clues to suggest an unnatural cause of death. The victim is most commonly a child under two years of age, although cases have been described in children up to five years of age and even in an adult (American Academy of Pediatrics Committee on Child Abuse and Neglect, 2001a; Pounder, 1997).

As already noted, a young child or infant is susceptible to injuries from shaking as the head is disproportionately heavy relative to the body, the neck muscles are weak, the brain is soft because many of the axons are unmyelinated, and the base of the skull is flat (Case *et al.*, 2001).

Shaking is often precipitated by crying or perceived misbehavior. As with child abuse in general, the initial history given is often either misleading or insufficient to explain the injuries. Common explanations for the child's condition include no predisposing event, minor falls, seizures, or spontaneous respiratory arrest (Bruce & Zimmerman, 1989; Ludwig & Warman, 1984; Peinkofer, 2002). A diagnosis of shaken infant syndrome based on clinical assessment was made in 11.3% of all abusive head injuries in Gilliland & Folberg's (1996) series and 57% of Brown & Minns' (1993) cases.

The type of shaking bringing about significant brain injury is caused by holding an infant by the thorax or extremity with violent shaking, forcing the head to whiplash back and forth, with repeated accelerations and decelerations in both directions (Brown & Minns, 1993; Caffey, 1974; Case *et al.*, 2001). It has been asserted that the shaking is so violent that it should be recognized by the perpetrator as harmful and likely to be injurious (American Academy of Pediatrics Committee on Child Abuse and Neglect, 2001a; Levin, 2000). Playfully tossing a child in the air and catching him or her does not cause this type of brain injury, neither does normal "wear and tear" activity.

In a non-fatally shaken infant or child, symptoms may include poor feeding, vomiting, lethargy, or irritability. In a severely shaken infant who dies, there will be alteration in conscious state followed by evidence of brainstem dysfunction (American Academy of Pediatrics Committee on Child Abuse and Neglect, 2001a; King *et al.*, 2003). This is not surprising as there may have been direct axonal injury of the medulla or upper spinal cord causing apnea and hypoventilation (Shannon & Becker, 2001; Shannon *et al.*, 1998).

Obvious external injuries are absent in up to half of the cases (Case *et al.*, 2001), especially if the child was clad at the time of the assault, or there may be finger and thumb grip contusions on the arms, chest, or back (Figure 3.12) where the infant was grasped. There may also be evidence of other forms of inflicted trauma (Alexander *et al.*, 1990a). Internal head injuries include subdural hemorrhage (usually bilateral), subarachnoid hemorrhage, and retinal hemorrhage. Hemorrhage tends to be maximal in the interhemispheric fissure (American Academy of Pediatrics Committee on Child Abuse and Neglect, 2001b). Subdural hemorrhage is nearly always minimal (no more than 5–10 ml on each side), does not cause a mass effect, and may be missed on CT scans (Case *et al.*, 2001).

Although subarachnoid hemorrhage in children is almost always traumatic in origin, occasional cases are due to vascular malformations and aneurysms. Spontaneous subarachnoid hemorrhage almost never occurs in infants (Newton, 1989).

Spinal cord injury may occur from abuse, although its frequency is difficult to determine as the spinal cord is often not examined routinely at autopsy (as it should be). Epidural hemorrhage and spinal cord contusion in the absence of vertebral fracture may result from severe lateral flexion, although most spinal cord injuries in battered infants are associated with spinal column fractures (Cullen, 1975; Gosnold & Sivaloganathan, 1980). Holding an infant by the head and shaking may cause the body to whiplash back and forth, also resulting in upper cord damage.

A common postmortem artifact that has been interpreted as evidence of shaking injury is hemorrhage around the lumbar spinal cord. However, this may occur in infants who have been left lying on their backs for some time after death, caused by postmortem pooling of blood that is released when the cord is taken out through a posterior approach. It is difficult to support a traumatic etiology in the

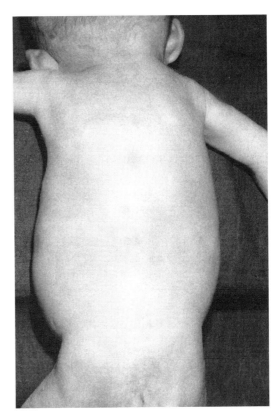

Figure 3.12 Subtle fingertip bruising along the spine in a nine-week-old boy with posterior fractured ribs

absence of injury to the spinal cord, vertebrae, and surrounding soft tissues.

Rarely reported injuries following shaking have included avulsion of portions of the spinous process of the thoracic and lumbar vertebrae, fractures of the cervical spine, anterior and posterior neck muscle hemorrhage, periadventitial vertebral artery hemorrhage with compression of the vertebral arteries, and pericallosal artery aneurysm (Gleckman, Kessler & Smith, 2000; Kleinman & Zito, 1984; McGrory & Fenichel, 1977; Saternus, Kernbach-Wighton & Oehmichon, 2000).

At autopsy in a case of possible lethal shaking, particular attention should be paid to soft tissue dissection of the chest and back for possible bruising caused by fingertip pressure. The brain and spinal cord should ideally be submitted for specialist neuropathological examination, and the eyeballs must be taken, sectioned, and stained routinely and for hemosiderin.

Death is the outcome in 15–38% of shaken infants who present with acute intracranial damage, 30–50% have neurologic sequelae, and about 30% will recover. Residual deficits include cortical blindness, microencephaly, spasticity, seizures, chronic subdural fluid collections, cerebral atrophy, and porencephalic cysts (Case *et al.*, 2001; American Academy of Pediatrics Committee on Child Abuse and Neglect, 2001b).

Since publication of the first edition of this book, controversy about the possibility of shaking causing significant craniocerebral injuries has continued. Certain authors believe that pure shaking rarely, if ever, causes severe cerebral injury, and that nearly all patients who have been shaken have also sustained blunt impact, either from being put down forcibly or from being struck deliberately (Bruce & Zimmerman, 1989; Duhaime *et al.*, 1987; Duhaime *et al.*, 1998; Ommaya, Goldsmith & Thibault, 2002; Plunkett, 1999). Duhaime and colleagues (1987) found that all 13 children in their study who died with a clinical diagnosis of shaking had evidence of blunt impact, including scalp contusions and skull fractures. They performed experiments using dolls with their heads filled with wet cotton to simulate the head weight of infants and found that shaking the dolls failed to generate enough tangential acceleration to theoretically cause injury, while impact, even against a padded surface, was associated with the potential for brain injury. Plunkett (1999) asserts that there are no scientific experiments to demonstrate fatal head injury in shaken infants, and Ommaya, Goldsmith & Thibault's (2002) theoretical calculations suggest that shaking does not generate sufficient force to cause injury.

Duhaime and colleagues' (1987) experiments have, however, been criticized, as doll heads do not resemble human infant heads, lacking the variable densities of brain parenchyma and surrounding cerebral spinal fluid (Case *et al.*, 2001). In the experiments, the dolls' heads were subjected to "repetitive violent shaking," but the exact force with which they were shaken was not stated. Dolls' heads also do not have active blood flow with potential for vascular rupture. Furthermore, in our own and others' experience, fatally head-injured children with subdural, subarachnoid, and retinal hemorrhages have been identified who have had no evidence of blunt impact to the head (Alexander *et al.*, 1990b; Brown & Minns, 1993; Carty & Ratcliffe, 1995; Gilliland & Folberg, 1996). In a case of witnessed shaking to which there were neutral observers, an infant has been documented to lose consciousness while being shaken, and in another case a perpetrator admitted shaking the child until death occurred: "I shook him, and I shook him and I shook him until he was no more" (Krous & Byard, 1999). Shaking is also not a precisely controlled exercise with regular accelerations and decelerations in one plane; descriptions suggest that complex angular rotation of the infant head can occur in a variety of directions over a short period of time.

Besides Duhaime and colleagues' (1987) doll model, Smith and colleagues (1998) have developed a rat model for shaken infant syndrome. As the animals were anesthetized and exposed to one episode of shaking per day for three successive days, the conditions to which shaken infants are exposed were not duplicated precisely.

Other studies have, however, further clarified our understanding of the biomechanics of shaking and head trauma by using experimental animal models (Adams, Graham & Gennarelli, 1981; Adams, Graham & Gennarelli, 1982; Adams, Gennarelli & Graham, 1982; Gennarelli, 1983; Gennarelli, 1993; Gennarelli *et al.*, 1982). Jenny and colleagues (2002) have developed a biomechanical model for shaken infant syndrome. Scenarios including violent shaking of the model for at least four seconds showed that the infant dummy experienced substantially greater linear and angular acceleration during shaking alone than has been reported previously, with less discrepancy between shaking alone versus slamming with or without shaking.

However, while we believe that it is possible for an adult to fatally shake an infant or young child, it is often impossible to separate shaking from impact injuries, as the resultant intracranial injuries may be similar. Focal injuries of the skull and soft tissues of the head indicate impact but do not exclude coexisting shaking. Conversely, in the absence of impact injuries, blunt trauma cannot be ruled out, as an impact may not leave visible injuries. Both impact and shaking may produce angular acceleration with subdural and subarachnoid hemorrhages, markers for the common underlying pathologic lesion, DAI. Rather than encourage protracted and often pointless courtroom debate, we believe that the best general diagnostic term for an inflicted head injury in an infant or child, whether from blunt impact or shaking, is craniocerebral trauma.

Geddes and colleagues (2003) have suggested a "unified hypothesis" in which hypoxia with brain swelling, rather than trauma, is considered to be the cause of subdural and retinal hemorrhages. However, the basis for this assertion is difficult to understand as their study of 50 infants and fetuses revealed only one case of subdural hemorrhage (which was attributed to sepsis and disseminated intravascular coagulation) and no retinal hemorrhages (as the eyes were not examined at autopsy). In fact, microscopically detectable intradural hemorrhage was the only significant pathology that was found. In our experience, retinal and subdural hemorrhages are not markers for hypoxic ischemic encephalopathy.

Finally, it has been proposed that immunization predisposes an infant to intracranial hemorrhage identical to that seen in shaken infant syndrome. The underlying mechanism is hypothesized to be thrombocytopenia from a delayed reaction to immunization that predisposes to soft tissue, intracranial, and retinal hemorrhages. An additional problem that diphtheria/pertussis/tetanus (DPT) vaccine has also been blamed for is induction of convulsions resulting in injury-producing falls. As there is no peer-reviewed literature to support either of these theories or to explain the lack of generalized interstitial hemorrhage, or how unwitnessed falls can occur in young infants incapable of walking, they should be firmly refuted whenever the opportunity arises (see section below on expert evidence).

Lucid interval

Assailants in cases of inflicted head injury in children often claim that a child was injured before being in their care, and that the injury took some time to manifest. However, head injury in infants and young children from a major mechanical force sufficient to result in death is usually accompanied by an immediate or rapid onset of neurologic symptoms (Duhaime et al., 1998). In adults, studies have shown that patients with severe DAI are unconscious from the time of impact (Blumbergs, Jones & North, 1989).

Willman and colleagues (1997) reviewed the medical charts of 95 accidentally injured children in order to determine whether an infant or young child who suffers a fatal head injury will look and act normally post-injury. The mean age was 8.5 years, with a range of 99 days to 16.2 years. In all but two cases, injuries derived from automobile accidents. Normal activity of an infant included eye contact, reaching, grasping, playing, smiling, feeding, and other activities appropriate for age. In older children, normal behaviour included usual speech, eating, or playing. Ninety-four children had no lucid interval, with the only exception being a child with an epidural hematoma. This study showed that a fatal cerebral injury that was not due to an epidural hematoma must have occurred some time after a child last exhibited normal behavior. It must, unfortunately, be noted that assessment of an infant's behavior as normal or abnormal may not always have been made under optimal conditions by an experienced observer. Thus, it may not always be possible to determine retrospectively the true state of a victim's demeanor at a particular time (Byard et al., 2000a).

Other authors have, however, reported lucid intervals after allegedly accidental head injuries that ultimately proved to be fatal. For example, in Plunkett's (2001) series, five patients aged between one and five years were autopsied. Of these, two had no history of lucid intervals, one had a lucid interval of 10 minutes, one had a lucid interval of 15 minutes, and the fifth child had a three-hour lucid interval. However, given that the latter child had an epidural hematoma, a lucid interval would be not unexpected. In addition, the child with the 10-minute lucid interval had a large subdural hematoma, and the child with the 15-minute lucid interval had complex fractures of the left frontal and both temporal bones, with small epidural and subdural hematomas and *contrecoup* contusions. Unfortunately, Plunkett (2001) did not define "lucid interval;" for example, he did not specify whether the lucid interval included children who were conscious but obtunded. Schaber and colleagues (2002) have pointed out that in all three of Plunkett's (2001) cases the lucid intervals were consistent with the neuropathologic findings at the time of autopsy.

Humphreys, Hendrick & Hoffmann (1990) described a four-year-old child who was fatally injured in an automobile accident. Initially he had decerebrate posturing, but then his mental status improved slightly prior to having a cardiac arrest. Although this is put forward as one of four cases of children who "talked and died," this child was never normal after the accident. One of the other children was also not normal after the fatal accident, and assessment of the remaining two cases is complicated by lack of autopsies. No infants were included in this series. Nashelsky & Dix (1995) reviewed the literature for descriptions of lucid intervals in fatally shaken babies. Although they found one child who was alleged to have had a four-day lucid interval, the only witness was the alleged perpetrator. Of 76 non-accidental head injury deaths in Gilliland's (1998) study of infants and young children, 22 were claimed to have lucid intervals lasting more than 24 hours. Of these children, 10 were described as lethargic or otherwise abnormal during the interval between injury and collapse, and the other 12 were in the care of the presumed perpetrator and, thus, the validity of the descriptions of the children's conditions is suspect. In summary, excluding cases with epidural hematomas and those with unverifiable histories, "an alert, well-appearing child has not already suffered a devastating acute injury that will become clinically obvious hours to days later" (Duhaime *et al.*, 1998). To quote Chadwick and colleagues (1998): "Infants simply do not suffer massive head injury, show no significant symptoms for days, then suddenly collapse and die."

Finally, spontaneous rebleeding from a prior head injury that occurred days to weeks earlier may occur but has not been reported as a cause of rapid deterioration following a lucid interval (Barnes & Robson, 2000; Hymel, Jenny & Block, 2002).

Brain imaging

CT scanning and magnetic resonance imaging (MRI) can accurately indicate intracranial pathology and should be reviewed by the pathologist before autopsy in consultation with a pediatric radiologist and child protection physician (American Academy of Pediatrics Section on Radiology, 1991a; Cohen *et al.*, 1986; Dykes, 1986). CT findings indicative of inflicted trauma include interhemispheric (perifalcine) subdural hemorrhage, subdural hemorrhage over the convexities, subdural hygroma associated with an intracranial hemorrhage, intracranial hemorrhage in the absence of a skull fracture, basal ganglia edema, and mixed high- and low-density extracerebral collections (Hymel *et al.*, 1997b; Vinchon *et al.*, 2002; Wells, Vetter & Laud, 2002). Ewing-Cobbs and colleagues (1998) also found evidence of pre-existing injury, such as cerebral atrophy, hydrocephalus ex-vacuo, and subdural hygroma in nearly half of children with inflicted brain injury but not in children with accidental brain injury.

A comment should be made about mixed-density collections on CT scans that have been considered evidence of repeated trauma. It has been shown in both accidentally and non-accidentally injured children that a mixed-density collection may be seen very soon after injury. The high-density portion represents clotted blood and the low-density component indicates unclotted blood or fluid. This may result from a variety of causes, including active bleeding, clot retraction with extrusion of serum, an arachnoid laceration with cerebrospinal fluid leak into the subdural space, or a combination of those factors. Cerebrospinal fluid accumulation in the subdural space may also occur because of impaired absorption in the arachnoid villi (Barnes & Robson, 2000; Hymel, Jenny & Block, 2002; Vinchon *et al.*, 2002).

MRI is of limited usefulness in the acute post-injury period since it requires the patient to be anesthetized, it takes a long time to perform, and the child may be unstable. In the subsequent days after trauma, however, MRI can be used effectively to demonstrate subacute or chronic hemorrhages. MRI is extremely useful in assessing a child presenting with unexplained neurologic signs that have lasted for several days (Chabrol, Decarie & Fortin, 1999; Vinchon *et al.*, 2002). Sato and colleagues (1989) found MRI to be superior to CT scanning in showing subdural hemorrhage, cortical contusions, and shearing injuries, although subarachnoid hemorrhage was detected more easily with CT scans. Relative sparing of the cerebellum and brainstem from the effects of hypoxia is seen on CT scan as the "white cerebellum" sign (Harwood-Nash, 1992). MRI examinations performed in the early postmortem period have correlated well with similar studies during life, and MRI has also been useful in directing attention to focal abnormal areas that may have otherwise been overlooked during brain cutting (Hart, Dudley & Zumwalt, 1996).

Small intraparenchymal tissue tear hemorrhages in the corpus callosum, dorsolateral quadrants of the rostral brainstem, and other central portions of the brain exposed to high strain, are considered to be radiologic markers of DAI (Hymel *et al.*, 1998). Importantly, it has been noted that determination of the precise timing of when an infant was injured should not be based on radiological changes in isolation (Dias *et al.*, 1998).

Skin and soft tissue injury

While not usually lethal in themselves, the pattern of skin and soft tissue injuries may be helpful in separating inflicted from non-inflicted injury (Chadwick, 1992; Ellerstein, 1979; Feldman, 1995). In accidentally injured young children, the most common injuries are bruises of the hands, feet, and lower legs. In intentionally injured children of the same age, injuries of the head and lumbar region predominate (Johnson & Showers, 1985; Roberton, Barbor & Hull,

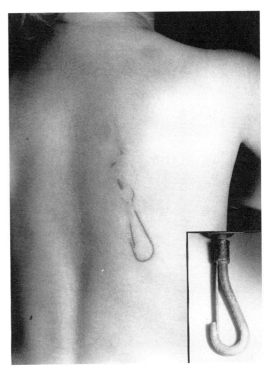

Figure 3.13 A patterned injury to the back of a child corresponding to a metal clasp (inset).

1982). Bruises are far more common than lacerations in children with inflicted injury (Pascoe *et al.*, 1979). Patterned injuries may result from being hit with an electrical cord or belt buckle, or may be due to pinching or biting, gagging of the mouth, or binding of the ankles and wrists with ligatures (Showers & Bandman, 1986; Raimer, Raimer & Hebeler, 1981). A variety of injury patterns are illustrated in Figures 3.13–3.26. Alopecia or subgaleal hematoma formation may follow vigorous hair pulling, and penile trauma should prompt careful investigation (Hamlin, 1968; Reece & Grodin, 1985; Slosberg *et al.*, 1978).

Although not widely recognized, it is possible to beat a child to death without causing fatal injury to internal organs. An example from Grand Rapids, USA, was a nine-year-old boy whose father beat him repeatedly with a looped cord. At autopsy, there were extensive contusions of the lower back and posterior thighs but no injuries to the central nervous

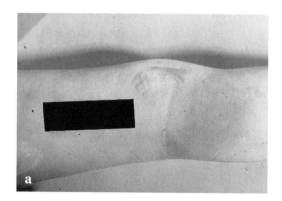 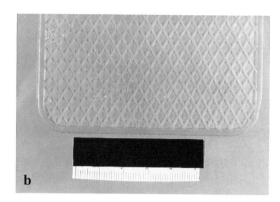

Figure 3.14 A patterned bruise behind the knee (a) corresponding to the mesh of a flyswatter (b).

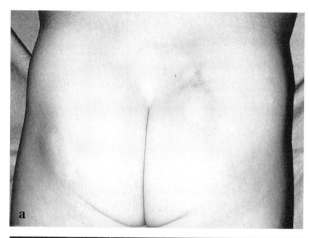

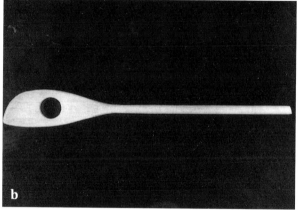

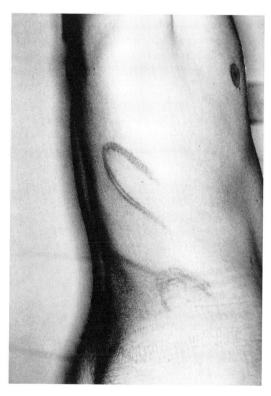

Figure 3.15 A patterned bruise on the buttock (a) corresponding to a similarly shaped kitchen implement (b).

Figure 3.16 Patterned curvilinear bruises after being struck with an electric flex.

system or to the thoracic or abdominal viscera. There was also extensive recent and old subcutaneous hemorrhage within the soft tissue of the lumbar region. Descriptions of such deaths are rare, and cases are probably underreported. Mechanisms of death include exsanguination from the accumulation of blood within subcutaneous tissue of the back, fat embolization, dehydration, gastric aspiration, and stress cardiomyopathy (Nichols, Corey & Davis, 1990). Life-threatening rhabdomyolysis with renal failure has also been described in a five-year-old boy arising from extensive inflicted soft tissue bruising (Mukherji & Siegel, 1987). Rarely, foreign bodies such as sewing needles may be inserted under the skin, with subsequent migration and sepsis (Ramu, 1977).

Demonstration of soft tissue injury to the back, buttocks, and legs requires "striping," i.e. making longitudinal incisions into the skin and soft tissues of the back, buttocks, and posterior thighs (Figure 3.27) (DiMaio & DiMaio, 2001; Sturner, 1998). Layer

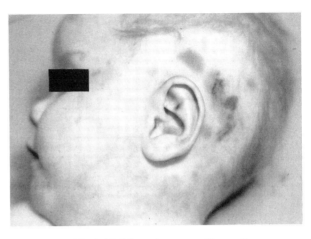

Figure 3.17 Bruising behind the ear in a young girl caused by a blow with a fist. A ring worn by the assailant caused the central linear abrasion.

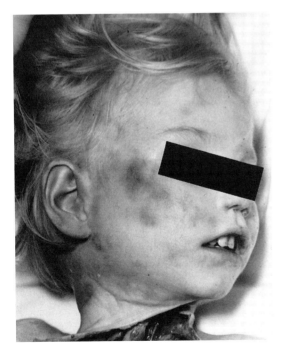
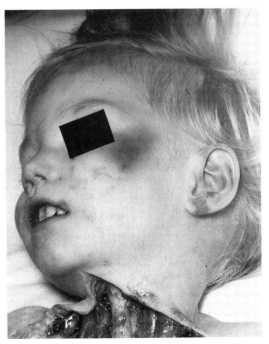

Figure 3.18 Symmetrical facial and ear bruises noted at autopsy in this fatally assaulted 18-month-old girl who also had recent and healing fractures of the ribs, and a rupture of the duodenum. Her father was subsequently convicted of manslaughter.

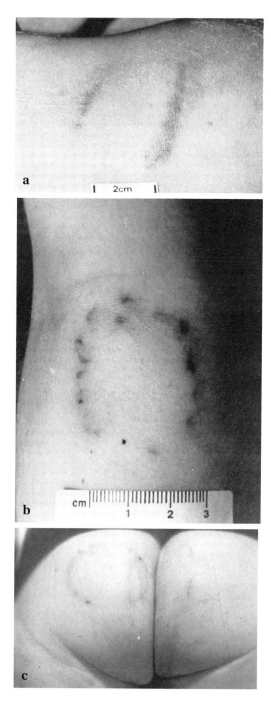

Figure 3.19 Adult bite marks on the shoulder (a), arm (b), and buttocks (c) of three children.

dissection of skin and muscles may also reveal occult injuries or define more clearly the extent of trauma (Figures 3.28 and 3.29). Incising possible bruises may be the only way to confirm their existence, particularly in dark-skinned children, or to differentiate them from postmortem lividity (Figures 3.30 and 3.31). Fat embolization may be best detected by post-fixing formalin-fixed tissue in osmium tetroxide before routine processing (Davison & Cohle, 1987).

Aging of bruises with any precision is usually a thankless task. Standard texts will give quite precise tables indicating that bruises are red, purple, and swollen in the first two days and then progress through green discoloration from four to seven days, to yellow from seven to 10 days, followed by resolution between 14 and 30 days. However, there is disagreement as to the precise sequence and timing of these color changes (Schwartz & Ricci, 1996; Stephenson & Bialas, 1996; Wilson, 1977). The development of bruises depends not only on the nature of the injury but also on the depth of the interstitial hemorrhage, the location of the injury, and the color of the overlying skin. Langlois & Gresham (1991) assert that the only statement that can be made reliably about the color of bruises is that a yellow bruise is at least 18 hours old. Having observed yellow bruises in adult victims of car accidents who died at the scene, the authors are not even sure that this can be relied upon. The authors have found that more important information involves the pattern of bruises, which is often lost after several days, and the presence of old and recent bruising in keeping with more than one episode of trauma (bearing in mind the above caveats). Histological sampling of representative bruises in homicide cases is required so that further confirmation of their existence can be provided. In addition, a vital reaction or hemosiderin deposition indicates that the injury occurred some time before death. The time taken for macrophages to convert ferritin into hemosiderin is approximately 24–72 hours (Gilliland *et al.*, 1991; Langlois & Gresham, 1991).

It is important not to confuse trauma from attempted cardiopulmonary resuscitation with child abuse (Figure 3.32). Similarly, certain folk-healing practices such as cupping or rubbing the body with coins may result in lesions of unusual appearance (*vide infra*) (Figures 3.33 and 3.34). Mongolian blue spots that are most commonly found over the sacrum or buttocks should not be mistaken for bruising, which can be excluded easily by incising affected skin and subcutaneous tissues (Figure 3.35).

Sexual assault

Evidence of possible sexual abuse (Figures 3.36–3.38), the features of which are summarized in Table 3.1, should be sought at all ages. Knowledge of the range of anatomical differences in immature anogenital tract morphology is essential to the evaluation of such cases. This will prevent overinterpretation of normal variants, such as exposure of the anal

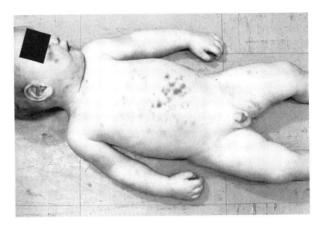

Figure 3.20 Bruising of the abdomen and lower chest due to being struck by a clenched fist in a 17-month-old boy who died from a ruptured liver.

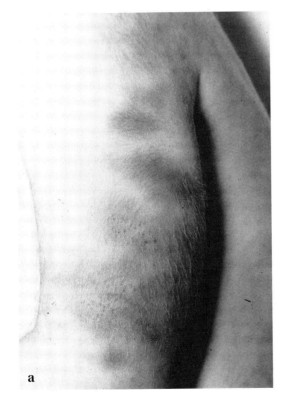

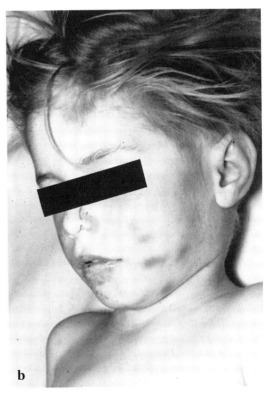

Figure 3.21 Bruising and abrasions of the upper arm corresponding to finger grip marks in a three-year-old boy who died as a result of a subdural hematoma (a). Linear bruises on the cheek correspond to finger slap marks (b).

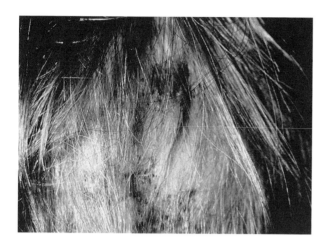

Figure 3.22 Scalp injuries from hair pulling.

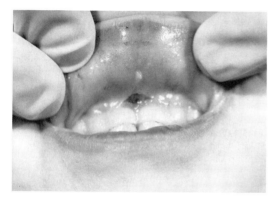

Figure 3.23 Torn frenulum with minimal abrasion and bruising of the upper lip following a blow to the mouth.

mucosa and pectinate line, and will enable the identification of subtle lesions (Emans, 1992; Gardner, 1992; McCann *et al.*, 1996; McCann, Voris & Simon, 1988; Paul, 1990).

The appearances of the hymen vary depending on age and technique of examination, with "considerable overlap" in the diameter of the hymenal opening between abused and non-abused children (Wissow, 1995). The anus is normally quite patulous in children at autopsy (Figure 3.39), and may be even more so in children with underlying medical conditions such as myotonic dystrophy or central nervous system injuries (McCann *et al.*, 1996;

Reardon *et al.*, 1992). It has been suggested that children with Crohn's disease or chronic constipation may also have anal dilation (Robinson, 1991). Anal dilation on its own therefore cannot be used as a marker for sexual abuse.

Colposcopic examination assists in the evaluation of sexual injuries by magnifying lesions and enabling photography and careful documentation (McCann, 1990). The exclusion of accidental trauma such as straddle and penetration injuries is also important (Figure 3.40) (Pierce & Robson, 1993; West, Davies & Fenton, 1989). Death may be physically unrelated to sexual assault, or it may be a direct result due to perforation of a small vagina or rectum with resultant hemorrhage or sepsis (Orr *et al.*, 1995). Small-intestinal evisceration through the anus has been described in a four-year-old boy most likely due to insertion of a rectal foreign body (Press *et al.*, 1991).

While genital warts (condylomata acuminata) in an infant or child may be an indicator of previous sexual contact, cases have been reported where infections with human papilloma virus causing these lesions have been due to non-sexual contact with family members, auto-inoculation, or a delayed result of transmission during delivery (Ross, Scott & Busuttil, 1993).

Protocols for the examination of the sexually abused child are widely available (American Academy of Pediatrics Committee on Child Abuse and Neglect, 1991b; Paradise, 1990), and involvement of a child protection physician in such cases is always very useful. Smears and swabs of the pharynx, mouth, labia, upper and lower vagina, anus and rectum, nipples, neck, and bite marks (if present) are required for DNA analyses, along with hair and fiber samples. Testing clothing for acid phosphatase may also help to direct DNA sampling for semen, as may screening with a Wood's lamp (Krugman, 1986).

Skeletal injury

Again, while not usually lethal in themselves, bone fractures may be another indication of occult child abuse, usually involving infants and younger children. Quite characteristic patterns of injury occur. Child abuse should be suspected if there is evidence of multiple or severe fractures without adequate explanation, fractures at different stages of healing, metaphyseal ("bucket handle" and "corner") fractures, or scapular or sternal fractures (Figures 3.41–3.47) (Table 3.1) (Kleinman, 1990; Leonidas, 1983). Complete body X-rays are a mandatory part of any infant autopsy, particularly where there is suspected child abuse, as bones in certain sites such as the limbs, hands, feet, pelvis, and vertebrae will not be visualized during routine dissection (Ellerstein & Norris, 1984; Evans & Roberts, 1989; Kleinman & Marks, 1992; Thomsen, Elle & Thomsen, 1997). If possible, this should be augmented with radionuclide bone scanning if the child was in hospital before death (Jaudes, 1984). Features differentiating accidental from intentional skull fractures are described in the section dealing with head injuries. Radiologists need to be familiar with the range of ossification times of other bones in infancy and childhood to prevent misinterpreting normal variants as possible fractures (Kleinman & Spevak, 1991).

Histological examination of fracture should be undertaken, mainly as an adjunct to detailed radiological investigation (Kleinman, Marks & Blackbourne, 1986). Dating of fractures histologically is difficult, and often the most useful information that can be provided is an assessment of whether fractures of different ages are present, indicating more than one episode of trauma.

Very occasionally, a medical condition or deficiency such as osteogenesis imperfecta, rickets, copper deficiency, or scurvy may cause bone changes or fractures; however, gross and histological differences are usually readily apparent (Brill & Winchester, 1987; Taitz, 1991) (Figures 3.48–3.50). Birth trauma may also cause fractures, particularly if there has been obstructed labor with shoulder dystocia, and so it is important to obtain a history of the labor and delivery (Barry & Hocking, 1993; Rizzolo & Coleman, 1989). Spontaneous fractures of long bones in children and adolescents with cerebral palsy have been attributed to underlying osteoporosis (Lingam & Joester, 1994), and the possibility of accidental injury must not be

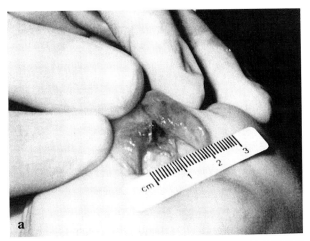

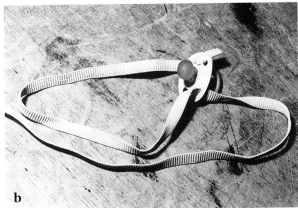

Figure 3.24 Ulceration of the frenulum of a two-month-old boy (a) due to gagging with a pacifier (b).

discounted in certain long bone fractures in highly mobile young children (Thomas *et al.*, 1991). Careful examination of skeletonized remains may also reveal evidence of inflicted trauma long after organs and soft tissues have decomposed (Walker, Cook & Lambert, 1997).

Chest and abdominal trauma

Compared with lethal head injuries, chest and abdominal injuries are less common and tend to occur at an older age. Dissipation of kinetic energy is

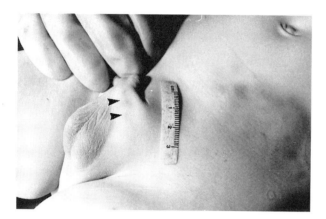

Figure 3.25 Subtle bruising to the base of the penis, in keeping with a pinching injury. There was also extensive bruising of the anterior abdominal wall.

the key to injury causation. Kinetic energy transfer to internal organs may cause injury by three different mechanisms: (i) by exceeding the longitudinal tensile strength of mobile structures, such as blood vessels; (ii) by exceeding the vertical tensile strength of fixed structures, such as vessels and intestines at their points of attachment; and (iii) by exceeding the compressive strength of structures such as bone and solid viscera (Templeton, 1993).

In blunt trauma, the depth of deformation and the speed of deformation (with both acceleration and deceleration) determine the extent of injury (Cooper & Taylor, 1989). The most extensive injuries occur when energy transfer is both focal and rapid. With a high rate of compression and low velocity, crush injury results. Low compression and high velocity characterize blast injury. The theory of viscous tolerance states that injuries can occur at lower levels of compression with increased rates of deformation (Templeton, 1993).

Chest injuries

The pediatric chest wall is more compliant than that of adults, and thus kinetic energy is transferred more easily to a child's thoracic viscera. Squeezing or punching the chest of a child can fracture ribs, although a great deal of kinetic energy, applied

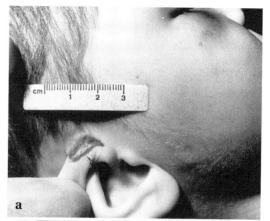

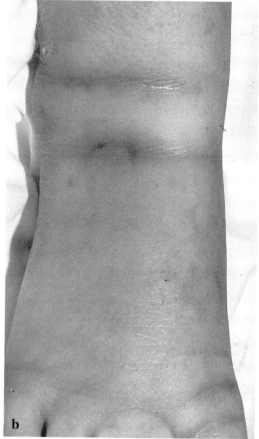

Figure 3.26 Laceration of the right ear resulting from a twisting/tugging injury (a). Ligature marks around the ankle (b).

locally or diffusely, is required. Mortality is increased 20-fold in a child with rib fractures compared with a child without rib fractures (Templeton, 1993). Most inflicted rib fractures are situated posteriorly next to the costovertebral junction, reflecting chest compression from encirclement (Merten, Radkowski & Leonidas, 1983).

Reported cases of fatal chest injury have included children with cardiac lacerations (Figure 3.51) (Cohle *et al.*, 1995; Cumberland, Riddick & McConnell, 1991). The ages of the nine children in these series ranged from nine weeks to three years, with a mean of 14 months (there were also three teenagers aged 15, 17, and 19 years). In Cohle and colleagues' (1995) series of six cases, five had right atrial lacerations and one had a left ventricular laceration. In the three cases with perpetrator confessions, one victim was kicked, one was struck with a fist, and one was stomped. Cumberland, Riddick & McConnell's (1991) three youngest victims were each struck in the abdomen, two with a foot and one with a fist, and each had right atrial lacerations. A five-year-old girl has been reported who survived a ruptured interventricular septum sustained from a kick in the chest from her stepfather (Rees *et al.*, 1975).

Mechanisms of cardiac laceration include compression of the heart between the sternum and vertebral column, compression of the abdomen or legs, deceleration or acceleration, puncture of the heart by a fractured rib, and rupture of a resolving contusion (Cohle *et al.*, 1995). The most common mechanism in Cohle and colleagues' (1995) series was compression of the heart between the spine and sternum. Cumberland, Riddick & McConnell (1991) attributed right atrial lacerations in their cases to transmission of hydrostatic pressure through the inferior vena cava to the right atrium from blows to the abdomen.

Commotio cordis is a concussive low-impact injury to the precordium that disrupts the electrical activity of the heart without cardiac contusion or laceration. The precordial impact causes collapse with cardiac arrhythmia that is highly resistant to resuscitation attempts (Denton & Kalelkar, 2000). Most deaths due to commotio cordis are accidental,

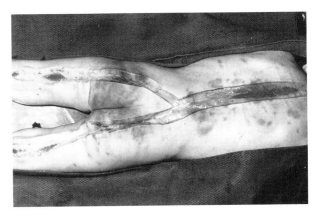

Figure 3.27 The extent of soft tissue injury demonstrated by extensive skin incision in a three-year-old boy who had multiple injuries elsewhere.

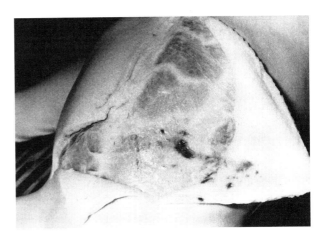

Figure 3.28 Bruising of abdominal wall musculature and subcutaneous tissues demonstrated after layer dissection in a nine-month-old boy who was found dead in his parents' bed.

usually resulting from the victim's chest being struck by a baseball, softball, or hockey puck (Maron, Mitten & Greene Burnett, 2002), but several homicides have been reported (Boglioli, Taff & Harleman, 1998). Denton & Kalelkar (2000) described two children, aged three years and 14 months, each of whom was hit in the chest by an adult male. An 11-year-old who died after his father gave him two "light disciplinary blows" during a tutorial session and a 14-year-old who was killed by five hard chest blows

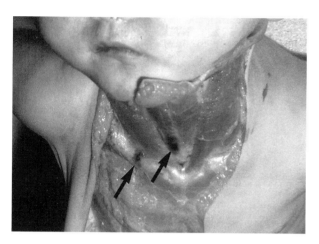

Figure 3.29 Two bruises (arrows) of subcutaneous tissues at the base of the neck in a one-year-old girl were revealed only after the skin had been reflected. The bruises could not be seen on external examination.

administered as part of a gang ritual have also been reported (Maron, Mitten & Greene Burnett, 2002). Ventricular tachyarrhythmias, especially ventricular fibrillation, were the most common substrates for death induced by commotio cordis in an experimental pig model (Link *et al.*, 1998).

Abdominal injuries

Blunt trauma to the abdomen may cause injury by laceration of solid or hollow viscera or the mesentery (Figures 3.52 and 3.53), or by compressing them between the intruding fist, elbow or knee and the vertebral column. Due to the distensibility of the abdominal wall, there may be minimal external evidence of trauma (Color Plate 4). Ultrasound and CT may help to identify solid organ injuries if a child has made it to hospital, while barium studies may be useful in identifying injuries to hollow viscera (Kleinman, Raptopoulos & Brill, 1981; Sivit, Taylor & Eichelberger, 1989). In Case & Nanduri's (1983) report, the abdomen of a two-year-old boy was forcibly rammed into the upraised knee of his stepfather, rupturing the child's stomach at two separate points. The child died from peritonitis 12 hours after the injury. We have investigated the case of a 19-month-

old boy who died shortly after his father's partner struck him twice in the abdomen with her fist. At autopsy, the child had a large mesenteric laceration, pancreatic contusion, and hemoperitoneum. Fossum & Descheneaux (1991) described a 2.5-year-old girl who had been struck many times in the abdomen by her babysitter over several months and who died of peritonitis from a ruptured jejunum. These authors cited two other cases from their experience of repeated abdominal trauma in which no signs or symptoms of ruptured viscera were elicited until shortly before death.

In Touloukian's (1968) series of five fatal cases, averaging 25 months in age, the most common injuries were mesenteric lacerations with retroperitoneal hematomas, duodenal hematomas, lacerations and contusions of the duodenum and jejunum, and hemorrhagic pancreatitis (Figures 3.54 and 3.55). Four cases had an alleged history of minor trauma, such as a short fall, and in one case a father admitted beating his child. Pancreatic pseudocyst formation may also follow blunt abdominal trauma (Pena & Medovy, 1973). Cooper and colleagues (1988) reported 22 children with inflicted abdominal trauma treated in emergency departments. The mortality was 45%, and the assailant was nearly always the child's father or the child's mother's partner. Injuries in the 10 fatal cases included liver and kidney lacerations, vena caval lacerations, retroperitoneal hematomas, and duodenal-jejunal rupture. The mechanism of death was shock due to massive intraperitoneal hemorrhage in nine cases and peritonitis due to small-intestinal rupture in the remaining case. The histories given to explain the injuries in hemodynamically unstable chidren were either "unknown" or a trivial episode of head trauma, often due to alleged falls from bed. All of the children in both series had additional abusive injuries, and in each series a delay in seeking treatment contributed to fatal outcomes (Cooper *et al.*, 1988; Touloukian, 1968).

Injuries from blunt abdominal trauma tend to occur at points of fixation of viscera to the abdominal wall, for example the ligament of Trietz. Consequences include blood loss, sepsis caused by peritoneal contamination (a late complication), and organ dysfunction, which may occur early or late (Ogata & Tsuganezawa, 1995; Ramenofsky, 1987). The stomach may rupture when compressed between the abdominal wall and the vertebral column by a sharp blow, with the likelihood of perforation increased if there is distension by food or air. Approximately half the total number of gastric lacerations that occur result from rapid deceleration, primarily in motor vehicle accidents, indicating the force necessary to rupture the stomach. Purported cases of spontaneous rupture of the stomach have occurred during the first two weeks of life and have been related to birth trauma, congenital defects of the stomach, peptic ulcer, gavage, septicemia, hypoxia, and oxygen therapy. Rarely, gastric rupture may occur during cardiopulmonary resuscitation, presumably secondary to distension of the stomach by air during ventilation with inappropriately placed chest compressions. The mortality of traumatic gastric rupture has been reported as 11% (Case & Nanduri, 1983). Buchino (1983) noted the importance of the surgical pathologist recognizing perforations in surgically removed intestines from children as possibly arising from inflicted injury.

Although chylous ascites is most often caused by congenital malformation of the lymphatic system, it may also be a manifestation of blunt abdominal trauma (Figure 3.56). Damage to the root of the mesentery may cause leakage of chyle into the peritoneal cavity from compromised or obstructed lymphatic channels (Olazagasti *et al.*, 1994). Thus, when this is found at autopsy, other manifestations of child abuse should be sought carefully.

Thermal injuries

While it is has been proposed that intentionally inflicted thermal injuries occur in 10% of all abused children and account for variable percentages (1.4–25%) of all burns and scalds in children (Montrey & Barcia, 1985; Purdue, Hunt & Prescott, 1988; Ryan, Shankowsky & Tredget, 1992), interpretation of the literature is difficult as cases have not always been clearly described or investigated. Inadequate super-

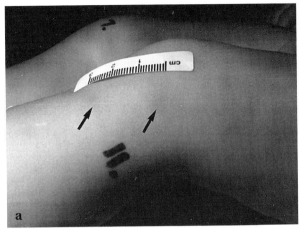

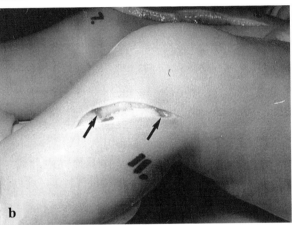

Figure 3.30 Two subtle bruises of the leg (arrows) (a) were confirmed by incising skin and subcutaneous tissues (arrows) (b).

vision rather than intentionally inflicted injury may be responsible for a number of such cases. In cases of inflicted thermal injury, the perpetrator is most often a poorly educated single parent (usually the mother), friend of a parent (usually the mother's partner), or babysitter (Showers & Garrison, 1988).

There are a number of different types of thermal injury (Hobbs, 1989b; McLoughlin & Crawford, 1985). Scalds are caused by hot liquids, whereas contact burns are caused by the body touching a hot object. Flame burns result in charred skin and singed hairs, while cigarette burns are typically round and crater-like. Electrical burns are small and often

a   b

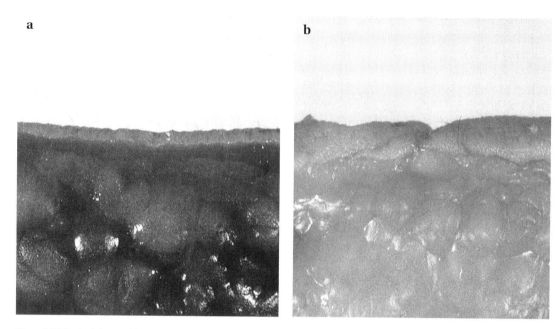

Figure 3.31 Bruised tissue with extensive subcutaneous hemorrhage (a) compared with paler dependent tissue in an area of lividity (b).

punctate, sometimes with two such burns present (entry and exit). "Friction burns" are simply abrasions, often caused by being dragged across a surface such as a carpeted floor. Chemical burns may stain and scar the skin, and radiant burns occur from fires or the sun. Scalds are the most frequent type of accidental and inflicted thermal injury in children, followed by contact and flame burns (Purdue, Hunt & Prescott,1988; Rossignol, Locke & Burke, 1990; Ryan, Shankowsky & Tredget, 1992).

Scalds may be divided into spill/splash or immersion. In abused children, scalds most often originate from hot water taps. Spills usually occur when a toddler or older infant pulls over a container of hot liquid and are characterized by irregular margins and a non-uniform depth of injury. Liquids flow downward, cooling with distance, resulting in progressively shallower and narrower injuries with an "arrowhead" pattern (Figures 3.57 and 3.58) (Purdue, Hunt & Prescott,1988). Accidental scalds usually involve the head, face, arms, and upper torso, while inflicted scalds are found more often on the buttocks,

perineum, hands, and feet (Montrey & Barcia, 1985; Hobbs, 1989b). Immersion scalds have a uniform depth and a distinct border or waterline (Figure 3.59 and Color Plate 5). If the hands or feet are scalded, then the pattern is often a "glove and stocking" type (Hobbs, 1986), with sparing of the soles of the feet where they come into contact with the relatively cool bottom of the bathtub. If the buttocks and perineum are immersed, there may be sparing of the medial aspect of the buttocks where they have contacted the bottom of the tub, in a "doughnut" pattern (Figure 3.60) (Hobbs, 1989b). Splash scalds are not seen in inflicted injury but occur in accidents because of the lack of restraint and movement of the child. Full-thickness injuries from scalding are more typical of inflicted injury (Hight, Bakalar & Lloyd, 1979).

At 49 °C (120 °F), water causes full-thickness scalds in adults after 10 minutes; at 52 °C (125 °F) it takes two minutes, at 60 °C (140 °F) six seconds, and at 66 °C (150 °F) two seconds. Since children have thinner skin, a shorter duration of exposure is required to cause scalds. Many home hot-water temperatures

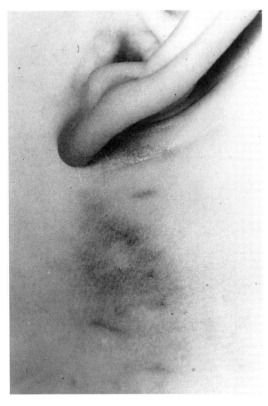

Figure 3.32 Bruising and linear abrasions under the ear resulting from trauma during attempted resuscitation.

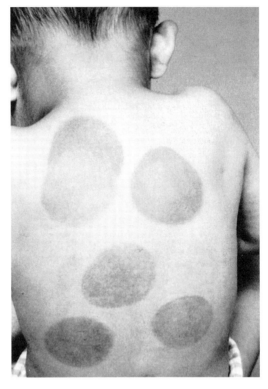

Figure 3.33 Skin lesions left after treatment with cupping in an oriental infant.

are set at 60 °C (140 °F), although 49 °C (120 °F) is sufficiently hot for most household needs (Feldman *et al.*, 1978).

Inflicted contact burns often have the shape of the hot object (Figures 3.61–3.63), whereas accidental contact burns often show no pattern because of withdrawal of the child from the painful stimulus. Inflicted contact burns are deeper, except in cases where a child has grasped a hot object and stuck to it, or has sat on a hot surface such as a vinyl car seat (Hobbs, 1989b; Schmitt, Gray & Britton, 1978). Inflicted burns of varying ages may also be present from repeated episodes of abuse. Perioral burns suggest attempted forcing of hot food or caustic substances, such as drain cleaner, into the mouth (Gillespie, 1965; Hobbs, 1989b).

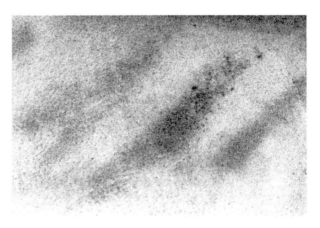

Figure 3.34 Parallel linear abrasions caused by coin rubbing (cạo gío).

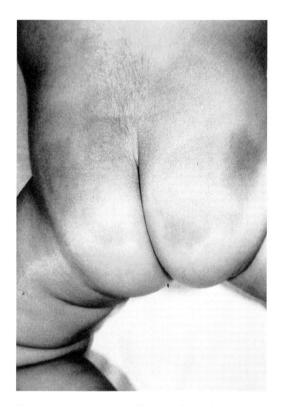

Figure 3.35 Large Mongolian blue spot of the right buttock.

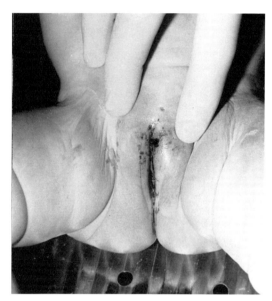

Figure 3.36 Recent hemorrhage around the vulva of a previously well three-month-old girl suggesting occult trauma.

Electric hairdryers may cause burns from hot air or patterned burns from contact with the protective grill (Prescott, 1990). Placing an infant in a microwave oven may cause well-defined burns in the skin at the point nearest the microwave-emitting device (Alexander, Surrell & Cohle, 1987). Histologic examination of such burns will reveal a pattern characteristic of microwave injury, with greater damage to tissues with high water content, such as muscle, compared with tissues with lower water content, such as fat (Reece, 1990).

Delay in seeking treatment is common in inflicted thermal injuries but rare in accidents. An abusive carer may show little guilt or concern over the child's injury, may provide a history incompatible with the injury, may deny that the injury is a burn or scald, or may blame the injury on a sibling. In assessing the likelihood of accidental thermal injury, the in-

vestigator should take into account the child's developmental ability and stature. Table 3.10 summarizes the important differences between accidental and intentional thermal injuries.

Death from thermal injuries may be immediate or protracted, resulting from sepsis with contributions from metabolic disturbances and dehydration (Ryan, Shankowsky & Tredget, 1992). Delay in seeking medical attention may be a factor hastening a burned child's death. While inflicted burns or scalds may not be a direct cause of death, they may also be present in infants or children who have died of other causes and thus may be the first indicator of abuse. In a case from Grand Rapids, USA, a two-year-old girl was immersed in hot water, sustaining partial-thickness injuries to her perineum, buttocks, and legs. She asphyxiated by aspirating vomitus as she lay obtunded in bed several hours after being burned. Isopropyl alcohol applied to inflicted immersion scalds has also been reported as a contributor to death in a four-year-old girl (Russo *et al.*, 1986).

Natural diseases simulating burns or scalds include epidermolysis bullosa, impetigo, papular

Table 3.10. Comparison of unintentional and inflicted thermal injuries

	Unintentional	Inflicted
"Glove and stocking" pattern	–	+
Water line	–	+
Location	Face, arms, upper trunk	Feet, hands, buttocks, perineum
Splash burns	+	–
Patterned burns	–	+
Depth of burn	Variable	Uniform
Delay in seeking treatment	–	+

urticaria, contact dermatitis, and severe diaper rash. Children with insensitivity to pain, which may be congenital or due to anesthesia, as well as children with spina bifida, mental disability, cerebral palsy, and epilepsy, are also more likely to be accidentally burned or scalded (Hobbs, 1989b).

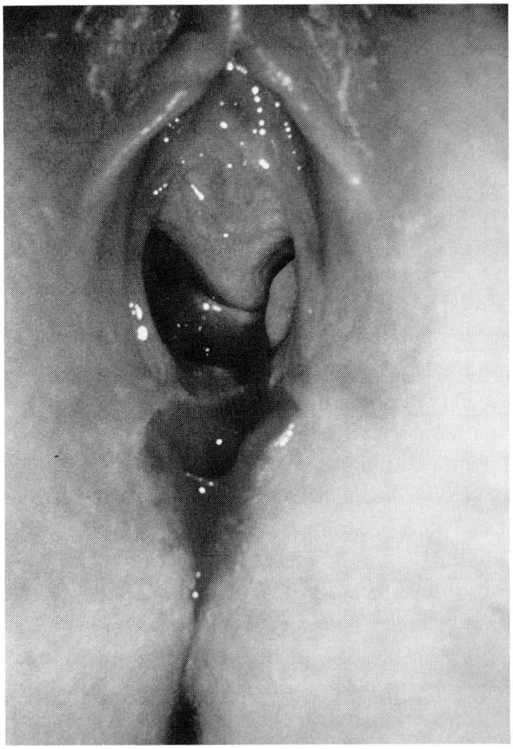

Subtle, unusual, and miscellaneous injuries and causes of death

Investigations into the deaths of infants continue to be of extremely variable quality, with significant

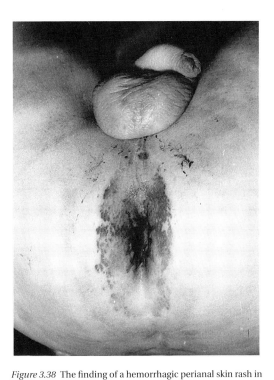

Figure 3.37 Posterior tear of the introitus in a young girl who had been sexually assaulted.

Figure 3.38 The finding of a hemorrhagic perianal skin rash in a toddler who hung himself from a door handle raised the possibility of anal trauma. However, colposcopic examination revealed no bruising or lacerations, with a clearly defined margin between the rash and normal anal mucosa; cultures grew streptococci.

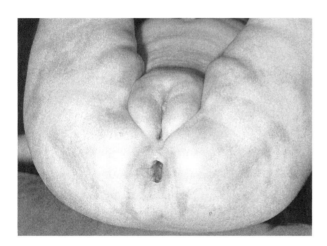

Figure 3.39 Patulous anus representing a normal postmortem change in an 18-month-old girl who died of pneumonia.

omissions occurring in both death scene and autopsy examinations (Wagner, 1986; Byard, 2001). Pathological findings are misinterpreted and homicides missed (Ewigman, Kivlahan & Land, 1993; Meadow, 1999; Rimsza *et al.*, 2002). Recent examples of mistakes in cases attributed incorrectly to homicide have included attributing normal retinal congestion to trauma-related hemorrhage and

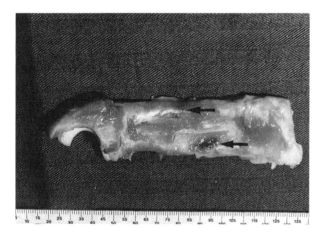

Figure 3.41 Dissection of fractured bones revealing surrounding soft tissue hemorrhage (arrows) in the case of greenstick fractures of the right radius and ulna from a nine-month-old boy.

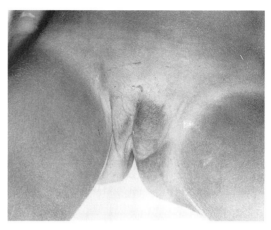

Figure 3.40 A vulval bruise typical of a straddle injury was found in a three-year-old girl. Disturbing features included being found dead face down in the bath with no history of epilepsy or fever. At autopsy, multiple other superficial bruises and abrasions were present, with no underlying organic diseases.

postmortem artefact to antemortem cerebral lacerations. Acute brain syndromes due to trauma have also been confused with metabolic disorders (Conradi & Brissie, 1986), and lethal organic illnesses have not been identified. Basic errors such as this have led to erroneous diagnoses with far-reaching consequences.

At other times, the autopsy will not be able to reveal an anatomic cause of death. Successful determination of the fatal event in these cases may therefore depend upon the history that is gathered. This is particularly important in young infants in order to separate a subtle homicide from SIDS (see Chapter 13) (Christoffel, Zieserl & Chiaramonte, 1985). One of the more recently defined types of subtle pediatric homicide, Munchausen syndrome by proxy, is discussed in detail later in this chapter.

Subtle fatal child abuse has been subdivided into (i) physical assault, including smothering, foreign body obstruction of airway and commotio cordis, or minor trauma in a child debilitated by disease; (ii) chemical assault, including poisoning or force-feeding noxious substances; and (iii) negligence, including starvation, failure to provide necessary

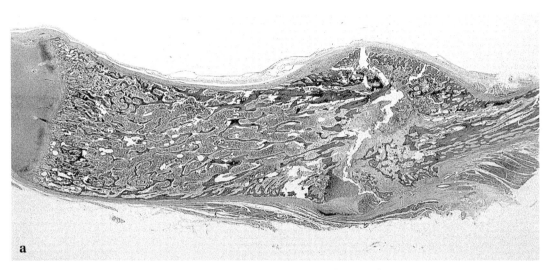

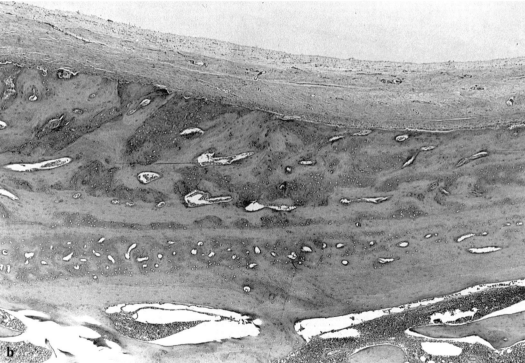

Figure 3.42 Elevation of the periosteum with thickened subcortical bone in two fractured ribs from a five-month-old girl (a and b) contrast with exuberant fibrous callous formation of an adjacent rib with a more recent fracture near the growth plate (c) (hematoxylin and eosin, whole mount, ×20).

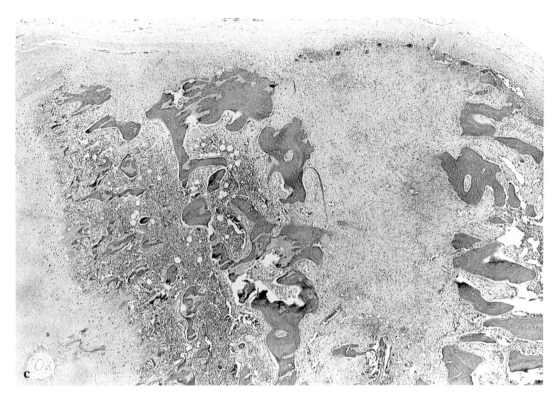

Figure 3.42 (cont.)

medical care, exposing a child to a dangerous environment, or exacerbating or triggering natural disease through neglect (Margolin, 1990; Zumwalt & Hirsch, 1980).

Examples include a 4.5-year-old child who died of dehydration after being tied to a bed overnight to punish her for bedwetting. Her usual habit had been to arise at night to get a drink of water. In addition to the ligature marks, she had multiple healing abrasions and contusions of the head, neck, and extremities. A five-year-old boy was also encountered who asphyxiated when his foster mother poured pepper down his throat as punishment for lying (Cohle, 1986). Seven other cases of homicidal pepper aspiration were subsequently documented (Cohle *et al.*, 1988). Other examples of unusual causes of death include hyperkalemia caused by forced intake of salt substitute containing potassium chloride; dehydration with intravascular sickling in a two-year-old with sickle cell trait who was bound by ligatures; hyperthermia and dehydration in a two-year-old boy who was locked in a car for 10 hours on a hot day; and hypothermia in a six-year-old boy who was tied to a bed clad only in underpants in an unheated house in winter (Zumwalt & Hirsch, 1980).

Starvation, failure to thrive, and neglect

There are a variety of possible causes of severe weight loss or failure to grow normally in a young infant or child. These include underlying organic illnesses, chronic exposure to drugs or toxins, rare metabolic disorders, and starvation.

Underlying organic illnesses

Malignancy, congenital heart disease, neurological disease, immunodeficiencies, and some forms of malabsorption syndrome may result in failure to thrive. Malignancies may be intra- or extracranial, the latter involving solid organs or hematopoietic tissues. Poor weight gain may result from underlying metabolic disturbances from a tumor, from nausea and disinterest in food, or from the side effects of therapies and prescribed medications/chemotherapy. Congenital cardiac diseases with or without chromosomal abnormalities may also delay growth. Children with certain neurological conditions such as cerebral palsy may have difficulty obtaining sufficient caloric intake to maintain growth due to problems with swallowing. Immunodeficiency disorders may also be associated with chronic infections and failure to thrive (see Chapter 4). All of these conditions should be reasonably obvious on history or autopsy examination. Death may also have occurred because of failure to provide adequate or appropriate medical care for children with these disorders.

A number of malabsorption states may occur in young children, including celiac disease, short gut syndrome, and mucosal enzyme deficiencies, in which there is a problem with the intestinal absorption of nutrients. Assessment of these conditions may be extremely difficult after death, as gut function has ceased and the surface of the intestine disintegrates rapidly. This may mean that a malabsorption state cannot be excluded on histological grounds. Children who suffer from malabsorption states, however, have histories of severe diarrhoea with bloating of the abdomen. Liquid malodorous feces may also be detected at autopsy.

Chronic exposure to toxins or drugs

Drugs such as amphetamines may be ingested in maternal milk, and in sufficient dosage may cause failure to thrive in infancy due to a combination of appetite suppression and elevation of basal metabolic rate (Figure 3.64). A history of possible family drug use with toxicological evaluation of blood levels of

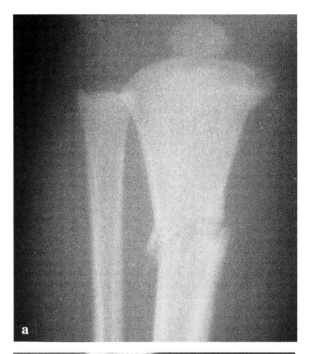

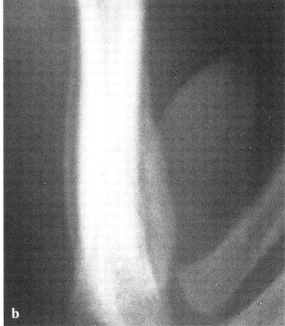

Figure 3.43 Radiographs showing recent fracture of the right tibia (a) with a healing fracture and callus formation of the left humerus (b) in a three-month-old girl.

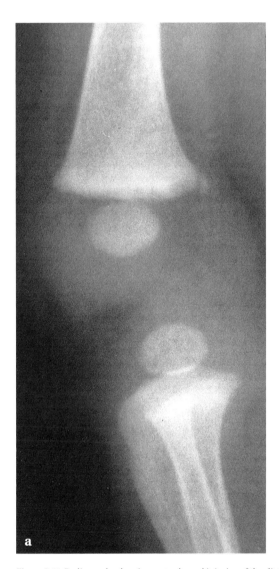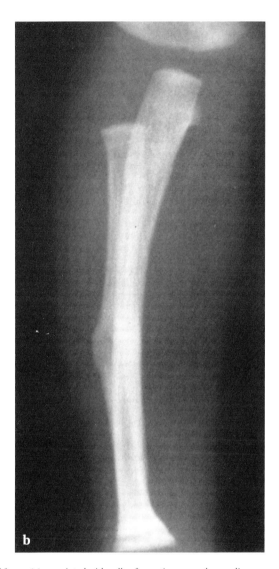

Figure 3.44 Radiographs showing metaphyseal injuries of the distal femur (a) associated with callus formation around an earlier injury involving the right radius (b) in a seven-month-old boy.

common drugs and toxins in the deceased may be useful in clarifying this issue.

Rare metabolic conditions

A variety of rare metabolic conditions discussed further in Chapter 11 may cause failure to thrive. Affected children may have had histories of hypotonia, psychomotor delay, seizures, unusual odours, vomiting, or diarrhea. There may be a family history of inherited metabolic disease or of previous infant or childhood deaths. Autopsy findings include cardiomegaly and fatty change in the liver, heart, muscle, and renal tubules, but are often non-specific.

While screening for metabolic disease is mandatory in cases of unexpected failure to thrive, problems may be encountered in the interpretation of results when children have been starved, i.e. results in young children who have had failure to thrive from inadequate caloric intake may be equivocal. Presumably this occurs because biochemical derangements associated with starvation produce abnormal laboratory profiles, thus preventing the exclusion of rare metabolic diseases.

Starvation

If the above disorders can be excluded, then the possibility of inadequate dietary intake should be considered (Sarvesvaran, 1992). Children who do not receive enough calories to sustain life may present with marked wasting and loss of muscle bulk (Davis, Rao & Valdes-Dapena, 1984). Failure to thrive may result from deficiencies in proteins, vitamins, trace metals, other specific nutrients, and hormones.

Failure to provide adequate nutrition for a child may be unintentional or intentional (Skuse, 1985). Unintentional starvation may occur with fad dieting or cult activity (Roberts *et al.*, 1979). Young, inexperienced, and socially isolated mothers may also simply not appreciate the significance of difficulties with poor feeding and inadequate weight gain. There may be a history of prior admission to hospital with negative investigations and significant weight gain during supervised feeding in hospital (Koel, 1969).

The postmortem assessment of cases of possible starvation is often not easy, as feeding histories may have been falsified and growth charts may not be available. Careful review of the birth and subsequent medical history is required with information on family stature. Most neglected children who die are under one year of age, and the autopsy shows thin, stretched skin over the face, with sunken eyes due to loss of periorbital fat and sometimes concomitant dehydration. The ribs are seen easily, and the abdomen is scaphoid, with prominent costal margins and iliac crests (see Figure 3.1). The limbs are thin, with wrinkling of skin due to loss of underlying muscle and subcutaneous adipose tissue. The skin is dry and may be infected. There may be skin ulcers and a diaper rash.

If deliberate withholding of food forms part of a pattern of inflicted injury, then there may be

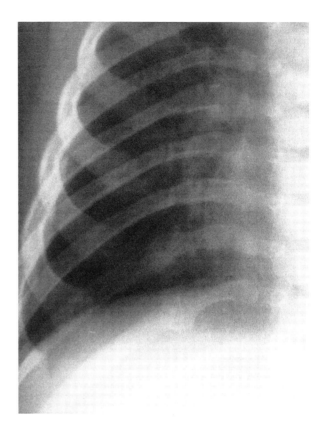

Figure 3.45 Radiograph showing recent and healing fractures of the ribs in a seven-month-old boy who was suffocated by a parent.

evidence of traumatic lesions, such as brain trauma or skeletal injuries, as it has been shown that children with non-organic failure to thrive have a four to five times greater risk of subsequent abuse or neglect than other infants (Skuse *et al.*, 1995).

Water deprivation in infants may cause hypernatremic dehydration, with recurrent vomiting, failure to thrive, and fitting. This may be due to deliberate withholding of water or to failure of breastfeeding, with sodium levels sometimes exceeding 200 mEq/l (Chesney & Brusilow, 1981; Coe, 1993; Ernst, Wynn & Schreiner, 1981; Kaplan, Siegler & Schmunk, 1998; Pickel, Anderson & Holliday, 1970). Hypernatremic dehydration may also be caused by feeding with improperly mixed formula or rehydration

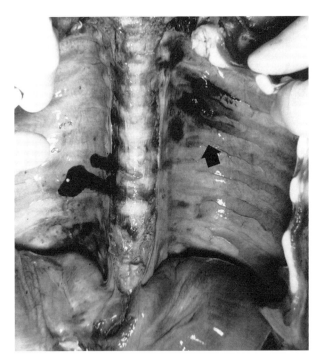

Figure 3.46 Retropleural hemorrhage from recent posterior rib fractures (arrow).

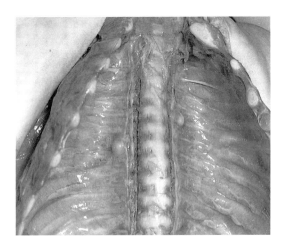

Figure 3.47 Callus formation at two separate sites involving healing of rib fractures on the right and left sides.

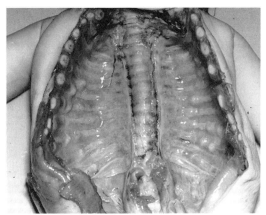

Figure 3.48 Multiple irregular fractures of the ribs in an infant with osteogenesis imperfecta.

solution, and may be a manifestation of Munchausen syndrome by proxy or maternal psychosis (Conley, 1990; Meadow, 1993a; Pickel, Anderson & Holliday, 1970). Failure to provide adequate fluid intake may occur in children with diarrhea (Huser & Smialek, 1986; Whitehead *et al.*,1996). There is no evidence that hypernatremia causes subdural hemorrhage, as was once proposed (Corey Handy *et al.*, 1999).

Starvation may result in kwashiorkor (protein deficiency) or marasmus (caloric deficiency), or often an overlapping syndrome. Autopsy findings in kwashiorkor include edema, depigmentation of the skin and hair, fatty change of the liver, and small-intestinal mucosal atrophy (Emery, 1978). In marasmus, the infant or child is markedly wasted, with a prematurely aged face, as noted above (see Figure 3.1). The changes in the small intestine and liver that occur in kwashiorkor are usually not found. General findings include atrophy of organs, with minimal food within the stomach (Kaschula, 1995; Sarvesvaran, 1992). While the heart usually also atrophies, deficiencies in trace elements such as copper and iron may cause anemia, with cardiac enlargement. Thiamine (vitamin B1) deficiency may also cause enlargement and dilation of the heart. Death usually results from infections, metabolic derangements, or cardiac failure. Although calculations have been used to determine the duration of starvation

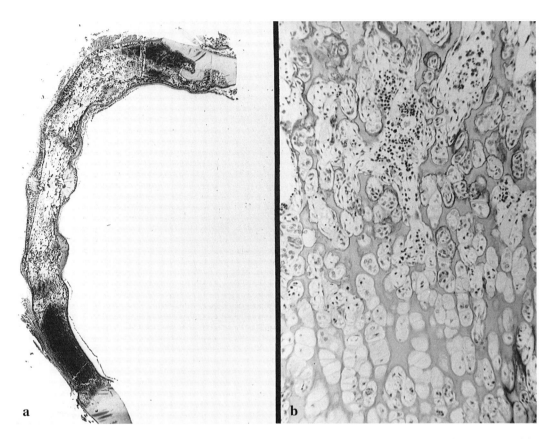

Figure 3.49 Whole mount of a rib demonstrating healing fractures (a), with microscopy revealing complete disorganization of the growth plate (b) in the preceding case of osteogenesis imperfecta (Figure 3.48) (hematoxylin and eosin, ×200).

from the estimated caloric deficit (Meade & Brissie, 1985), these are based on a number of premises that may not be applicable to the case being studied. Assessment of percentile charts, if available, may provide more useful information on the time course of malnutrition (Wehner, Schieffer & Wehner, 1999).

Drowning

Details of the autopsy investigation and findings in cases of drowning may be found in Chapter 2. While the majority of drowning deaths in childhood are unintentional, occasional homicides occur, many of which take place in household bathtubs (Nixon & Pearn, 1977). In a review of 32 infants and children under two years of age in South Australia, two (6%) cases were found where the carer's description of events did not match the physical capabilities of the infants (Byard & Lipsett, 1999). In another study of 205 submersion deaths in childhood, 16 (8%) cases were judged to have been inflicted (Gillenwater, Quan & Feldman, 1996). The ease with which an infant can be held under water means that the autopsy findings may not differ between inflicted and unintentional drownings. However, older children may have bruising around the wrists or ankles from being restrained, or there may be bruising of the back or head if sufficient force has been used to hold the struggling child under water. Layer dissection of subcutaneous tissues may be required to confirm the presence of such bruising.

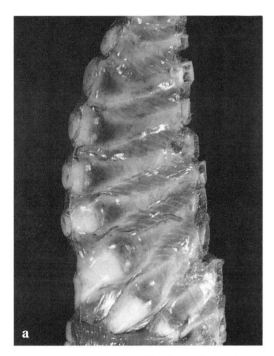 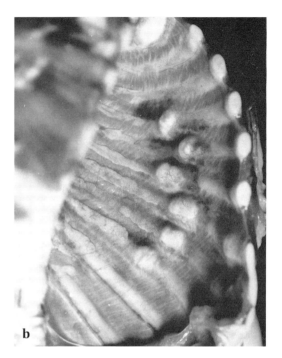

Figure 3.50 Regular expansion of the rib growth plates in a case of rickets (a), contrasting with irregular callus formation following fractures (b).

Poisoning

Poisoning generally leaves no anatomic signs, and the diagnosis therefore requires scene investigation, a thorough history, and a drug screen. Forcing material into the mouth of a child may cause injuries to the buccal mucosa and the frenula of the upper and lower lips, which should be examined carefully in suspected cases.

Poisoning is an uncommon type of inflicted injury, accounting for a minority of childhood deaths (Campbell & Collins, 2001; Dine, 1965; Dine & McGovern, 1982; Fischler, 1983; Lansky, 1974; Lorber, Reckless & Watson, 1980). For example, Rivara, Kamitsuka & Quan (1988) found only five of 156 patients under one year of age who died of poisoning. Three of these deaths were accidental, and only two were intentional. Nevertheless, poisoning may be a component of Munchausen syndrome by proxy (Zumwalt & Hirsch, 1987) or may be a sign of neglect.

For example, Case, Short & Poklis (1983) described a five-year-old who drank perfume and died of ethanol and aspirin poisoning after his parents failed to take him for treatment. Infant death may also occur if there has been miscalculation in the amount of a drug, such as amitriptyline, that is being used as a sedative to quieten a child (Perrot, 1988).

It must be borne in mind that cardioactive drugs such as digoxin accumulate in the heart during life and are released into heart blood after death, resulting in a spuriously high level if cardiac blood is used for a drug screen. For this reason, peripheral blood is preferred for analysis of cardiac drugs, although it may not be possible to obtain this in infants. Vitreous humor may also be a source for more accurate levels of drugs such as digoxin. It is important not to confuse endogenous digoxin-like immunoreactivity found in the sera of infants dying of a number of conditions with exogenously administered digoxin (Couper, Aldis & Byard, 1998).

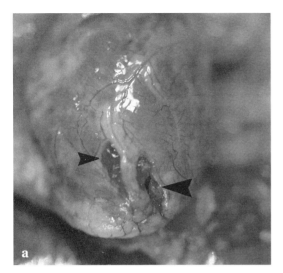

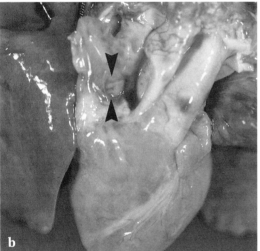

Figure 3.51 Transmural laceration of the left ventricle near the apex of the heart (larger arrowhead) associated with a hemopericardium following blunt injury to the chest in a 2.5-year-old girl. A superficial laceration of the right ventricle is nearby (smaller arrowhead) (a). Right atrial laceration (arrowheads) associated with a hemopericardium following striking of the chest of a nine-week-old infant. The atrial appendage has been reflected to demonstrate the injury; the underlying atrial wall can be seen through the defect (b).

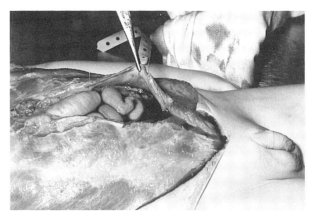

Figure 3.52 Filling of the peritoneal cavity with fluid blood following inflicted blunt abdominal trauma with extensive laceration of the liver in a three-year-old boy.

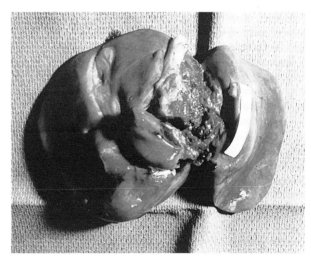

Figure 3.53 Splitting of the liver in a three-year-old boy following a blow to the abdomen.

If it is suspected that a drug or toxin has been injected, sampling of tissues at the injection site may be useful for drug quantitation or, in the case of insulin, for immunohistochemical staining (Hood *et al.*, 1986). Control tissue is required from an area other than the suspected injection site if quantitation is to be undertaken.

Forced ingestion of any substance in sufficient quantities may result in coma or even death.

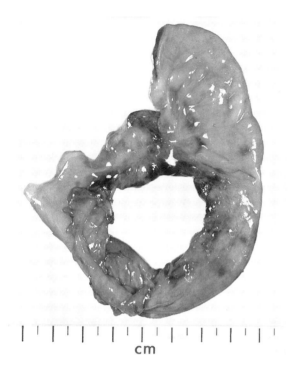

Figure 3.54 Mesenteric tear following inflicted blunt abdominal trauma, with fatal intraperitoneal hemorrhage.

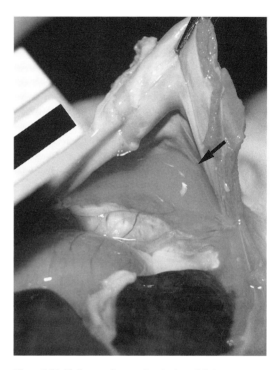

Figure 3.56 Chylous ascites pooling in the pelvis in a one-month-old infant.

Hyponatremia from acute water intoxication has been reported in a 4.5-year-old boy who was being forced to drink from a hose (Mortimer, 1980). Acute water intoxication with seizures has also been documented in infants from feeding mismanagement by young, poorly educated mothers (Partridge *et al.*, 1981). Hypernatremia from excessive salt ingestion has been reported in abused children (Reece & Grodin, 1985).

Electrocution

Homicidal electrocutions are uncommon and usually involve adults, although occasional cases have been reported where children have been victims (Al-Alousi, 1990). Depending on the circumstances, there may be little present at autopsy other than characteristic contact lesions that have central blistering surrounded by a blanched area with a hyperemic rim. Sparking between the body and

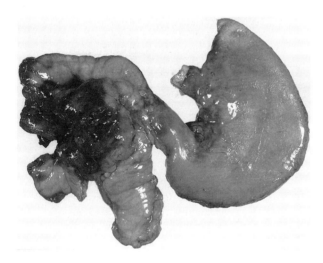

Figure 3.55 Pancreatic and duodenal rupture in a 4.5-year-old boy following inflicted blunt trauma to the abdomen.

another object may produce nodules of burnt keratin (Byard *et al.*, 2003). If the victim has had wire ligatures applied, there may be patterned burns, as in the case of a one-year-old boy who was intentionally electrocuted by his father (Al-Alousi, 1990). Unusual circumscribed skin lesions have also been described in a seven-month-old infant who died following repeated shocking with a stun gun by his foster mother (Turner & Jumbelic, 2003). Unfortunately, if electrocution takes place while the victim is immersed in water, such as in a bath or swimming pool, no electrical markings may be present as water will lower both skin resistance and current density, as well as cool tissues that current is passing through (Goodson, 1993).

Neonaticide

A variety of terms have been used to classify the killing of very young children, including infanticide for deaths between one month and one year of age, and neonaticide for deaths under 24 hours, or less than 28–30 days, depending on the jurisdiction (Adelson, 1991; Marks & Kumar, 1996; Pitt & Bale, 1995). Practically, most neonaticides occur immediately after birth. There are several typical scenarios, often involving mothers who have either concealed their pregnancies and subsequent deliveries, or who were unaware that they were pregnant (Wissow, 1998). The mothers are usually young, single, and poorly educated, with no criminal record (Overpeck *et al.*, 1998). They have rarely attempted to obtain an abortion. The infants have been delivered in secrecy and have either been allowed to die by omitting adequate supportive care, such as feeding or failing to tie the umbilical cord, or been killed by an overt act, such as smothering, strangling, head trauma, or drowning (Mendlowicz *et al.*, 1999; Pitt & Bale, 1995; Saunders, 1989).

Neonaticide has a long tradition, having been used to propitiate the gods by many tribal groups, including the Gauls, Celts, and Vikings (Kellett, 1992). In some cultures, and at some points in history, it has also been an accepted way to remove "deformed" or "sickly" infants or those who might burden the

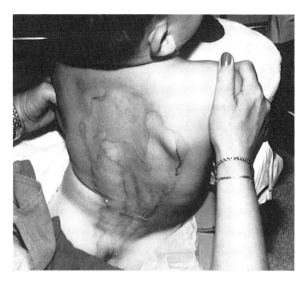

Figure 3.57 "Arrow" pattern of scalding on the back of a child who was held under a running hot tap.

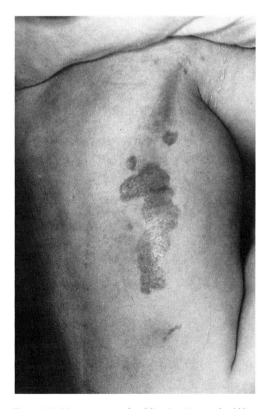

Figure 3.58 Linear pattern of scalding in a 20-month-old boy from a running hot tap.

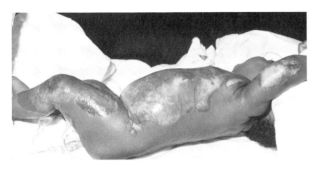

Figure 3.59 Lateral aspect of an infant who had hot water poured on to her anterior body surface.

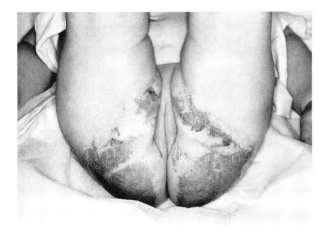

Figure 3.60 Healing scalds around the perineum and buttocks from a "dunking injury."

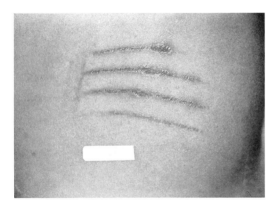

Figure 3.61 Radiator grill burns.

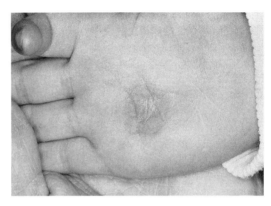

Figure 3.62 Recent cigarette burn of the palm.

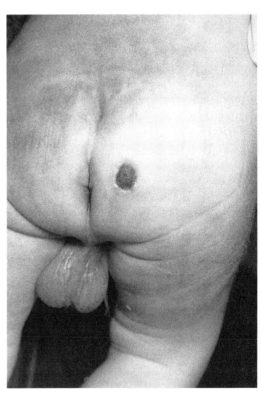

Figure 3.63 Healing circular full-thickness burn on the buttock of a three-month-old boy who was found unresponsive on a waterbed. Subsequent full-body radiographs revealed recent bilateral parietal bone fractures, recent rib fractures, and healing posterior rib fractures.

financial resources of a family or community (Ober, 1986). Despite a recent relative increase in percentages of infanticide cases since the numbers of SIDS deaths have fallen, there is no indication that absolute rates are increasing (Krous *et al.*, 2002).

Reasons for neonaticide include fear of job loss, not wanting to raise a child, waiting too long for an abortion, poverty, and psychosis. Young single women may fear revealing the pregnancy to their families because of shame or fear of punishment or rejection, and married women may wish to eliminate an unwanted extramarital pregnancy (Pitt & Bale, 1995; Saunders, 1989). Some authors (Mendlowicz *et al.*, 1999) believe that perpetrators of neonaticide are not mentally ill, while others (Spinelli, 2001) have found that nearly all of these women experience symptoms such as depersonalization, dissociative hallucinations, and intermittent amnesia at delivery. Mothers may appear indifferent, may deny having been pregnant, and often describe "watching" themselves during the birth. In the UK a mother may be presumed to be mentally ill with legislation stating that a mother may have "the balance of her mind . . . disturbed by reason of her not having fully recovered from the effect of giving birth to the child or by reasons of the effect of lactation consequent on the birth of the child" (Kellett, 1992; Marks & Kumar, 1996). However, to *a priori* assume mental illness seems unwarranted given the lengths to which some mothers may go to conceal the pregnancy, the delivery, and the body of the dead neonate. Multiple neonaticides have been reported with one mother who killed nine infants (Funayama *et al.*, 1994).

Bodies are often dumped in rubbish bins or public washrooms, or are concealed in woodlands (Figures 3.65 and 3.66). Different cultures utilize different methods of disposal, depending on availability, with perpetrators in Japan dumping infant bodies in coin-operated railway lockers (Kouno & Johnson, 2001). The percentage of infanticides where these type of lockers were used was as high as 10–13% before 1980 but has declined in recent years (Kouno, 2000).

Neonaticides are difficult cases to investigate as injuries may be extremely subtle or non-existent and proof of live birth may not be possible. The point at

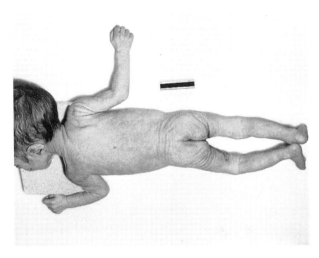

Figure 3.64 Marked wasting of the buttocks of a nine-week-old infant with failure to thrive associated with positive blood toxicology for amphetamines.

which an infant becomes a "person" with independent existence depends on legal definition and varies from one jurisdiction to another, with different criteria specifying evidence of heart rate, respiratory effort, and/or complete expulsion from the birth canal.

The pathologist conducting the investigation of a neonaticide has several goals. These include establishing the gestational age of the infant, determining whether the infant was live-born, helping to establish the identity of the mother, and establishing the cause and manner of death (Kellett, 1992).

Gestational age

An estimate of the gestational age can be made from examining the fetus and the placenta. Methods of estimating gestational age from examination of the fetus include measuring the crown–rump length, the crown–heel length, the chest circumference, the head circumference, the foot length, and the weight. Standard tables for correlating gestational age with these measurements are widely available in texts and on various Internet sites (Keeling, 1987). The infant's body should also be radiographed in order to determine ossification centers, in consultation with a radiologist. Placental chorionic villi mature along with

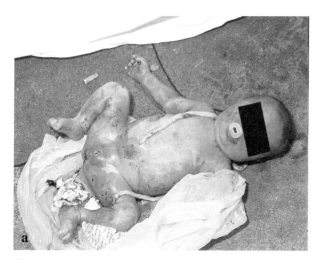

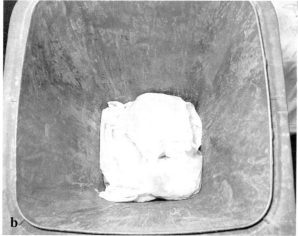

Figure 3.65 Body of a recently delivered infant smeared with blood from delivery, with vernix caseosa visible in the groin folds. The umbilical cord had been cut but not tied. A plastic airway from attempted resuscitation was present in the mouth (a). The body had been placed in a plastic bag and hidden in a garbage bin (b). Both exsanguination and suffocation were possible causes of death.

the fetus and can be studied microscopically to assess gestational age, although this is not precise.

The viability of a fetus increases with greater gestational age, and nowadays most infants without severe life-threatening conditions born after 28 weeks gestation would be expected to survive. In Britain,

the minimum age for viability is taken to be 24 weeks' gestation (Knight, 1996).

Live birth

Determining that an infant was expelled completely from the birth canal and was capable of independent existence based on autopsy findings is an extremely difficult exercise and is often not possible. The medical literature has numerous warnings about the problems, with recommendations that extreme caution should be taken before live birth is diagnosed.

If an infant has been dead for some time within the uterus, then changes will develop that indicate that death preceded delivery (Figure 3.67). During this process of sterile tissue breakdown, or maceration, the fetus will develop reddened skin, with skin slippage and peeling approximately 6–12 hours after death. After 24 hours, blistering of the skin will be seen, with purple mottling, and after 48 hours reddish fluid will accumulate within the chest and abdominal cavities. The joints become hyperextensible, and after several days the skull begins to collapse with overriding of cranial bones (Keeling, 1987).

Vernix caseosa is white material that is normally adherent to the skin of a fetus (see Figure 3.65a). The presence of vernix and blood merely indicates that delivery has occurred recently; their absence may simply mean that the infant had been cleaned after birth.

Flotation test

Radiographs may show aeration of the lungs and a gas bubble in the stomach (Figure 3.68). The commonly used, and controversial, method at autopsy is the flotation test. First described by Swammerdam in 1667 and called "docimasy" or "hydrostasy," this test involves placing the lungs in water to determine whether they float (Figure 3.69) (Kellett, 1992). Knight (1996) advocates floating the block of tissue containing the heart and lungs as more indicative of lung expansion than floating just the lungs themselves.

The principle of the test is that the lungs will be expanded and will float if the infant has breathed and will appear spongy and salmon pink in color, with expansion of the distal airspaces. This compares with the lungs of a stillborn infant, which feel quite dense and heavy, are collapsed, and appear dark red in color (Knight, 1996).

Caveats for interpreting a positive test are several. Gas production from decomposition and air introduced during cardiopulmonary resuscitation (CPR) may cause a positive flotation test (Kellett, 1992; Knight, 1996). Although infants born in extremis due to birth asphyxia may gasp agonally, this usually produces either no change in the lungs or a mottled pattern with variable areas of expansion adjacent to collapsed non-aerated areas. However, the lungs of stillborns may float and the lungs of live-born infants may sink. Histologically, lungs that are uniformly expanded occur in an infant who has been breathing spontaneously or who has had effective resuscitation attempted. Problems in separating stillbirth from live birth arise mainly when there are admixed areas of aeration and collapse.

The presence of milk within the stomach indicates that the infant had been alive for long enough to feed. Air/gas may also be present in the stomach and adjacent small intestine if the infant has swallowed air after delivery (i.e. live birth), has had air forced into the stomach during attempted resuscitation, or has had gas produced by bacteria due to putrefaction (Figure 3.70). Other compelling evidence of live birth is the mother (or, preferably, an independent witness) reporting the infant to be crying, moving, or exhibiting other signs of life. Evidence of strangulation, stabbing, or certain forms of head trauma also suggests that the infant was alive after delivery and suffered a lethal assault (Figure 3.71).

Identity of mother
Although tissue sampling of the neonate and/or placenta is necessary to enable DNA testing if a possible mother is found, the circumstances of these cases may make identification unlikely.

Cause and manner of death
The most common cause of death in neonaticide is neglect/inattention/exposure, followed by asphyxia (mainly suffocation and strangulation) and blunt

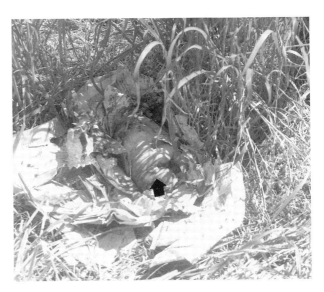

Figure 3.66 Body of a recently delivered infant (arrowhead) found wrapped in paper and hidden in scrubland.

head trauma. Less common causes of death include stabbing and throwing infants out of windows or on to roadways. Midwives have been reported who killed neonates by inserting needles under the eyelids or through the fontanelles (Funayama *et al.*, 1994; Kellett, 1992; Pitt & Bale, 1995; Mendlowicz *et al.*, 1999).

Signs of smothering or drowning in infants may not be discernible at autopsy, in which case a confession may be the only method of determining the cause of death. Strangulation may be manual or by ligature. Fingernail marks on the infant's neck may, however, have come from the mother's attempt to deliver the baby by pulling on the infant's head and neck, rather than from strangulation. The resultant elongated linear abrasions are often found under the chin and sides of the neck of the infant. Apparent ligature abrasions must not be mistaken for a postmortem artifact from winding of the umbilical cord around the neck (Kellett, 1992).

Accidental injuries may also occur during the birth process in prolonged and difficult labors, or where there is malpresentation of a fetus such as in a breech delivery. Distinguishing these lesions from inflicted

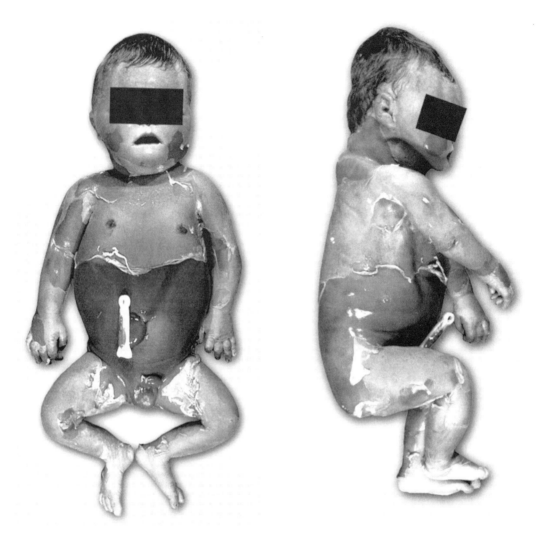

Figure 3.67 Typical changes of maceration in a near-term infant, with extensive skin slippage resulting from separation of the epidermis from the underlying darker shiny dermis. Changes of maceration indicate that death has occurred *in utero*.

injuries requires careful documentation of the pattern of injuries, the likely type of presentation (i.e. head versus breech), and a history of the labor. Unfortunately, much of this information may not be available. Asphyxia may occur in large fetuses due to impaction, or in small fetuses from precipitate labor.

Injuries resulting from delivery include trauma to the head, such as caput succedaneum (bleeding and edema within the soft tissues of the scalp) and cephalhematoma (bleeding under the periosteum). These two forms of injury are not uncommon and are not life-threatening. Extradural hemorrhage may occur but is usually minimal and associated with skull fracture. Subdural hemorrhage may also result. Skull fractures are uncommon and are usually linear fractures of the parietal bones occurring during difficult forceps deliveries. Separation of parts of the occipital bone at the back of the skull (occipital osteodiastasis) during

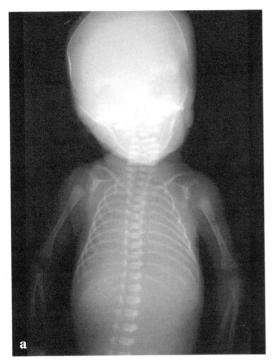 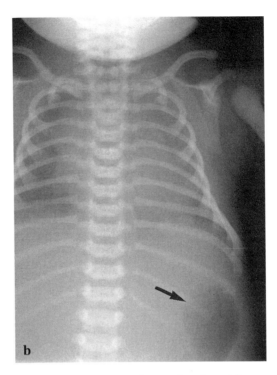

Figure 3.68 Radiograph from a stillborn infant, showing dense lungs and no air in the stomach (a). Close-up of a radiograph from a term infant who was allegedly stillborn, showing a gastric air bubble (arrow) and aerated lungs (b). As the infant was not putrefactive and resuscitation had not been attempted, the findings were those of live birth.

a difficult breech delivery may result in significant and sometimes fatal injuries to the back of the brain, with tearing of venous sinuses causing marked subdural hemorrhage and laceration of the cerebellum (Keeling, 1987). Head injuries may also occur with precipitate delivery if the mother was standing and the cord was of sufficient length to allow the infant to strike the floor.

Birth injuries may occur to other parts of the body, with fractures of long bones and the clavicles, spinal injuries during breech deliveries, and damage to internal organs such as the liver, spleen, and kidneys. Drowning may occur if an infant was delivered into a toilet (Mitchell & Davis, 1984).

A full-term infant who has died from asphyxia during delivery may show evidence of prior chronic stress, with poor growth, reduced subcutaneous fat, and meconium staining of the fingernails or skin. Acute asphyxia during delivery may result in small hemorrhages over the thymus gland, heart, and lungs, and microscopically the lungs may show hemorrhage into the smaller airways, which may contain meconium and shed fetal skin ("squames") (Keeling, 1987).

Maternal conditions that predispose to fetal asphyxia include heart and kidney disease, diabetes mellitus, anemia, essential hypertension, hypertension of pregnancy (pre-eclampsia), a high number of previous pregnancies, and prolonged gestation (greater than 42 weeks). Many of these conditions will be associated with poor fetal growth.

Conditions may also be present that are incompatible with life or that require urgent medical intervention for survival. These include anencephaly, diaphragmatic hernias, severe congenital cardiac defects, sepsis, and certain metabolic disorders. These should be documented clearly in the autopsy report.

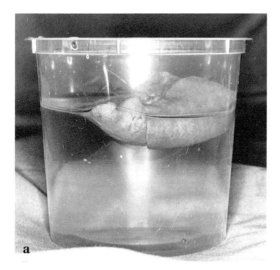

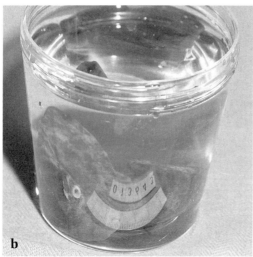

Figure 3.69 Uniformly well-inflated lungs floating in water of a term infant who was allegedly stillborn. The infant was not putrefactive and resuscitation had not been attempted. The mother later pleaded guilty to manslaughter (a). Lungs from a genuine stillbirth for comparison sinking to the bottom of a container (b).

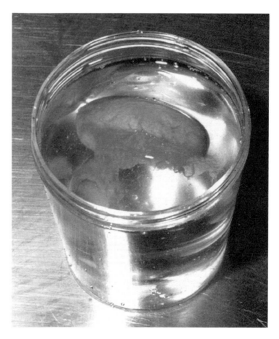

Figure 3.70 Floating stomach from an alleged stillbirth, demonstrating filling of the stomach with air. Resuscitation had not been attempted.

Placenta

Examination of the placenta may be extremely useful (Ito, Tsuda & Kimura, 1989) and may reveal a possible cause of death in the form of:

- severe bleeding behind the placenta due to premature separation from the uterus (placental abruption), resulting in loss of the fetal blood supply (Figure 3.72). Similar catastrophic bleeding may occur if the placenta or cord are lying over the entrance to the birth canal (placenta or vasa previa);
- tearing of the umbilical cord due to insertion of the cord into the membranes rather than the body of the placenta (velamentous insertion), causing fetal hemorrhage (mortality rate 60–70%) (Figure 3.73);
- lack of blood supply to the placenta causing infarction, or infections resulting in inflammation of the placenta (villitis), or the cord and membranes (funisitis and chorioamnionitis), may also be associated with fetal death.

Detailed examination of the cord should also be undertaken to look for:

- the presence or absence of a vital reaction, i.e. if an infant has survived for more than 24–48 hours, the portion of cord attached to the abdominal wall

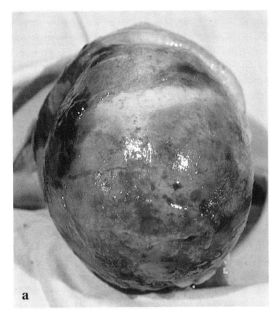

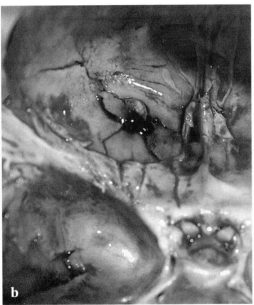

Figure 3.71 Relatively minor subgaleal hematomas of the right frontal and left temporal regions (a) of a newborn infant who suffered fatal head injuries inflicted by a shovel. There were associated complex fractures of the left orbital plate (b), in addition to the left frontal bone, right orbital plate, and both parietal bones.

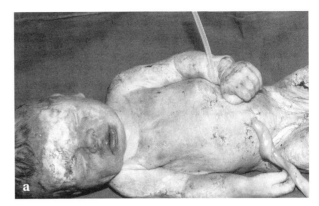

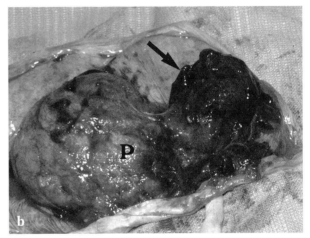

Figure 3.72 A 35-week gestation infant who was delivered into a toilet bowl (a). Examination of the placenta (P) revealed extensive retroplacental blood clot in keeping with placental abruption (arrow) (b).

will begin to show signs of separation, with reddening and desiccation. Histologically there may be evidence of an inflammatory cell reaction at the cut end of the cord after a number of hours. Unfortunately, in deaths occurring soon after delivery neither of these changes are present;

• the length of the cord. The average umbilical cord measures between 54 and 61 cm, although this is extremely variable. It has been proposed that abnormally short umbilical cords (less than 30 cm) may result in asphyxia during delivery due to excessive traction. Conversely, cords of more than 100 cm

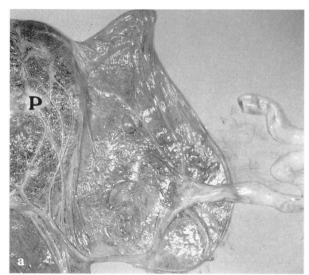

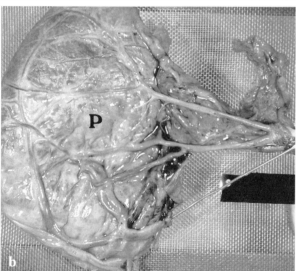

Figure 3.73 Two cases of velamentous insertion of the umbilical cord, with vessels running through the membranes prior to insertion into the placental discs (P). A probe in (b) demonstrates a ruptured vessel.

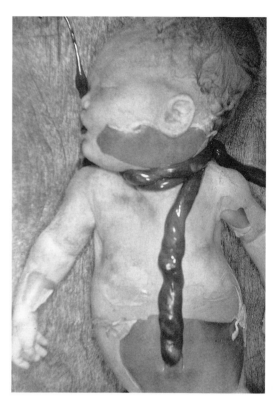

Figure 3.74 A macerated infant following intrauterine death. The cord is wound tightly around the neck.

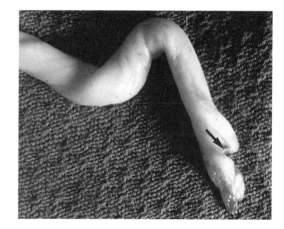

Figure 3.75 Irregular cutting of the umbilical cord (arrow) without clamping in a case of concealed pregnancy and delivery followed by death of the infant.

in length have been associated with problems from knotting, wrapping around the neck, torsion, and prolapse (Keeling, 1987). Interpretation of knotting may be difficult. A significant lesion consists of a tight knot with grooving of the cord and narrowing

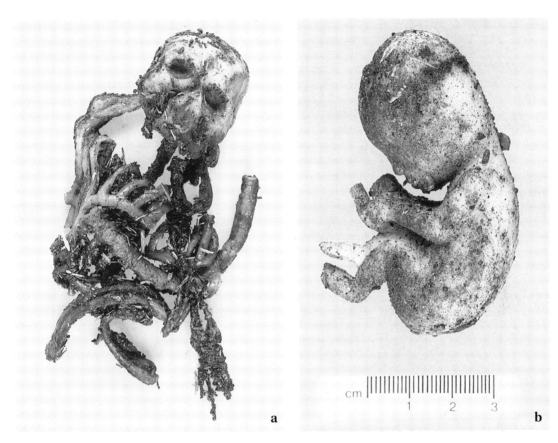

Figure 3.76 A plastic fetal skeleton (a) that had been buried for some time before being unearthed by a family dog. A rubber fetus (b) that was found at a refuse site. The cases were initially treated by police officers and hospital personnel as possible concealed stillbirths or infanticides. Sections of "cord" had even been submitted for tissue studies in specimen (b) (before consultation with a pathologist).

of vessels, associated with congestion and edema of the cord on one side and pallor on the other. There may be thrombosis within the vessels. Significant torsion or twisting should result in the cord remaining twisted after death, with congestion and edema. Wrapping of the cord around the neck is not an uncommon finding at delivery in infants with long cords. To be considered significant, the cord should have remained wrapped tightly around the neck after delivery (Figure 3.74), although it may have been removed by attendants or the mother;
• the ends of the cord. Examination of the severed ends of the cord will show whether the cord was cut (Figure 3.75), or whether the ends were torn, possibly indicating a precipitate delivery.

Conclusion

The investigation of cases of alleged stillbirth and concealed birth must be performed by individuals with experience in this area, as fundamental mistakes can easily be made (Figure 3.76). It must also be realized that in many infants the question of live birth simply cannot be answered definitively, and in these cases stillbirth should be assumed.

Inflicted asphyxia

Asphyxia occurs when tissues do not receive sufficient oxygen for metabolic purposes. It can be caused by deprivation of oxygen, or by interference with oxygen use at the cellular level by chemicals such as cyanide. Deprivation of oxygen may occur from strangling, when external pressure to the neck from a ligature or the application of hands cuts off the blood and air supply. The features at autopsy in infants and children are much the same as in adults, with parchmented ligature marks around the neck or deep and superficial bruising from fingertip pressure, and abrasions from fingernails. Damage to the thyroid cartilage and hyoid bone occur less often in children than in adults due to the flexible nature of these cartilaginous structures in the young.

Oxygen deprivation may also occur from suffocation due to obstruction of the external airways in smothering, obstruction of the internal airways in choking, pressure on the chest preventing respiration in mechanical asphyxia, deprivation of environmental oxygen in entrapment, or replacement of oxygen by inert gases (Byard & Wilson, 1992). Several of these scenarios have been dealt with in Chapter 2.

A problem occurs in infants and young children who have been intentionally suffocated as no specific autopsy findings may be present. Holding a hand, or particularly a pillow, over an infant's face and mouth will usually leave no markings. Even when pressure is applied to an infant's chest there may be no findings, for example when an infant is compressed between a pillow and a mattress or squeezed tightly in adult arms (Boos, 2000). This may result in several deaths occurring in the same family, as has been seen in Munchausen syndrome by proxy (*vide infra*). Homicidal hanging is rare in pediatric populations (Wyatt *et al.*, 1998).

Features of concern at autopsy that suggest asphyxia are facial and conjunctival petechiae and subconjunctival hemorrhages (Figure 3.77). Conjunctival petechiae are uncommon in infants and do not occur in SIDS (Byard & Krous, 1999a; Matsumura & Ito, 1996). Conversely, they may occur after a fit or after forceful vomiting or coughing (Betz, Penning & Keil, 1994). They may also be part of a more gen-

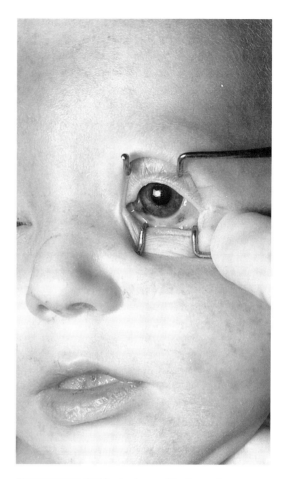

Figure 3.77 Petechial hemorrhages of the face and conjunctivae, with subconjunctival hemorrhages in a previously well seven-month-old boy who was found moribund by his mother's partner. No explanation could be offered for the asphyxial features.

eralized bleeding disturbance, with infections such as meningococcemia. In children with dark skin and meningococcal sepsis, the conjunctiva may be the only place where petechiae can be observed.

Cutaneous petechiae are much less common at autopsy in infants then in adults, who not infrequently have petechial hemorrhages in dependent or congested areas. If no plausible explanation is forthcoming, then strangulation or mechanical asphyxia due to pressure on the chest must be considered. On occasion, the diagnosis will not be difficult if there has been constant pressure on the chest as this may have caused extensive petechial hemorrhages over the face and neck, with cervicofacial cyanosis and subconjunctival hemorrhages, the so-called "masque ecchymotique" (Perrot, 1989).

While serosanguinous oronasal secretions are not uncommon in infant deaths, most likely related to terminal pulmonary edema, the presence of frank blood is unusual. In the absence of trauma related to attempts at cardiopulmonary resuscitation, oronasal blood raises the possibility of accidental or inflicted suffocation (Becroft, Thompson & Mitchell, 2001). Careful inspection of mucosal surfaces or the nose and mouth with an otoscope may reveal sites of trauma or may identify other lesions such as hemangiomas, tumors, or infections (Krous *et al.*, 2001).

Intra-alveolar hemorrhage has been proposed as a marker of airway obstruction from smothering in a study by Yukawa and colleagues (1999). However, the study was not blinded and details of the sampling protocol were not provided. In addition, intra-alveolar hemorrhage is a common finding in infants that may be influenced by a number of factors, including prolonged postmortem intervals, maturity of lungs, attempts at resuscitation, and the position of the infant's body after death (Berry, 1999; Hanzlick, 2001). Tissue sampling from dependent areas may also introduce bias. Thus, intra-alveolar hemorrhage is a not uncommon finding in infants dying from a number of conditions, and its significance should not be overinterpreted.

Hemosiderin within macrophages has also been used as a marker for previous imposed suffocation (Becroft & Lockett, 1997; Green, 1998; Milroy, 1999). However, again it is not a specific finding as it may occur in typical SIDS cases. Hemosiderin was found in one study within the lung tissues in nearly a fifth of cases that had been attributed to SIDS after full investigations (Byard *et al.*, 1997).

Ritual abuse

The exact incidence of child abuse and homicide occurring in cults who engage in "satanic" practices is uncertain, despite occasional media reports of adolescents who disappear into such groups, and stories of infant sacrifices (Johnson, 1990). Child prostitution and pornography are more likely reasons for the existence of such "cults" . More commonly, children who are found in circumstances with bizarre and pseudo-religious paraphernalia, who may have been tattooed or had crosses cut into their skin, are usually the victims of a psychotic parent (Johnson, 1994).

Self-inflicted injuries

A variety of diverse conditions may be associated with self-inflicted injuries in childhood and adolescence that can create confusion with inflicted injury. Behavioral disturbances such as headbanging and self-biting may be found in severely mentally retarded children, and self-injurious behavior may occur in children with developmental disorders such as autism or in children exhibiting tantrum behavior. Certain genetic and metabolic conditions such as Lesch–Nyan syndrome, Cornelia–Delange syndrome and familial dysautonomia are characterized by intellectual impairment and self-harm. Children with Lesch–Nyan syndrome, an X-linked disorder of purine metabolism, are particularly prone to self-mutilation and often lose digits, lips, and portions of the tongue. Adolescents with personality disorders or factitious illness behavior may induce injuries, and self-harm may also be a manifestation of depressive illness or eating disorders, such as pica, anorexia nervosa, or bulimia (Putnam & Stein, 1985).

Iatrogenic homicide

Iatrogenic homicides present a challenge for the death investigator (James & Leadbeatter, 1997). For example, a series of unexpected deaths and cardiorespiratory arrests in a San Antonio pediatric intensive care ward were linked to a nurse after an epidemiologic investigation had been performed. Several of the deaths were thought to be caused by drug intoxication, including digoxin, potassium, phenytoin, chloral hydrate, and phenobarbital, either singly or in combination. Although the nurse was not charged with any of the deaths, she was later convicted of injuring a child in that hospital by an overdose of unprescribed heparin (Istre *et al.*, 1985). In a Toronto children's hospital, an unusually high number of deaths was attributed to intravenous digoxin intoxication that had an apparent temporal association with the duty times of a particular nurse (Buehler *et al.*, 1985), although subsequent investigations failed to identify the perpetrator. Recommendations for the prevention of such cases have included limiting access to critical areas, with swipe-card access for staff and surveillance cameras in patient areas (Buchino, Corey & Montgomery, 2002). Formal protocols for the evaluation and assessment of complaints against hospital staff have also been advocated (Feldman, Mason & Shugerman, 2001).

Munchausen syndrome by proxy

Munchausen syndrome by proxy, or Munchausen by proxy, or factitious illness by proxy, is a disorder in which an adult either simulates or causes an illness in a child and brings it to the attention of the medical profession in order to obtain ill-understood gratification (Byard & Beal, 1993; Mitchell *et al.*, 1993; Schreier, 2002). The essential features described by Rosenberg (1987) are:

- the production of a spurious or genuine illness in a child by a carer (usually the mother). The term "illness" is used to denote chronicity in the behavior, rather than a single episode in isolation;
- repetitive attendance for medical assessment, investigation, and treatment;
- complete absence of symptoms and signs, or dramatic resolution of the illness, in the absence of the offending parent;
- denial by the perpetrator of the cause of the child's illness;
- a significant mortality rate.

The initial use of the term "Munchausen" in the medical literature occurred when Asher (1951) coined the name "Munchausen's syndrome" to described individuals who continually seek hospital admission and treatment by fabricating complex medical histories and clinical symptoms. The name derives from an eighteenth-century German soldier, Baron Hieronymus von Munchhausen (sic), a famous raconteur who was known widely for his colorful stories. The tall tales told by hospital-addicted patients who suffer from the syndrome that now bears his name are thought to be reminiscent of his "embellished" travels.

In 1977, Meadow described a far more disturbing disorder in which an adult guardian or parent achieves close medical contact not by submitting themselves to investigation and treatment but instead by using their child as a proxy. Symptoms and signs in a child victim are either falsified, resulting in extensive and often invasive medical investigations, or are created deliberately (in 75% of published cases) in an effort to obtain that "curious sense of purpose and safety in the midst of the disasters which they themselves have created" (Meadow, 1985; Rosenberg, 1987). The marked morbidity and possibility of sudden death in this "syndrome by proxy" quickly dispel all but the most superficial connection between this most sinister disorder and the entertaining Baron (Alexander, Smith & Stevenson, 1990; Byard, 1992). For example, Meadow (1990) reported a mortality rate of 33% in a series of 27 infants who were repetitively suffocated by their mothers, with 18 previous deaths noted in the 33 older siblings of these infants (a mortality rate of 55%). A mortality rate in siblings in another series was 11%, with 39% also having had illnesses fabricated by their mothers (Bools, Neale & Meadow, 1992). Cases have now been reported from a variety of countries (Feldman & Brown, 2002), and victims have included fetuses and adults in care. A similar syndrome has also been described in pet owners who repeatedly create illness and injury in their animals to obtain veterinary attention (Munro & Thrusfield, 2001a; Munro & Thrusfield, 2001b).

"Polle syndrome" is a term that has been used in varied fashion in the literature, initially to refer to cases of Munchausen by proxy inflicted by a parent with Munchausen syndrome (Verity *et al.*, 1979). Later it was used synonymously with the term "Munchausen by proxy" (Clark *et al.*, 1984) or even as the tautological "child abuse variant of Munchausen by proxy" (Liston, Levine & Anderson, 1983). The name derives from the incorrect idea that the baron had a son named Polle who died at an early age (Burman & Stevens, 1977). As detailed investigation by Meadow & Lennert (1984) has shown that the baron did not have a son, and that the name "Polle" refers instead to the town of origin of his second wife, the use of this confusing term should be discouraged.

The range of possible presentations of Munchausen by proxy is extraordinarily varied and has resulted from such diverse activities as adding blood to urine or feces, falsifying sweat tests and stool fat analyses, injecting insulin or petroleum distillates, administering psychotropic drugs, injecting saliva, vaginal secretions, or feces, poisoning, anticoagulating with warfarin, scratching or pricking the skin, exsanguinating, and manual suffocation (Halsey *et al.*, 1983; Hvizdala & Gellady, 1978; Kohl, Pickering & Dupree, 1978; Lee, 1979; Malatack *et al.*, 1985; Orenstein & Wasserman, 1986; Samuels & Southall, 1992; Saulsbury, Chobanian & Wilson, 1984; Shnaps *et al.*, 1981; White, Voter & Perry, 1985). Thus, the pathologist may receive tissues from the living patient from a variety of sites, such as the liver to exclude rare metabolic disorders, or the skin to help clarify an unusual rash. Two of the striking features that may be noted on review of the hospital record are the number of clinical services that have been consulted about the patient and the general puzzlement that exists over the possible etiology of the observed changes. Hospital staff may also become unwitting participants in the process if Munchausen by proxy has not been suspected (Donald & Jureidini, 1996; Jureidini, Shafer & Donald, 2003; Zitelli, Seltman & Shannon, 1987). Perpetrators have falsely claimed that their child has serious epilepsy, allergies, or reflux, or is the victim of sexual abuse (Barber & Davis, 2002; Meadow, 1993b).

In general, children who are victims of Munchausen by proxy are older than infants who succumb from SIDS, with the average age at diagnosis being a little over three years. Although patients who have suffered lethal suffocation tend to be younger, resulting in confusion with SIDS, there is still a significant difference in the average age at death, in that infants with spurious apnea usually survive for 6–12 months following the first episode, which tends

Table 3.11. Characteristics of infants dying of SIDS compared with those dying from non-accidental suffocation in Munchausen syndrome by proxy (MSBP)

Clinical features	SIDS infants (%)	MSBP infants (%)
Age >6 months	<15	55
History of apnea	<10	90
History of unexplained illness	<5	44
Previous death of a sibling	2	48

Adapted from Meadow (1990).

to occur between one to three months of age. Table 3.11 lists the features that may help to differentiate SIDS from Munchausen by proxy (Meadow, 1990).

All of the 117 victims of the syndrome reviewed by Rosenberg (1987) suffered short-term morbidity, nine suffered some form of permanent disability, and 10 (9%) died. In this latter group, the two major causes of death were poisoning in five (three due to salt poisoning) and suffocation in four. The most common symptoms prior to death were apnea, decreased level of consciousness, fitting, bleeding, and diarrhea. Survivors may have brain damage from repeated hypoxic episodes or from drugs or poisons administered by the perpetrator. There may also be considerable morbidity associated with unnecessary medications, investigations, and operations (Meadow, 1984a).

Apart from a small number of cases involving fathers (Makar & Squier, 1990; Meadow, 1998; Morris, 1985; Samuels *et al.*, 1992), virtually all reported cases have shown the abusing adult to be the victim's mother (Meadow, 1984b; Meadow, 1990). However, in some cases it seems likely that there was paternal collusion. The abusing mother usually gets on well with hospital staff and appears to have some medical knowledge. Although a history of child abuse in the mother may not always be found (Rosenberg, 1987), this may reflect lack of detailed investigation, as Samuels and colleagues (1992) documented emotional, physical, or sexual abuse in the perpetrator in 11 of 14 cases of imposed upper-airway obstruction. While it appears that there is rarely any evidence of psychosis, an understanding of the psychological profile of the offending parent is difficult due to the contradictory and patchy nature of psychiatric investigations reported in the literature (Emery, 1986). For example, while all of the abusing parents in Samuel and colleagues' (1992) series were diagnosed as suffering from "personality disorders," Rosenberg (1987) describes personality disorders as being present in only some of the cases. In a quarter to a half of reported cases in both of these papers, there have been at least some elements of Munchausen syndrome or abnormal illness behavior present, suggesting a definite link between the two syndromes (Meadow, 2002). Others have described depressive illness, emotional disturbances, and drug addiction (Souid, Keith & Cunningham, 1998). Of some importance is the fact that occasionally the perpetrator will asphyxiate not only her own children but also relatives' and neighbors' children, and even adopted children, as was the case of a woman reported by DiMaio & Bernstein (1974), who fatally asphyxiated seven infants over a 23-year period. The occurrence of five deaths in a family attributed to SIDS in another report must raise the likelihood of inflicted asphyxia, particularly given that two of the children were aged 13 months and two years, respectively (Diamond, 1986). The wide range of presentations and great variation in perpetrator psychopathology has led to proposals to abandon the term "Munchausen by proxy" in favor of diagnoses more specific to individual cases (Fisher & Mitchell, 1995; Morley, 1995). Others have suggested terms such as "pediatric condition falsification" (PCF) and "factitious disorder by proxy" (FDP) as components of Munchausen by proxy (Ayoub et al., 2002; Shreier, 2002).

A disturbing point made by Rosenberg (1987) is that 20% of the reported children who subsequently died had been identified correctly as being victims of Munchausen by proxy but had been discharged from hospital still in the care of their parents. A high incidence of unusual sibling deaths (9–55%) (Rosenberg, 1987; Meadow, 1990) in these families also included a number that had been attributed to SIDS, which in retrospect must be viewed with skepticism. It is now believed that the two fatal cases described by Steinschneider (1972) that linked repetitive

apneic episodes with SIDS were in reality homicides occurring in a family in which three other sibling deaths had occurred in children under the age of 28 months (DiMaio, 1988; Firstman & Talan, 1997; Little & Brooks, 1994). This issue had been raised many years before by Hick (1973).

Detection of cases may be difficult, as the parent will characteristically deny any knowledge of the basis of the child's illness or death. Unfortunately, observation in hospital is not guaranteed to either detect or prevent the behavior (Berger, 1979), and it has been estimated that in 95% of cases the presenting illness has been reproduced successfully during admission.

In cases where review of the current and previous histories has suggested the possibility of Munchausen by proxy, in-hospital covert video surveillance has been used to document the presence or absence of abusive behaviour (Hall et al., 2000). Although this technique has been used successfully to identify a number of cases of Munchausen by proxy in the USA, Great Britain, and Australia, there has been considerable debate as to its ethical status (Anonymous, 1994; Byard & Burnell, 1994; Epstein et al., 1987; Foreman & Farsides, 1993; Rosen et al., 1983; Shabde & Craft, 1999; Shinebourne, 1996; Southall et al., 1987; Southall et al., 1997; Williams & Bevan, 1988). Criteria for the implementation of covert surveillance have been reported (Samuels et al., 1992), in addition to guidelines for the forensic evaluation of possible cases (Sanders & Bursch, 2002).

Rosenberg (1987) found the legal outcome of this behavior reported in only 13% of cases, with no conviction being recorded in 5% and a criminal conviction occurring in the remaining 8% of perpetrators.

One of the most common presentations to the pathologist of this syndrome in its lethal form is of an infant with a history of apneic episodes who has died suddenly, ostensibly from SIDS. The underlying pathology is not, of course, with the infant but resides instead with the parent, who has been repeatedly suffocating the child to produce significant apneic spells that will lead to medical concern and investigation (Light & Sheridan, 1990; Mitchell et al., 1993).

Whether the final episode results from a genuine desire to murder the infant, or is a miscalculation resulting from an attempt to gradually escalate the severity of the symptoms, is difficult to determine. Certainly one of the features distinguishing Munchausen by proxy from standard child abuse is the secondary gain achieved by the sublethal harmful actions; however, reported ambivalence in maternal feelings toward the victim suggest that there is a complex mix of psychopathological processes contributing to the overall behavior (Meadow, 1995).

Unfortunately, even with a strong degree of suspicion, the autopsy in isolation may not be able to establish whether the death was due to natural causes or to homicide (Dix, 1998). If suffocation without undue force was used in an infant, then the findings will be identical to those of SIDS, with no evidence of trauma, and petechial hemorrhages only within the thoracic cavity (Mitchell, Krous & Byard, 2002; Moore & Byard, 1993; Valdes-Dapena, 1982). The non-specificity of autopsy findings is believed, therefore, to have led to erroneous diagnoses of SIDS in the past in a number of infants who may have been suffocated by their parents. However, although the diagnosis of SIDS has sometimes been made too readily in the past (Emery, Gilbert & Zugibe, 1988), the authors would not agree with the statement that up to 10% (or more) of infants whose deaths were attributed to SIDS were smothered by their mothers (Meadow, 1989). It should be stated clearly that these cases are infrequent and are less likely to be missed if there has been a careful interview of the parents by trained personnel, with formal death scene investigation and performance of the autopsy according to standard protocols by a pathologist, preferably with pediatric forensic experience (American Academy of Pediatrics Committee on Child Abuse and Neglect, 2001b; Byard & Krous, 1999b; Smialek & Lambros, 1988). Unfortunately, the corollary of this statement is that there is going to be a certain number of cases that will remain unproven or undetected, in spite of the most rigorous of investigations.

The relatively high incidence of poisoning in fatal cases of Munchausen by proxy will necessitate the taking of body fluids and tissue samples for evaluation. Given cases of lethal salt poisoning, biochemical analysis of serum, vitreous humor, and gastric content electrolytes may also be informative (Coe, 1993). Parental medications may provide a clue to the type of overdose that has been administered; poisoning has been described with a wide variety of drugs, such as antidepressants, barbiturates, phenothiazines, insulin, warfarin, laxatives, and antidiarrheal agents.

Munchausen by proxy is a complex disorder that is being increasingly recognized. The relative plausibility of the abusing parent and lack of specificity that is often present in histologic and autopsy findings may render it a particularly difficult problem for the pathologist. The repetitive nature of the abusive behavior, often with a lethal outcome in subsequent infants, however, makes accuracy of diagnosis of paramount importance.

Injuries caused by cardiopulmonary resuscitation

In some cases of unexpected childhood death, there may be confusion between deliberately inflicted trauma and that caused by cardiopulmonary resuscitation (see Figure 3.32). While the most common injuries in adults and animal models resulting from cardiopulmonary resuscitation include fractured ribs, pulmonary edema or contusion, hemothorax, and liver laceration (Kern *et al.*, 1986), cardiopulmonary resuscitation-induced injuries and lesions in children are very uncommon (except for venipuncture wounds, lesions caused by endotracheal tubes, and impressions left by electrocardiograph or defibrillator pads). Tibial fractures may be caused by intra-osseous lines, and shaving of hair prior to the insertion of an intravenous line may subsequently be confused with an abrasion. While facial petechiae may occur after attempted resuscitation in adolescents and adults (Hood, Ryan & Spitz, 1988), it is not a finding that the authors have encountered in infants.

Facial injuries may include nasal and perinasal fingernail injury from attempted mouth-to-mouth resuscitation, abrasions over the cheeks, bridge of nose, lips, and chin from plastic masks, and lacerations of the lips from intubation (Kaplan & Fossum, 1994). Similar injuries may of course occur from inflicted suffocation, and so they must be taken in the context of a clear description of the resuscitative efforts (Minford, 1981).

The occurrence of retinal hemorrhage following cardiopulmonary resuscitation is controversial and unfortunately complicated by the lack of details in older reports, which interferes with evaluation of their conclusions. For example, Weedn, Mansour & Nichols (1990) reported retinal hemorrhage in a four-month-old infant who died 30 hours after receiving allegedly accidental burns and repeated cardiopulmonary resuscitation. No comment on possible DAI was made, and the infant was also septic, with death due to a *Klebsiella* sp. bronchopneumonia. Goetting & Sowa (1990) found retinal hemorrhage in three of 21 infants and children who had been resuscitated. One patient had one hemorrhage, another had two hemorrhages, and the third had multiple large bilateral hemorrhages. Although Kirschner & Stein (1985) reported a case of retinal hemorrhage following vigorous chest compressions performed by the father of a three-month-old infant whose death was ultimately ruled as SIDS, there is no mention of postmortem radiographs, microbiology, toxicology, or soft tissue dissections to enable occult trauma, sepsis, or poisoning to be excluded. Kanter (1986) performed fundoscopic examinations on 54 infants and young children who had undergone cardiopulmonary resuscitation. Of the six patients who had retinal hemorrhages, four had central nervous system injuries from abuse and one was a pedestrian hit by a car. The remaining patient had no evidence of trauma and had been found at home having a seizure, with subsequent arterial hypertension of 190/120 mm Hg. A 17-month-old girl who was documented to develop retinal hemorrhages after resuscitation also had sepsis in the form of lethal adenovirus gastroenteritis (Kramer & Goldstein, 1993).

More recent studies have supported the concept that retinal hemorrhages occur rarely, if ever, from cardiopulmonary resuscitation. Gilliland & Luckenbach (1993) found no retinal hemorrhages in 70 children who had cardiopulmonary resuscitation. Of the children in their series who did have retinal hemorrhages and cardiopulmonary resuscitation, all but one had recognized causes of retinal hemorrhage, such as head trauma, sepsis, or central nervous system disease. The possibility of inflicted injury was present in the remaining case. Similarly, no retinal hemorrhages were identified in Bush and colleagues' (1996) 211 cases. Thus, although cardiopulmonary resuscitation may be a very rare cause of retinal hemorrhage, other conditions, particularly inflicted head injury, are far more likely.

While it has been proposed that cardiopulmonary resuscitation may rarely cause rib fractures in children (Dorfman & Paradise, 1995), Feldman & Brewer (1984) found no cases of rib fracture in children who had undergone cardiopulmonary resuscitation, compared with 15% of abused children. In the latter cases, the fractures also tended to be multiple, to be of different ages, and to involve adjacent ribs. Similarly, Spevak and colleagues (1994) did not find any cardiopulmonary resuscitation-induced rib fractures in 91 infants. Bush and colleagues (1996) identified only one patient out of 211 children under 12 years of age with fractures of the ribs following resuscitation attempts. Rib fractures appear to occur from compressive, encircling forces that occur when the chest is squeezed, rather than from intermittant direct anteroposterior compression that characterizes cardiopulmonary resuscitation (Boos, 2000; Gunther, Symes & Berryman, 2000; Kleinman, 1998). Thus, bilateral posterior rib fractures should be considered to be due to sustained, compressive pressure on the chest until proven otherwise.

Reardon and colleagues (1987) reported a case of right atrial laceration allegedly due to cardiopulmonary resuscitation in a four-year-old child who was taken to hospital following a seizure. Three days after admission, he developed cardiac tamponade and at surgery was found to have the atrial laceration. At that time, his father admitted to performing chest compressions at the time of the seizure. We would consider that recollection of the performance of cardiopulmonary resuscitation only after the discovery of the cardiac laceration suggests inflicted injury rather than a genuine resuscitation attempt. Pancreatic contusion was reported by Waldman, Walters & Grunau (1984) in an eight-year-old girl who had cardiopulmonary resuscitation with interposed abdominal compressions following cardiopulmonary arrest from a ruptured intracerebral arteriovenous malformation. No intra-abdominal injuries were found following attempted resuscitation in 324 infants and children aged 10 years and under who died of natural causes (Price *et al.*, 2000).

When making a judgment about whether cardiopulmonary resuscitation might have caused an injury, a detailed history of the collapse, the type of resuscitation that was attempted, the equipment used, the type of ventilation attempted, the precise site on the body where compressions were applied, and the degree of force used is essential (Leadbeatter, 2001). The best way to assess this is to ask the person (or people) who performed cardiopulmonary resuscitation to demonstrate using a doll.

"Pseudoabuse"

As noted previously, some natural diseases, folk customs, and accidental injuries can mimic abuse. Lesions of the skin simulating inflicted bruising may occur with hemophilia, hypersensitivity vasculitis, platelet aggregation disorders, disseminated intravascular coagulation, purpura fulminans, phytophotodermatitis, erythema multiforme, rickettsial infection, measles, streptococcal toxic shock syndrome, postmortem lividity, and intradermal nevi (Mongolian blue spots) (see Figure 3.35). Eczema around the neck may be mistaken for a ligature mark if it is severe and excoriated. Subgaleal hemorrhage may occur from vigorous hair combing, and dermatorrhexis with prominent scar formation in Ehlers–Danlos syndrome may simulate the features of abuse (Evans, 2001; Kirschner & Stein, 1985; Kaplan, 1986; Nields *et al.*, 1998; Owen & Durst, 1984). An infant has been reported with an ulcerated vulval hemangioma that was initially thought to be due to abusive burns (Levin & Selbst, 1988), and impetigo, staphylococcal

"scalded skin syndrome," Henoch–Schönlein purpura, mechanical abrasions, and car seat burns may also be misinterpreted as intentional burns (Brown & Melinkovich, 1986; Wheeler & Hobbs, 1988).

Bone lesions with the potential to simulate abuse can be divided into several different categories. Nutritional and metabolic defects include scurvy, rickets, secondary hyperparathyroidism, Menkes kinky hair syndrome, and mucolipidosis II. Bone disorders caused by drugs include methotrexate osteopathy and hypervitaminosis A. Congenital syphilis and osteomyelitis are infections of bone that can mimic inflicted injuries. Skeletal dysplasias include osteogenesis imperfecta and infantile cortical hyperostosis (Caffey disease) (Radkowski, 1983).

Folk customs that may produce lesions that can be confused with abuse include cupping, or moxibustion, which consists of placing heated containers on the skin surface to cause a localized suction effect. The body may also be rubbed with coins (*cạo gío* or *kua-sha*) (see Figures 3.33 and 3.34) (Gellis & Feingold, 1976). Both of these practices are found in oriental populations and are not harmful. Coins are usually dipped in aromatic oils, water, or wine and scraped backwards and forwards over the skin until petechiae and bruises occur. Rubbing may be accompanied by pinching of the skin in the form of a counter-irritant to the presenting symptoms. Favored areas for rubbing include the chest following the intercostal spaces, the bridge of the nose, the mid-forehead, the front and back of the neck, and the cubital and popliteal fossae (Hulewicz, 1994). Burns may be caused by naturopathic remedies or the prolonged application of herbal poultices (Garty, 1993).

Subdural hematomas may result from trauma associated with a Latin American folk remedy, *caida de mollera*, used for sunken fontanelle most likely caused by dehydration. Traditional healers, or *curanderos*, will attempt to elevate a sunken fontanelle by taking a mouthful of warm water and sucking over the fontanelle, or by suspending an infant with his or her head in boiling water while shaking or slapping the soles of the feet (Guarnaschelli, Lee & Pitts, 1972). Despite extensive knowledge of

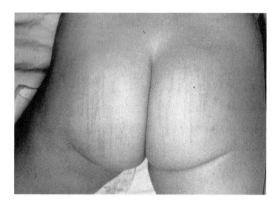

Figure 3.78 Linear scarring of the buttocks of uncertain origin attributed by carers to the results of a folk remedy.

herbal remedies, simple surgical procedures, and magico-religious rites (Byard, 1988; Sharon, 1978), folk healers in traditional communities may persist with counterproductive techniques such as this. The use of folk remedies does not exclude coincident abuse, and although folk remedies may be blamed for causing injury or scarring, odd lesions should always prompt careful and full investigation (Figure 3.78).

Obstetrical trauma may cause fractures, especially of the clavicle, and resolving cephalhematomas may simulate healing skull fractures. Osteoporosis from disuse atrophy can predispose bones to fracture with minor trauma. Finally, normal skull variants such as atypical parietal sutures may appear to be fractures (Radkowski, 1983; Kirschner & Stein, 1985; Kaplan, 1986; Wheeler & Hobbs, 1988).

Glutaric aciduria type I can predispose an infant or child to subdural hemorrhage from minor trauma, as frontal-temporal atrophy associated with this condition causes elongation of bridging veins (Kohler & Hoffman, 1998). Similarly, infants with cerebral atrophy from other causes may develop regional subdural hemorrhage following an injury such as a minor fall. There is, however, no evidence to suggest that infants with benign expansion of the subarachnoid space are predisposed to subdural bleeding (Hymel, Jenny & Block, 2002). Subdural hematomas may also occur in Menkes syndrome, an X-linked disorder of copper absorption (Nassogne *et al.*, 2002).

Murder–suicide

Murder–suicide, homicide–suicide, or so-called "dyadic deaths" refer to cases where a perpetrator commits suicide following a homicide (Milroy, 1993). Situations where children have been the victims have not been investigated extensively, but there appear to be certain differences in the profile of such cases (Byard *et al.*, 1999).

Murder–suicides at all ages are uncommon events compared with suicides and homicides, with homicide rates in Atlanta, USA (from 1988 to 1991) and Kentucky, USA (from 1985 to 1990) of 38.8 and five per 100,000, respectively, compared with murder–suicide rates in those locations of 0.46 and 0.3 per 100,000, respectively. Although there is considerable geographic variation in homicide rates, the ratio of homicides to murder–suicides remains high. For example, homicide and murder–suicide rates per 100,000 in Australia from 1989 to 1991 were two and 0.16, in Scotland from 1986 to 1990 were 1.75 and 0.05, and in England and Wales from 1980 to 1990 were 1.11 and 0.07 (Milroy, 1995a), i.e. there were between 13 and 84 times as many homicides compared with murder–suicides in these areas. Murder–suicides account for a higher percentage of all homicides in countries with low homicide rates, e.g. 42% of homicides in Denmark, where the homicide rate is low, are murder–suicides, compared with 2–4% in the USA, where the homicide rate is much higher (Coid, 1983; Copeland, 1985; Felthous & Hempel, 1995).

Murder–suicides have been subdivided into extrafamilial, spousal/consortial, and familial subgroups. Extrafamilial cases include disgruntled ex-employees, cult deaths, and pseudocommando attacks. Spousal murder–suicides usually involve either couples in whom advancing age, physical disability, or terminal illness provoke the event, or a "possessive" type, where the event is initiated by a rejected spouse or lover – the "Othello syndrome" (Hanzlick & Koponen, 1994; Marzuk, Tardiff & Hirsch, 1992; Milroy, 1995b; Milroy, Dratsas & Ranson, 1997).

Familial murder–suicides occur in situations of marital breakdown and tend to involve a depressed

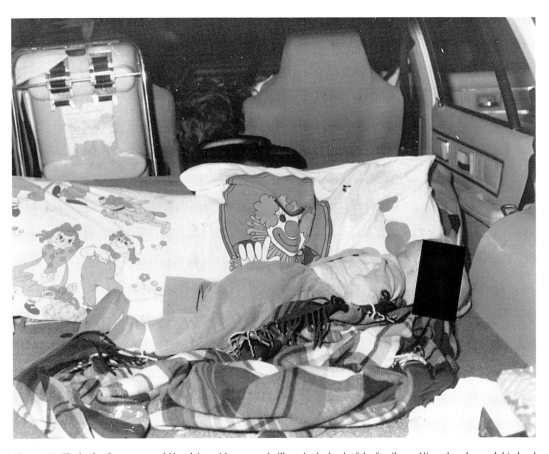

Figure 3.79 The body of a one-year-old boy lying with a rug and pillows in the back of the family car. His carboxyhemoglobin level was 55%. The bodies of his brother, sister, and mother were in the front of the car. A pipe was connected from the exhaust to the cabin.

parent who murders his or her children and then commits suicide afterwards. This makes the investigation of cases difficult as not only is the perpetrator dead but so are those who were closest to him or her and who may have been able to provide some reason for the attack. Infanticide–suicides are distinctly uncommon, although cases have been reported from Japan and Canada (Berman, 1979; Buteau, Lesage & Kiely, 1993).

Studies have shown a higher percentage of female perpetrators, who generally murder only their own children. This contrasts with males, who tend to murder not only their own children but also other children, their spouse, and sometimes even family pets.

The term "family annihilator" has been coined for these individuals (Milroy, 1995a).

Mothers have tended to use less violent methods than fathers to kill their children (Figures 3.79 and 3.80). This, combined with the known higher incidence of depression among perpetrators, has led to the suggestion that murder–suicides represent an extension of suicide, and that a parent may perceive their behavior to be altruistic in "saving" their children from the problems of life (Palermo *et al.*, 1997; Somander & Rammer, 1991). The use by mothers of less violent methods and sedation would support this contention (Byard *et al.*, 1999). Cases where more violent methods have been used by mothers have

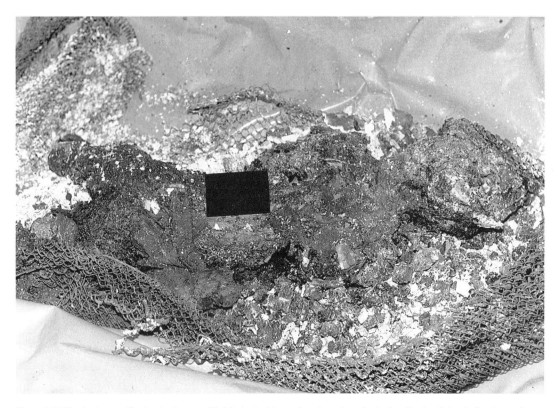

Figure 3.80 The incinerated body of a six-year-old girl who had been shot three times in the head by her father before he set fire to the house. One other sister and her mother had also been shot fatally; the father then shot himself fatally.

been associated with psychiatric disturbance and access to weapons (Figure 3.81).

Suicide

Suicide is now the major cause of violent death in a number of countries, with higher rates than motor vehicle accidents and homicides (Byard *et al.*, 2000b). Considerable variation occurs among countries in the demographic characteristics of victims and in the methods that are utilized. In addition, conflicting data have been presented regarding the contribution of "youth" suicide to overall suicide numbers.

Despite studies that have shown an increase in suicide in the young (Lee, Collins & Burgess, 1999; Roesler, 1997), this is fortunately not a generalized

trend (Males, 1994). National Injury Surveillance Unit data in Australia showed no increase in the suicide rate of males aged 15–24 years from 1990 to 1995 (Harrison, Moller & Bordeaux, 1995), and Australian Bureau of Statistics data from 1881 to 1995 showed that the suicide rates for both males and females aged under 14 years have remained stable in that country for over a century (Australian Bureau of Statistics, 1996; Hassan, 1995). A joint study from California and South Australia demonstrated that suicide under the age of 17 years accounted for only 1.6–2% of all suicides (Figure 3.82), with no increase in numbers between 1985 and 1997 (Byard *et al.*, 2000b). More recent data from South Australia have shown that suicides under the age of 20 years accounted for only 3.4% of the total number of 444 suicides for the years 1998 and 1999 (Byard, Eitzen & James, 2000).

A particular problem in interpreting apparently conflicting data lies in the use of the term "youth," with some reports using the term for victims up to the age of 29 years (Goldney, 1993). It has also been stated correctly that media reports have "unfortunately overemphasized the contribution of youth suicides to all suicides" (Bell & Clark, 1998).

Despite assertions to the contrary (Baume & McTaggart, 1998), methods of suicide used by the young have differed from older victims. Whereas hanging, inhalation of carbon monoxide, gunshot wounds, and drug overdoses represent more than 90% of the total number of suicides in Australia, they account for only 73% of methods in the young. A greater incidence of uncommon methods of self-destruction has also been found (Byard *et al.*, 2000b). This may be a reflection of accessibility to certain lethal activities and lack of familiarity with others. For example, the effects of carbon monoxide and medication toxicity may be less obvious to an adolescent than the effects of self-immolation, inhaling

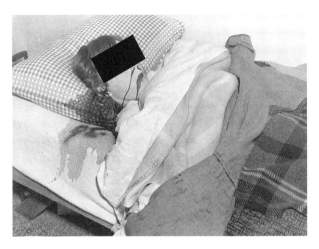

Figure 3.81 A sleeping 13-year-old girl had been shot once in the head by her mother, who then committed suicide by ingesting strychnine. The mother had a recent history of "odd" behavior and lived in a rural area in South Australia with access to firearms.

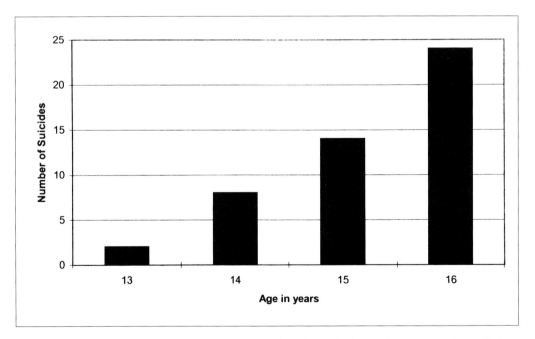

Figure 3.82 Number of suicides per year of age in adolescents and children under the age of 17 years in South Australia from 1985 to 1997.

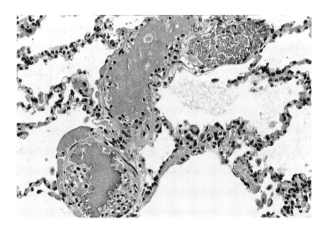

Figure 3.83 Histologic examination of lung tissue from a 14-year-old girl who injected herself with hair conditioner, showing distention of small arteries by foreign material (hematoxylin and eosin, ×200).

insecticide, jumping from heights, or standing in front of a train (Klitte *et al.*, 2001). Greater numbers of firearm suicides in the USA are most likely due to accessibility to weapons. Distinguishing attention-seeking behavior from a genuine suicide attempt may be difficult, particularly if an unusual method has been used (Figure 3.83) (Knight *et al.*, 1998).

Expert evidence

In recent years, there has been a number of high-profile cases of alleged infant and child homicides in which the validity of the evidence and opinions by medical experts has been questioned. Unfortunately, most physicians who have attended court for such cases would have witnessed examples where opinions have been forcefully espoused based on questionable data. Weintraub (1995) has deemed this a "corruption of science."

Chadwick & Krous (1997) have listed criteria to identify individuals who give irresponsible medical testimony. These include absence of proper qualifications, use of unique theories of causation, use of unique or very unusual interpretations of the medical findings, proposing non-existent medical findings, misquoting of the literature, making false statements, and deliberately omitting important facts. Additional problems arise when the significance of important literature is deliberately downplayed or published hypotheses are elevated to the level of fact. Unfortunately, courts and juries are particularly vulnerable to the opinions of individuals who are presented to them as experts, and usually have no effective mechanisms for dealing with incorrectly submitted material and opinion. For this reason, it has been suggested by Chadwick & Krous (1997) that experts should be able to clearly demonstrate certain points. These include training and experience in childhood inflicted injuries and neglect, specific training and experience related to the case being tried, membership of relevant professional organizations, presentations and attendance at child abuse and neglect conferences, and relevant professional publications. In addition, an expert should be able to demonstrate current involvement in the field.

If the role and criteria for the assessment of the medical expert are not addressed, then this unacceptable situation will continue to beset courts. It is a particular problem in cases of inflicted injury, in infants, as the findings may be very subtle or non-existent, and precise mechanisms of death may not yet be understood, as has been demonstrated clearly in this chapter. The high levels of uncertainty in many facets of these cases provide fertile ground for those who would rather muddy the waters than assist the court.

REFERENCES

Adams, J. H., Doyle, D., Ford, I., *et al.* (1989). Diffuse axonal injury and head injury: definition, diagnosis and grading. *Histopathology*, **15**, 49–59.

Adams, J. H., Gennarelli, T. A. & Graham, D. I. (1982). Brain damage in non-missile head injury: observations in man and in subhuman primates. In *Recent Advances in Neuropathology*, ed. R. Smith & J. Cavanagh. Edinburgh: Churchill Livingston, pp. 165–90.

Adams, J. H., Graham, D. I. & Gennarelli, T. A. (1981). Acceleration induced head injury in the monkey. II. Neuropathology. *Acta Neuropathologica*, **7** (Suppl), 26–8.

Adams, J. H., Graham, D. I. & Gennarelli, T. A. (1982). Neuro-pathology of acceleration-induced head injury in the sub-human primate. In *Seminars in Neurological Surgery: Proceedings of the 4th Annual Conference on Neural Trauma*, ed. R. Grossman. New York: Raven Press, pp. 141–52.

Adelson, L. (1991). Pedicide revisited. The slaughter continues. *American Journal of Forensic Medicine and Pathology*, **12**, 16–26.

Adesunkanmi, A. R., Oseni, S. A. & Bodru, O. S. (1999). Severity and outcome of falls in children. *West African Journal of Medicine*, **18**, 281–5.

Al-Alousi, L. M. (1990). Homicide by electrocution. *Medicine, Science and the Law*, **30**, 239–46.

Alexander, R., Crabbe, L., Sato, Y., Smith, W. & Bennett, T. (1990a). Serial abuse in children who are shaken. *American Journal of Diseases of Children*, **144**, 58–60.

Alexander, R., Sato, Y., Smith, W. & Bennett, T. (1990b). Incidence of impact trauma with cranial injuries ascribed to shaking. *American Journal of Diseases of Children*, **144**, 724–6.

Alexander, R., Smith, W. & Stevenson, R. (1990). Serial Munchausen syndrome by proxy. *Pediatrics*, **86**, 581–5.

Alexander, R. C., Surrell, J. A. & Cohle, S. D. (1987). Microwave oven burns to children: an unusual manifestation of child abuse. *Pediatrics*, **79**, 255–60.

American Academy of Pediatrics Committee on Child Abuse and Neglect (1991). Guidelines for the evaluation of sexual abuse of children. *Pediatrics*, **87**, 254–60.

American Academy of Pediatrics Committee on Child Abuse and Neglect (2001a). Shaken baby syndrome: rotational cranial injuries–technical report. *Pediatrics*, **108**, 206–10.

American Academy of Pediatrics Committee on Child Abuse and Neglect (2001b). Distinguishing sudden infant death syndrome from child abuse fatalities. *Pediatrics*, **107**, 437–41.

American Academy of Pediatrics Section on Radiology (1991). Diagnostic imaging of child abuse. *Pediatrics*, **87**, 262–4.

Anonymous (1994). Spying on mothers. *Lancet*, **343**, 1373–4.

Arnholz, D., Hymel, K. P., Hay, T. C. & Jenny, C. (1998). Bilateral pediatric skull fractures: accident or abuse? *Journal of Trauma*, **45**, 172–4.

Asher, R. (1951). Munchausen's syndrome. *Lancet*, **1**, 339–41.

Australian Bureau of Statistics (1996). Causes of Death, Australia, 1995. Catalogue no. 3303.0. Canberra: Australian Government Publishing Service.

Ayoub, C. C., Alexander, R., Beck, D., *et al.* (2002). Position paper: definitional issues in Munchausen by proxy. *Child Maltreatment*, **7**, 105–11.

Ball, D. J. & King, K. L. (1991). Playground injuries: a scientific appraisal of popular concerns. *Journal of the Royal Society of Health*, **111**, 134–7.

Barber, M. A. & Davis, P. M. (2002). Fits, faints, or fatal fantasy? Fabricated seizures and child abuse. *Archives of Disease in Childhood*, **86**, 230–33.

Barlow, B., Niemirska, M., Gandhi, R. P. & Leblanc, W. (1983). Ten years of experience with falls from a height in children. *Journal of Pediatric Surgery*, **18**, 509–11.

Barnes, P. D. & Robson, C. D. (2000). CT findings in hyperacute nonaccidental brain injury. *Pediatric Radiology*, **30**, 74–81.

Barry, P. W. & Hocking, M. D. (1993). Infant rib fracture – birth trauma or non-accidental injury. *Archives of Disease in Childhood*, **68**, 250.

Baume, P. & McTaggart, P. (1998). Suicides in Australia. In *Suicide Prevention. The Global Context*, ed. R. J. Kosky, H. S. Eshkevari, R. D. Goldney & R. Hassan. New York: Plenum Press, pp. 67–78.

Becroft, D. M. & Lockett, B. K. (1997). Intra-alveolar pulmonary siderophages in sudden infant death: a marker for previous imposed suffocation. *Pathology*, **29**, 60–63.

Becroft, D. M., Thompson, J. M. & Mitchell, E. A. (2001). Nasal and intrapulmonary hemorrhage in sudden infant death syndrome. *Archives of Disease in Childhood*, **85**, 116–20.

Bell, C. C. & Clark, D. C. (1998). Adolescent suicide. *Pediatric Clinics of North America*, **45**, 365–80.

Berger, D. (1979). Child abuse simulating "near-miss" sudden infant death syndrome. *Journal of Pediatrics*, **95**, 554–6.

Berman, A. L. (1979). Dyadic death: murder-suicide. *Suicide and Life Threatening Behaviour*, **9**, 15–23.

Berry, P. J. (1999). Intra-alveolar haemorrhage in sudden infant death syndrome: a cause for concern? *Journal of Clinical Pathology*, **52**, 553–4.

Betz, P., Penning, R. & Keil, W. (1994). The detection of petechial haemorrhages of the conjunctivae in dependency on the post-mortem interval. *Forensic Science International*, **64**, 61–7.

Betz, P., Püschel, K., Miltner, E., Lignitz, E. & Eisenmenger, W. (1996). Morphometrical analysis of retinal hemorrhages in the shaken baby syndrome. *Forensic Science International*, **78**, 71–80.

Billmire, M. E. & Myers, P. A. (1985). Serious head injury in infants: accident or abuse? *Pediatrics*, **75**, 340–42.

Blumbergs, P. C., Jones, N. R. & North, J. B. (1989). Diffuse axonal injury in head trauma. *Journal of Neurology, Neurosurgery and Psychiatry*, **52**, 838–41.

Boglioli, L. R., Taff, M. L. & Harleman, G. (1998). Child homicide caused by commotio cordis. *Pediatric Cardiology*, **19**, 436–8.

Bools, C. N., Neale, B. A. & Meadow, S. R. (1992). Co-morbidity associated with fabricated illness (Munchausen syndrome by proxy). *Archives of Disease in Childhood*, **67**, 77–9.

Boos, S. C. (2000). Constrictive asphyxia: a recognizable form of child abuse. *Child Abuse and Neglect*, **24**, 1503–7.

Brill, P. W. & Winchester, P. (1987). Differential diagnosis of child abuse. In *Diagnostic Imaging of Child Abuse*, ed. P. K. Kleinman. Baltimore: Williams & Wilkins, pp. 221–41.

Brown, J. & Melinkovich, P. (1986). Schönlein–Henoch purpura misdiagnosed as suspected child abuse. A case report and literature review. *Journal of the American Medical Association*, **256**, 617–18.

Brown, J. K. & Minns, R. A. (1993). Non-accidental head injury, with particular reference to whiplash shaking injury and medico-legal aspects. *Developmental Medicine and Child Neurology*, **35**, 849–69.

Bruce, D. A., Alavi, A., Bilaniuk, L., *et al.* (1981). Diffuse cerebral swelling following head injuries in children: the syndrome of "malignant brain edema". *Journal of Neurosurgery*, **54**, 170–78.

Bruce, P. A. & Zimmerman, R. A. (1989). Shaken impact syndrome. *Pediatric Annals*, **18**, 482–94.

Buchino, J. J. (1983). Recognition and management of child abuse by the surgical pathologist. *Archives of Pathology and Laboratory Medicine*, **107**, 204–5.

Buchino, J. J., Corey, T. S. & Montgomery, V. (2002). Sudden unexpected death in hospitalized children. *Journal of Pediatrics*, **140**, 461–5.

Buehler, J. W., Smith, L. F., Wallace, E. M., *et al.* (1985). Unexplained deaths in a children's hospital. An epidemiologic assessment. *New England Journal of Medicine*, **313**, 211–16.

Burman, D. & Stevens, D. (1977). Munchausen family. *Lancet*, **ii**, 456.

Bush, C. M., Jones, J. S., Cohle, S. D. & Johnson, H. (1996). Pediatric injuries from cardiopulmonary resuscitation. *Annals of Emergency Medicine*, **28**, 40–44.

Buteau, J, Lesage A. D. & Kiely, M. C. (1993). Homicide followed by suicide: a Quebec case series, 1988–1990. *Canadian Journal of Psychiatry*, **38**, 552–6.

Byard, R. (1988). Traditional medicine of aboriginal Australia. *Canadian Medical Association Journal*, **139**, 792–4.

Byard, R. W. (1992). Factitious patients with fictitious disorders: a note on Munchausen's syndrome. *Medical Journal of Australia*, **156**, 507–8.

Byard, R. W. (2001). Inaccurate classification of infant deaths in Australia: a persistent and pervasive problem. *Medical Journal of Australia*, **175**, 5–7.

Byard, R. W. & Beal, S. M. (1993). Munchausen syndrome by proxy: repetitive infantile apnoea and homicide. *Journal of Paediatrics and Child Health*, **29**, 77–9.

Byard, R. W. & Burnell, R. H. (1994). Covert video surveillance in Munchausen syndrome by proxy – ethical compromise or essential technique? *Medical Journal of Australia*, **160**, 352–6.

Byard, R. W. & Krous, H. F. (1999a). Petechial hemorrhages and unexpected infant death. *Legal Medicine*, **1**, 193–7.

Byard, R. W. & Krous, H. F. (1999b). Suffocation, shaking or sudden infant death syndrome: can we tell the difference? *Journal of Paediatrics and Child Health*, **35**, 432–3.

Byard, R. W. & Lipsett, J. (1999). Drowning deaths in toddlers and preambulatory children in South Australia. *American Journal of Forensic Medicine and Pathology*, **20**, 328–32.

Byard, R. W. & Wilson, G. W. (1992). Death scene gas analysis in suspected methane asphyxia. *American Journal of Forensic Medicine and Pathology*, **13**, 69–71.

Byard, R. W., Donald, T. & Chivell, W. (1999). Non-lethal and subtle inflicted injury and unexpected infant death. *Journal of Law and Medicine*, **7**, 47–52.

Byard, R. W., Donald, T., Hilton, J. N. & Krous, H. F. (2000a). Shaking-impact syndrome and lucidity. *Lancet*, **355**, 758.

Byard, R. W., Eitzen, D. & James, R. A. (2000). Suicide trends: adolescence and beyond. *Medical Journal of Australia*, **172**, 461–2.

Byard, R. W., Hanson, K. A., Gilbert, J. D., *et al.* (2003). Death due to electrocution in childhood and early adolescence. *Journal of Paediatrics and Child Health*, **39**, 46–8.

Byard, R. W., Knight, D., James, R. A. & Gilbert, J. (1999), Murder-suicides involving children. *American Journal of Forensic Medicine and Pathology*, **20**, 323–7.

Byard, R. W., Markopoulos, D., Prasad, D., *et al.* (2000b). Early adolescent suicide: a comparative study. *Journal of Clinical Forensic Medicine*, **7**, 6–9.

Byard, R. W., Stewart, W. A., Telfer, S. & Beal, S. M. (1997). Assessment of pulmonary and intrathymic hemosiderin deposition in sudden infant death syndrome. *Pediatric Pathology and Laboratory Medicine*, **17**, 275–82.

Caffey, J. (1974). The whiplash shaken infant syndrome: manual shaking by the extremities with whiplash-induced intracranial and intraocular bleedings, linked with residual permanent brain damage and mental retardation. *Pediatrics*, **54**, 396–403.

Calder, I. M., Hill, I. & Scholtz, C. L. (1984). Primary brain trauma in non-accidental injury. *Journal of Clinical Pathology*, **37**, 1095–100.

Campbell, T. A. & Collins, K. A. (2001). Pediatric toxicologic deaths. A 10-year retrospective study. *American Journal of Forensic Medicine and Pathology*, **22**, 184–7.

Campbell-Hewson, G. L., D'Amore, A. & Busuttil, A. (1998). Non-accidental injury inflicted on a child with an air weapon. *Medicine, Science and the Law*, **38**, 173–6.

Carty, H. & Ratcliffe, J. (1995). The shaken infant syndrome. *British Medical Journal*, **310**, 344–5.

Case, M. E. S. & Nanduri, R. (1983). Laceration of the stomach by blunt trauma in a child: a case of child abuse. *Journal of Forensic Sciences*, **28**, 496–501.

Case, M. E., Graham, M. A., Corey Handy, T., Jentzen, J. M. & Monteleone, J. A. (2001). Position paper on fatal abusive head injuries in infants and young children. *American Journal of Forensic Medicine and Pathology*, **22**, 112–22.

Case, M. E. S., Short, C. D. & Poklis, A. (1983). Intoxication by aspirin and alcohol in a child. A case of child abuse by medical neglect. *American Journal of Forensic Medicine and Pathology*, **4**, 149–51.

Chabrol, B., Decarie, J.-C. & Fortin, G. (1999). The role of cranial MRI in identifying patients suffering from child abuse and presenting with unexplained neurological findings. *Child Abuse and Neglect*, **23**, 217–28.

Chadwick, D. L. (1992). The diagnosis of inflicted injury in infants and young children. *Pediatric Annals*, **21**, 477–83.

Chadwick, D. L. & Krous, H. F. (1997). Irresponsible testimony by medical experts in cases involving the physical abuse and neglect of children. *Child Maltreatment*, **2**, 313–21.

Chadwick, D. L. & Salerno, C. (1993). Likelihood of death of an infant or young child in a short fall of less than 6 vertical feet. *Journal of Trauma*, **35**, 968.

Chadwick, D. L., Chin, S., Salerno, C., Landsverk, J. & Kitchen L. (1991). Deaths from falls in children: how far is fatal? *Journal of Trauma*, **31**, 1353–5.

Chadwick, D. L., Kirschner, R. H., Reece, R. M., *et al.* (1998). Shaken baby syndrome – a forensic pediatric response. *Pediatrics*, **101**, 321–3.

Chesney, R. W. & Brusilow, S. (1981). Extreme hypernatremia as a presenting sign of child abuse and psychosocial dwarfism. *Johns Hopkins Medical Journal*, **148**, 11–13.

Chiaviello, C. T., Christoph, R. A. & Bond, G. R. (1994). Stairway-related injuries in children. *Journal of Pediatrics*, **94**, 679–81.

Christian, C. W., Taylor, A. A., Hertle, R. W. & Duhaime, A. C. (1999). Retinal hemorrhages caused by accidental household trauma. *Journal of Pediatrics*, **135**, 125–7.

Christoffel, K. K. (1990). Violent death and injury in U.S. children and adolescents. *American Journal of Diseases of Children*, **144**, 697–706.

Christoffel, K. K., Zieserl, E. J. & Chiaramonte, J. (1985). Should child abuse and neglect be considered when a child died unexpectedly? *American Journal of Diseases of Children*, **139**, 876–80.

Clark, G. D., Key, J. D., Rutherford, P. & Bithoney, W. G. (1984). Munchausen's syndrome by proxy (child abuse) presenting as apparent autoerythrocyte sensitization syndrome: an unusual presentation of Polle syndrome. *Pediatrics*, **74**, 1100–102.

Coe, J. I. (1993). Postmortem chemistry update. Emphasis on forensic application. *American Journal of Forensic Medicine and Pathology*, **14**, 91–117.

Cohen, R. A., Kaufman, R. A., Myers, P. A. & Towbin, R. B. (1986). Cranial computed tomography in the abused child with head injury. *American Journal of Roentgenology*, **146**, 97–102.

Cohle, S. D. (1986). Homicidal asphyxia by pepper aspiration. *Journal of Forensic Sciences*, **31**, 1475–8.

Cohle, S. D., Hawley, D. A., Berg, K. K., Kiesel, E. L. & Pless, J. E. (1995). Homicidal cardiac lacerations in children. *Journal of Forensic Sciences*, **40**, 212–18.

Cohle, S. D., Trestrail, J. D., Graham, M. A., *et al.* (1988). Fatal pepper aspiration. *American Journal of Diseases of Children*, **142**, 663–6.

Coid, J. (1983). The epidemiology of abnormal homicide and murder followed by suicide. *Psychological Medicine*, **13**, 855–60.

Collins, K. A. & Nichols, C. A. (1999). A decade of pediatric homicide. A retrospective study at the Medical University of South Carolina. *American Journal of Forensic Medicine and Pathology*, **20**, 169–72.

Colombani, P. M., Buck, J. R., Dudgeon, D. L., Miller, D. & Haller, J. A., Jr (1985). One-year experience in a regional pediatric trauma center. *Journal of Pediatric Surgery*, **20**, 8–13.

Conley, S. B. (1990). Hypernatremia. *Pediatric Clinics of North America*, **37**, 365–72.

Conradi, S. & Brissie, R. (1986). Battered child syndrome in a four year old with previous diagnosis of Reye's syndrome. *Forensic Science International*, **30**, 195–203.

Cooper, G. J. & Taylor, D. E. M. (1989). Biophysics of impact injury to the chest and abdomen. *Journal of the Royal Army Medical Corps*, **135**, 58–67.

Cooper, A., Floyd, T., Barlow, B., *et al.* (1988). Major blunt abdominal trauma due to child abuse. *Journal of Trauma*, **28**, 1483–7.

Copeland, A. R. (1985). Dyadic death revisited. *Journal of the Forensic Science Society*, **25**, 181–8.

Corey Handy, T., Hanzlick, R., Shields, L. B. E., Reichard, R. & Goudy, S. (1999). Hypernatremia and subdural hematoma in the pediatric age group: is there a causal relationship? *Journal of Forensic Sciences*, **44**, 1114–18.

Cory, C. Z., Jones, M. D., James, D. S., Leadbeatter, S. & Nokes, L. D. M. (2001). The potential and limitations of utilizing head impact injury models to assess the likelihood of significant head injury in infants after a fall. *Forensic Science International*, **123**, 89–106.

Couper, R. T. L., Aldis, J. J. E. & Byard, R. W. (1998). Digoxin-like immunoreactivity in early infant death. *Medicine, Science and the Law*, **38**, 52–6.

Cullen, J. (1975). Spinal lesions in battered babies. *Journal of Bone and Joint Surgery – British Volume*, **57**, 364–6.

Cumberland, G. D., Riddick, L. & McConnell, C. F. (1991). Intimal tears of the right atrium of the heart due to blunt force injuries to the abdomen. Its mechanisms and implications. *American Journal of Forensic Medicine and Pathology*, **12**, 102–4.

Curran, W. J., McGarry, A. L., & Petty, C. S. (ed.) (1980). *Modern Legal Medicine, Psychiatry and Forensic Science*. Philadelphia: F.A. Davis.

Davis, J. H., Rao, V. J. & Valdes-Dapena, M. (1984). A forensic science approach to a starved child. *Journal of Forensic Sciences*, **29**, 663–9.

Davison, P. R. & Cohle, S. D. (1987). Histologic detection of fat emboli. *Journal of Forensic Sciences*, **32**, 1426–30.

De Silva, S. & Oates, R. K. (1993). Child homicide – the extreme of child abuse. *Medical Journal of Australia*, **158**, 300–301.

Denton, J. S. & Kalelkar, M. B. (2000). Homicidal commotio cordis in two children. *Journal of Forensic Sciences*, **45**, 734–5.

Diamond, E. F. (1986). In five consecutive siblings sudden infant death. *Illinois Medical Journal*, **170**, 33–4.

Dias, M. S., Backstrom, J., Falk, M. & Li, V. (1998). Serial radiography in the infant shaken impact syndrome. *Pediatric Neurosurgery*, **29**, 77–85.

DiMaio, V. J. M. (1988). SIDS or murder? *Pediatrics*, **81**, 747.

DiMaio, V. J. M. & Bernstein, C. G. (1974). A case of infanticide. *Journal of Forensic Sciences*, **19**, 744–54.

DiMaio, D. J. & DiMaio, V. J. M. (2001). *Forensic Pathology*, 2nd edn. New York: Elsevier, p. 339.

Dine, M. S. (1965). Tranquilizer poisoning: an example of child abuse. *Pediatrics*, **36**, 782–5.

Dine, M. S. & McGovern, M. E. (1982). Intentional poisoning of children – an overlooked category of child abuse: report of seven cases and review of the literature. *Pediatrics*, **70**, 32–5.

Division of Injury Control. Centers for Disease Control. (1990). Childhood injuries in the United States. *American Journal of Diseases of Children*, **144**, 627–46.

Dix, J. (1998). Homicide and the baby-sitter. *American Journal of Forensic Medicine and Pathology*, **19**, 321–3.

Dolinak, D., Smith, C. & Graham, D. I. (2000). Global hypoxia per se is an unusual cause of axonal injury. *Acta Neuropathologica*, **100**, 553–60.

Donald, T. & Jureidini, J. (1996). Munchausen syndrome by proxy. Child abuse in the medical system. *Archives of Pediatric and Adolescent Medicine*, **150**, 753–8.

Dorfman, D. H. & Paradise, J. E. (1995). Emergency diagnosis and management of physical abuse and neglect of children. *Current Opinion in Pediatrics*, **7**, 297–301.

Duhaime, A. C., Alario, A. J., Lewander, W. J., *et al.* (1992). Head injury in very young children: mechanisms, injury types, and ophthalmologic findings in 100 hospitalized patients younger than 2 years of age. *Pediatrics*, **90**, 179–85.

Duhaime, A. C., Christian, C. W., Rorke, L. B. & Zimmerman, R. A. (1998). Nonaccidental head injury in infants – the "shaken-baby syndrome". *New England Journal of Medicine*, **338**, 1822–9.

Duhaime, A. C., Gennarelli, T. A., Thibault, L. E., *et al.* (1987). The shaken baby syndrome. A clinical, pathological and biomechanical study. *Journal of Neurosurgery*, **66**, 409–15.

Dykes, L. J. (1986). The whiplash shaken infant syndrome: what has been learned? *Child Abuse and Neglect*, **10**, 211–21.

Elder, J. E., Taylor, R. G. & Klug, G. L. (1991). Retinal haemorrhage in accidental head trauma in childhood. *Journal of Paediatrics and Child Health*, **27**, 286–9.

Ellerstein, N. S. (1979). The cutaneous manifestations of child abuse and neglect. *American Journal of Diseases of Children*, **133**, 906–9.

Ellerstein, N. S. & Norris, K. J. (1984). Value of radiologic skeletal survey in assessment of abused children. *Pediatrics*, **74**, 1075–8.

Ellis, P. S. J. (1997). The pathology of fatal child abuse. *Pathology*, **29**, 113–21.

Emans, S. J. (1992). Sexual abuse in girls: what have we learned about genital anatomy? *Journal of Pediatrics*, **120**, 258–60.

Emery, J. L. (1978). The deprived and starved child. *Medicine, Science and the Law*, **18**, 138–42.

Emery, J. L. (1986). Families in which two or more cot deaths have occurred. *The Lancet*, **1**, 313–15.

Emery, J. L., Gilbert, E. F. & Zugibe, F. (1988). Three crib deaths, a babyminder and probable infanticide. *Medicine, Science and the Law*, **28**, 205–11.

Epstein, M. A., Markowitz, R. L., Gallo, D. M., Holmes, J. W. & Gryboski, J. D. (1987). Munchausen syndrome by proxy: considerations in diagnosis and confirmation by video surveillance. *Pediatrics*, **80**, 220–24.

Ernst, J. A., Wynn, R. J. & Schreiner, R. L. (1981). Starvation with hypernatremic dehydration in two breast-fed infants. *Journal of the American Dietetic Association*, **79**, 126–30.

Evans, M. J. (2001). Mimics of non-accidental injury in children. In *Essentials of Autopsy Practice*, vol. 1, ed. G. N. Rutty. London: Springer, pp. 121–42.

Evans, K. T. & Roberts, G. M. (1989). Radiological aspects of child abuse. In *Paediatric Forensic Medicine and Pathology*, ed. J. K. Mason. London: Chapman & Hall, pp. 288–306.

Ewigman, B., Kivlahan, C & Land, G. (1993). The Missouri Child Fatality Study: underreporting of maltreatment fatalities among children younger than five years of age, 1983 through 1986. *Pediatrics*, **91**, 330–37.

Ewing-Cobbs, L., Kramer, L., Prasad, M., *et al.* (1998). Neuroimaging, physical and developmental findings after inflicted and non-inflicted traumatic brain injury in young children. *Pediatrics*, **102**, 300–307.

Feldman, K. W. (1992). Patterned abusive bruises of the buttocks and the pinnae. *Pediatrics*, **90**, 633–6.

Feldman, K. W. (1995). Confusion of innocent pressure injuries with inflicted dry contact burns. *Clinical Pediatrics*, **34**, 114–15.

Feldman, K. W. & Brewer, D. K. (1984). Child abuse, cardiopulmonary resuscitation, and rib fractures. *Pediatrics*, **73**, 339–42.

Feldman, M. D. & Brown, R. M. (2002). Munchausen by proxy in an international context. *Child Abuse and Neglect*, **26**, 509–24.

Feldman, K. W., Bethel, R., Shugerman, R. P., *et al.* (2001). The cause of infant and toddler subdural hemorrhage: a prospective study. *Pediatrics*, **108**, 636–46.

Feldman, M. D., Mason, C. & Shugerman, R. P. (2001). Accusations that hospital staff have abused pediatric patients. *Child Abuse and Neglect*, **25**, 1555–69.

Feldman, K. W., Schaller, R. T., Feldman, J. A. & McMillon, M. (1978). Tap water scald burns in children. *Pediatrics*, **62**, 1–7.

Felthous, A. R. & Hempel, A. (1995). Combined homicide-suicides: a review. *Journal of Forensic Sciences*, **40**, 846–57.

Finnie, J. W. (2001). Animal models of traumatic brain injury: a review. *Australian Veterinary Journal*, **79**, 628–33.

Firstman, R. & Talan, J. (1997). *The Death of Innocents*. New York: Bantam Books.

Fischler, R. S. (1983). Poisoning: a syndrome of child abuse. *American Family Physician*, **28**, 103–8.

Fisher, G. C. & Mitchell, I. (1995). Is Munchausen syndrome by proxy really a syndrome? *Archives of Disease in Childhood*, **74**, 530–34.

Foreman, D. M. & Farsides, C. (1993). Ethical use of covert videoing techniques in detecting Munchausen syndrome by proxy. *British Medical Journal*, **307**, 611–14.

Fornes, P., Druilhe, L. & Lecomte, D. (1995). Childhood homicide in Paris, 1990–1993: a report of 81 cases. *Journal of Forensic Sciences*, **40**, 201–4.

Fossum, R. M. & Descheneaux, K. A. (1991). Blunt trauma of the abdomen in children. *Journal of Forensic Sciences*, **36**, 47–50.

Funayama, M., Ikeda, T., Tabata, N., Azumi, J.-I. & Morita, M. (1994). Case report: repeated neonaticides in Hokkaido. *Forensic Science International*, **64**, 147–50.

Gardner, J. J. (1992). Descriptive study of genital variation in healthy, nonabused premenarchal girls. *Journal of Pediatrics*, **120**, 251–7.

Garrettson, L. K. & Gallagher, S. S. (1985). Falls in children and youth. *Pediatric Clinics of North America*, **32**, 153–62.

Garty, B.-Z. (1993). Garlic burns. *Pediatrics*, **91**, 658–9.

Geddes, J. F., Hackshaw, A. K., Vowles, G. H., Nickols, C. D. & Whitwell, H. L. (2001a). Neuropathology of inflicted head injury in children I. Patterns of brain damage. *Brain*, **124**, 1290–98.

Geddes, J. F., Tasker, R. C., Hackshaw, A. K., *et al.* (2003). Dural haemorrhage in non-traumatic infant deaths: does it explain the bleeding in "shaken baby syndrome"? *Neuropathology and Applied Neurobiology*, **29**, 14–22.

Geddes, J. F., Vowles, G. H., Hackshaw, A. K., *et al.* (2001b). Neuropathology of inflicted head injury in children II. Microscopic brain injury in infants. *Brain*, **124**, 1299–1306.

Geddes, J. F., Whitwell, H. L. & Graham, D. I. (2000). Traumatic axonal injury: practical issues for diagnosis in medicolegal cases. *Neuropathology and Applied Neurobiology*, **26**, 105–16.

Gellis, S. S. & Feingold, M. (1976). Picture of the Month. Cạo gío (pseudo-battering in Vietnamese children). *American Journal of Diseases of Children*, **130**, 857–8.

Gennarelli, T. A. (1983). Head injury in man and experimental animals: clinical aspects. *Acta Neurochirurgica Supplement*, **32**, 1–13.

Gennarelli, T. A. (1993). Mechanisms of brain injury. *Journal of Emergency Medicine*, **11** (suppl 1), 5–11.

Gennarelli, T. A., Thibault, L. E., Adams, J. H., *et al.* (1982). Diffuse axonal injury and traumatic coma in the primate. *Annals of Neurology*, **12**, 564–74.

Gillenwater, J. M., Quan, L. & Feldman, K. W. (1996). Inflicted submersion in childhood. *Archives of Pediatric and Adolescent Medicine*, **150**, 298–303.

Gilles, E. E. & Nelson, M. D. (1998). Cerebral complications of nonaccidental head injury in childhood. *Pediatric Neurology*, **19**, 119–28.

Gillespie, R. W. (1965). The battered child syndrome: thermal and caustic manifestations. *Journal of Trauma*, **5**, 523–33.

Gilliland, M. G. (1998). Interval duration between injury and severe symptoms in nonaccidental head trauma in infants and young children. *Journal of Forensic Sciences*, **43**, 723–5.

Gilliland, M. G. F. & Folberg, R. (1996). Shaken babies – some have no impact injuries. *Journal of Forensic Sciences*, **41**, 114–16.

Gilliland, M. G. F. & Luckenbach, M. W. (1993). Are retinal hemorrhage found after resuscitation attempts? *American Journal of Forensic Medicine and Pathology*, **14**, 187–92.

Gilliland, M. G. F., Luckenbach, M. W. & Chenier, T. C. (1994). Systemic and ocular findings in 169 prospectively studied child deaths: retinal hemorrhages usually mean child abuse. *Forensic Science International*, **68**, 117–32.

Gilliland, M. G. F., Luckenbach, M. W., Massicotte, S. J. & Folberg, R. (1991). The medicolegal implications of detecting hemosiderin in the eyes of children who are suspected of being abused. *Archives of Ophthalmology*, **109**, 321–2.

Gleckman, A. M., Bell, M. D., Evans, R. J. & Smith, T. W. (1999). Diffuse axonal injury in infants with nonaccidental craniocerebral trauma: enhanced detection by beta-amyloid precursor protein immunohistochemical staining. *Archives of Pathology and Laboratory Medicine*, **123**, 146–51.

Gleckman, A. M., Kessler, S. C. & Smith, T. W. (2000). Periadventitial extracranial vertebral artery hemorrhage in a case of shaken baby syndrome. *Journal of Forensic Sciences*, **45**, 1151–3.

Goetting, M. G. & Sowa, B. (1990). Retinal hemorrhage after cardiopulmonary resuscitation in children: an etiologic re-evaluation. *Pediatrics*, **85**, 585–8.

Goldney, R. D. (1993). Suicide in the young. *Journal of Paediatrics and Child Health*, **29** (suppl 1), S50–52.

Goodson, M. E. (1993). Electrically induced deaths involving water immersion. *American Journal of Forensic Medicine and Pathology*, **14**, 330–33.

Gosnold, J. K. & Sivaloganathan, S. (1980). Spinal cord damage in a case of non-accidental injury in children. *Medicine, Science and the Law*, **20**, 54–7.

Green, M. A. (1998). A practical approach to suspicious death in infancy – a personal view. *Journal of Clinical Pathology*, **51**, 561–3.

Green, M. A., Lieberman, G., Milroy, C. M. & Parsons M. A. (1996). Ocular and cerebral trauma in non-accidental injury in infancy: underlying mechanisms and implications for paediatric practice. *British Journal of Ophthalmology*, **80**, 282–7.

Guarnaschelli, J., Lee, J. & Pitts, F. W. (1972). "Fallen fontanelle" (caida de Mollera). A variant of the battered child syndrome. *Journal of the American Medical Association*, **222**, 1545–6.

Gunther, W. M., Symes, S. A. & Berryman, H. E. (2000). Characteristics of child abuse by anteroposterior manual compression versus cardiopulmonary resuscitation. Case reports. *American Journal of Forensic Medicine and Pathology*, **21**, 5–10.

Hall, D. E., Eubanks, L., Meyyazhagan, S., Kenney, R. D. & Johnson, S. C. (2000). Evaluation of covert video surveillance in the diagnosis of Munchausen syndrome by proxy: lessons from 41 cases. *Pediatrics*, **105**, 1305–12.

Hall, J. R., Reyes, H. M., Horvat, M., Meller, J. L. & Stein, R. (1989). The mortality of childhood falls. *Journal of Trauma*, **29**, 1273–5.

Halsey, N. A., Tucker, T. W., Redding J., *et al.* (1983). Recurrent nosocomial polymicrobial sepsis secondary to child abuse. *Lancet*, **ii**, 558–60.

Hamlin, H. (1968). Subgaleal hematoma caused by hair-pull. *Journal of the American Medical Association*, **204**, 129.

Hanigan, W. C., Peterson, R. A. & Njus, G. (1987) Tin ear syndrome: rotational acceleration in pediatric head injuries. *Pediatrics*, **80**, 618–22.

Hanzlick, R. (2001). Pulmonary hemorrhage in deceased infants. Baseline data for further study of infant mortality. *American Journal of Forensic Medicine and Pathology*, **22**, 188–92.

Hanzlick, R. & Koponen, M. (1994). Murder-suicide in Fulton County, Georgia: comparison with a recent report and proposed typology. *American Journal of Forensic Medicine and Pathology*, **15**, 168–73.

Harcourt, B. & Hopkins, D. (1971). Ophthalmic manifestations of the battered-baby syndrome. *British Medical Journal*, **3**, 398–401.

Hargrave, D. R. & Warner, D. P. (1992). A study of child homicide over two decades. **32**, 247–50.

Harley, R. D. (1980) Ocular manifestations of child abuse. *Journal of Pediatric Opthalmology and Strabismus*, **17**, 5–13.

Harrison, J., Moller, J. & Bordeaux, S. (1995). Youth suicide and self-injury Australia. *Australian Injury Prevention Bulletin*, **15** (suppl).

Hart, B. L., Dudley, M. H. & Zumwalt, R. E. (1996). Postmortem cranial MRI and autopsy correlation in suspected child abuse. *American Journal of Forensic Medicine and Pathology*, **17**, 217–24.

Harwood-Nash, D. C. (1992). Abuse to the pediatric central nervous system. *American Journal of Neuroradiology*, **13**, 569–75.

Hassan, R. (1995). *Suicide Explained: The Australian Experience*. Melbourne: Melbourne University Press, p. 50.

Helfer, R. E., Slovis, T. L. & Black, M. (1977). Injuries resulting when small children fall out of bed. *Pediatrics*, **60**, 533–5.

Hick, J. F. (1973). Sudden infant death syndrome and child abuse. *Pediatrics*, **52**, 147–8.

Hight, D. W., Bakalar, H. R. & Lloyd, J. R. (1979). Inflicted burns in children. *Journal of the American Medical Association*, **242**, 517–20.

Hiss, J. & Kahana, T. (1995). The medicolegal implications of bilateral cranial fractures in infants. *Journal of Trauma*, **38**, 32–4.

Hobbs, C. J. (1984). Skull fracture and the diagnosis of abuse. *Archives of Disease in Childhood*, **59**, 246–52.

Hobbs, C. J. (1986). When are burns not accidental? *Archives of Disease in Childhood*, **61**, 357–61.

Hobbs, C. J. (1989a). Head injuries. *British Medical Journal*, **298**, 1169–70.

Hobbs, C. J. (1989b). Burns and scalds. *British Medical Journal*, **298**, 1302–5.

Holloway, M., Bye, A. M. E. & Moran, K. (1994). Non-accidental head injury in children. *Medical Journal of Australia*, **160**, 786–9.

Hood, I., Mirchandani, H., Monforte, J. & Stacer, W. (1986). Immunohistochemical demonstration of homicidal insulin injection site. *Archives of Pathology and Laboratory Medicine*, **110**, 973–4.

Hood, I., Ryan, D. & Spitz, W. U. (1988). Resuscitation and petechiae. *American Journal of Forensic Medicine and Pathology*, **9**, 35–7.

Hulewicz, B. S. F. (1994). Coin-rubbing injuries. *American Journal of Forensic Medicine and Pathology*, **15**, 257–60.

Humphreys, R. P., Hendrick, E. B. & Hoffman, H. J. (1990). The head-injured child who "talks and dies". A report of 4 cases. *Child's Nervous System*, **6**, 139–42.

Huser, C. J. & Smialek, J. E. (1986). Diagnosis of sudden death in infants due to acute dehydration. *American Journal of Forensic Medicine and Pathology*, **7**, 278–82.

Hutson, H. R., Anglin, D. & Pratts, M. J. (1994). Adolescents and children injured or killed in drive-by shootings in Los Angeles. *New England Journal of Medicine*, **330**, 324–7.

Hvizdala, E. V. & Gellady, A. M. (1978). Intentional poisoning of two siblings by prescription drugs. *Clinical Pediatrics*, **17**, 480–82.

Hymel, K. P., Abshire, T. C., Luckey, D. W. & Jenny, C. (1997a). Coagulopathy in pediatric abusive head trauma. *Pediatrics*, **99**, 371– 5.

Hymel, K. P., Bandak, F. A., Partington, M. D. & Winston, K. R. (1998). Abusive head trauma? A biomechanics-based approach. *Child Maltreatment*, **3**, 116–28.

Hymel, K. P., Jenny, C. & Block, R. W. (2002). Intracranial hemorrhage and rebleeding in suspected victims of head trauma: addressing the forensic controversies. *Child Maltreatment*, **7**, 329–48.

Hymel, K. P., Rumack, C. M., Hay, T. C., Strain, J. D. & Jenny, C. (1997b). Comparison of intracranial computed tomographic (CT) findings in pediatric abusive and accidental head trauma. *Pediatric Radiology*, **27**, 743–7.

Istre, G. R., Gustafson, T. L., Baron, R. C., Martin, D. L. & Orlowski, J. P. (1985). A mysterious cluster of deaths and cardiopulmonary arrests in a pediatric intensive care unit. *New England Journal of Medicine*, **313**, 205–11.

Ito, Y., Tsuda, R. & Kimura, H. (1989). Diagnostic value of the placenta in medico-legal practice. *Forensic Science International*, **40**, 79–84.

James, D. S. & Leadbeatter, S, (1997). Detecting homicide in hospital. *Journal of the Royal College of Physicians of London*, **31**, 296–8.

Jaudes, P. K. (1984). Comparison of radiography and radionuclide bone scanning in the detection of child abuse. *Pediatrics*, **73**, 166–8.

Jenny, C., Fukuda, T., Rangarajan, N., & Shams, T. (2002). A biomechanical model of abusive infant head trauma. Paper presented to Fourth National Conference on Shaken Baby Syndrome, Salt Lake City, Utah, September 12.

Joffe, M. & Ludwig, S. (1988). Stairway injuries in children. *Pediatrics*, **82**, 457–61.

Johnson, C. F. (1990). Inflicted injury versus accidental injury. *Pediatric Clinics of North America*, **37**, 791–814.

Johnson, C. F. (1994). Symbolic scarring and tattooing. *Clinical Pediatrics*, **33**, 46–9.

Johnson, C. F. & Showers, J. (1985). Injury variables in child abuse. *Child Abuse and Neglect*, **9**, 207–15.

Johnson, D. L., Braun, D. & Friendly, D. (1993). Accidental head trauma and retinal hemorrhage. *Neurosurgery*, **33**, 231–5.

Jureidini, J. N., Shafer, A. T. & Donald, T. G. (2003). "Munchausen by proxy syndrome": not only pathological parenting but also problematic doctoring? *Medical Journal of Australia*, **178**, 130–32.

Kanter, R. K. (1986). Retinal hemorrhage after cardiopulmonary resuscitation or child abuse. *Journal of Pediatrics*, **108**, 430–32.

Kaplan, J. A. & Fossum, R. M. (1994). Patterns of facial resuscitation injury in infancy. *American Journal of Forensic Medicine and Pathology*, **15**, 187–91.

Kaplan, J. A., Siegler, R. W. & Schmunk, G. A. (1998). Fatal hypernatremic dehydration in exclusively breast-fed newborn infants due to maternal lactation failure. *American Journal of Forensic Medicine and Pathology*, **19**, 19–22.

Kaplan, J. M. (1986). Pseudoabuse – the misdiagnosis of child abuse . *Journal of Forensic Sciences*, **31**, 1420–28.

Kaschula, R. O. C. (1995). Malnutrition and intestinal malabsorption. In *Tropical Pathology*, vol. 8, 2nd edn, ed. W. Doerr & G. Seifest. Berlin: Springer-Verlag, pp. 985–1030.

Keeling, J. (1987). *Fetal and Neonatal Pathology*. London: Springer-Verlag.

Kellett, R. J. (1992). Infanticide and child destruction – the historical, legal and pathological aspects. *Forensic Science International*, **53**, 1–28.

Kempe, C. H., Silverman, F. N., Steele, B. F., Droegemueller, W. & Silver, H. K. (1962). The battered-child syndrome. *Journal of the American Medical Association*, **181**, 105–12.

Keogh, S., Gray, J. S., Kirk, C. J. C., Coats, T. J. & Wilson, A. W. (1996). Children falling from a height in London. *Injury Prevention*, **2**, 188–91.

Kern, K. B., Carter, A. B., Showen, R. L., *et al.* (1986). CPR-induced trauma: comparison of three manual methods in an experimental model. *Annals of Emergency Medicine*, **15**, 674–9.

King, W. J., Mackay, M., Sirnick, A. & the Canadian Shaken Baby Study Group (2003). Shaken baby syndrome in Canada: clinical characteristics and outcomes of hospital cases. *Canadian Medical Association Journal*, **168**, 155–9.

Kirschner, R. H. & Stein, R. J. (1985). The mistaken diagnosis of child abuse. A form of medical abuse? *American Journal of Diseases of Children*, **139**, 873–5.

Kleinman, P. K. (1990). Diagnostic imaging in infant abuse. *American Journal of Roentgenology*, **155**, 703–12.

Kleinman, P. K. (1998). Bony thoracic trauma. In *Diagnostic Imaging of Child Abuse*, ed. P. K. Kleinmann. Baltimore: Williams & Wilkins, pp. 67–89.

Kleinman, P. K. & Marks, S. C. (1992). Vertebral body fractures in child abuse. Radiologic-histopathologic correlates. *Investigative Radiology*, **27**, 715–22.

Kleinman, P. K. & Spevak, M. R. (1991) Variations in acromial ossification simulating infant abuse in victims of sudden infant death syndrome. *Radiology*, **180**, 185–7.

Kleinman, P. K. & Zito, J. L. (1984). Avulsion of the spinous processes caused by infant abuse. *Radiology*, **151**, 389–91.

Kleinman, P. K., Marks, S. C. & Blackbourne, B. (1986). The metaphyseal lesion in abused infants: a radiologic-histopathologic study. *American Journal of Roentgenology*, **146**, 895–905.

Kleinman, P. K., Raptopoulos, V. D. & Brill, P. W. (1981). Occult nonskeletal trauma in the battered-child syndrome. *Radiology*, **141**, 393–6.

Klitte, Å., Gilbert, J. D., Lokan, R. & Byard, R. W. (2001). Adolescent suicide due to inhalation of insect spray. *Journal of Clinical Forensic Medicine*, **8**, 22–4.

Knight, B. (1986). The history of child abuse. *Forensic Science International*, **30**, 135–41.

Knight B. (1996). *Forensic Pathology*, 2nd edn. London: Arnold Press.

Knight, D. M., James, R. A., Sims, D. N., *et al.* (1998). Sudden death due to intravenous infusion of hair conditioner. *American Journal of Forensic Medicine and Pathology*, **19**, 252–4.

Koel, B. S. (1969). Failure to thrive and fatal injury as a continuum. *American Journal of Diseases of Children*, **118**, 565–7.

Kohl, S., Pickering, L. K. & Dupree, E. (1978). Child abuse presenting as immunodeficiency disease. *Journal of Pediatrics*, **93**, 466–8.

Kohler, M. & Hoffmann, G. F. (1998). Subdural haematoma in a child with glutaric aciduria type I. *Pediatric Radiology*, **28**, 582.

Kouno, A. (2000). Coin-operated locker babies: murder of unwanted infants and child abuse in Japan. In *Child Suffering in the World. Child Maltreatment by Parents, Culture and Governments in Different Countries and Cultures*, ed. J. A. Marvasti. Manchester, Conn: Sexual Trauma Center Publication, pp. 285–98.

Kouno, A. & Johnson, C. F. (2001). Japan. In *Child Abuse – A Global View*, ed. B. M. Schwartz-Kenney, M. McCauley & M. A. Epstein. Westport, Conn.: Greenwood Press, pp. 99–116.

Kramer, K. & Goldstein, B. (1993). Retinal hemorrhages following cardiopulmonary resuscitation. *Clinical Pediatrics*, **32**, 366–8.

Krous, H. F. & Byard, R. W. (1999). Shaken infant syndrome: selected controversies. *Pediatric and Developmental Pathology*, **2**, 497–8.

Krous, H. F., Nadeau, J., Byard, R. W. & Blackbourne, B. D. (2001). Oronasal blood in sudden infant death. *American Journal of Forensic Medicine and Pathology*, **22**, 346–51.

Krous, H. F., Nadeau, J. M., Silva, P. D. & Byard, R. W. (2002). Infanticide: is its incidence among postneonatal infant deaths increasing? An 18-year population-based analysis in California. *American Journal of Forensic Medicine and Pathology*, **23**, 127–31.

Krugman, R. D. (1986). Recognition of sexual abuse in children. *Pediatrics in Review*, **8**, 25–30.

Langlois, N. E. I. & Gresham, G. A. (1991). The ageing of bruises: a review and study of the colour changes with time. *Forensic Science International*, **50**, 227–38.

Lansky, L. L. (1974). An unusual case of childhood chloral hydrate poisoning. *American Journal of Diseases of Children*, **127**, 275–6.

Leadbeater, S. (2001). Resuscitation injuries. In *Essentials of Autopsy Practice*, vol. 1, ed. G. N. Rutty. London: Springer-Verlag, pp 43–62.

Lee, C. J., Collins, K. A. & Burgess, S. E. (1999). Suicide under the age of eighteen. A 10-year retrospective study. *American Journal of Forensic Medicine and Pathology*, **20**, 27–30.

Lee, D. A. (1979). Munchausen syndrome by proxy in twins. *Archives of Disease in Childhood*, **54**, 646–7.

Leonidas, J. C. (1983). Skeletal trauma in the child abuse syndrome. *Pediatric Annals*, **12**, 875–81.

Levene, S. & Bonfield, G. (1991). Accidents on hospital wards. *Archives of Disease in Childhood*, **66**, 1047–9.

Levin, A. V. (2000). Retinal haemorrhages and child abuse. In *Recent Advances in Paediatrics*, ed. T. J. David. London: Churchill Livingstone, pp. 151–219.

Levin, A. V. & Selbst, S. M. (1988). Vulvar hemangioma simulating child abuse. *Clinical Pediatrics*, **27**, 213–5.

Light, M. J. & Sheridan, M. S. (1990). Munchausen syndrome by proxy and apnea (MBPA). A survey of apnea programs. *Clinical Pediatrics*, **29**, 162–8.

Lindenberg, R. & Freytag, E. (1969). Morphology of brain lesions from blunt trauma in early infancy. *Archives of Pathology*, **87**, 298–305.

Lingam, S. & Joester, J. (1994). Spontaneous fractures in children and adolescents with cerebral palsy. *British Medical Journal*, **309**, 265.

Link, M. S., Wang, P. J., Pandian, N. G., *et al.* (1998). An experimental model of sudden death due to low-energy chest-wall impact (commotio cordis). *New England Journal of Medicine*, **338**, 1805–11.

Liston, T. E., Levine, P. L. & Anderson, C. (1983). Polymicrobial bacteremia due to Polle syndrome: the child abuse variant of Munchausen by proxy. *Pediatrics*, **72**, 211–13.

Little, G. A. & Brooks J. G. (1994). Accepting the unthinkable. *Pediatrics*, **94**, 748–9.

Lorber, J., Reckless, J. P. D. & Watson, J. B. G. (1980). Nonaccidental poisoning: the elusive diagnosis. *Archives of Disease in Childhood*, **55**, 643–7.

Ludwig, S. & Warman, M. (1984). Shaken baby syndrome: a review of 20 cases. *Annals of Emergency Medicine*, **13**, 104–7.

Lyons, T. J. & Oates, R. K. (1993). Falling out of bed: a relatively benign occurrence. *Pediatrics*, **92**, 125–7.

Macgregor, D. M. (2000). Injuries associated with falls from beds. *Injury Prevention*, **6**, 291–2.

Makar, A. F. & Squier, P. J. (1990). Munchausen syndrome by proxy: father as a perpetrator. *Pediatrics*, **85**, 370–73.

Malatack, J. J., Wiener, E. S., Gartner, J. C., Zitelli, B. J. & Brunetti, E. (1985). Munchausen syndrome by proxy: a new complication of central venous catheterization. *Pediatrics*, **75**, 523–5.

Males, M. (1994). California's suicide decline, 1970–1990. *Suicide and Life Threatening Behaviour*, **24**, 24–37.

Margolin, L. (1990). Fatal child neglect. *Child Welfare*, **59**, 309–19.

Marks, M. N. & Kumar, R. (1996). Infanticide in Scotland. *Medicine, Science and the Law*, **36**, 299–305.

Maron, B. J., Gohman, T. E., Kyle, S. B., Estes, N. A., III & Link, N. S. (2002). Clinical profile and spectrum of commotio cordis. *Journal of the American Medical Association*, **287**, 1142–6.

Maron, B. J., Mitten, M. J., & Greene Burnett, C. (2002). Criminal consequences of commotio cordis. *American Journal of Cardiology*, **89**, 210–13.

Marshall, W. N., Jr, Puls, T. & Davidson, C. D. (1988). New child abuse spectrum in an era of increased awareness. *American Journal of Diseases of Children*, **142**, 664–7.

Marzuk, P. M., Tardiff, K. & Hirsch, C. S. (1992). The epidemiology of murder-suicide. *Journal of the American Medical Association*, **267**, 3179–83.

Matsumura, F. & Ito, Y. (1996). Petechial hemorrhage of the conjunctiva and histological findings of the lung and pancreas in infantile asphyxia – evaluation of 85 cases. *Kurume Medical Journal*, **43**, 259–66.

Maxeiner, H. (1997). Detection of ruptured cerebral bridging veins at autopsy. *Forensic Science International*, **89**, 103–10.

Maxeiner, H. (2001). Demonstration and interpretation of bridging vein ruptures in cases of infantile subdural bleedings. *Journal of Forensic Sciences*, **46**, 82–90.

Mayr, J. M., Seebacher, U., Schimpl, G. & Fiala, F. (1999). Highchair accidents. *Acta Paediatrica*, **88**, 319–22.

McCann, J. (1990). Use of the colposcope in childhood sexual abuse examinations. *Pediatric Clinics of North America*, **37**, 863–80.

McCann, J., Reay, D., Siebert, J., Stephens, B. G. & Wirtz, S. (1996). Postmortem perianal findings in children. *American Journal of Forensic Medicine and Pathology*, **17**, 289–98.

McCann, J., Voris, J. & Simon, M. (1988). Labial adhesions and posterior fourchette injuries in childhood sexual abuse. *American Journal of Diseases in Childhood*, **142**, 659–63.

McClain, P. W., Sacks, J. J, Froehlke, R. G. & Ewigman, B. G. (1993). Estimates of fatal child abuse and neglect, United States, 1979 through 1988. *Pediatrics*, **91**, 338–43.

McGrory, B. E. & Fenichel, G. M., (1977). Hangman's fracture subsequent to shaking in an infant. *Annals of Neurology*, **2**, 82.

McLellan, N. J., Prasad, R. & Punt, J. (1986). Spontaneous subhyaloid and retinal haemorrhages in an infant. *Archives of Disease in Childhood*, **61**, 1130–32.

McLoughlin, E. & Crawford, J. D. (1985). Burns. *Pediatric Clinics of North America*, **32**, 61–75.

McNeese, M. C. & Hebeler, J. R. (1977). The abused child, a clinical approach to identification and management. *Ciba Clinical Symposia*, **29**, 1–36.

Meade, J. L. & Brissie, R. M. (1985). Infanticide by starvation: calculation of caloric deficit to determine degree of deprivation. *Journal of Forensic Sciences*, **30**, 1263–8.

Meadow, R. (1977). Munchausen syndrome by proxy. The hinterland of child abuse. *Lancet*, **2**, 343–5.

Meadow, R. (1984a). Munchausen by proxy and brain damage. *Developmental Medicine and Child Neurology*, **26**, 672–4.

Meadow, R. (1984b). Factitious illness – the hinterland of child abuse. In *Recent Advances in Paediatrics*, no. 7, ed. R. Meadow. New York: Churchill Livingstone, pp. 217–32.

Meadow, R. (1985). Management of Munchausen syndrome by proxy. *Archives of Disease in Childhood*, **60**, 385–93.

Meadow, R. (1989). Suffocation. *British Medical Journal*, **298**, 1572–3.

Meadow, R. (1990). Suffocation, recurrent apnea, and sudden infant death. *Journal of Pediatrics*, **117**, 351–7.

Meadow, R. (1993a). Non-accidental salt poisoning. *Archives of Disease in Childhood*, **68**, 448–52.

Meadow, R. (1993b). False allegations of abuse and Munchausen syndrome by proxy. *Archives of Disease in Childhood*, **68**, 444–7.

Meadow, R. (1995). What is, and what is not, "Munchausen syndrome by proxy"? *Archives of Disease in Childhood*, **72**, 534–8.

Meadow, R. (1998). Munchausen syndrome by proxy abuse perpetrated by men. *Archives of Disease in Childhood*, **78**, 210–16.

Meadow, R. (1999). Unnatural sudden infant death. *Archives of Disease in Childhood*, **80**, 7–14.

Meadow, R. (2002). Different interpretations of Munchausen syndrome by proxy. *Child Abuse and Neglect*, **26**, 501–8.

Meadow, R. & Lennert, T. (1984). Munchausen by proxy or Polle syndrome: which term is correct? *Pediatrics*, **74**, 554–6.

Medana, I. M. & Esiri, M. M. (2003). Axonal damage: a key predictor of outcome in human CNS diseases. *Brain*, **126**, 515–30.

Mendlowicz, M. V., Jean-Louis, G., Gekker, M. & Rapaport, M. H. (1999). Neonaticide in the city of Rio de Janeiro: forensic and psycholegal perspectives. *Journal of Forensic Sciences*, **44**, 741–5.

Merten, D. F., Radkowski, M. A. & Leonidas, J. C. (1983). The abused child: a radiological reappraisal. *Radiology*, **146**, 377–81.

Meservy, C. J., Towbin, R., McLaurin, R. L., Myers, P. A. & Ball, W. (1987). Radiographic characteristics of skull fractures resulting from child abuse. *American Journal of Roentgenology*, **149**, 173–5.

Milroy, C. M. (1993). Homicide followed by suicide (dyadic death) in Yorkshire and Humberside. *Medicine, Science and the Law*, **33**, 167–71.

Milroy, C. M. (1995a). The epidemiology of homicide-suicide (dyadic death). *Forensic Science International*, **71**, 117–22.

Milroy, C. M. (1995b). Reasons for homicide and suicide in episodes of dyadic death in Yorkshire and Humberside. *Medicine, Science and the Law*, **35**, 213–17.

Milroy, C. M. (1999). Munchausen syndrome by proxy and intra-alveolar haemosiderin. *International Journal of Legal Medicine*, **112**, 309–12.

Milroy, C. M., Dratsas, M. & Ranson, D. L. (1997). Homicide-suicide in Victoria, Australia. *American Journal of Forensic Medicine and Pathology*, **18**, 369–73.

Minford, A. M. B. (1981). Child abuse presenting as apparent "near-miss" sudden infant death syndrome. *British Medical Journal*, **282**, 521.

Mitchell, E. K & Davis, J. H. (1984). Spontaneous births into toilets. *Journal of Forensic Sciences*, **29**, 591–6.

Mitchell, I., Brummitt, J., DeForest, J. & Fisher, G. (1993). Apnea and factitious illness (Munchausen syndrome) by proxy. *Pediatrics*, **92**, 810–14.

Mitchell, E., Krous, H. F. & Byard, R. W. (2002). Pathological findings in overlaying. *Journal of Clinical Forensic Medicine*, **9**, 133–5.

Montrey, J. S. & Barcia, P. J. (1985). Nonaccidental burns in child abuse. *Southern Medical Journal*, **78**, 1324–6.

Moore, L. & Byard, R. W. (1993). Pathological findings in hanging and wedging deaths in infants and young children. *American Journal of Forensic Medicine and Pathology*, **14**, 296–302.

Morley, C. J. (1995). Practical concerns about the diagnosis of Munchausen syndrome by proxy. *Archives of Disease in Childhood*, **72**, 528–38.

Morris, B. (1985). Child abuse manifested as factitious apnea. *Southern Medical Journal*, **78**, 1013–14.

Mortimer, J. C. (1980). Acute water intoxication as another unusual manifestation of child abuse. *Archives of Disease in Childhood*, **55**, 401–3.

Mukherji, B. K. & Siegel, M. J. (1987). Rhabdomyolysis and renal failure in child abuse. *American Journal of Roentgenology*, **148**, 1203–4.

Munger, C. E., Peiffer, R. L., Bouldin, T. W., Kylstra, J. A. & Thompson, R. L. (1993). Ocular and associated neuropathologic observations in suspected whiplash shaken infant syndrome. *American Journal of Forensic Medicine and Pathology*, **14**, 193–200.

Munro, H. M. C. & Thrusfield, M. V. (2001a). 'Battered pets': features that raise suspicion of non-accidental injury. *Journal of Small Animal Practice*, **42**, 218–26.

Munro, H. M. C. & Thrusfield, M. V. (2001b). 'Battered pets': Munchausen syndrome by proxy (factitious illness by proxy). *Journal of Small Animal Practice*, **42**, 385–9.

Murray, J. A., Chen, D., Velmahos, G. C., *et al.* (2000). Pediatric falls: is height a predictor of injury and outcome? *American Surgeon*, **66**, 863–5.

Musemeche, C. A., Barthel, M., Cosentino, C. & Reynolds, M. (1991). Pediatric falls from heights. *Journal of Trauma*, **31**, 1347–9.

Nashelsky, M. B. & Dix, J. D. (1995). The time interval between lethal infant shaking and onset of symptoms. A review of the shaken baby syndrome literature. *American Journal of Forensic Medicine and Pathology*, **16**, 154–7.

Nassogne, M. C., Sharrard, M., Hertz-Pannier, L., *et al.* (2002). Massive subdural haematomas in Menkes disease mimicking shaken baby syndrome. *Child's Nervous System*, **18**, 729–31.

Newton, R. W. (1989). Intracranial haemorrhage and non-accidental injury. *Archives of Disease in Childhood*, **64**, 188–90.

Nichols, G. R., Corey, T. S. & Davis, G. J. (1990). Case report: nonfracture-associated fatal fat embolism in a case of child abuse. *Journal of Forensic Sciences*, **35**, 493–9.

Nields, H., Kessler, S. C., Boisot, S. & Evans, R. (1998). Streptococcal toxic shock syndrome presenting as suspected child abuse. *American Journal of Forensic Medicine and Pathology*, **19**, 93–7.

Niess, C., Grauel, U., Toennes, S. W., & Bratzke, H. (2002). Incidence of axonal injury in human brain tissue. *Acta Neuropathologica*, **104**, 79–84.

Nimityongskul, P. & Anderson, L. D. (1987). The likelihood of injuries when children fall out of bed. *Journal of Pediatric Orthopedics*, **7**, 184–6.

Nixon, J. & Pearn, J. (1977). Non-accidental immersion in bath-water: another aspect of child abuse. *British Medical Journal*, **i**, 271–2.

Ober, W. B. (1986). Infanticide in eighteenth-century England. William Hunter's contribution to the forensic problem. *Pathology Annual*, **21**, 311–19.

Oehmichen, M., Meissner, C., Schmidt, V., Pedal, I. & Konig, H. G. (1999). Pontine axonal injury after brain trauma and nontraumatic hypoxic-ischemic brain damage. *International Journal of Legal Medicine*, **112**, 261–7.

Ogata, M. & Tsuganezawa, O. (1995). An isolated perforation of the jejunum caused by child abuse. *American Journal of Forensic Medicine and Pathology*, **16**, 17–20.

O'Hare, A. E. & Eden, O. B. (1984). Bleeding disorders and non-accidental injury. *Archives of Disease in Childhood*, **69**, 860–64.

Olazagasti, J. C., Fitzgerald, J. F., White, S. J. & Chong, S. K. F. (1994). Chylous ascites: a sign of unsuspected child abuse. *Pediatrics*, **94**, 737–9.

Ommaya, A. K., Goldsmith, W. & Thibault, L. (2002). Biomechanics and neuropathology of adult and paediatric head injury. *British Journal of Neurosurgery*, **16**, 220–42.

Ophthalmology Child Abuse Working Party. (1999). Child abuse and the eye. *Eye*, **13**, 3–10.

Orenstein, D. M. & Wasserman, A. L. (1986). Munchausen syndrome by proxy simulating cystic fibrosis. *Pediatrics*, **78**, 621–4.

Orr, C. J., Clark, M. A., Hawley, D. A., *et al.* (1995). Fatal anorectal injuries: a series of four cases. *Journal of Forensic Sciences*, **40**, 219–21.

Osmond, M. H., Brennan-Barnes, M. & Shephard, A. L. (2002). A 4-year review of severe pediatric trauma in eastern Ontario: a descriptive analysis. *Journal of Trauma*, **52**, 8–12.

Overpeck, M. D., Brenner, R. A., Trumble, A. C., Trifiletti, L. B. & Berendes, H. W (1998). Risk factors for infant homicide in the United States. *New England Journal of Medicine*, **339**, 1211–16.

Owen, S. M. & Durst, R. D. (1984). Ehlers–Danlos syndrome simulating child abuse. *Archives of Dermatology*, **120**, 97–101.

Palermo, G. B., Smith, M. B., Jentzen, J. M., *et al.* (1997). Murder-suicide of the jealous paranoia type. A multicenter statistical pilot study. *American Journal of Forensic Medicine and Pathology*, **18**, 374–83.

Paradise, J. E. (1990). The medical evaluation of the sexually abused child. *Pediatric Clinics of North America*, **37**, 839–62.

Partridge, J. C., Payne, M. L., Leisgang, J. J., Randolph, J. F. & Rubinstein, J. H. (1981). Water intoxication secondary to feeding mismanagement. A preventable form of familial seizure disorder in infants. *American Journal of Diseases of Children*, **135**, 38–41.

Pascoe, J. M., Hildebrandt, H. M., Tarrier, A. & Murphy, M. (1979). Patterns of skin injury in nonaccidental and accidental injury. *Pediatrics*, **64**, 245–7.

Paul, D. M. (1990). The pitfalls which may be encountered during an examination for signs of sexual abuse. *Medicine, Science and the Law*, **30**, 3–11.

Peinkofer, J. R. (2002). *Silenced Angels. The Medical, Legal, and Social Aspects of Shaken Baby Syndrome*. Westport, Conn: Auburn House.

Pena, S. D. J. & Medovy, H. (1973). Child abuse and traumatic pseudocyst of the pancreas. *Journal of Pediatrics*, **83**, 1026–8.

Perrot, L. J. (1988). Amitriptyline overdose versus sudden infant death syndrome in a two-month-old white female. *Journal of Forensic Sciences*, **33**, 272–5.

Perrot, L. J. (1989). Masque echymotique. Specific or nonspecific indicator for abuse. *American Journal of Forensic Medicine and Pathology*, **10**, 95–7.

Pickel, S., Anderson, C. & Holliday, M. A. (1970). Thirsting and hypernatremic dehydration – a form of child abuse. *Pediatrics*, **45**, 54–9.

Pierce, A. M. & Robson, W. J. (1993). Genital injury in girls – accidental or not? *Pediatric Surgery International*, **8**, 239–43.

Pitt, S. E. & Bale, E. M. (1995). Neonaticide, infanticide and filicide: a review of the literature. *Bulletin of the American Academy of Psychiatry and Law*, **23**, 375–86.

Plunkett, J. (1999). Shaken baby syndrome and the death of Matthew Eappen. A forensic pathologist's response. *American Journal of Forensic Medicine and Pathology*, **20**, 17–21.

Plunkett, J. (2001). Fatal pediatric head injuries caused by short-distance falls. *American Journal of Forensic Medicine and Pathology*, **22**, 1–12.

Pounder, D. J. (1997). Shaken adult syndrome. *American Journal of Forensic Medicine and Pathology*, **18**, 321–4.

Prescott, P. R. (1990). Hair dryer burns in children. *Pediatrics*, **86**, 692–7.

Press, S., Grant, P., Thompson, V. T. & Milles, K. L. (1991). Small bowel evisceration: unusual manifestation of child abuse. *Pediatrics*, **88**, 807–9.

Price, E. A., Rush, L. R., Perper, J. A. & Bell, M. D. (2000). Cardiopulmonary resuscitation-related injuries and homicidal blunt abdominal trauma in children. *American Journal of Forensic Medicine and Pathology*, **21**, 307–10.

Purdue, G. F., Hunt, J. L. & Prescott, P. R. (1988). Child abuse by burning – an index of suspicion. *Journal of Trauma*, **28**, 221–4.

Putnam, N. & Stein, M. (1985). Self-inflicted injuries in childhood. A review and diagnostic approach. *Clinical Pediatrics*, **24**, 514–18.

Radkowski, M. A. (1983). The battered child syndrome: pitfalls in radiological diagnosis. *Pediatric Annals*, **12**, 894–903.

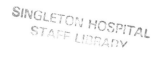

Raimer, B. G., Raimer, S. S. & Hebeler, J. R. (1981). Cutaneous signs of child abuse. *Journal of the American Academy of Dermatology*, **5**, 203–12.

Ramenofsky, M. L. (1987). Pediatric abdominal trauma. *Pediatric Annals*, **16**, 318–26.

Ramu, M. (1977). Needles in a child's body (a case report). *Medicine, Science and the Law*, **17**, 259–60.

Rao, N., Smith R. E., Choi, J. H., Xiaohu, X. & Kornblum, R. N. (1988). Autopsy findings in the eyes of fourteen fatally abused children. *Forensic Science International*, **39**, 293–9.

Reardon, M. J., Gross, D. M., Vallone, A. M., Weiland, A. P. & Walker, W. E. (1987). Atrial rupture in a child from cardiac massage by his parent. *Annals of Thoracic Surgery*, **43**, 557–8.

Reardon, W., Hughes, H. E., Green, S. H., Woolley, V. L. & Harper, P. S. (1992). Anal abnormalities in childhood myotonic dystrophy – a possible source of confusion in child sexual abuse. *Archives of Disease in Childhood*, **67**, 527–8.

Reece, R. M. (1990). Unusual manifestations of child abuse. *Pediatric Clinics of North America*, **37**, 905–21.

Reece, R. M & Grodin, M. A. (1985). Recognition of nonaccidental injury. *Pediatric Clinics of North America*, **32**, 41–60.

Reece, R. M. & Sege, R. (2000). Childhood head injuries: accidental or inflicted? *Archives of Pediatric and Adolescent Medicine*, **154**, 11–15.

Rees, A., Symons, J., Joseph, M. & Lincoln, C. (1975). Ventricular septal defect in a battered child. *British Medical Journal*, **1**, 20–21.

Reiber, G. D. (1993). Fatal falls in childhood. How far must children fall to sustain fatal head injury? Report of cases and review of the literature. *American Journal of Forensic Medicine and Pathology*, **14**, 201–7.

Riffenburgh, R. S. & Sathyavagiswaran, L. (1991). The eyes of child abuse victims: autopsy findings. *Journal of Forensic Sciences*, **36**, 741–7.

Rimsza, M. E., Schackner, R. A., Bowen, K. A. & Marshall W. (2002). Can child deaths be prevented? The Arizona Child Fatality Review Program experience. *Pediatrics*, **110** (1 part 1), e11.

Rivara, F. P., Kamitsuka, M. D. & Quan, L. (1988). Injuries to children younger than 1 year of age. *Pediatrics*, **81**, 93–7.

Rizzolo, P. J. & Coleman, P. R. (1989). Neonatal rib fracture: birth trauma or child abuse? *Journal of Family Practice*, **29**, 561–3.

Roberton, D. M., Barbor, P. & Hull, D. (1982). Unusual injury? Recent injury in normal children and children with suspected non-accidental injury. *British Medical Journal*, **285**, 1399–401.

Roberts, I. F., West, R. J., Ogilvie, D. & Dillon M. J. (1979). Malnutrition in infants receiving cult diets: a form of child abuse. *British Medical Journal*, **ii**, 296–8.

Robinson, R. (1991). Physical signs of sexual abuse in children. *British Medical Journal*, **302**, 863–4.

Roesler, J. (1997). The incidence of child suicide in Minnesota. *Minnesota Medicine*, **80**, 45–7.

Root, I. (1992). Head injuries from short distance falls. *American Journal of Forensic Medicine and Pathology*, **13**, 85–7.

Rosen, C. L., Frost, J. D., Jr, Bricker, T., *et al.* (1983). Two siblings with recurrent cardiorespiratory arrest: Munchausen syndrome by proxy or child abuse? *Pediatrics*, **71**, 715–20.

Rosenberg, D. A. (1987). Web of deceit: a literature review of Munchausen syndrome by proxy. *Child Abuse and Neglect*, **11**, 547–63.

Roshkow, J. E., Haller, J. O., Hotson, G. C., *et al.* (1990). Imaging evaluation of children after falls from a height: review of 45 cases. *Radiology*, **175**, 359–63.

Ross, J. D. C., Scott, G. R. & Busuttil, A. (1993). Condylomata acuminata in pre-pubertal children. *Medicine, Science and the Law*, **33**, 78–82.

Rossignol, A. M., Locke, J. A. & Burke, J. F. (1990). Paediatric burn injuries in New England, USA. *Burns*, **16**, 41–8.

Russo, S., Taff, M. I., Mirchandani, H. G., Monforte, J. R. & Spitz, W. U. (1986). Scald burns complicated by isopropyl alcohol intoxication. A case of fatal child abuse. *American Journal of Forensic Medicine and Pathology*, **7**, 81–3.

Ryan, C. A., Shankowsky, H. A. & Tredget, E. E. (1992). Profile of the paediatric burn patient in a Canadian burn center. *Burns*, **18**, 267–72.

Samuels, M. P. & Southall, D. P. (1992). Munchausen syndrome by proxy. *British Journal of Hospital Medicine*, **47**, 759–62.

Samuels, M. P., McClaughlin, W., Jacobson, R. R., Poets, C. F. & Southall, D. P. (1992). Fourteen cases of imposed upper airway obstruction. *Archives of Disease in Childhood*, **67**, 162–70.

Sanders, M. J. & Bursch, B. (2002). Forensic assessement of illness falsification, Muchausen by proxy, and factitious disorder, NOS. *Child Maltreatment*, **7**, 112–24.

Sarvesvaran, E. R. (1992). Homicide by starvation. *American Journal of Forensic Medicine and Pathology*, **13**, 264–7.

Saternus, K.-S., Kernbach-Wighton, G. & Oehmichen, M. (2000). The shaking trauma in infants – kinetic chains. *Forensic Science International*, **109**, 203–13.

Sato, Y., Yuh, W. T., Smith, W. L., *et al.* (1989). Head injury in child abuse: evaluation with MR imaging. *Radiology*, **173**, 653–7.

Saulsbury, F. T., Chobanian, M. C. & Wilson, W. G. (1984). Child abuse: parenteral hydrocarbon administration. *Pediatrics*, **73**, 719–22.

Saunders E. (1989). Neonaticides following 'secret' pregnancies: seven case reports. *Public Health Reports*, **104**, 368–72.

Schaber, B., Hart, A. P., Armbrustmacher, V. & Hirsch, C. S. (2002). Fatal pediatric head injuries caused by short distance falls.

American Journal of Forensic Medicine and Pathology, **23**, 101–3.

Schloff, S., Mullaney, P. B., Armstrong, D. C., *et al.* (2002). Retinal findings in children with intracranial hemorrhage. *Ophthalmology*, **109**, 1472–6.

Schmitt, B. D., Gray, J. D. & Britton, H. L. (1978). Car seat burns in infants: avoiding confusion with inflicted burns. *Pediatrics*, **62**, 607–9.

Schreier, H. (2002). Munchausen by proxy defined. *Pediatrics*, **110**, 985–8.

Schwartz, A. J. & Ricci, L. R. (1996). How accurately can bruises be aged in abused children? Literature review and synthesis. *Pediatrics*, **97**, 254–7.

Selbst, S. M., Baker, M. D. & Shames, M. (1990). Bunk bed injuries. *American Journal of Diseases in Children*, **144**, 721–3.

Shabde, N. & Craft, A. W. (1999). Covert video surveillance: an important investigative tool or a breach of trust? *Archives of Disease in Childhood*, **82**, 291–4.

Shannon, P. & Becker, L. (2001). Mechanisms of brain injury in infantile child abuse. *Lancet*, **358**, 686–7.

Shannon, P., Smith, C. R., Deck, J., *et al.* (1998). Axonal injury and the neuropathology of shaken baby syndrome. *Acta Neuropathologica*, **95**, 625–31.

Sharon, D. (1978). *Wizard of the Four Winds. A Shaman's Story.* New York: The Free Press.

Shinebourne, E. A. (1996). Covert video surveillance continues to provoke debate. *Journal of Medical Ethics*, **22**, 351.

Shnaps, Y., Frand, M., Rotem, Y. & Tirosh, M. (1981). The chemically abused child. *Pediatrics*, **68**, 119–21.

Showers, J. & Bandman, R. L. (1986). Scarring for life: abuse with electric cords. *Child Abuse and Neglect*, **10**, 25–31.

Showers, J. & Garrison, K. M. (1988). Burn abuse: a four-year study. *Journal of Trauma*, **28**, 1581–3.

Shugerman, R. P., Paez, A., Grossman, D. C., Feldman, K. W. & Grady, M. S. (1996). Epidural hemorrhage: is it abuse? *Pediatrics*, **97**, 664–8.

Sivit, C. J., Taylor, G. A. & Eichelberger, M. R. (1989). Visceral injury in battered children: a changing perspective. *Radiology*, **173**, 659–61.

Skuse, D. H. (1985). Non-organic failure to thrive: a reappraisal. *Archives of Disease in Childhood*, **60**, 173–8.

Skuse, D. H., Gill, D., Reilly, S., Wolke, D. & Lynch, M. A. (1995). Failure to thrive and the risk of child abuse: a prospective population survey. *Journal of Medical Screening*, **2**, 145–9.

Slosberg, E. J., Ludwig, S., Ducket, J. & Mauro, A. E. (1978). Penile trauma as a sign of child abuse. *American Journal of Diseases of Children* **132**, 719–21.

Smialek, J. E. & Lambros, Z. (1988). Investigation of sudden infant deaths. *Pediatrician*, **15**, 191–7.

Smith, S. L., Andrus, P. K., Gleason, D. D. & Hall, E. D. (1998). Infant rat model of the shaken baby syndrome: preliminary characterization and evidence for the role of free radicals in cortical hemorrhaging and progressive neuronal degeneration. *Journal of Neurotrauma*, **15**, 693–705.

Smith, M. D., Burrington, J. D. & Woolf, A. D. (1975). Injuries in children sustained in free falls: an analysis of 66 cases. *Journal of Trauma*, **15**, 987–91.

Smith, G. A., Dietrich, A. M., Garcia, C. T. & Shields, B. J. (1996). Injuries to children related to shopping carts. *Pediatrics*, **97**, 161–5.

Somander, L. K. H, Rammer, L. M. (1991). Intra- and extra-familial child homicide in Sweden, 1971–1980. *Child Abuse and Neglect*, **15**, 45–5.

Souid, A.-K., Keith, D. V. & Cunningham, A. S. (1998). Munchausen syndrome by proxy. *Clinical Pediatrics*, **37**, 497–504.

Southall, D. P., Plunkett, M. C. B., Banks, M. W., Falkov, A. F. & Samuels, M. P. (1997). Covert video recordings of life-threatening child abuse: lessons for child protection. *Pediatrics*, **100**, 735–60.

Southall, D. P., Stebbens, V. A., Rees, S. V., *et al.* (1987). Apnoeic episodes induced by smothering: two cases identified by covert video surveillance. *British Medical Journal*, **294**, 1637–41.

Spaide, R. F., Swengel, R. M., Scharre, D. W. & Mein, C. E. (1990). Shaken baby syndrome. *American Family Physician*, **41**, 1145–52.

Spevak, M. R., Kleinman, P. K., Belanger, P. L., Primack, C. & Richmond, J. M. (1994). Cardiopulmonary resuscitation and rib fractures in infants. A postmortem radiologic-pathologic study. *Journal of the American Medical Association*, **272**, 617–18.

Spinelli MG. (2001). A systemic investigation of 16 cases of neonaticide. *American Journal of Psychiatry*, **158**, 811–13.

Spitz, W. U. & Fisher, R. S. (1980). *Medicolegal Investigation of Death*, 2nd edn. Springfield, Ill. Charles Thomas.

Starling, S. P., Holden, J. R. & Jenny, C. (1995). Abusive head trauma: the relationship of perpetrators to their victims. *Pediatrics*, **95**, 259–62.

Steinschneider, A. (1972). Prolonged apnea and the sudden infant death syndrome: clinical and laboratory observations. *Pediatrics*, **50**, 646–54.

Stephenson, T. & Bialas, Y. (1996). Estimation of the age of bruising. *Archives of Disease in Childhood*, **74**, 53–5.

Sturner, W. Q. (1998). Common errors in forensic pediatric pathology. *American Journal of Forensic Medicine and Pathology*, **19**, 317–20.

Taitz, L. S. (1991). Child abuse and metabolic bone disease: are they often confused? *British Medical Journal*, **302**, 1244.

Tarantino, C. A., Dowd, M. D. & Murdock, T. C. (1999). Short vertical falls in infants. *Pediatric Emergency Care*, **15**, 5–8.

Taylor, D. (2000). Unnatural injuries. *Eye*, **14**, 123–50.

Templeton, J. M. (1993). Mechanism of injury: biomechanics. In *Pediatric Trauma*, ed. M. R. Eichelberger. St Louis: Mosby, pp. 20–36.

Thomas, S. A., Rosenfield, N. S., Leventhal, J. M. & Markowitz, R. I. (1991). Long-bone fractures in young children: distinguishing accidental injuries from child abuse. *Pediatrics*, **88**, 471–6.

Thomsen, T. K., Elle, B. & Thomsen, J. L. (1997). Post-mortem radiological examination in infants: evidence of child abuse? *Forensic Science International*, **90**, 223–30.

Tomasi, L. G. & Rosman, N. P. (1975). Purtscher retinopathy in the battered child syndrome. *American Journal of Diseases of Children*, **129**, 1335–7.

Touloukian, R. J. (1968). Abdominal visceral injuries in battered children. *Pediatrics*, **42**, 642–6.

Turner, M. S. & Jumbelic, M. I. (2003). Stun gun injuries in the abuse and death of a seven-month-old infant. *Journal of Forensic Sciences*, **48**, 180–82.

Valdes-Dapena, M. (1982). The pathologist and the sudden infant death syndrome . *American Journal of Pathology*, **106**, 118–31.

Verity, C. M., Winckworth, C., Burman, D., Stevens, D. & White, R. J. (1979). Polle syndrome: children of Munchausen. *British Medical Journal*, **2**, 422–3.

Vinchon, M., Noizet, O., Defoort-Dhellemmes, S., Soto-Ares, G. & Dhellemmes, P. (2002). Infantile subdural hematomas due to traffic accidents. *Pediatric Neurosurgery*, **37**, 245–53.

Wagner, G. N. (1986). Crime scene investigation in child-abuse cases. *American Journal of Forensic Medicine and Pathology*, **7**, 94–9.

Waldman, P. J., Walters, B. L. & Grunau, C. F. (1984). Pancreatic injury associated with interposed abdominal compressions in pediatric cardiopulmonary resuscitation. *American Journal of Emergency Medicine*, **2**, 510–12.

Walker, P. L., Cook, D. C. & Lambert, P. M. (1997). Skeletal evidence for child abuse: a physical anthropological perspective. *Journal of Forensic Sciences*, **42**, 196–207.

Wang, M. Y., Kim, K. A., Griffith, P. H., *et al.* (2001). Injuries from falls in the pediatric population: an analysis of 729 cases. *Journal of Pediatric Surgery*, **36**, 1528– 34.

Warrington, S. A., Wright, C. M. & the ALSPAC Study Team (2001). Accidents and resulting injuries in premobile infants: data from the ALSPAC study. *Archives of Disease in Childhood*, **85**, 104–7.

Weedn, V. W., Mansour, A. M. & Nichols, M. M. (1990). Retinal hemorrhage in an infant after cardiopulmonary resuscitation.

American Journal of Forensic Medicine and Pathology, **11**, 79–82.

Wehner, F., Schieffer, M. C. & Wehner, H.-D. (1999). Percentile charts to determine the duration of child abuse by chronic malnutrition. *Forensic Science International*, **102**, 173–80.

Weintraub, M. I. (1995). Expert witness testimony: a time for self-regulation. *Neurology*, **45**, 855–8.

Wells, R. G., Vetter, C. & Laud, P. (2002). Intracranial hemorrhage in children younger than 3 years: prediction of intent. *Archives of Pediatric and Adolescent Medicine*, **156**, 252–7.

West, R., Davies, A & Fenton, T. (1989). Accidental vulval injuries in childhood. *British Medical Journal*, **298**, 1002–3.

Wheeler, D. M. & Hobbs, C. J. (1988). Mistakes in diagnosing non-accidental injury: 10 years' experience. *British Medical Journal*, **296**, 1233–6.

Wheeler, D. S. & Shope, T. R. (1997). Depressed skull fracture in a 7-month old who fell from bed. *Pediatrics*, **100**, 1033–4.

White, S. T., Voter, K. & Perry, J. (1985). Surreptitious warfarin ingestion. *Child Abuse and Neglect*, **9**, 349–2.

Whitehead, F. J., Couper, R. T. L., Moore, L., Bourne, A. J. & Byard, R. W. (1996). Dehydration deaths in infants and children. *American Journal of Forensic Medicine and Pathology*, **17,** 73–8.

Wilkinson, W. S., Han, D. P., Rappley, M. D. & Owings, C. L. (1989). Retinal hemorrhage predicts neurologic injury in the shaken baby syndrome. *Archives of Ophthalmology*, **107**, 1472–4.

Willging, J. P., Bower, C. M. & Cotton, R. T. (1992). Physical abuse of children. A retrospective review and an otolaryngology perspective. *Archives of Otolaryngology and Head and Neck Surgery*, **118**, 584–90.

Williams, R. A. (1991). Injuries in infants and small children resulting from witnessed and corroborated free falls. *Journal of Trauma*, **31**, 1350–52.

Williams, C. & Bevan, V. T. (1988). The secret observation of children in hospital. *Lancet*, **1**, 780–81.

Willman, K. Y., Bank, D. E., Senac, M. & Chadwick, D. L. (1997). Restricting the time of injury in fatal inflicted head injuries. *Child Abuse and Neglect*, **21**, 929–40.

Wilson, E. F. (1977). Estimation of the age of cutaneous contusions in child abuse. *Pediatrics*, **60**, 750–52.

Wissow, L. S. (1995). Child abuse and neglect. *New England Journal of Medicine*, **332**, 1425–31.

Wissow, L. S. (1998). Infanticide. *New England Journal of Medicine*, **339**, 1239–41.

Wyatt, J. P., Wyatt, P. W., Squires, T. J. & Busutill, A. (1998). Hanging deaths in children. *American Journal of Forensic Medicine and Pathology*, **19**, 343–6.

Yoshino, E., Yamaki, T., Higuchi, T., Horikawa, Y. & Hirakawa, K. (1985). Acute brain edema in fatal head injury: analysis by dynamic CT scanning. *Journal of Neurosurgery*, **63**, 830–39.

Yukawa, N., Carter, N., Rutty, G. & Green, M. A. (1999). Intra-alveolar haemorrhage in sudden infant death syndrome: a cause for concern? *Journal of Clinical Pathology*, **52**, 581–7.

Zitelli, B. J., Seltman, M. F. & Shannon, R. M. (1987). Munchausen's syndrome by proxy and its professional partici-pants. *American Journal of Diseases of Children*, **141**, 1099–102.

Zumwalt, R. E. & Hirsch, C. S. (1980). Subtle fatal child abuse. *Human Pathology*, **11**, 167–74.

Zumwalt, R. E. & Hirsch, C. S. (1987). Pathology of fatal child abuse and neglect. In *The Battered Child*, 4th edn, ed. R. E. Helfer & R. S. Kemp. Chicago: University of Chicago Press, pp. 247–85.

Part IV

Natural disease

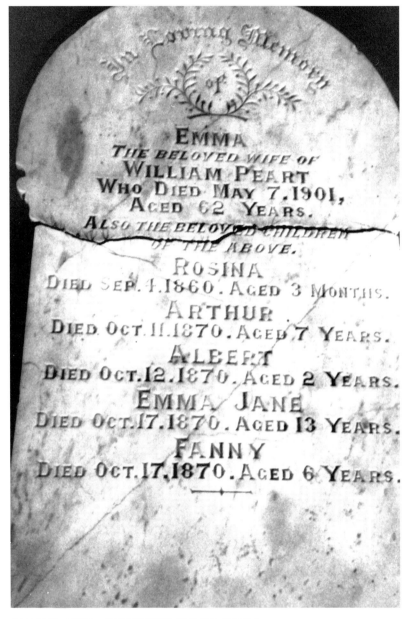

A tombstone located in the corner of a cemetery in Wynyard, North Western Tasmania, showing the devastating effects that epidemics had in previous years. Four children from the same family aged between two and 13 years died within one week in 1870, most likely from complications of infectious disease.

Infectious conditions

Introduction

Sudden death is a well-recognized sequel to infections from a wide variety of agents. The outcome of a particular infection depends on the age of the infant or child, the virulence of the organism, and the immunological status of the host. For example, certain bacteria such as *Neisseria meningitidis* are capable of producing a fulminant septicemia in previously healthy children, with death within hours, whereas *Aspergillus* sp. is generally only of concern in children who are immunodeficient.

In spite of the possibility of a lethal outcome from many "rare" organisms in immunocompromised hosts, this chapter tends to concentrate on more usual clinical syndromes, with only occasional reference to more obscure entities. The format reflects the sequence followed in other chapters of the book, with a discussion of infections based on particular organ systems or mechanisms rather than on specific classes of infectious agents.

On review of pediatric autopsy cases, the most common causes of rapid death are bacterial pneumonias, airway infections (including acute epiglottitis), meningitis, septicemias, viral myocarditis, and gastroenteritis. Table 4.1 lists possible microbiological causes of sudden death in childhood and Appendix VII summarizes the types of microbiological specimens that can be taken in the work-up of a septic case at autopsy.

Cardiovascular conditions

Myocarditis

Myocarditis is a well-known cause of sudden and unexpected death in children of all ages and may be found in infants who present in a similar manner to SIDS (deSa, 1986; Wentworth, Jentz & Croal, 1979).

Clinical features

Although some children may have symptoms and signs of heart failure (deMello *et al.*, 1990), a significant number of cases will have non-specific clinical features, giving no indication of a primary cardiac problem prior to autopsy (Haas, 1988). In children, a history of exercise-related collapse may suggest myocardial disease, and a clinical diagnosis of acute myocardial infarction may have been considered (Hoyer & Fischer, 1991). Sudden death results from an arrhythmia or acute cardiac decompensation.

Etiology

Myocarditis may be caused by a variety of non-infectious agents (see Chapter 5), but it is due most commonly to microbiological agents, in particular coxsackie B viruses (Kaplan *et al.*, 1983). Other viruses such as coxsackie A, polio, Echo, influenza A, adeno, cytomegalovirus, human immunodeficiency virus (HIV), and parvovirus may also cause myocarditis and death due to cardiac involvement (Dettmeyer *et al.*, 2003; Murry, Jerome & Reichenbach, 2001; Sánchez, Neches & Jaffe, 1982; Sun &

Table 4.1. Types of infectious illnesses associated with sudden pediatric death

Cardiovascular	Respiratory	Central nervous system	Hematological	Gastrointestinal	Genitourinary	Generalized
Myocarditis	Tonsillitis					
Rheumatic fever	Retropharyngeal abscess	Meningitis	Malaria	Gastroenteritis	Pyelonephritis	Septicemia
Endocarditis	Posterior lingual abscess	Encephalitis		Botulism	Hemolytic uremic syndrome	Viremia
Aortitis	Acute epiglottitis	Poliomyelitis		Primary peritonitis		Endotoxemia
Arteritis	Acute laryngotracheobronchitis			Hydatid disease		
	Bacterial tracheitis					
	Diphtheria					
	Acute bacterial pneumonia					
	Interstitial pneumonitis					
	Bronchiolitis					
	Tuberculosis					
	Infectious mononucleosis					
	Laryngeal papillomatosis					

Smith, 1984). Table 4.2 lists a variety of possible microbiological causes of myocardial infection.

Pathological features

On inspection at autopsy, the heart may not show any distinctive features, although cardiomegaly is often present, with dilated cardiac chambers and a pale, discolored myocardium (Smith *et al.*, 1992) (Figure 4.1).

The requirements for the diagnosis of myocarditis are an inflammatory cell infiltrate with myocyte necrosis (Aretz *et al.*, 1986) (Figure 4.2). Myocyte necrosis is specified in addition to inflammation, as there is normally a population of lymphocytes within the myocardium at all ages (Tazelaar & Billingham, 1986; Virmani & Roberts, 1987). For example, studies have demonstrated lymphocytic infiltrates in the conduction tracts in completely healthy children who died of trauma (Noren *et al.*, 1977).

Microscopically, the degree of inflammation in affected hearts is variable, with some cases showing

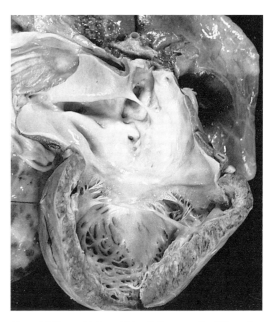

Figure 4.1 Opened left ventricle of a four-month-old boy who suddenly collapsed and died, revealing mottling of the myocardium due to extensive myocarditis.

Table 4.2. Infectious causes of myocarditis

Viruses	Chlamydia	Rickettsia	Mycoplasma	Bacteria	Fungi	Protozoa	Metazoa
Coxsackie A & B	*Chlamydia psittaci*	*Rickettsia typhi*	*Mycoplasma*	Diphtheria	*Aspergillus*	*Trypanosoma*	*Trichinella*
Echo	(psittacosis)	(typhus)	*pneumoniae*	*Salmonella*	*Candida*	*Toxoplasma*	*Echinococcus*
Polio	*Chlamydia*	*Rickettsia*		*Brucella*	*Blastomyces*		
Influenza A and B	*pneumoniaea*	*tsutsugamushi*		Streptococci	*Cryptococci*		
Cytomegalovirus		(scrub typhus)		(β-hemolytic)	*Coccidioidomyces*		
Mumps				Staphylococci			
Rubeola				*Clostridium*			
Rubella				*perfringens*			
Epstein–Barr				*Neisseria meningitidis*			
Adenovirus				*Borrelia burgdorferi*			
HIV							
Varicella zoster							
Variola							
Vaccinia							
Hepatitis B							
Yellow fever							

Adapted from Savoia & Oxman (1990) and Cotran, Kumar & Robbins (1989).

widespread myocyte necrosis with a florid interstitial inflammatory infiltrate composed of lymphocytes, eosinophils, or neutrophils. In other cases, the microscopic changes are more focal. Given the variable distribution of inflammation and necrosis, adequate sampling is required (Hauck, Kearney & Edwards, 1989), although the diagnosis is usually less of a problem with autopsy specimens due to the greater amount of material that is available for examination. Other histologic features in established cases may include myocyte hypertrophy and interstitial fibrosis with scarring (Gravanis & Sternby, 1991). The extent of myocardial damage may occasionally appear out of proportion to the relatively unimpressive clinical symptoms.

Scattered giant cells in some cases arise from degenerating myocytes in so-called giant-cell or Fiedler myocarditis. There is evidence to suggest that this may be an autoimmune disorder dependent on CD-4 positive T-lymphocytes (Cooper, Berry & Shabetai, 1997). Although it is generally a disorder of older individuals and is characterized by congestive cardiac failure, sudden death may occur in both children and adults (Piette & Timperman, 1990); such was the case in a 13-year-old schoolboy who collapsed and died following an apparently mild febrile illness (Figure 4.3). Eosinophilic myocarditis has also been described as a cause of sudden childhood death, possibly triggered by viral infection (Aoki *et al.*, 1996).

Autopsy investigation

An important step in any autopsy in which myocarditis is suspected is the taking of blood and cardiac tissue for microbiological and/or DNA hybridization studies, looking particularly for evidence of coxsackie B viruses (Bowles *et al.*, 1986). Detection of coxsackie B virus-specific immunoglobulin M (IgM) may also be helpful in arriving at a diagnosis (El-Hagrassy, Banatvala & Coltart, 1980). Interpretation of the significance of myocarditis must be undertaken cautiously, however, as studies have also demonstrated genuine myocarditis in apparently well children who suffered sudden death that was unrelated to any form of cardiac disease (Byard, 1997; Claydon, 1989).

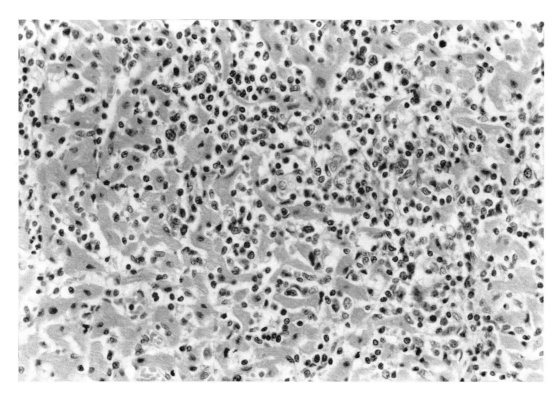

Figure 4.2 Established myocarditis showing a diffuse chronic inflammatory cell infiltrate with associated myocyte necrosis (hematoxylin and eosin, ×280).

Rheumatic fever

Clinical features

Rheumatic fever is a recurrent febrile illness of childhood characterized by subcutaneous nodules, erythema marginatum of the skin, chorea, migratory polyarthralgia, and carditis. It is uncommon nowadays.

Etiology

Rheumatic fever follows a group A streptococcal infection and is believed to be due to immunological cross-reactivity between tissue and streptococcal antigens. In recent years, the incidence of rheumatic fever has declined markedly in Western countries (Taubert, Rowley & Shulman, 1991).

Pathological features

On gross examination, the heart is often enlarged, with dilated chambers and typical vegetations along the margins of the valve leaflets (Figure 4.4). Microscopically, the most characteristic lesions are Aschoff bodies, which consist of round to oval nodules with central fibrinoid degeneration and a surrounding rim of cardiac histiocytes (Lie, 1989). Anitschkow cells are also characteristic and are distinguished by oval vesicular nuclei with centrally aggregated ribbons of chromatin (Josselson, Bagnall & Virmani, 1984). They are also known as "caterpillar cells" (Figure 4.5).

Occurrence of sudden death

Sudden death is a rare complication of rheumatic fever that may occur from early childhood to late

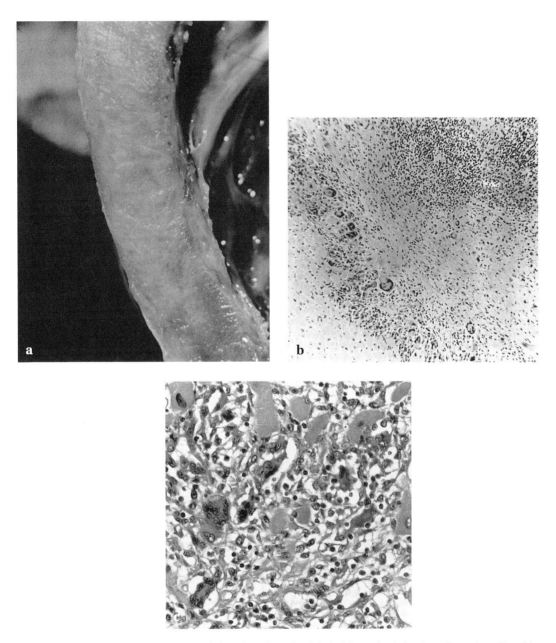

Figure 4.3 Giant cell myocarditis in a 13-year-old boy who collapsed and died while at school, showing pallor and mottling of the myocardium (a), with myocyte necrosis, chronic inflammation, and characteristic giant cell formation (b and c) (hematoxylin and eosin, ×150 and ×440, respectively).

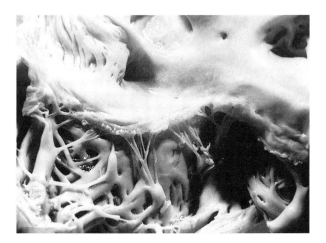

Figure 4.4 Tiny, bead-like valvular vegetations on the tricuspid valve in a 13-year-old girl who died suddenly from acute rheumatic fever.

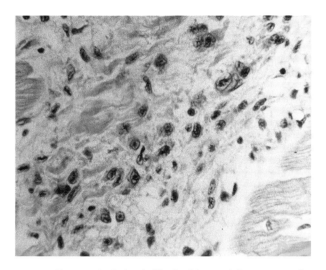

Figure 4.5 Typical Aschoff body of rheumatic fever composed of aggregated cells with vesicular nuclei containing a central ribbon of condensed chromatin, so-called Anitschkow cells (hematoxylin and eosin, ×440).

adolescence. For example, an 18-year-old youth with acute rheumatic valvulitis and myocarditis developed an acute myocardial infarct attributed to embolization of friable valvular vegetations (Josselson, Bagnall & Virmani, 1984; Phillips *et al.*, 1986), and

a three-year-old boy with rheumatic fever died suddenly due to involvement of his coronary arteries (Rae, 1937). A six-year-old girl with florid myocarditis due to rheumatic fever also died suddenly with an embolus into the left anterior descending coronary artery (Figure 4.6).

Endocarditis

Endocarditis is caused by infection of the endocardium or heart valves by a variety of microbiological agents, resulting in vegetation formation.

Etiology

Endocarditis in children usually occurs in those who have underlying defects such as tetralogy of Fallot, ventricular septal defect with aortic incompetence, or left ventricular outflow obstructions, with or without corrective surgery (Atkinson & Virmani, 1987). It also occurs in children who have had rheumatic fever or valve replacements, but it may also be found in children with normal hearts. Endocarditis may be associated with sepsis elsewhere or with in-dwelling vascular catheters. Most cases (>70%) are caused by *Staphylococcus aureus* and *Streptococcus viridans* (Coutlee *et al.*, 1990; Parras *et al.*, 1990).

Clinical features

While early symptoms and signs tend to be relatively non-specific, occasional cases may pursue a fulminant course, with fever, heart failure, and embolic phenomena (Cohle *et al.*, 1989). This is particularly so with staphylococcal endocarditis, where there may be significant valvular damage, erosion of conduction tracts precipitating arrhythmias, or embolization resulting in pulmonary, cerebral, or myocardial infarction. Embolization may also occur with other types of infective endocarditis (Schwöbel & Stauffer, 1983).

Pathological features

At autopsy, the classic lesions of endocarditis of splinter hemorrhages under the nails, subcutaneous

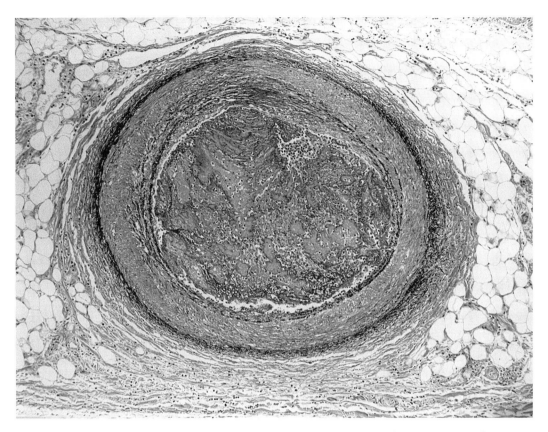

Figure 4.6 Embolized fragment of left ventricular mural thrombus in the left anterior descending coronary artery of a six-year-old girl with florid acute rheumatic fever (hematoxylin and eosin, ×45).

nodules in the fingers and toes (Osler's nodes), and hemorrhagic lesions on the palms and soles (Janeway lesions) are often not visible. Within the heart, the mitral valve is most often affected. Lesions include vegetations, valve perforations, annular abscesses, and rupture of the chordae (Dreyfus *et al.*, 1990).

The gross appearance of vegetations varies depending on the type of endocarditis present (Patterson, Donnelly & Dehner, 1992); however, in bacterial infections they often consist of friable masses of variable size adherent to the valve cusps or leaflets (Figure 4.7). Microscopically, vegetations consist of aggregated cellular debris, fibrin, bacterial colonies, and white blood cells.

Occurrence of sudden death

Death from embolic myocardial infarction has been reported occasionally in infants and older children with endocarditis (Bor, 1969), making careful examination of the coronary arteries important in such cases. A related mechanism of sudden death was demonstrated in an eight-year-old boy with a stenotic bicuspid aortic valve, who developed bacterial infection of the aortic valve cusps and died of an acute myocardial infarct following occlusion of a coronary artery ostium (Figure 4.8).

Death may also occur due to infiltration of inflammatory cells into the underlying myocardium, as in a 12-year-old girl with a permanent pacemaker for postsurgical complete heart block who

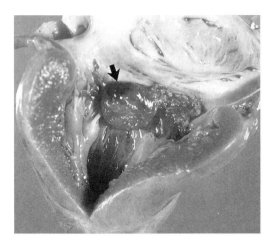

Figure 4.7 Large vegetation (arrow) on the anterior leaflet of the mitral valve of a nine-month old girl with *Staphylococcus aureus* infective endocarditis.

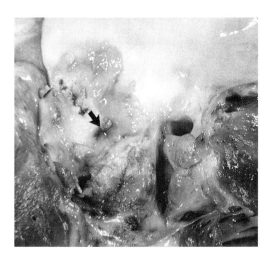

Figure 4.8 Vegetations containing bacteria adherent to the thickened cusp of a dysplastic bicuspid aortic valve in an eight-year-old boy. Involvement of the coronary artery ostium (arrow) resulted in death from an acute myocardial infarct.

died suddenly following several hours of mild, non-specific symptoms. At autopsy, there was a large vegetation containing Gram-positive cocci surrounding the pacemaker lead, with inflammation of the adjacent right atrial wall (Figure 4.9). Her pacemaker tested normally.

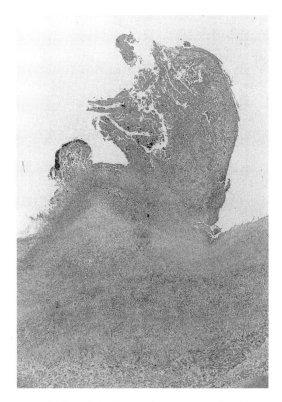

Figure 4.9 Necrotic debris, acute inflammatory cells, and bacterial colonies forming a collar surrounding a pacemaker lead within the right atrium in a 12-year-old girl who died suddenly following an apparently minor febrile illness (hematoxylin and eosin, ×45).

Aortitis

Bacterial infection with vegetation formation, so-called "intimitis," may also involve the aorta in areas of flow disturbance, such as within a patent ductus arteriosus or associated with coarctation (Figure 4.10). Symptoms of infection may be quite non-specific, and sudden death can occur unexpectedly due to rupture of an eroded vessel wall. Death results from hypovolemic shock, or from cardiac tamponade if the aortic root is involved.

Occasionally, the etiology of the inflammation may be uncertain, as was the case of a six-year-old girl who died suddenly from a ruptured ascending aorta following several hours of non-specific malaise and fever (Figure 4.11). At autopsy, focal acute inflammation of the aortic arch was found, with abscess formation and rupture. No organisms were found on microbiological culture or within tissues on Gram and periodic acid Schiff (PAS) staining.

Arteritis

Coronary artery inflammation with thrombosis, myocardial infarction, and death may occur in children with rheumatic fever, syphilis, or endocarditis with abscess formation (Neufeld & Blieden, 1975).

Respiratory conditions

Tonsillitis

Infection of the tonsils by a variety of viral and bacterial agents may result in enlargement, with the potential for upper-airway occlusion. The tonsils may also act as a portal for the entry of a variety of common and less common bacteria, including *Clostridium perfringens* (Gerber, 2001), or as a source of infection for spread to adjacent tissues with abscess formation. This demonstrates the need for careful examination of the upper aerodigestive tract in all cases of unexpected infant and childhood deaths.

Retropharyngeal abscess

Retropharyngeal abscess may result from infection following a penetrating injury to the posterior pharyngeal wall, or in early childhood as a sequel to pharyngitis or tonsillitis. Obstruction to the airway and even sudden death can occur if infection is severe (Regan, 1978; Voigt & Wright, 1974).

Posterior lingual abscess

Acute inflammation in the posterior portion of the tongue may result in occlusion of the upper airway, with unexpected death. A case of sudden death in

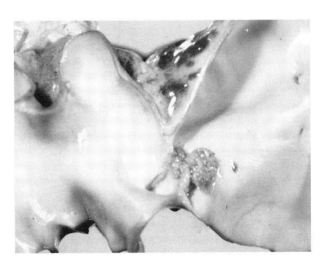

Figure 4.10 Vegetations at the site of coarctation of the aorta.

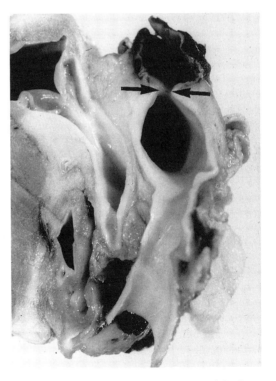

Figure 4.11 Rupture of the aortic arch (arrows) with focal acute inflammation in a six-year-old girl with minimal preceding symptoms. No structural abnormalities or migrated foreign bodies were present. The pulmonary outflow tract is adjacent.

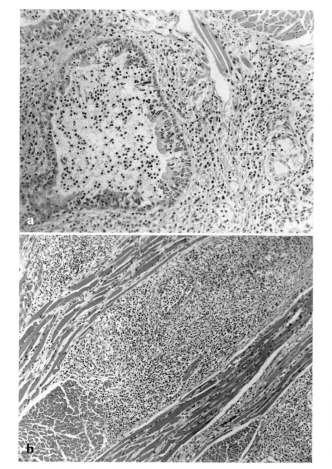

Figure 4.12 Infiltration of mucinous gland ducts by neutrophils in a five-month-old boy with upper-airway obstruction from a posterior lingual abscess (a) (hematoxylin and eosin, ×280). Adjacent tissues showed separation of muscle bundles of the tongue by the inflammatory infiltrate (b) (hematoxylin and eosin, ×110).

a five-month-old boy has been reported where extensive acute inflammation of the base of the tongue caused fatal upper-airway obstruction. The cause of the inflammation was uncertain, although infection of an underlying thyroglossal duct cyst remnant or a retention mucocele was considered (Byard & Silver, 1993) (Figure 4.12).

Acute epiglottitis

While many pediatricians and pathologists have had cases of sudden and unexpected death due to acute bacterial infection of the epiglottis, cases are now quite rare since the introduction of *Hemophilus influenzae* type B immunization.

Clinical features

The clinical course of the infection is often fulminant, with rapid development of fever, respiratory distress, odynophagia, and drooling, prior to respiratory obstruction and terminal cardiovascular arrest (Addy, Ellis & Turk, 1972). Occasionally, symptoms may be relatively non-specific, consisting of low-grade fever and sore throat (Bass *et al.*, 1985), or the child may be found dead in bed. Although it is considered to be primarily a disease of children aged between one and seven years, it does occur occasionally in older individuals and has been reported in late adolesence (Molander, 1982).

Occurrence of sudden death

Sudden death may occur if an attempt has been made to examine the epiglottis with a tongue depressor, as this may precipitate airway obstruction. The mortality rate for children in whom obstruction occurs is around 20%, even with prompt treatment (Bass, Steele & Wiebe, 1974; Rapkin, 1973). Fatal septic shock may also be a complication.

Etiology

The causative organism is almost invariably *Hemophilus influenzae* type B, although some cases are due to pneumococci, staphylococci, or streptococci (Sendi & Crysdale, 1987).

Pathological features

At autopsy, the epiglottis is characteristically red, swollen, and edematous (Color Plate 6). Microscopic examination will reveal marked submucosal edema and acute inflammation with surface ulceration (Figure 4.13).

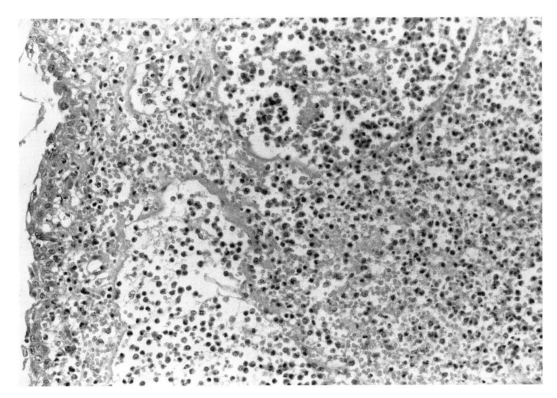

Figure 4.13 Submucosal edema and acute inflammation in acute epiglottitis (hematoxylin and eosin, ×280).

Autopsy investigation

Blood cultures are an important part of the postmortem work-up to determine the etiologic agent; they have been reported as positive in 50–75% of cases (Zalzal, 1989).

Other epiglottal lesions

Due to the vulnerability of the airway to obstruction at the laryngeal inlet, any condition that causes expansion of the submucosa of the epiglottis and surrounding tissues may result in lethal airway obstruction. The case of a one-year-old girl with neuroblastoma and *Pseudomonas* septicemia who developed stridor and died suddenly from marked interstitial hemorrhage around the laryngeal inlet underscores this point.

Acute laryngotracheobronchitis

Most cases of acute laryngotracheobronchitis occur in the form of epidemic croup due to parainfluenza and influenza viruses. The clinical course of croup is less severe than acute bacterial epiglottitis and it usually has an excellent prognosis. However, occasional cases occur where airway obstruction is severe enough to warrant endotracheal intubation (Zalzal, 1989). Respiratory arrest may also result if the child or infant is recumbent with the head tilted forward (Strife, 1988).

Although there has been debate over the likelihood of croup causing sudden death, Segard & Koneman (1968) have concluded that "laryngotracheobronchitis is a common and acceptable anatomic cause of death in children dying suddenly and

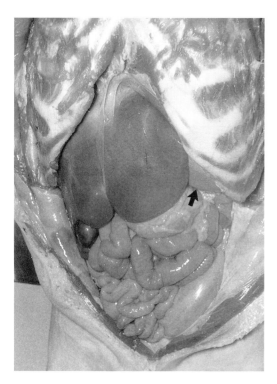

Figure 4.14 Ptosis of abdominal organs caused by a tension pneumothorax complicating staphylococcal pneumonia in a 12-year-old girl. The bulging diaphragm can be seen beneath the left costal margin (arrow).

unexpectedly." An additional problem that may result in death due to airway obstruction in children with viral laryngotracheobronchitis is secondary infection with *Staphylococcus aureus* producing thick pseudomembranes (McKenzie *et al.*, 1984).

Bacterial tracheitis

Acute bacterial tracheitis is most often due to staphylococci, is less acute in onset than bacterial epiglottitis, and usually has a favorable outcome. Unfortunately, some cases do occur in which acute airway obstruction results from impaction of tenacious mucopurulent membranes (Han, Dunbar & Striker, 1979), although no deaths were recorded in this paper.

Diphtheria

Pharyngeal infection with *Corynebacterium diphtheriae* affects unvaccinated children aged between two and 15 years. The bacteria produces an exotoxin that causes epithelial inflammation and necrosis, with the formation of an inflammatory pseudomembrane composed of necrotic mucosal cells and debris (Pappenheimer & Gill, 1973). Sudden death may occur from acute airway obstruction due to impaction of the dislodged pharyngeal pseudomembrane in the lower airway. Alternatively, sudden death may result from cardiac damage due to an exotoxin (*vide infra*).

Acute bacterial pneumonia

Clinical features

Symptoms and signs of acute bacterial pneumonia in older children are similar to those in adults, with fever, cough, and pleuritic chest pain. In infants, the diagnosis may not be as obvious, with mild fever and non-specific malaise preceding the sudden onset of respiratory distress.

Etiology

In children, the most common serious lower-respiratory tract infection is acute lobar pneumonia due to *Streptococcus pneumoniae*, accounting for 90% of cases. Fulminant respiratory infections also occur with *Hemophilus influenzae* and *Staphylococcus aureus*, the latter being associated with abscess formation and tension pneumothoraces (Figure 4.14).

Pathological features

The appearance of the lungs depends on whether the underlying process is an acute lobar or lobular (broncho-) pneumonia. In acute lobar pneumonia, confluent areas of pneumonic consolidation are present, which appear solid and airless. In acute bronchopneumonia, the lungs are mottled, with scattered areas of patchy consolidation. On cut section, these appear as discrete, pale, and firm areas throughout both lung fields.

Microscopically, alveoli are filled with neutrophils, fibrin, and necrotic debris. In lobar pneumonia, the stage of "red hepatization" is marked microscopically by extravasation of red blood cells into confluent alveoli filled with pus. This progresses to the stage of gray hepatization, as the inflammatory and red blood cells disintegrate. In acute bronchopneumonia, the acute inflammatory infiltrate is bronchocentric.

Autopsy investigation

Although tissue and blood cultures may reveal pathogenic bacteria, prior antibiotic treatment may result in sterile cultures.

Diagnostic problems

Assessing how well established a disease has to be to result in a lethal outcome is a problem that arises not infrequently at autopsy, i.e. "how much is enough?" Unfortunately, a preceding history of fever is of minimal use in establishing the diagnosis of lethal acute bronchopneumonia given the number of febrile illnesses of childhood. It is important, therefore, not to attribute death to lesions that are of doubtful significance and that would probably be overlooked except when the presentation is of sudden, unexpected death of uncertain etiology (Byard & Krous, 1995). This is particularly so if a plausible mechanism of death cannot be established.

In cases of sudden and unexpected death involving young children or infants, it is possible to have a very non-specific history and yet still find a marked interstitial and intra-alveolar acute inflammatory infiltrate at autopsy due to bacterial infection. In cases where there is either diffuse involvement of lung fields by the inflammatory process (Figures 4.15 and 4.16), or in which there is abscess formation with microbiological and histological evidence of disseminated sepsis, then establishing the cause of death as infective is not difficult. Other less well established cases are not as straightforward, and it may simply not be possible to determine where the cut-off point lies between an infection that is relatively innocuous and one that is lethal.

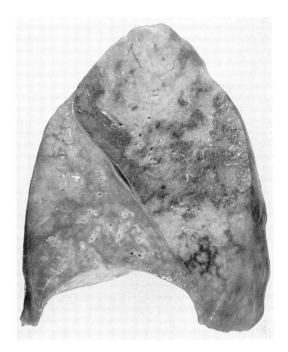

Figure 4.15 Fulminant pneumonia in a 16-month-old girl being treated for mild "croup" who was found dead 30 minutes after being placed in bed to sleep.

Interstitial pneumonitis

Interstitial pneumonitis is usually caused by viruses that result in a patchy interstitial chronic inflammatory infiltrate within the alveolar septae. Although often self-limiting, a fulminant course may occur in infants or in immunocompromised children. A similar histological picture can result from a number of other organisms, including mycoplasmas, rickettsiae, and chlamydiae (Yip, Sein & Lung, 1987). Polymerase chain reaction (PCR) of formalin-fixed paraffin-embedded material has been used to correctly identify the causative agent, as in the case of a seven-month-old boy who died unexpectedly due to infection with human herpesvirus-6 (Hoang *et al.*, 1999).

Again, the problem arises as to what degree of interstitial inflammation can be accepted as significant. This is even more difficult than in cases of acute bacterial inflammation, since there is normally

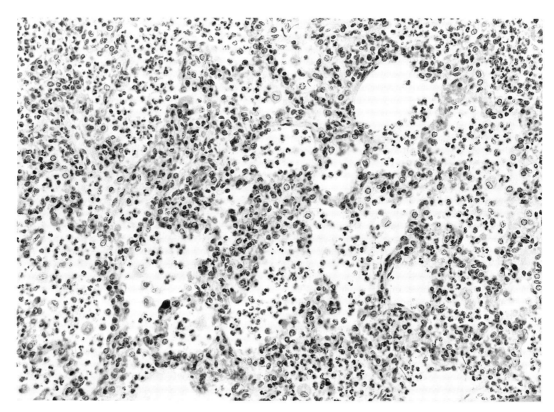

Figure 4.16 Florid acute bacterial bronchopneumonia in an infant with an unremarkable history of mild fever who was found unexpectedly dead one morning (hematoxylin and eosin, ×220).

a population of peribronchial lymphocytes present in the lungs. In the past, SIDS deaths were occasionally attributed to interstitial pneumonitis because of the presence of mildly increased numbers of peribronchial chronic inflammatory cells (Grice & McGlashan, 1978). However, a recent study has shown no differences in chronic inflammatory infiltrate in lung sections from SIDS infants and controls (Krous *et al.*, 2003). Microscopic features of interstitial pneumonitis in cases of sudden death have been described by Yip, Sein & Lung (1987).

Bronchiolitis

The major cause of bronchiolitis in infants under six months of age is respiratory syncytial virus (RSV). Other causative agents are adeno, parain-fluenza, and influenza viruses, *Bordetella pertussis*, and *Mycoplasma pneumoniae*. Microscopically, there is a diffuse mononuclear inflammatory cell infiltrate around bronchi and bronchioles extending into the surrounding parenchyma. The airway lumena are also infiltrated by mononuclear cells and are filled with mucus and necrotic debris.

RSV infection may cause apneic episodes, plugging of distal bronchioles with mucus and inflammatory debris, air trapping within the lungs, and sudden death (Aherne, 1972; Bruhn, Mokrohisky & McIntosh, 1977).

Tuberculosis

Infection by *Mycobacterium tuberculosis* usually involves the lungs, but any tissue or organ may be affected. Individuals with established disease are often undernourished, with respiratory symptoms, including hemoptysis. With increasing drug resistance and immunodeficiency states, there has been an increase in tuberculosis reported in certain groups in Western countries (Alkhuja & Miller, 2001).

While sudden death is a rare but recognized complication of tuberculosis that usually occurs in the elderly, cases involving children have been reported (Arthur, 1995; Hassan & Hanna, 1984). Mechanisms of death in children could theoretically involve fulminant bronchopneumonia or massive hemoptysis with aspiration. Less commonly, death may be due to tuberculous myocarditis or infiltration of the adrenal glands, with an Addisonian crisis (Alkhuja & Miller, 2001; Dada et al., 2000).

Histologically, there is characteristic necrotizing granulomatous inflammation with caseation and acid-fast bacilli demonstrable on Ziehl–Neelson or fluorescent dye staining. On occasion, when organisms are not found, it may be possible to detect mycobacterial DNA by using a ligase chain reaction technique (Dada et al., 2000).

Infectious mononucleosis

Infectious mononucleosis, or glandular fever, is an acute viral illness characterized by fever, pharyngitis, lymphadenopathy, splenomegaly, and hepatitis. While most cases are relatively benign, a mortality rate of one in 3000 has been reported associated with splenic rupture, neurological complications, and upper-airway obstruction (Boglioli & Taff, 1998; Byard, 2002; Johnsen, Katholm & Stangerup, 1984). Myocarditis, nasopharyngeal hemorrhage, and fatal secondary infections may also occur (McCurdy, 1975; Penman, 1970).

Rupture of the spleen (see Figure 9.20) may follow only minor trauma such as coughing, vomiting, or straining at stool, and has even been reported following medical examination (Bell & Mason, 1980; Springate & Adelson, 1966).

Neurological complications may result in motor paralysis from Guillain–Barré syndrome and meningoencephalitis. While it has often been assumed that respiratory arrest in infected individuals was due to upper-airway obstruction, bulbar palsy or Guillain–Barré syndrome may be more common (Wolfe & Rowe, 1980). Respiratory embarrassment or sudden death may certainly result from upper-airway obstruction due to enlargement of the tonsils and adenoids, with edema of the uvula and epiglottis, sometimes with the added complication of pertitonsillar abscess formation (Byard, 2002; Gewirtz et al., 1982; Woolf & Diedericks, 1989). A pseudomembrane may form, causing airway occlusion, mimicking diphtheria (Ch'en & Teng, 1941). Figure 4.17 shows an obstructed upper airway due to massive tonsillar enlargement in a 14-year-old boy with infectious mononucleosis who died suddenly in hospital.

Laryngeal papillomatosis

This condition is characterized by recurrent spreading papillomas that grow around the glottis, within the larynx, and along the posterior wall of the pharynx. The lesions are exophytic and cause vocal changes and sometimes shortness of breath in affected children. The lesions have a viral etiology, with human papilloma virus types 6 and 11 being isolated from infected tissues. Rapid growth may occur, with compromise of airway patency. Rarely, this may cause sudden death, as in a 23-month-old girl who was found dead in bed by her mother. At autopsy, the larynx was markedly narrowed by papillomas (Sperry, 1994).

Central nervous system conditions

Meningitis

Bacterial infection of the meninges may result in fulminant disease and sudden death in children before symptoms are obvious and in spite of antibacterial therapy. Rupture of intracerebral abscesses into the subarachnoid space is another situation that results in extensive purulent meningitis, with rapid death

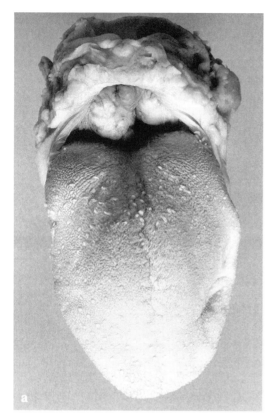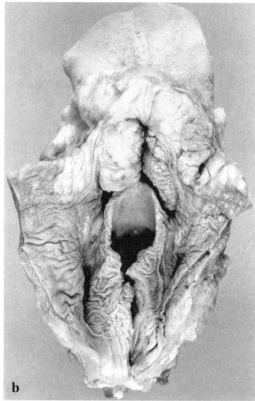

Figure 4.17 Marked enlargement of the tonsils in a previously healthy 14-year-old boy with infectious mononucleosis and acute upper-airway obstruction: (a) anterior view; (b) posterior view, demonstrating virtual occlusion of the pharynx due to tonsillar hypertrophy.

(Friede, 1989), in addition to extension of infections from the middle ear or orbit (Figures 4.18 & 4.19).

Etiology

Causative organisms vary depending on age, with *Streptococcus* group B and enterobacteria being more common in neonates. In children up to 12 years of age, the most common bacterial pathogens causing meningitis are *Hemophilus influenzae* type B, *Streptococcus pneumoniae*, and *Neisseria meningitidis*; after this age, *Streptococcus pneumoniae* and *Neisseria meningitidis* are more significant. Fulminant bacterial meningitis may also be caused by other agents, such as *Listeria monocytogenes* (Kilpi *et al.*, 1991).

Clinical features

Children with bacterial infection of the meninges may have several days' history of nausea, vomiting, and photophobia, followed by alteration in conscious state and nuchal rigidity. However, infants may have minimal or non-specific symptoms and signs.

Infection with *Neisseria meningitidis* in children usually causes minimal or no inflammation at the site of entry within the upper airway. The clinical history is of a febrile illness followed by skin rash (Color Plate 7) and collapse (Bausher & Baker, 1986). Death occurs most commonly in children under the age of two years who present with rapid deterioration, including coma or shock (Rimar, Fox & Goschke,

1985), but it may occur at any age in a previously well individual.

Pathological features

At autopsy, inflammation of the meninges and skin rash may not be apparent on visual inspection due to the rapid clinical course of the infection (Arey & Sotos, 1956), although this is variable (Figure 4.20), i.e. death may occur from septicemia before meningitis develops (Welsby & Golledge, 1990). Bilateral intra-adrenal hemorrhage, so-called Waterhouse–Friderichson syndrome, may be present (Knight, 1980) (Color Plate 8), most commonly associated with *Neisseria meningitidis* but also found with other types of bacteria such as *Hemophilus influenzae* (Tepper, Overman & Parker, 1993). Microscopy will reveal a polymorphonuclear cell infiltrate of the meninges (Figure 4.21) and cultures of cerebrospinal fluid should yield bacteria unless prior antibiotic therapy has occurred.

Cerebral infarction has been documented in approximately 5% of children with *Hemophilus influenzae* meningitis (Taft, Chusid & Sty, 1986), possibly due to arteritis with spasm. Necrotizing cerebral vasculitis occurs with group B streptococcal, rickettsial, fungal, and viral central nervous system infections (Caldarelli, 1992). Viral infections include congenital rubella and herpes zoster. Vascular stenosis following meningitis may also occur in the absence of thrombosis due to a reactive fibrointimal reparative process (Yamashima *et al.*, 1985).

Occurrence of sudden death

Lethal effects derive from septicemia and/or meningitis, both of which may have a very fulminant course. Septicemic shock found in cases of meningococcemia is thought to be caused by a circulating endotoxin that also acts on the myocardium and adrenal glands (Boucek *et al.*, 1984).

Myocarditis may be found in a significant number of cases of meningococcal sepsis, sometimes with involvement of the atrioventricular node (Hardman, 1968; Robboy, 1972). Other lethal mechanisms involve cerebral edema due to increased capillary permeability, with brainstem herniation, vascular

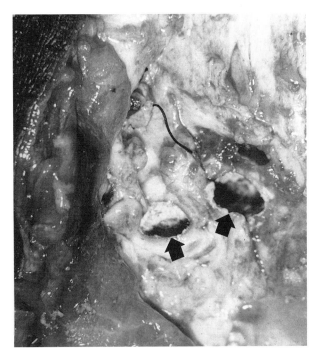

Figure 4.18 Extension of otitis media through petrous temporal bone (arrows) into the cranial cavity of a young child, with resultant meningitis and intracerebral abscess formation.

inflammation with thrombosis, and decreased cerebral perfusion due to hypotension (Ashwal *et al.*, 1992; Quagliarello & Scheld, 1992). Fatal cerebral herniation may also follow lumbar puncture in children with meningitis (Rennick, Shann & de Campo, 1993).

Autopsy investigation

Cerebrospinal fluid (CSF) aspirates should be obtained aseptically before opening the skull, either through the fontanelle or through the posterior atlanto-occipital membrane. CSF may also be taken posteriorly through the lower spine, or anteriorly after evisceration. Swabs for microbiological assessment should also be taken from areas of meningeal congestion or suppuration. Blood cultures are routine in such cases.

As infection may spread from adjacent areas such as the middle ear, these should be examined carefully at autopsy, and microbiological swabs should

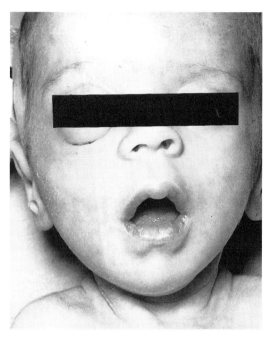

Figure 4.19 Orbital cellulitis, with swelling of right periorbital tissues, retrograde extension, and subsequent fatal intracranial sepsis.

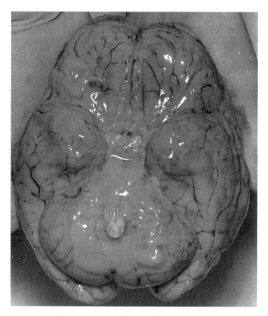

Figure 4.20 Suppuration of the meninges in established pneumococcal meningitis.

be taken if necessary. It may also be appropriate to check for skull fractures and CSF leakage in cases of recurrent meningitis.

Encephalitis

Certain viruses may infect the substance of the brain, resulting in inflammation, necrosis, and edema. For example, Herpes simplex virus may infect predominantly the temporal and frontal lobes in the child/adult type of encephalitis, or act more diffusely in the neonatal form. Rapid death may occur in children with these types of infections.

Poliomyelitis

Poliomyelitis is caused by an enterovirus that produces paralysis through infection of motor neurons. As with a number of other infections, epidemics are rare in Western countries since the introduction of immunization programs. Death in affected children may occur from respiratory paralysis, which may be sudden, mimicking the presentation of SIDS. At autopsy, the findings are relatively non-specific, although destruction of motor neurons, particularly of the anterior horns of the spinal cord, may be seen on microscopy (Dunne, Harper & Hilton, 1984).

Hematological conditions

Malaria

Almost any infectious cause of splenomegaly increases the risk of rupture from relatively minor trauma. In Western countries, infection with Epstein–Barr virus causing infectious mononucleosis is probably the most common microbiological cause of fatal rupture (Bell & Mason, 1980), whereas malaria is of greater significance in endemic areas.

Malaria is an acute febrile illness caused by *Plasmodium* spp. and transmitted by mosquito vectors. *Plasmodium falciparum* infection is the most severe form and may result in sudden death in adults from cerebral involvement (Ette *et al.*, 2002), with vascular thrombosis and localized ischemia, or, more rarely, from splenic rupture. At autopsy,

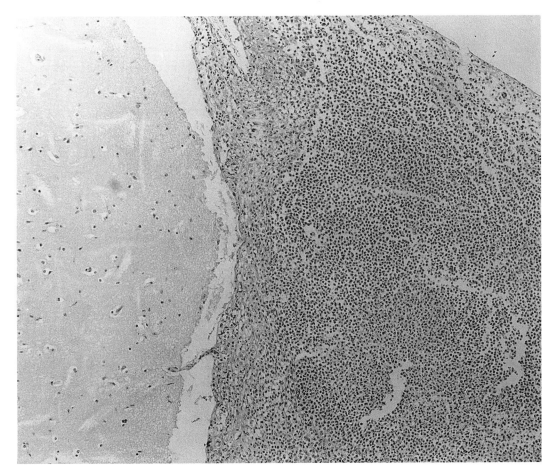

Figure 4.21 Infiltration of the meninges by acute inflammatory cells in bacterial meningitis (hematoxylin and eosin, ×110).

hepatosplenomegaly may be present, with plugging of congested cerebral vessels with red blood cells in which malarial parasites can be seen on microscopy (Edington, 1967).

Sickle cell disease

The clinicopathological features of sickle cell disease are dealt with in Chapter 9. One of the complications of sickle cell disease is reduced splenic function, which predisposes to fulminant infections, particularly by encapsulated bacteria. Infectious agents include *Streptococcus pneumoniae, Hemophilus influenzae, Salmonella* sp., *Escherichia coli*, and *Staphylococcus aureus*.

Affected children have a higher rate than normal children of generalized sepsis, osteomyelitis, and meningitis.

Gastrointestinal infections

Gastroenteritis

Dehydration from any cause may result in electrolyte imbalances, with the attendant risk of sudden death. In children, fulminant gastroenteritis is one of the most important causes of rapid clinical deterioration if fluid balance is not maintained. Infants are at particular risk as watery diarrhea may be mistaken for urine, leading to underestimation of the severity

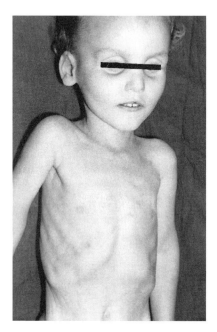

Figure 4.22 Deeply sunken eyes are evidence of marked dehydration in a two-year-old boy with gastroenteritis.

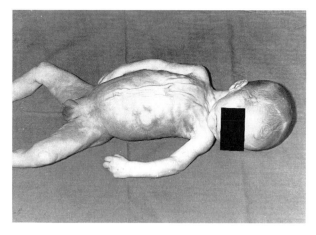

Figure 4.23 Wrinkling of the skin and depression of the fontanelle in a male infant with marked dehydration from gastroenteritis.

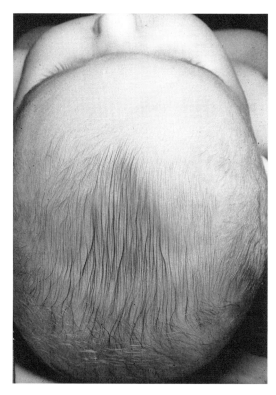

Figure 4.24 Sunken fontanelle in a five-month-old girl due to dehydration following gastroenteritis. This was associated with basal subarachnoid hemorrhage (see Figure 4.27).

of the condition. Neglected children who develop gastroenteritis are also vulnerable to lethal consequences due to parental inattention and the late seeking of medical care. However, poorly educated parents may genuinely fail to appreciate the severity of a child's illness. The effects of excessive fluid loss may also be exacerbated in areas with a hot climate, especially in the middle of summer (Whitehead *et al.*, 1996).

Pathological features

Evidence of marked dehydration may be obvious at autopsy, with sunken eyes, a depressed fontanelle in infants, dry mucous membranes and internal organs, and decreased skin turgor (Figures 4.22–4.25), but this is not invariable (Whitehead *et al.*, 1996). Reflection of the scalp will demonstrate a sunken fontanelle more clearly (Figure 4.26). As the clinical history may be equivocal and microbiological investigations unhelpful, postmortem analysis of vitreous humor should be performed in all cases

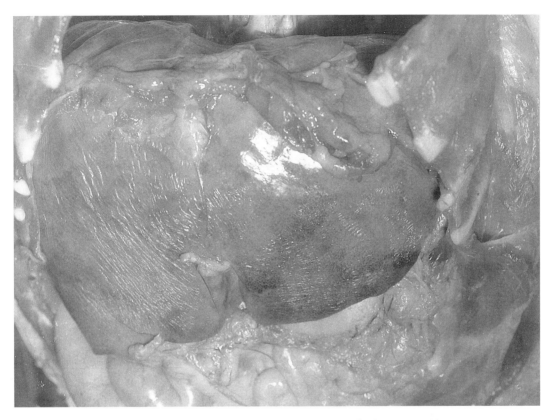

Figure 4.25 Shrinkage of the liver capsule in a severely dehydrated six-month-old girl with gastroenteritis.

of unexplained infant death as this may reveal elevation in sodium and urea nitrogen levels (Huser & Smialek, 1986). Knight (1997) cites levels of vitreous sodium >155 mmol/l, chloride >135 mmol/l, and urea >40 mmol/l as reliable markers of antemortem dehydration. This may be of particular significance if the possibility of parental neglect exists.

Occurrence of sudden death

The cause of sudden death in these cases may be hyperkalemic cardiac arrhythmia, or cerebral hemorrhage or infarction from venous thrombosis (Friede, 1989) (Figures 4.27–4.29). Renal vein thrombosis may also occcur (Figure 4.30).

Occasionally, sudden death may occur without dehydration, as was the case in a four-month-old boy who had apparently recovered from gastroenteritis

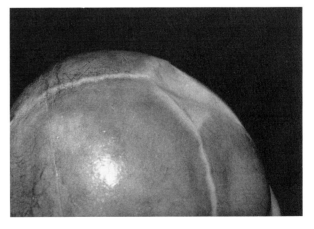

Figure 4.26 Reflecting the scalp demonstrates more clearly the degree of fontanelle depression that occurs with significant dehydration.

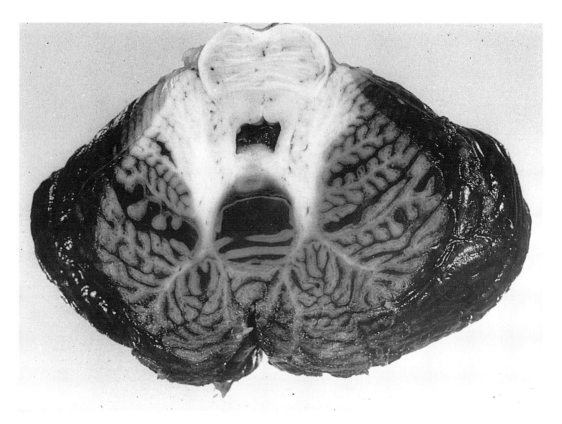

Figure 4.27 Diffuse subarachnoid hemorrhage of the cerebellum, causing sudden death in a five-month-old girl with acute gastroenteritis and dehydration.

but who had *Salmonella virchow* isolated from the gut, middle ear, and cerebrospinal fluid, with organisms identified on immunohistochemical staining of the liver (Bignardi & Khong, 1989).

Botulism

Infantile botulism is a recognized cause of sudden death due to the actions of a potent neurotoxin that interferes with respiration (Midura & Arnon, 1976). Further details are discussed in the section later in this chapter.

Primary peritonitis

Infants may die suddenly after the development of primary peritonitis, symptoms of which are vomiting, diarrhea, and acute prostration. Causative organisms include *Pneumococcus*, *Streptococcus*, and *Escherichia coli*. At autopsy, purulent ascitic fluid will be identified, with no demonstrable focus of infection.

Hydatid disease

Hydatid disease is found in sheep-raising communities where children become infected following ingestion of the eggs of *Echinococcus granulosus* from the feces of infected dogs. Hydatid cysts develop in various parts of the body, most commonly in the liver and lungs.

Sudden death may be due to anaphylaxis following rupture of a cyst (Franquet, Lecumberri & Joly, 1984),

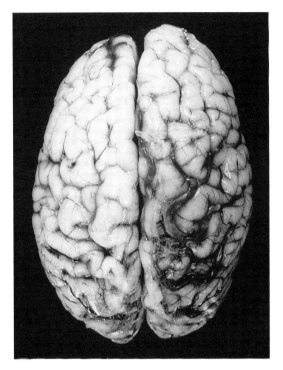

Figure 4.28 Cerebral venous thromboses over the right hemisphere of the brain in a case of dehydration.

or more rarely to acute vessel occlusion from cerebral or pulmonary embolism (Buris, Takacs & Varga, 1987; Byard & Bourne, 1991) (Figure 4.31). Cyst rupture may be precipitated by trauma (Kök, Yurtman & Aydin, 1993). At autopsy, cysts are typically surrounded by a thickened fibrous capsule with a laminated outer layer on microscopy.

Genitourinary conditions

Pyelonephritis

The majority of cases of acute bacterial pyelonephritis present with fever and loin pain. Cases in which sudden death is purported to have occurred may represent examples of parental inattention or of underestimation of the severity of symptoms by attending physicians.

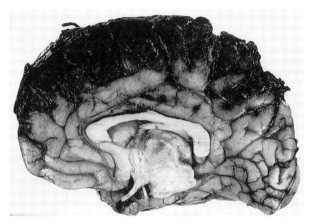

Figure 4.29 Cerebral venous thromboses with cerebral infarction in a nine-month-old boy with acute gastroenteritis and dehydration.

Hemolytic-uremic syndrome

Hemolytic-uremic syndrome is a condition characterized by microangiopathic hemolytic anemia, thrombocytopenia, and renal failure. Although the precise etiology is uncertain, it is associated with certain strains of toxigenic *Escherichia coli*, which produce Shiga toxins, resulting in widespread endothelial damage (Henning *et al.*, 1998). Outbreaks have occurred following food contamination. While recovery is usual, sudden death can result from intracranial hemorrhage (Manton, Smith & Byard 2000). Further details may be found in Chapter 10.

Generalized conditions

Septicemia

Generalized bacterial sepsis may cause sudden deterioration and death in infancy and childhood (Sharief, Khan & Conlan, 1993). For example, group B streptococcal infection is a major cause of sudden death within the first two months of life due to pneumonia, meningitis, and generalized sepsis. Fever may not have been marked, and the presentation may be similar to SIDS (Barnham & Henderson, 1987; Berry, 1989). At autopsy, a focus for the infection

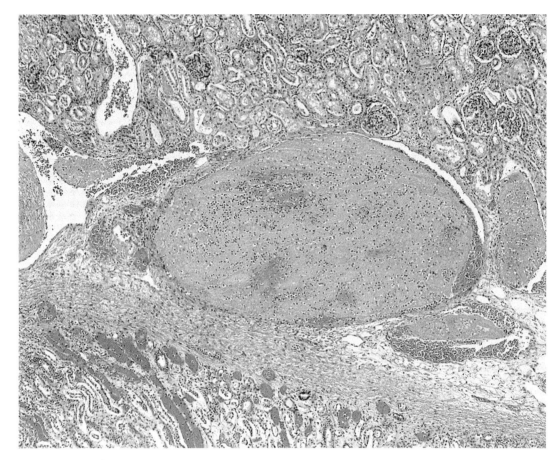

Figure 4.30 Section of kidney showing a thrombosed vein in a three-month-old boy who collapsed at home following a febrile illness. He was found to be profoundly dehydrated, with a vitreous humor sodium of 158 mmol/l and bilateral renal vein thromboses (hematoxylin and eosin, ×80).

may be discernible in some cases, although other cases may have no apparent source of the pathogenic agent. The mechanism of death in children who die suddenly from septicemia is not always clear (Arey & Sotos, 1956).

In the absence of a clear-cut history of antemortem sepsis, the diagnosis of lethal septicemia in cases of sudden death requires positive blood cultures and/or isolation of the same organism from multiple sites, preferably with microscopic evidence of disseminated sepsis (Barnham & Henderson, 1987). Histologic evidence of sepsis may include areas of localized acute inflammation, such as an acute pneumonia, or hemorrhage and intravascular

fibrin thrombi from disseminated intravascular coagulation (Usón, Melicow & Pascal, 1976). In the absence of these findings, the possibility of external contamination, agonal sepsis, or postmortem overgrowth must be considered (du Moulin & Paterson, 1985). No histologic changes may be discernible in cases of dissemination of lethal toxin-producing bacteria.

Viremia

Disseminated infection with organisms other than bacteria may also result in sudden and unexpected cardiac arrest. Examples include adenovirus,

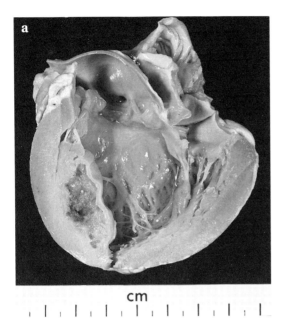 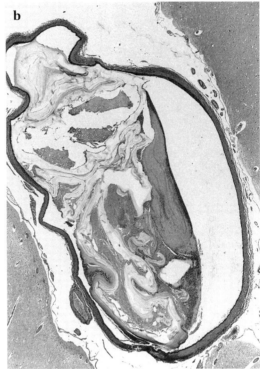

Figure 4.31 Cross-section of the heart of a seven-year-old boy who collapsed at school, revealing a ruptured intraventricular hydatid cyst (a). Middle cerebral artery containing embolized laminated hydatid material (b) (hematoxylin and eosin, ×50).

rhinovirus, and herpes simplex virus (Cantor, Pipas & McCabe, 1990; Traisman *et al.*, 1988). Although it was once proposed that disseminated cytomegalovirus infection was associated with some cases of SIDS, based on the finding of viral inclusions within salivary glands (Figure 4.32) and brainstem microglial nodules (Variend, 1990), this had been discounted (Smith, Telfer & Byard, 1992).

Endotoxemia

A variety of locally invasive bacteria may cause effects due to the elaboration of systemically acting potent toxins in the absence of histologically detectable tissue changes.

Staphylococcus aureus
Toxin-producing *Staphylococcus aureus* may cause sudden death in infants and children following

relatively minor skin or upper respiratory infections (Bentley *et al.*, 1997; Whitley *et al.*, 1982). A similar syndrome, known as "toxic shock syndrome," has occurred in menstruating adolescent and young adult women (Chesney *et al.*, 1981), the staphylococci being present in contaminated tampons (Morris, 1983). Antemortem symptoms of vomiting, sore throat, and skin rash with fever may progress rapidly to shock, with renal and cardiac failure (Paris *et al.*, 1982). Staphylococcal enterotoxins may be involved in some cases that have presented as SIDS (Malam *et al.*, 1992) (see Chapter 13). Exotoxins produced by *Streptococcus pyogenes* may also result in toxic shock syndrome. The mortality is higher than with staphylococcal disease, and victims tend to be older.

Corynebacterium diphtheriae
The exotoxin derived from *Corynebacterium diphtheriae* not only causes local changes in the form

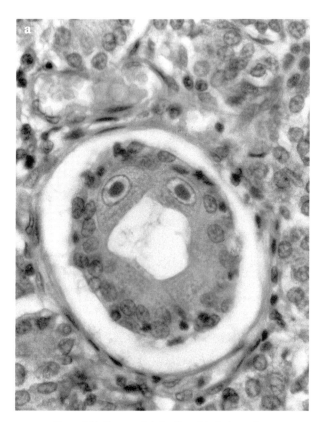

Figure 4.32 Characteristic "owl's eye" inclusions of cytomegalovirus in a salivary gland duct (a). Electron microscopy demonstrating viral particles (b).

of epithelial necrosis with pseudomembrane formation in the pharynx, but may also result in myocardial damage. The intensity of myocarditis varies, with 10 to over 80% of affected patients demonstrating clinical evidence of cardiac disease (Boyer & Weinstein, 1948; Morgan, 1963). Involvement of conduction tracts may lead to heart block and sudden death from arrhythmia. At autopsy, fatty change within the myocardium, liver, and kidneys may be observed.

Escherichia coli

Escherichia coli may produce an enterotoxin that is considered by some researchers to be associated with SIDS (Bettelheim *et al.*, 1990), although this has not been verified.

Clostridium sp.

Both *Clostridium tetani* and *Clostridium botulinum* produce potent neurotoxins that may result in sudden death. Tetanus is characterized by progressive stiffness of voluntary muscles, with the development of respiratory failure or laryngeal spasm (Weinstein, 1973). Occasionally, the clinical course may be fulminant, and death can occur rapidly, particularly in children with sickle cell disease (Akpede, 1992). Changes at autopsy are relatively non-specific, with local inflammation at the site of infection and swelling of motor neurons in the brainstem and spinal cord.

Botulism occurs in children and adults when the neurotoxin produced by *Clostridium botulinum* is ingested. Clinical symptoms and signs usually evolve over some time and consist of vomiting and diarrhea progressing to respiratory paralysis. In infants and neonates, botulism may present with sudden respiratory arrest (Hurst & Marsh, 1993). Examination of the bowel at autopsy is important, as a case of pseudomembranous colitis due to *Clostridium difficile* has been reported in a three-month-old boy presenting as SIDS (Scopes, Smith & Beach, 1980). *Clostridium welchii* toxin has been associated with outbreaks of rapidly lethal necrotizing enterocolitis (*pig bel*) in children in the highlands of Papua New Guinea following the ingestion of large amounts of pork at traditional ceremonies (Byard, 1988).

Immunodeficiency states

A heterogeneous variety of primary and secondary immunodeficiency states exist (Burgio & Ugazio, 1982; Rosen, Cooper & Wedgwood, 1984a; Rosen, Cooper & Wedgwood, 1984b), only some of which are associated with the occurrence of fulminant infections and death. Affected children may have been investigated for failure to thrive.

Primary immunodeficiency states

X-linked agammaglobulinemia of Bruton is one of the most common types of heritable immunodeficiencies. In severe forms, it is characterized

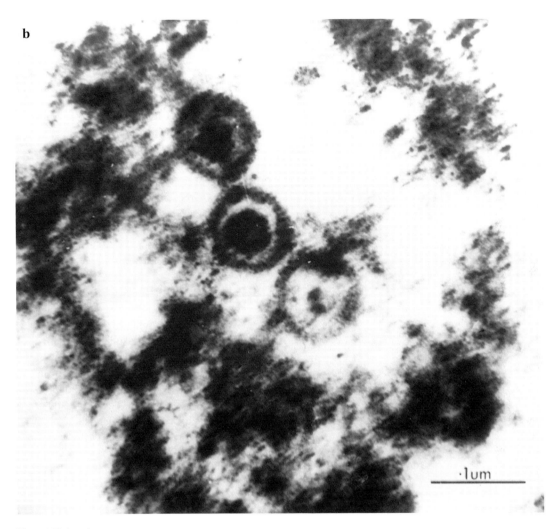

·1um

Figure 4.32 (cont.)

by marked reduction or absence of serum immunoglobulins, resulting in recurrent pyogenic infections from an early age. Findings at autopsy include a lack of germinal centers in lymph nodes and
the spleen, with rudimentary tonsils and an absence
of plasma cells on microscopy.

Severe combined immunodeficiency is a heterogeneous disorder characterized by defects in both hu-
moral and cell-mediated immunity (Stephan *et al.*,
1993). Death usually occurs in early life from
overwhelming *Pseudomonas* sp. or viral infections.

At autopsy, the thymus is not found within the anterior mediastinum, but is higher up in the neck,
and on microscopy is found to be devoid of lymphoid cells and Hassal's corpuscles. Affected children often lack erythrocyte and leukocyte adenosine
deaminase, an enzyme that can be tested for on fresh
samples.

Common variable immunodeficiency represents
the most frequent form of serious heritable immunodeficiency. This condition is characterized by reduced blood immunoglobulin levels, resulting in

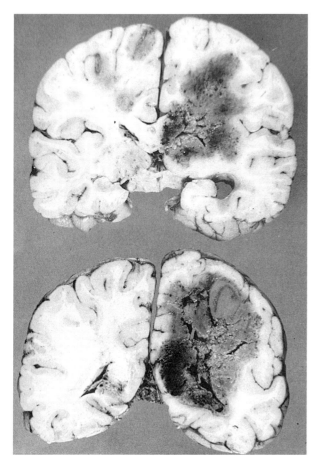

Figure 4.33 Necrotizing vasculitis with cerebral infarction caused by *Aspergillus* infection in a 12-year-old boy with leukemia.

recurrent pyogenic infections. Examination of lymph nodes reveals hyperplastic lymphoid follicles, in contrast to X-linked agammaglobulinemia.

DiGeorge syndrome results from third and fourth pharyngeal pouch anomalies, such as aplasia, hypoplasia, or ectopia of derived tissues, including the thymus and parathyroid glands. Sudden death in infants and children with this disorder may also occur due to associated cardiovascular abnormalities (discussed in greater detail in Chapter 6).

Wiskott–Aldrich syndrome is an X-linked recessive condition characterized by eczema, thrombo-cytopenia, and variable T- and B-cell defects that result in recurrent infections. Sudden death may occur due to the low number of circulating platelets, as occurred in a five-month-old boy with Wiskott–Aldrich syndrome who died rapidly soon after hospital admission and was found at autopsy to have had an intracranial hemorrhage.

Congenital asplenia may occur on its own or may be part of a more extensive syndrome involving cardiovascular anomalies (Katcher, 1980). The clinical presentation of cases in which other congenital malformations are present (90%) tends to be overshadowed by cardiovascular problems in early infancy. However, in children who survive early life, there is still the ever-present risk of fulminant sepsis (Singer, 1973; Waldman *et al.*, 1977), which may result in sudden and unexpected death (Dyke, Martin & Berry, 1991; Moore, 1991). Although *Hemophilus influenzae* infection and intra-adrenal hemorrhages were present in five of the six cases in these reports (all of which pursued a fulminant course, with death often within 12 hours of the onset of symptoms), pneumococcal sepsis is more usual (Kanthan, Moyana & Nyssen, 1999). Familial cases of congenital hyposplenism have been reported (Kevy *et al.*, 1968).

If a hypoplastic or absent spleen is noted on initial examination of the abdominal cavity at autopsy, then not only should complex cardiovascular abnormalities be looked for but full microbiological examination should be conducted. This is particularly so if hemorrhagic adrenal glands are also present.

Other forms of immunodeficiency syndromes include defects in the complement system and defects in macrophage/neutrophil function, such as chronic granulomatous disease.

Secondary immunodeficiency states

Iatrogenic

Children who have received chemotherapy for malignancies are at increased risk of developing fulminant infections due to opportunistic organisms. These may be multiple and result in disseminated intravascular coagulation.

Sudden death due to fungal thromboembolism may occur in children infected with angio-invasive fungi such as *Aspergillus* sp. (Figures 4.33–4.35 and Color Plate 9). In these children, sometimes it may be difficult to identify fungi in tissue sections unless sampling is extensive, as angio-invasion with infarction may have caused widespread tissue necrosis. Sampling of venous blood may not detect fungus as hyphae may not have passed through the capillary bed (Byard, 1989). An autopsy sampling protocol for fungi that includes arterial blood collection is outlined in Appendix VII. A wide variety of other organisms may also be found in the tissues of immunocompromised children, including viruses and nematodes (Byard *et al.*, 1993) (Figure 4.36).

Acquired immunodeficiency syndrome

It could be suggested that one of the particularly unpleasant features of acquired immunodeficiency syndrome (AIDS) is the prolonged clinical course that sufferers are forced to endure. However, while sudden and unexpected death does not stand out as a particularly obvious presentation, it may occur.

In adults with AIDS, cardiac lesions have included myocarditis, endocarditis, pericardial effusions, left ventricular hypokinesia, mitral incompetence, and right ventricular dilation (D'Cruz *et al.*, 1986; Fink, Reichek & St John Sutton, 1984; Roldan, Moskowitz & Hensley, 1987). Clinical studies of children with AIDS have also demonstrated abnormalities in left ventricular function, sometimes caused by dilated cardiomyopathy (Issenberg, Charytan & Rubinstein, 1985; Joshi, 1989) or by cytomegalovirus infection (Brady *et al.*, 1988).

Vascular lesions found in children with AIDS may also precipitate sudden death. For example, involvement of the coronary arteries with aneurysm formation has been reported as a cause of death from myocardial infarction in a 32-month-old girl with AIDS (Joshi *et al.*, 1987). Microscopically, vessels show intimal and medial fibrosis, with disruption of elastin fibers and medial calcification. These fibrocalcific vascular lesions are similar to those found in idiopathic arterial calcification of infancy.

Vasculitis and perivasculitis of the cerebral vessels may be associated with intracerebral hemorrhage and ischemic lesions in infected individuals

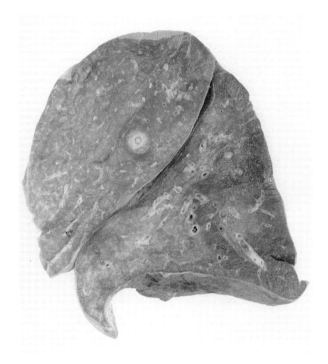

Figure 4.34 Pulmonary infarction and a "target" lesion of *Aspergillus* infection in a six-year-old girl with acute lymphoblastic leukemia.

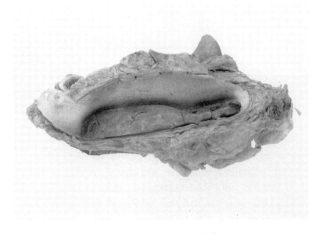

Figure 4.35 Thrombosis of the aorta due to an infective embolus in disseminated aspergillosis.

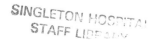

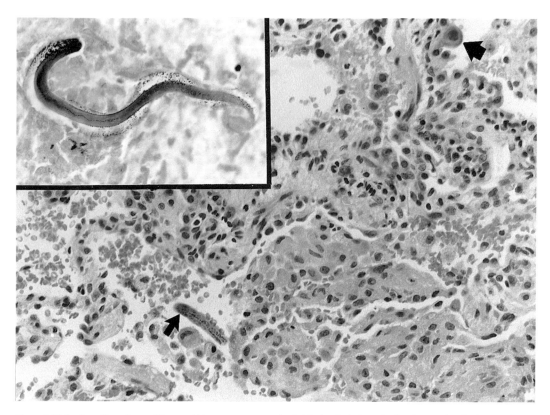

Figure 4.36 Section of lung from a 12-year-old immunocompromised girl who died of sepsis, showing an alveolar lining cell with a cytomegalovirus inclusion (large arrow) and a portion of a *Strongyloides* larva within an alveolus (small arrow). Inset shows a complete *Strongyloides* larva within sputum (hematoxylin and eosin, ×300).

(Mizusawa *et al.*, 1988). Vasculitis may result in cerebral artery aneurysm formation (Husson *et al.*, 1992), and vascular calcification has been found in the basal ganglia of infants and children with AIDS (Belman *et al.*, 1986).

A case of sudden death in an eight-year-old boy with AIDS following massive gastrointestinal tract hemorrhage has been reported, but unfortunately further comment is not possible as permission for autopsy was not granted (Balbi *et al.*, 1989).

Children with AIDS are also at much higher risk for developing a variety of other opportunistic infections, the features of which have been documented in several reviews (Arpadi & Caspe, 1990; Frenkel & Gaur, 1991; Prober & Gershon, 1991; Sun, 1988).

REFERENCES

Addy, M. G., Ellis, P. D. M. & Turk, D. C. (1972). Haemophilus epiglottitis: nine recent cases in Oxford. *British Medical Journal*, **1**, 40–42.

Aherne, W. (1972). The pathology of sudden unexpected death in childhood. *Journal of the Forensic Science Society*, **12**, 585–6.

Akpede, G. O. (1992). Unusually severe course of tetanus in a vaccinated child with sickle cell disease. *Lancet*, **340**, 981–2.

Alkhuja, S. & Miller, A. (2001). Tuberculosis and sudden death: a case report and review. *Heart and Lung*, **30**, 388–91.

Aoki, Y., Nata, M., Hashiyada, M. & Sagisaka, K. (1996). Sudden unexpected death in childhood due to eosinophilic myocarditis. *International Journal of Legal Medicine*, **108**, 221–4.

Aretz, H. T., Billingham, M. E., Edwards, W. D., *et al.* (1986). Myocarditis. A histopathologic definition and classification. *American Journal of Cardiovascular Pathology*, **1**, 3–14.

Arey, J. B. & Sotos, J. (1956). Unexpected death in early life. *Journal of Pediatrics*, **49**, 523–39.

Arpadi, S. & Caspe, W. B. (1990). Diagnosis and classification of HIV infection in children. *Pediatric Annals*, **19**, 409–36.

Arthur, J. T. (1995). Sudden deaths: cardiac and non-cardiac in children in Accra. *West African Journal of Medicine*, **14**, 108–11.

Ashwal, S., Tomasi, L., Schneider, S., Perkin, R. & Thompson, J. (1992). Bacterial meningitis in children: pathophysiology and treatment. *Neurology*, **42**, 739–48.

Atkinson, J. B. & Virmani, R. (1987). Infective endocarditis: changing trends and general approach for examination. *Human Pathology*, **18**, 603–8.

Balbi, H. J., McAbee, G., Annunziato, D. & Johnson, G. M. (1989). Fatal gastrointestinal tract hemorrhage in a child with AIDS. *Journal of the American Medical Association*, **262**, 1470.

Barnham, M. & Henderson, D. C. (1987). Group B streptococcal infection presenting as sudden death in infancy. *Archives of Disease in Childhood*, **62**, 419–20.

Bass, J. W., Fajardo, J. E., Brien, J. H., Cook, B. A. & Wiswell, T. E. (1985). Sudden death due to acute epiglottis. *Pediatric Infectious Disease*, **4**, 447–9.

Bass, J. W., Steele, R. W. & Wiebe, R. A. (1974). Acute epiglottis. A surgical emergency. *Journal of the American Medical Association*, **229**, 671–5.

Bausher, J. C. & Baker, R. C. (1986). Early prognostic indicators in acute meningococcemia: implications for management. *Pediatric Emergency Care*, **2**, 176–9.

Bell, J. S. & Mason, J. M. (1980). Sudden death due to spontaneous rupture of the spleen from infectious mononucleosis. *Journal of Forensic Sciences*, **25**, 20–24.

Belman, A. L., Lantos, G., Horoupian, D., *et al.* (1986). AIDS: calcification of the basal ganglia in infants and children. *Neurology*, **36**, 1192–9.

Bentley, A. J., Zorgani, A. A., Blackwell, C. C., Weir, D. M. & Busuttil, A. (1997). Bacterial toxins and sudden unexpected death in a young child. *Forensic Science International*, **88**, 141–6.

Berry, C. L. (1989). Causes of sudden natural death in infancy and childhood. In *Paediatric Forensic Medicine and Pathology*, ed. J. K. Mason. London: Chapman & Hall Medical, pp. 165–77.

Bettelheim, K. A., Goldwater, P. N., Dwyer, B. W., Bourne, A. J. & Smith, D. L. (1990). Toxigenic *Escherichia coli* associated with sudden infant death syndrome. *Scandinavian Journal of Infectious Diseases*, **22**, 467–76.

Bignardi, G. E. & Khong, T. Y. (1989). Immunohistological demonstration of *Salmonella virchow* in a case of infant death. *Journal of Clinical Pathology*, **42**, 329–30.

Boglioli, L. R. & Taff, M. L. (1998). Sudden asphyxial death complicating infectious mononucleosis. *American Journal of Forensic Medicine and Pathology*, **19**, 174–7.

Bor, I. (1969). Myocardial infarction and ischaemic heart disease in infants and children. Analysis of 29 cases and review of the literature. *Archives of Disease in Childhood*, **44**, 268–81.

Boucek, M. M., Boerth, R. C., Artman, M., Graham, T. P., Jr & Boucek, R. J., Jr (1984). Myocardial dysfunction in children with acute meningococcemia. *Journal of Pediatrics*, **105**, 538–42.

Bowles, N. E., Olsen, E. G. J., Richardson, P. J. & Archard, L. C. (1986). Detection of coxsackie-B-virus-specific RNA sequences in myocardial biopsy samples from patients with myocarditis and dilated cardiomyopathy. *Lancet*, **i**, 1120–22.

Boyer, N. H. & Weinstein, L. (1948). Diphtheritic myocarditis. *New England Journal of Medicine*, **239**, 913–19.

Brady, M. T., Reiner, C. B., Singley, C., Roberts, W. H., III & Sneddon, J. M. (1988). Unexpected death in an infant with AIDS: disseminated cytomegalovirus infection with pancarditis. *Pediatric Pathology*, **8**, 205–14.

Bruhn, F. W., Mokrohisky, S. T. & McIntosh, K. (1977). Apnea associated with respiratory syncytial virus infection in young infants. *Journal of Pediatrics*, **90**, 382–6.

Burgio, G. R. & Ugazio, A. G. (1982). Immunodeficiency and syndromes: a nosographic approach. *European Journal of Pediatrics*, **138**, 288–92.

Buris, L., Takacs, P. & Varga, M. (1987). Sudden death caused by hydatid embolism. *Zeitschrift fur Rechtsmedizin*, **98**, 125–8.

Byard, R. W. (1988). Health care in the highlands of Papua New Guinea. *Canadian Family Physician*, **34**, 709–14.

Byard, R. W. (1989). Arterial blood cultures in disseminated fungal disease. *Pediatric Infectious Disease Journal*, **8**, 728–9.

Byard, R. W. (1997). Significant coincidental findings at autopsy in accidental childhood death. *Medicine, Science and the Law*, **37**, 259–62.

Byard, R. W. (2002). Unexpected death due to infectious mononucleosis. *Journal of Forensic Sciences*, **47**, 202–4.

Byard, R. W. & Bourne, A. J. (1991). Cardiac echinococcosis with fatal intracerebral embolism. *Archives of Disease in Childhood*, **66**, 155–6.

Byard, R. W. & Krous, H. F. (1995). Minor inflammatory lesions and sudden infant death: cause, coincidence or epiphenomena? *Pediatric Pathology*, **15**, 649–54.

Byard, R. W. & Silver, M. M. (1993). Sudden infant death and acute posterior lingual inflammation. *International Journal of Pediatric Otorhinolaryngology*, **28**, 77–81.

Byard, R. W., Bourne, A. J., Matthews, N., *et al.* (1993). Pulmonary strongyloidiasis in a child diagnosed on open lung biopsy. *Surgical Pathology*, **5**, 55–62.

Caldarelli, M. (1992). Inflammatory conditions. In *Cerebrovascular Diseases in Children*, ed. A. J. Raimondi, M. Choux & C. Di Rocco. New York: Springer-Verlag, pp. 216–26.

Cantor, R., Pipas, L. & McCabe, J. (1990). Emergency department evaluation of the etiology of pediatric cardiac arrest: the role of post mortem cultures. *Pediatric Emergency Care*, **6**, 223.

Ch'en, K-C. & Teng, C-T. (1941). Infectious mononucleosis in a Chinese simulating laryngeal diphtheria with laryngeal obstruction. *Chinese Medical Journal*, **59**, 116–30.

Chesney, P. J., Davis, J. P., Purdy, W. K., Wand, P. J. & Chesney, R. W. (1981). Clinical manifestations of toxic shock syndrome. *Journal of the American Medical Association*, **246**, 741–8.

Claydon, S. M. (1989). Myocarditis as an incidental finding in young men dying from unnatural causes. *Medicine, Science and the Law*, **29**, 55–8.

Cohle, S. D., Graham, M. A., Sperry, K. L. & Dowling, G. (1989). Unexpected death as a result of infective endocarditis. *Journal of Forensic Sciences*, **34**, 1374–86.

Cooper, L. T., Jr, Berry, G. J. & Shabetai, R. (1997). Idiopathic giant-cell myocarditis – natural history and treatment. *New England Journal of Medicine*, **336**, 1860–66.

Cotran, R. S., Kumar, V. & Robbins, S. L. (1989). *Robbins Pathologic Basis of Disease*, 4th edn. Philadelphia: W. B. Saunders.

Coutlee, F., Carceller, A-M., Deschamps, L., *et al.* (1990). The evolving pattern of pediatric endocarditis from 1960 to 1985. *Canadian Journal of Cardiology*, **6**, 164–70.

Dada, M. A., Lazarus, N. G., Kharsany, A. B. M. & Sturm, A. W. (2000). Sudden death caused by myocardial tuberculosis. Case report and review of the literature. *American Journal of Forensic Medicine and Pathology*, **21**, 385–8.

D'Cruz, I. A., Sengupta, E. E., Abrahams, C., Reddy, H. K. & Turlapati, R. V. (1986). Cardiac involvement, including tuberculous pericardial effusion, complicating acquired immune deficiency syndrome. *American Heart Journal*, **112**, 1100–102.

DeMello, D. E., Liapis, H., Jureidini, S., *et al.* (1990). Cardiac localization of eosinophil-granule major basic protein in acute necrotizing myocarditis. *New England Journal of Medicine*, **323**, 1542–5.

DeSa, D. J. (1986). Isolated myocarditis as a cause of sudden death in the first year of life. *Forensic Science International*, **30**, 113–17.

Dettmeyer, R., Kandolf, R., Baasner, A., *et al.* (2003). Fatal parvovirus B19 myocarditis in an 8-year-old boy. *Journal of Forensic Sciences*, **48**, 183–6.

Dreyfus, G., Serraf, A., Jebara, V. A., *et al.* (1990). Valve repair in acute endocarditis. *Annals of Thoracic Surgery*, **49**, 706–13.

Du Moulin, G. C. & Paterson, D. G. (1985). Clinical relevance of postmortem microbiologic examination: a review. *Human Pathology*, **16**, 539–48.

Dunne, J. W., Harper, C. G. & Hilton, J. M. N. (1984). Sudden infant death syndrome caused by poliomyelitis. *Archives of Neurology*, **41**, 775–7.

Dyke, M. P., Martin, R. P. & Berry, P. J. (1991). Septicaemia and adrenal haemorrhage in congenital asplenia. *Archives of Disease in Childhood*, **66**, 636–7.

Edington, G. M. (1967). Pathology of malaria in West Africa. *British Medical Journal*, **1**, 715–18.

El-Hagrassy, M. M. O., Banatvala, J. E. & Coltart, D. J. (1980). Coxsackie-B-virus-specific IgM responses in patients with cardiac and other diseases. *Lancet*, **ii**, 1160–62.

Ette, H. Y., Koffi, K., Botti, K., *et al.* (2002). Sudden death caused by parasites. Postmortem cerebral malaria discoveries in the African endemic zone. *American Journal of Forensic Medicine and Pathology*, **23**, 202–7.

Fink, L., Reichek, N. & St John Sutton, M. G. (1984). Cardiac abnormalities in acquired immune deficiency syndrome. *American Journal of Cardiology*, **54**, 1161–3.

Franquet, T., Lecumberri, F. & Joly, M. (1984). Hyatid heart disease. *British Journal of Radiology*, **57**, 171–3.

Frenkel, L. D. & Gaur, S. (1991). Pediatric human immunodeficiency virus infection and disease. *Current Opinion in Pediatrics*, **3**, 867–73.

Friede, R. L. (1989). *Developmental Neuropathy*, 2nd edn. Berlin: Springer-Verlag.

Gerber, J. E. (2001). Acute necrotizing bacterial tonsillitis with *Clostridium perfringens*. *American Journal of Forensic Medicine and Pathology*, **22**, 177–9.

Gewirtz, J. M., Caspe, W. B., Daley, T. J. & DiCarlo, S. (1982). Airway obstruction in infectious mononucleosis in young children. *Clinical Pediatrics*, **21**, 370–72.

Gravanis, M. B. & Sternby, N. H. (1991). Incidence of myocarditis. A 10-year autopsy study from Malmo, Sweden. *Archives of Pathology and Laboratory Medicine*, **115**, 390–92.

Grice, A. C. & McGlashan, N. D. (1978). Sudden death in infancy in Tasmania, 1970–1976. *Medical Journal of Australia*, **2**, 177–80.

Haas, J. E. (1988). Case 5. Myocarditis and sudden, unexpected death in childhood. *Pediatric Pathology*, **8**, 443–6.

Han, B. K., Dunbar, J. S. & Striker, T. W. (1979). Membranous laryngotracheobronchitis (membranous croup). *Annals of Otology, Rhinology and Laryngology*, **133**, 53–8.

Hardman, J. M. (1968). Fatal meningococcal infections: the changing pathologic picture in the '60s. *Military Medicine*, **133**, 951–64.

Hassan, D. N. & Hanna, A. J. Y. (1984). Tuberculosis and sudden death in Baghdad. *American Journal of Forensic Medicine and Pathology*, **5**, 169–74.

Hauck, A. J., Kearney, D. L. & Edwards, W. D. (1989). Evaluation of postmortem endomyocardial biopsy specimens from 38 patients with lymphocytic myocarditis: implications for role of sampling error. *Mayo Clinic Proceedings*, **64**, 1235–45.

Henning, P. H., Tham, E. B. C., Martin, A. A., Beare, T. H. & Jureidini, K. F. (1998). Haemolytic-uraemic syndrome outbreak caused by *Eschericia coli* O111:H-: clinical outcomes. *Medical Journal of Australia*, **168**, 552–5.

Hoang, M. P., Ross, K. F., Dawson, D. B., Scheuermann, R. H. & Rogers, B. B. (1999). Human herpesvirus-6 and sudden death in infancy: report of a case and review of the literature. *Journal of Forensic Sciences*, **44**, 432–7.

Hoyer, M. H. & Fischer, D. R. (1991). Acute myocarditis simulating myocardial infarction in a child. *Pediatrics*, **87**, 250–53.

Hurst, D. L. & Marsh, W. W. (1993). Early severe infantile botulism. *Journal of Pediatrics*, **122**, 909–11.

Huser, C. J. & Smialek, J. E. (1986). Diagnosis of sudden death in infants due to acute dehydration. *American Journal of Forensic Medicine and Pathology*, **7**, 278–82.

Husson, R. N., Saini, R., Lewis, L. L., *et al.* (1992). Cerebral artery aneurysms in children infected with human immunodeficiency virus. *Journal of Pediatrics*, **121**, 927–30.

Issenberg, H. J., Charytan, M. & Rubinstein, A. (1985). Cardiac involvement in children with acquired immune deficiency. *American Heart Journal*, **110**, 710.

Johnsen, T., Katholm, M. & Strangerup, S.-E. (1984). Otolaryngological complications of infectious mononucleosis. *Journal of Laryngology and Otology*, **98**, 999–1001.

Joshi, V. V. (1989). Pathology of AIDS in children. *Pathology Annual*, **24** (part 1), 355–81.

Joshi, V. V., Pawel, B., Connor, E., *et al.* (1987). Arteriopathy in children with acquired immune deficiency syndrome. *Pediatric Pathology*, **7**, 261–75.

Josselson, A., Bagnall, J. W. & Virmani, R. (1984). Acute rheumatic carditis causing sudden death. *American Journal of Forensic Medicine and Pathology*, **5**, 151–4.

Kanthan, R., Moyana, T. & Nyssen, J. (1999). Asplenia as a cause of sudden unexpected death in childhood. *American Journal of Forensic Medicine and Pathology*, **20**, 57–9.

Kaplan, M. H., Klein, S. W., McPhee, J. & Harper, R. G. (1983). Group B coxsackie virus infections in infants younger than three months of age: a serious childhood illness. *Reviews of Infectious Diseases*, **5**, 1019–32.

Katcher, A. L. (1980). Familial asplenia, other malformations, and sudden death. *Pediatrics*, **65**, 633–5.

Kevy, S. V., Tefft, M., Vawter, G. F. & Rosen, F. S. (1968). Hereditary splenic hypoplasia. *Pediatrics*, **42**, 752–7.

Kilpi, T., Anttila, M., Kallio, M. J. T. & Peltola, H. (1991). Severity of childhood bacterial meningitis and duration of illness before diagnosis. *Lancet*, **338**, 406–9.

Knight, B. (1980). Sudden unexpected death from adrenal haemorrhage. *Forensic Science International*, **16**, 227–9.

Knight, B. (1997). *Forensic Pathology*, 2nd edn. London: Arnold.

Kök, A. N., Yurtman, T. & Aydin, N. E. (1993). Sudden death due to ruptured hydatid cyst of the liver. *Journal of Forensic Sciences*, **38**, 978–80.

Krous, H. F., Nadeau, J. M., Silva, P. D. & Blackbourne, B. D. (2003). A comparison of respiratory symptoms and inflammation in sudden infant death syndrome and in accidental or inflicted infant death. *American Journal of Forensic Medicine and Pathology*, **24**, 1–8.

Lie, J. T. (1989). Diagnostic histology of myocardial disease in endomyocardial biopsies and at autopsy. *Pathology Annual*, **24** (part 2), 255–91.

Malam, J. E., Carrick, G. F., Telford, D. R. & Morris, J. A. (1992). Staphylococcal toxins and sudden infant death syndrome. *Journal of Clinical Pathology*, **45**, 716–21.

Manton, N., Smith, N. M. & Byard, R. W. (2000). Unexpected childhood death due to hemolytic uremic syndrome. *American Journal of Forensic Medicine and Pathology*, **21**, 90–92.

McCurdy, J. A., Jr (1975). Life-threatening complications of infectious mononucleosis. *Laryngoscope*, **85**, 1557–63.

McKenzie, M., Norman, M. G., Anderson, J. D. & Thiessen, P. N. (1984). Upper respiratory tract infection in a 3-year-old girl. *Journal of Pediatrics*, **105**, 129–33.

Midura, T. F. & Arnon, S. S. (1976). Infant botulism: identification of clostridium botulinum and its toxins in faeces. *Lancet*, **ii**, 934–5.

Mizusawa, H., Hirano, A., Llena, J. F. & Shintaku, M. (1988). Cerebrovascular lesions in acquired immune deficiency syndrome (AIDS). *Acta Neuropathologica*, **76**, 451–7.

Molander, N. (1982). Sudden natural death in later childhood and adolescence. *Archives of Disease in Childhood*, **57**, 572–6.

Moore, L. M. (1991). Septicaemia and adrenal haemorrhage in congenital asplenia. *Archives of Disease in Childhood*, **66**, 1366–7.

Morgan, B. C. (1963). Cardiac complications of diphtheria. *Pediatrics*, **32**, 549–57.

Morris, J. A. (1983). Tampon associated staphylococcal infection and sudden death. *Lancet*, **2**, 772.

Murry, C. E., Jerome, K. R. & Reichenbach, D. D. (2001). Fatal parvovirus myocarditis in a 5-year-old girl. *Human Pathology*, **32**, 342–5.

Neufeld, H. N. & Blieden, L. C. (1975). Coronary artery disease in children. In *Progress in Cardiology*, ed. P. N. Yu & J. F. Goodwin. Philadelphia: Lea & Febiger, pp. 119–49.

Noren, G. R., Staley, N. A., Bandt, C. M. & Kaplan, E. L. (1977). Occurrence of myocarditis in sudden death in children. *Journal of Forensic Sciences*, **22**, 188–96.

Pappenheimer, A. M., Jr & Gill, D. M. (1973). Diphtheria. Recent studies have clarified the molecular mechanisms involved in its pathogenesis. *Science*, **182**, 353–8.

Paris, A. L., Herwaldt, L. A., Blum, D., *et al.* (1982). Pathologic findings in twelve fatal cases of toxic shock syndrome. *Annals of Internal Medicine*, **96**, 852–7.

Parras, F., Bouza, E., Romero, J., *et al.* (1990). Infectious endocarditis in children. *Pediatric Cardiology*, **11**, 77–81.

Patterson, K., Donnelly, W. H. & Dehner, L. P. (1992). The cardiovascular system. In *Pediatric Pathology*, vol. 1, ed. J. T. Stocker & L. P. Dehner. Philadelphia: J. B. Lippincott, pp. 575–652.

Penman, H. G. (1970). Fatal infectious mononucleosis: a critical review. *Journal of Clinical Pathology*, **23**, 765–71.

Phillips, M. M., Robinowitz, M., Higgins, J. R., *et al.* (1986). Sudden cardiac death in air force recruits. A 20-year review. *Journal of the American Medical Association*, **256**, 2696–9.

Piette, M. & Timperman, J. (1990). Sudden death in idiopathic giant cell myocarditis. *Medicine, Science and the Law*, **30**, 280–84.

Prober, C. G. & Gershon, A. A. (1991). Medical management of newborns and infants born to human immunodeficiency virus-seropositive mothers. *Pediatric Infectious Disease Journal*, **10**, 684–95.

Quagliarello, V. & Scheld, W. M. (1992). Bacterial meningitis: pathogenesis, pathophysiology, and progress. *New England Journal of Medicine*, **327**, 864–72.

Rae, M. V. (1937). Coronary aneurysms with thrombosis in rheumatic carditis. *Archives of Pathology*, **24**, 369–76.

Rapkin, R. H. (1973). Tracheostomy in epiglottis. *Pediatrics*, **52**, 426–9.

Regan, W. A. (1978). Mononucleosis patient dies of asphyxiation. *Hospital Progress*, **59**, 80–82.

Rennick, G., Shann, F. & de Campo, J. (1993). Cerebral herniation during bacterial meningitis in children. *British Medical Journal*, **306**, 953–5.

Rimar, J. M., Fox, L. & Goschke, B. (1985). Fulminant meningococcemia in children. *Heart & Lung*, **14**, 385–90.

Robboy, S. J. (1972). Atrioventricular-node inflammation – mechanism of sudden death in protracted meningococcemia. *New England Journal of Medicine*, **286**, 1091–3.

Roldan, E. O., Moskowitz, L. & Hensley, G. T. (1987). Pathology of the heart in acquired immunodeficiency syndrome. *Archives of Pathology and Laboratory Medicine*, **111**, 943–6.

Rosen, F. S., Cooper, M. D. & Wedgwood, R. J. P. (1984a). The primary immunodeficiencies (first of two parts). *New England Journal of Medicine*, **311**, 235–42.

Rosen, F. S., Cooper, M. D. & Wedgwood, R. J. P. (1984b). The primary immunodeficiencies (second of two parts). *New England Journal of Medicine*, **311**, 300–310.

Sánchez, G. R., Neches, W. H. & Jaffe, R. (1982). Myocardial aneurysm in association with disseminated cytomegalovirus infection. *Pediatric Cardiology*, **2**, 63–5.

Savoia, M. C. & Oxman, M. N. (1990). Myocarditis, pericarditis and mediastinitis. In *Principles and Practice of Infectious Diseases*, 3rd edn, ed. G. L. Mandell, R. G. Douglas & J. E. Bennett. New York: Churchill Livingstone, pp. 721–30.

Schwöbel, M. & Stauffer, U. G. (1983). Pulmonary embolism in children. *Zeitschrift fur Kinderchirurgie*, **38** (suppl), 30–32.

Scopes, J. W., Smith, M. F. & Beach, R. C. (1980). Pseudomembranous colitis and sudden infant death. *Lancet*, **1**, 1144.

Segard, E. C. & Koneman, E. W. (1968). Laryngotracheobronchitis and sudden death in children. *American Journal of Clinical Pathology*, **50**, 695–9.

Sendi, K. & Crysdale, W. S. (1987). Acute epiglottitis: decade of change – a 10 year experience with 242 children. *Journal of Otolaryngology*, **16**, 196–202.

Sharief, N., Khan, K. & Conlan, P. (1993). Overwhelming sepsis presenting as sudden unexpected death. *Archives of Disease in Childhood*, **69**, 381–3.

Singer, D. B. (1973). Postsplenectomy sepsis. In *Perspectives in Pediatric Pathology*, vol. 1, ed. H. S. Rosenberg & R. P. Bolande. Chicago: Year Book Medical Publishers, pp. 285–311.

Smith, N. M., Bourne, A. J., Clapton, W. K. & Byard, R. W. (1992). The spectrum of presentation at autopsy of myocarditis in infancy and childhood. *Pathology*, **24**, 129–31.

Smith, N. M., Telfer, S. M. & Byard, R. W. (1992). A comparison of the incidence of cytomegalovirus inclusion bodies in submandibular and tracheobronchial glands in SIDS and non-SIDS autopsies. *Pediatric Pathology*, **12**, 185–90.

Sperry K. (1994). Lethal asphyxiating juvenile laryngeal papillomatosis. A case report with human papillomavirus *in situ* hybridization analysis. *American Journal of Forensic Medicine and Pathology*, **15**, 146–50.

Springate II, C. S. & Adelson, L. (1966). Sudden and unexpected death due to splenic rupture in infectious mononucleosis. *Medicine, Science and the Law*, **6**, 215–16.

Stephan, J. L., Vlekova, V., Le Deist, F., *et al.* (1993). Severe combined immunodeficiency: a retrospective single-center study of clinical presentation and outcome in 117 patients. *Journal of Pediatrics*, **123**, 564–72.

Strife, J. L. (1988). Upper airway and tracheal obstruction in infants and children. *Radiologic Clinics of North America*, **26**, 309–22.

Sun, C.-C. J. & Smith, T. (1984). Sudden infant death with congenital cytomegalic inclusion disease. *American Journal of Forensic Medicine and Pathology*, **5**, 65–7.

Sun, T. (1988). Opportunistic parasitic infections in patients with acquired immunodeficiency syndrome. *Pathology Annual*, **23** (part 2), 1–23.

Taft, T. A., Chusid, M. J. & Sty, J. R. (1986). Cerebral infarction in *Hemophilus influenzae* type B meningitis. *Clinical Pediatrics*, **25**, 177–80.

Taubert, K. A., Rowley, A. H. & Shulman, S. T. (1991). Nationwide survey of Kawasaki disease and acute rheumatic fever. *Journal of Pediatrics*, **119**, 279–82.

Tazelaar, H. D. & Billingham, M. E. (1986). Myocardial lymphocytes. Fact, fancy, or myocarditis? *American Journal of Cardiovascular Pathology*, **1**, 47–50.

Tepper, S. L., Overman, J. & Parker, J. R. (1993). Invasive *Haemophilus influenzae* type B disease. *Journal of Forensic Sciences*, **38**, 94–7.

Traisman, E. S., Young, S., Lifschultz, B. D., *et al.* (1988). Sudden death in a neonate as a result of herpes simplex infection. *Journal of Forensic Sciences*, **33**, 267–71.

Usón, A. C., Melicow, M. M. & Pascal, R. R. (1976). Pathology of gram-negative sepsis and septicemic shock. *Antibiotics and Chemotherapy*, **21**, 66–8.

Variend, S. (1990). Infant mortality, microglial nodules and parotid CMV-type inclusions. *Early Human Development*, **21**, 31–40.

Virmani, R. & Roberts, W. C. (1987). Sudden cardiac death. *Human Pathology*, **18**, 485–92.

Voigt, G. C. & Wright, J. R. (1974). Cyanotic congenital heart disease and sudden death. *American Heart Journal*, **87**, 773–82.

Waldman, J. D., Rosenthal, A., Smith, A. L., Shurin, S. & Nadas, A. S. (1977). Sepsis and congenital asplenia. *Journal of Pediatrics*, **90**, 555–9.

Weinstein, L. (1973). Tetanus. *New England Journal of Medicine*, **289**, 1293–6.

Welsby, P. D. & Golledge, C. L. (1990). Meningococcal meningitis. A diagnosis not to be missed. *British Medical Journal*, **300**, 1150–51.

Wentworth, P., Jentz, L. A. & Croal, A. E. (1979). Analysis of sudden unexpected death in southern Ontario, with emphasis on myocarditis. *Canadian Medical Association Journal*, **120**, 676–706.

Whitehead, F. J., Couper, R. T. L., Moore, L., Bourne, A. J. & Byard, R. W. (1996). Dehydration deaths in infants and children. *American Journal of Forensic Medicine and Pathology*, **17**, 73–8.

Whitley, C. B., Thompson, L. R., Osterholm, M. T., *et al.* (1982). Toxic shock syndrome in a newborn infant. *Pediatric Research*, **16**, 254A.

Wolfe, J. A. & Rowe, L. D. (1980). Upper airway obstruction in infectious mononucleosis. *Annals of Otology*, **89**, 430–33.

Woolf, D. C. S. & Diedericks, R. J. (1989). Airway obstruction in infectious mononucleosis. *South African Medical Journal*, **75**, 584–5.

Yamashima, T., Kashihara, K., Ikeda, K., Kubota, T. & Yamamoto, S. (1985). Three phases of cerebral arteriopathy in meningitis: vasospasm and vasodilation followed by organic stenosis. *Neurosurgery*, **16**, 546–53.

Yip, D. C. P., Sein, K. K. & Lung, H. K. (1987). A retrospective study of interstitial pneumonitis ("viral pneumonia") as a cause of sudden and unexpected natural death. *Medicine, Science and the Law*, **27**, 79–84.

Zalzal, G. H. (1989). Stridor and airway compromise. *Pediatric Clinics of North America*, **36**, 1389–401.

5

Cardiac conditions

Introduction

Cardiac disease is one of the major causes of sudden and unexpected death in children and adolescents. Myocarditis, hypertrophic cardiomyopathy, congenital aortic stenosis, and cyanotic congenital heart disease with pulmonary obstruction are among the most common medical conditions that cause sudden death in this age group. This contrasts with adults, in whom atherosclerotic coronary artery disease is a far more usual finding. Additionally, there are many rarer entities that may also result in sudden cardiac decompensation and death in childhood. Determination of the precise incidence of a number of these rarer entities is difficult because of subtle autopsy findings and variable standards of postmortem investigation (Byard, 2002).

A number of cases of sudden death in children are associated with exercise and may have been heralded by palpitations, dyspnea, chest pain, or syncope, although this is not always the case (Byard, James & Gilbert, 2002; Liberthson, 1996). Causes of sudden cardiac death in childhood are listed in Table 5.1, many of which now have established complex gene linkages.

The author has noted a decline in the number of cases of congenital heart disease presenting to autopsy in recent years, presumably reflecting improvements in antenatal and clinical diagnoses and the efficacy of subsequent cardiac surgery. Unfortunately, this may also be a reflection of prevailing low hospital autopsy rates.

Infections and related disorders

Myocarditis

Myocarditis is a major cause of sudden death in childhood. Affected children may be ill with fever and heart failure, or may show only minimal signs and symptoms of disease despite extensive cardiac involvement (Bonadio & Losek, 1987). Inflammation of the myocardium with myocyte necrosis may be caused by a range of infectious and non-infectious agents, including viruses, bacteria, chlamydia, rickettsiae, fungi, protozoa, helminths, drugs, hypersensitivity reactions, metabolic disorders, and radiation (Hohn & Stanton, 1987; Markus *et al.*, 1989) (Table 5.2). The finding of myocarditis does not automatically suggest a cause of death, however, and assessment of other autopsy findings, the history, and the circumstances of death is important as myocarditis may be quite incidental to the mechanisms responsible for the lethal episode (Byard, 1997).

The most common causative agents in childhood are viruses. These include coxsackie A, influenza, polio, and enteroviruses, with the group B coxsackie viruses predominating. Myocarditis also occurs in rheumatic fever and in Kawasaki disease and has also been found not infrequently at autopsy in AIDS patients (Anderson *et al.*, 1988). Other cases, such as giant cell myocarditis, are of unknown etiology.

Death may be due to inflammation and necrosis of the myocardium and conduction tracts during the

Table 5.1. Cardiac causes of sudden pediatric death

Infections and related disorders
   Myocarditis
   Endocarditis
   Rheumatic fever
Congenital cardiac defects
   Before and after surgery
Cardiomyopathies
   Hypertrophic
   Dilated
   Restrictive
   Right ventricular
   Histiocytoid
   Spongy myocardium
Valvular abnormalities
   Aortic stenosis
   Mitral valve prolapse syndrome
   Tricuspid valve prolapse
Subaortic stenosis
Tumors
Conduction defects
Miscellaneous

Table 5.2. Etiology of myocarditis

Infective	Non-infective	Idiopathic
Viruses	Connective tissue	Giant cell myocarditis
Bacteria	disease	Kawasaki disease
Chlamydia	Drugs	
Rickettsiae	Hypersensitivity	
Protozoa	reactions	
Helminths	Metabolic disorders	
	Radiation	

acute stages of the disease with arrhythmias. Alternatively, sudden death may occur some time later due to fibrous scarring, which predisposes to electrical instability, re-entry circuits, and rhythm disturbance (Lecomte *et al.*, 1993). (Further discussion of the role of myocarditis in the causation of sudden death may be found in Chapter 4.)

Endocarditis

Bacterial infection of the endocardium usually occurs in children with congenital cardiac defects and results in friable vegetations, which may cause sudden death due to embolization to the coronary or carotid circulations (see Chapter 4).

Rheumatic fever

Rheumatic fever is a febrile illness in which pancarditis may follow an acute streptococcal infection. It is believed to be due to immunological cross-reactivity between cardiac myocyte and streptococcal antigens. Sudden death may occur secondary to conduction abnormalities, valve compromise, and coronary embolism (see Chapter 4).

Congenital cardiac defects

A variety of congenital cardiac defects, including cyanotic, acyanotic, and obstructive conditions, may result in sudden and unexpected death in infancy and childhood (Lambert *et al.*, 1974). Among the most commonly encountered are tetralogy of Fallot and transposition of the great vessels. The following discussion focuses on classical malformations, although different lesions may overlap and some patients may present with extremely complex anomalies. Several of these conditions, including secundum atrial septal defects, subvalvular aortic stenosis, ventricular septal defects, tetralogy of Fallot, and pulmonary atresia, may be autosomal dominantly inherited associated with conduction tract disturbances and mutations in the gene encoding the homeobox transcription factor NKX2-5 on chromosome 5q35 (Schott *et al.*, 1998). There is also a strong association between congenital cardiac defects and the trisomy syndromes (Strauss & Johnson, 1996).

Sudden death is an unusual occurrence in children with only mild cardiac disease (Anonymous, 1975). However, the immediate clinical history may not be of use in directing the autopsy, as children with unoperated congenital cardiac defects often die in their sleep (Gillette & Garson, 1992) with minimal

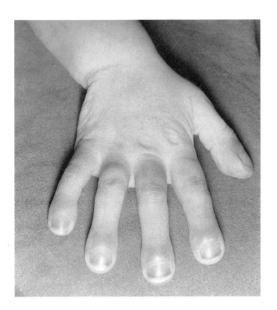

Figure 5.1 Marked clubbing of the fingers in a two-year-old girl with known cyanotic congenital heart disease.

preceding symptoms. One-third of sudden cardiac deaths in a series of individuals under the age of 35 years were attributed to congenital structural defects (Basso *et al.*, 1995).

Finger clubbing (Figure 5.1) or poly- or asplenia (Figure 5.2) may be useful indicators of the presence of extensive cardiovascular anomalies early in the autopsy that should prompt careful examination and dissection of the heart and its connections (Kiuchi, Kawachi & Kimura, 1988). Detailed radiographic and dissection techniques for examining the heart and coronary vessels at autopsy have been described (Devine, Debich & Anderson, 1991; Virmani, Ursell & Fenoglio, 1987). In mortuaries and laboratories where there may not be expertise in congenital cardiac conditions, access to a pediatric cardiologist, or facilities to process such cases, referral to a cardiac pathologist may be required.

Complications of cyanotic congenital heart disease

Cerebral infarction is a serious complication of cyanotic congenital heart disease and may follow bacterial endocarditis, cardiac catheterization, or surgery (Terplan, 1973). The reported incidence of cerebrovascular disease in children with cyanotic congenital heart disease varies between 1.6 and 3.8%, with a mortality rate of 10%. Predisposing factors are anemia and dehydration in infants, and polycythemia and hypoxemia in older children (Pellegrino, Zanesco & Battistella, 1992; Phornphutkul *et al.*, 1973). Most cases of cerebral infarction occur in children with transposition of the great vessels or with tetralogy of Fallot, the two most prevalent forms of cyanotic heart disease. Both arterial and venous thromboses may occur, the latter being more common in younger children (Cottrill & Kaplan, 1973).

Myocardial infarction may occur in children with congenital heart disease, either from reduced arterial perfusion associated with polycythemia or from hypoxemia (Franciosi & Blanc, 1968). Coronary artery thromboembolism also occurs. Studies have demonstrated that a high percentage of children with congenital cardiac defects have areas of cardiac necrosis, particularly in cases of ventricular outflow obstruction (Russell, 1992; Russell & Berry, 1989). The location of a significant percentage of infarcts in the subendocardium and within the papillary muscles in these children (Pesonen, 1974) makes sampling of these areas important at the time of autopsy. As myocardial infarcts may be difficult to detect on visual inspection of the heart in children, and as infarcts may involve the atria, samples should be taken routinely from all four cardiac chambers.

Postsurgical sudden death

Children who have undergone surgical repair of congenital cardiac defects are at increased risk of sudden and unexpected death, although the risk is small. The two most common entities with this association are repaired tetralogy of Fallot and transposition of the great vessels (Basso *et al.*, 1995; Murphy *et al.*, 1993; Rosenthal, 1993). Other types of surgically corrected congenital cardiac defects, such as atrial septal defect (primum and secundum), double outlet right ventricle, and ventricular septal defect, may also, rarely, be associated with late sudden death (Meijboom *et al.*, 1994).

Frequency

Sudden death has been documented in 3–10% of patients following repair of a tetralogy and in 2–8% of patients after repair of transposition (Deanfield, McKenna & Hallidie-Smith, 1980; Gillette & Garson, 1992; Quattlebaum *et al.*, 1976).

Etiology

Major mechanisms of sudden death following cardiac surgery are heart block and arrhythmias (Silka, Kron & McAnulty, 1992), with rarer complications including rupture of prosthetic valves and foreign body coronary artery embolism (Lambert *et al.*, 1974). Sudden death occurs in 60–80% of patients who develop complete heart block following surgery if pacemaker therapy is not instituted (Vetter, 1985).

Electrocardiographic changes in patients with ventricular septal defect (with and without tetralogy of Fallot) demonstrate particular vulnerability to damage of the right bundle branch and left superior division of the left branch during surgery, and to involvement in fibrous scar formation after surgery (Kulbertus, Coyne & Hallidie-Smith, 1969). Right bundle branch, left anterior hemiblock, and complete heart block are all observed, the latter possibly accounting for the increased incidence of sudden death.

Ventricular tachyarrhythmia may also be responsible for unexpected cardiac arrest following intraventricular surgery. Although it has been reported that the risk of sudden death is highest in the first few years after surgery (Murphy *et al.*, 1993), death may be delayed until years after the corrective procedure (Bharati & Lev, 1983; Silka *et al.*, 1998). In the series of James, Kaplan & Chou (1975), sudden death occurred in three patients with tetralogy of Fallot up to 15 years after successful surgical correction. All of the patients were considered to be well, and only one was exercising, although all had demonstrated premature ventricular contractions on postoperative electrocardiograms.

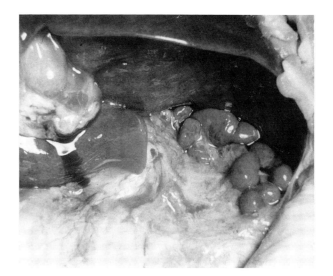

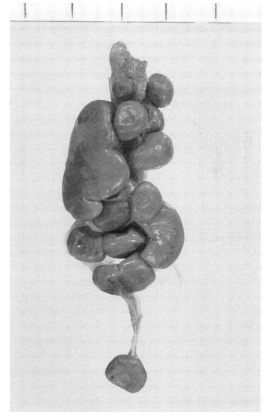

Figure 5.2 Polysplenia may be a clue to the presence of complex congenital cardiac disease.

Patients with tetralogy of Fallot are also at risk of developing arrhthymias from ectopic foci emanating from hypertrophic myocytes around the ventriculotomy scar, from fibrosed areas within the right ventricle, or from any other scarred areas (Davies, 1992; Deanfield, McKenna & Rowland, 1985). Sudden death may, therefore, occur in patients with tetralogy of Fallot due to these features despite technically excellent surgery (Dunnigan *et al.*, 1984).

Another factor that may predispose children with surgically corrected tetralogy of Fallot to sudden death is the increasing incidence of pulmonary insufficiency with age (Garson, 1991). Right ventricular function may be markedly impaired, with dilation and reduced contractility. Ventricular dilation may also affect the pre-existing surgical scar, resulting in arrhythmogenic foci.

Children who have had Mustard or Senning procedures for transposition of the great vessels are also at increased risk for arrhythmias and sudden death. Most rhythm disturbances are bradyarrhythmias; however, 10–15% of patients develop tachyarrhythmias, and it is this group that has a stronger association with sudden death (Gillette & Garson, 1992). The Fontan procedure in children with single functioning ventricles is associated with an increased risk of sudden death, believed to be caused by atrial tachycardia, with rapid conduction through the atrioventricular node (Berger, Dhala & Friedberg, 1999).

Autopsy findings

Due to the rapidity with which death can occur from lethal arrhythmia or heart block, autopsy investigation in these patients may not reveal acute changes. The cause of death may therefore have to be deduced from an assessment of the presenting history and an analysis of the type of malformation and corrective surgery. Autopsy should include a careful examination of conduction pathways and tissue surrounding the sinoatrial and atrioventricular nodes for evidence of fibrous scarring (Bharati *et al.*, 1979b).

Tetralogy of Fallot

Tetralogy of Fallot, one of the most common forms of cyanotic congenital heart disease, is characterized by ventricular septal defect, infundibular pulmonary

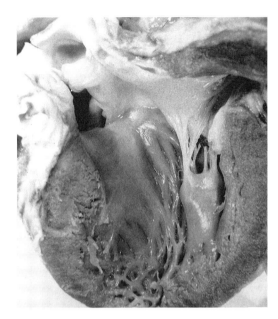

Figure 5.3 Tetralogy of Fallot, demonstrating ventricular septal defect with overriding aorta.

stenosis, an overriding aorta, and right ventricular hypertrophy. It is a well known cause of sudden death both before and after corrective surgery (*vide supra*) (Denfield & Garson, 1990) (Figure 5.3).

Eisenmenger syndrome

In this malformation, pulmonary hypertension results from a reversal of flow through an atrial or ventricular septal defect or through a patent ductus arteriosus (Rutledge & Boor, 1989). Usual symptoms are of marked cyanotic congestive cardiac failure; however, sudden and unexpected death may occur. In a multicenter study of sudden and unexpected death from cardiovascular disease (Lambert *et al.*, 1974), Eisenmenger syndrome accounted for 15% of cases. Pregnancy greatly increases the risk of cardiac decompensation in affected females (Colman *et al.*, 2000; Siu & Colman, 2001).

Ventricular septal defect

Ventricular septal defect is the most common congenital cardiac defect, accounting for as many as

43% of all isolated congenital cardiac malformations (Bower & Ramsay, 1994; Samanek, Goetzova & Benesova, 1985). While uncomplicated ventricular septal defect has been associated only rarely with sudden pediatric death (Arey & Sotos, 1956; Byard, 1994; Byard, Bourne & Adams, 1990; Lambert *et al.*, 1974; Smith & Ho, 1994) (Figure 5.4), serious arrhythmias have been reported in 16–31% of patients (Cohle, Balraj & Bell, 1999). In one report, the largest group presenting as sudden death were Down syndrome children with endocardial cushion defects (Gillette & Garson, 1992). In infancy, it may be impossible to exclude SIDS as a cause of death, and the possibility of a purely coincidental association with death should always be considered, particularly if there is no significant cardiomegaly. Bacterial endocarditis and pulmonary hypertension are associated complications that may also result in sudden death (Bloomfield, 1964; Cohle *et al.*, 1989).

A case of unexpected death occurring in a three-month-old boy with a ventricular septal defect is shown in Figure 5.5. There was significant cardiomegaly and pulmonary venous congestion, with scattered hemosiderin-laden macrophages within the lungs. The absence of any other lesion that could have resulted in these changes makes the ventricular septal defect, with possible associated aortic valve leaflet compromise, the most likely cause of death due to cardiac hypertrophy with arrhythmia (Byard, Bourne & Adams, 1990).

Hypoplastic left heart syndrome

This is characterized by hypoplasia or absence of the left ventricle, with aortic arch hypoplasia and aortic valve hypoplasia, stenosis, or atresia (Norwood, 1989) (Figures 5.6 and 5.7). Systemic blood flow depends on a patent ductus arteriosus. While the usual manifestations are of severe heart failure in the neonatal period, some infants may survive for weeks and then present either with fulminant cardiac failure or with sudden death. Hypoplastic left heart syndrome usually occurs as an isolated phenomenon, but it may be associated with genetic disorders including trisomies 13, 18, and 21, Turner syndrome, and Smith–Lemli–Opitz syndrome. Dysmorphic

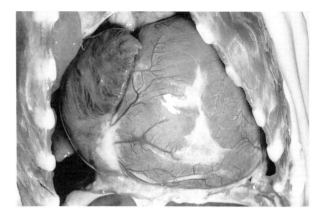

Figure 5.4 Marked cardiomegaly in a 2.5-year-old boy who collapsed and died with an undiagnosed large membranous ventricular septal defect.

features should, therefore, be looked for in such cases. Isolated rare familial cases have been reported (Kojima *et al.*, 1969).

Cor triatriatum

In this condition, the pulmonary veins empty into a chamber that is separated from the left atrium by a fibromuscular membrane (Color Plate 10) (Gheissari *et al.*, 1992). Cor triatriatum is believed to result from stenosis of the common pulmonary vein and has a variety of anatomical subtypes (Hammon & Bender, 1990). While symptoms and signs during life are usually of significant pulmonary venous obstruction, sudden death may occur in association with pulmonary hypertension.

Cardiomyopathies

Cardiomyopathies may be primary diseases of the heart related to specific gene defects or may be phenomena occurring secondarily to underlying metabolic conditions. The latter disorders are described in further detail in Chapter 11 and include systemic metabolic conditions, such as the mucopolysaccharidoses, GM_1 gangliosidosis, galactosialidosis, lysosomal and glycogen storage diseases, and fatty acid mitochondrial β-oxidation

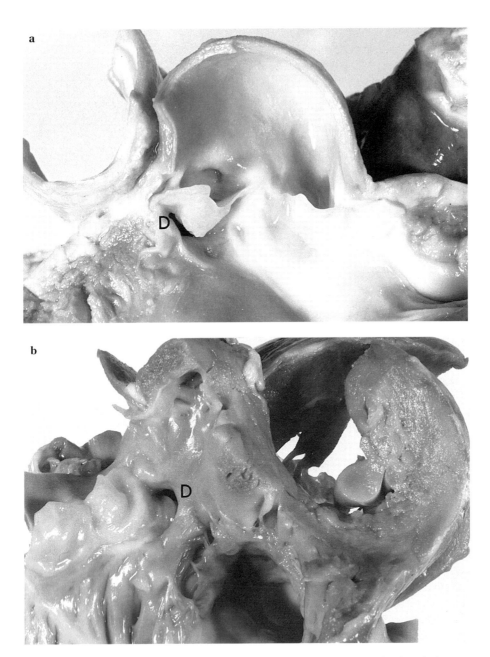

Figure 5.5 Subvalvular ventricular septal defect (D) beneath the aortic valve (a) associated with marked cardiomegaly (b) in an apparently well three-month-old boy who was found dead in his crib.

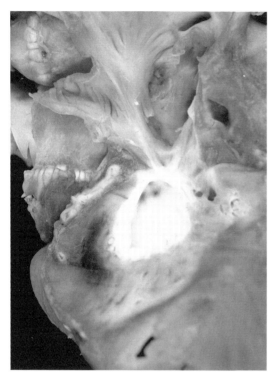

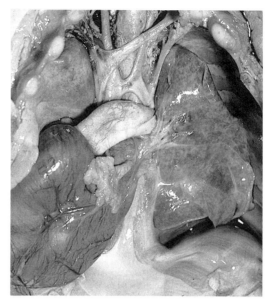

Figure 5.7 Hypoplasia of the left ventricle, with associated hypolastic aortic arch.

Figure 5.6 Marked endocardial fibroelastosis and reduction in the size of the left ventricular cavity in left ventricular hypoplasia.

defects, such as carnitine transport defects and long-chain acyl coenzyme A dehydrogenase deficiency (Guertl, Noehammer & Hoefler, 2000; Kelly & Strauss, 1994; Schwartz *et al.*, 1996).

Hypertrophic cardiomyopathy

This primary disorder of the myocardium is characterized by a profound increase in size and weight of the heart due to myocyte hypertrophy. It is also known as asymmetric septal hypertrophy, hypertrophic subaortic stenosis, and obstructive cardiomyopathy.

Clinical features

There is considerable heterogeneity in the clinical and pathological presentations, even within the

same family. Manifestations may appear in infancy (Maron, Roberts & Epstein, 1982) caused by obstruction of the left ventricular outflow tract, mitral valve incompetence due to distortion of the valve annulus, or left ventricular failure. Mural thrombus formation with systemic embolization and bacterial endocarditis of the abnormal mitral valve may also be found. Inheritance may be autosomal dominant or recessive (Bryant, 1999; Landing *et al.*, 1994).

Etiology

There is marked heterogeneity in the inheritance of hypertrophic cardiomyopathy, with mutations being identified on a range of chromosomes, including 1q3, 3p21.2-3p21.3, 7q3, 11p13-q13, 12q23-q24.3, 14q1, 14q11-q12, 15q2, 15q14, and 19p13.2-q13.2. These genes, including the beta-myosin heavy chain and the alpha-cardiac actin (ACTC) genes, code for proteins or cytoskeletal components that are involved in myocyte contractility (Anderson, 1995; Branzi *et al.*, 1985; Bhavsar *et al.*, 1996; Carrier *et al.*, 1993; Curfman, 1992; Epstein *et al.*, 1992; Jarcho *et al.*, 1989; MacRae *et al.*, 1995; Maron *et al.*, 1987a; Mogensen *et al.*, 1999; Thierfelder *et al.*, 1993; Towbin & Bowles, 2001; Watkins *et al.*, 1992; Watkins *et al.*, 1993). Mutations in either the essential or regulatory light chains of myosin have also been identified in a subset of families with hypertrophic cardiomyopathy (Poetter *et al.*, 1996).

Pathological features

Disproportionate hypertrophy of the interventricular septum is the usual morphologic feature of this disorder. However, the term "asymmetric septal hypertrophy" may be confusing, as the myocardial hypertrophy is not always asymmetrical (see below). Similarly, the name "obstructive cardiomyopathy" may also be misleading, as not all cases demonstrate significant obstruction (Maron *et al.*, 1982).

On gross examination, there is obvious cardiomegaly, with heart weights in infants often two to three times greater than the upper limit of normal. Four patterns of hypertrophy have been identified:

1 Hypertrophy limited to the anterior portion of the intraventricular septum.
2 Hypertrophy of the anterior and posterior portions of the intraventricular septum.
3 Hypertrophy of both the intraventricular septum and the free wall of the left ventricle.
4 Hypertrophy of the posterior portion of the intraventricular septum, the anterolateral portion of the left ventricular free wall, or the apical portion of the septum (Ciró, Nichols & Maron, 1983).

Transverse sectioning of the ventricles will usually reveal marked reduction in size of the left ventricular cavity (Figure 5.8), and in adults there may be mitral valve thickening associated with prolapse and endocardial plaques (Roberts, 1978). The main features in children are greater thickening of the interventricular septum compared with the ventricular free wall, narrowed ventricular cavities, disorganization of myofibers within the interventricular septum, and abnormal intramural arteries (Roberts, 1980).

Endocardial fibroelastosis may be present, and individual myocytes may show considerable glycogen accumulation. There may also be patchy interstitial myocardial fibrosis (Okoye, Congdon & Mueller, 1985). Significant thickening of the walls of intramural coronary arteries due to intimal and medial proliferation has been found at all ages, even in infancy, and may exacerbate myocardial ischemia (Maron *et al.*, 1989).

Myocyte hypertrophy and disorganization with loss of the usual parallel orientation may be obvious microscopically, even in very early infancy (Maron *et al.*, 1974) (Figure 5.9). However, extensive myofiber disarray may not be present in some infants despite the presence of gross cardiomegaly and the screening of multiple histologic sections. In these instances, correlation of the clinical history with the presence of profound cardiomegaly (in the absence of an alternative cause such as aortic obstruction) may be necessary to establish the diagnosis.

Occurrence of sudden death

Overall, there is a higher rate of sudden death reported in afflicted individuals under the age of 30 years, with sudden death occurring in 6–8% of affected children and 2–4% of affected adults (Gow, 1996; Maron *et al.*, 1987b; Maron, Roberts & Epstein, 1982). Hypertrophic cardiomyopathy has been cited as the most common finding in young athletes who die suddenly and unexpectedly (Maron *et al.*, 1980), although not all series of sudden death in the young have shown this (Basso *et al.*, 1995). Sudden death is a well recognized occurrence, even in asymptomatic children (Gourdie, Robertson & Busuttil, 1989). The yearly mortality rate of 5–6% in affected children (Edwards, 1991) reduces to 2% after successful surgical myomectomy (McKenna & Deanfield, 1984). Early presentation with clinical symptoms such as exertional syncope and a family history of sudden death are markers for a child at increased risk (Bryant, 1999; Wilkinson, 1994), in addition to ventricular ectopy on ambulatory recording and evidence of myocardial ischemia (Yetman *et al.*, 1998).

Pathophysiology

The mechanism of sudden death in children with any of the forms of outflow obstruction is believed to be lethal arrhythmia associated with left ventricular hypertrophy, or reflex bradycardias and arrhythmias

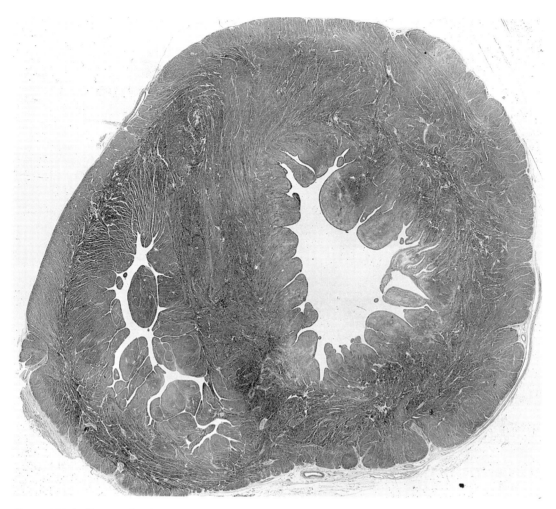

Figure 5.8 Marked hypertrophy of the left ventricle and in particular of the interventricular septum in a nine-month-old girl with hypertrophic cardiomyopathy (Masson Trichrome stain, ×3).

caused by activation of left ventricular barorecep-tors. Impaired ventricular filling results in profound hypotension (Maron & Fananapazir, 1992; Silka *et al.*, 1990). Myocardial ischemia in diastole results from compression of intramural coronary arteries by in-creased end-diastolic pressures. In systole, ischemia results from decreased coronary artery blood flow due to compression of arteries from increased mus-cle bulk (Cohle *et al.*, 1988). Left ventricular hypertro-phy is an independent risk factor for sudden death in adult populations and also for high-grade ventricular

ectopy (Chambers, 1995; Dunn, Burns & Hornung, 1991; Messerli, 1990; Pringle *et al.*, 1992).

Associated features

Hypertrophic cardiomyopathy may be associated with a range of heritable and other conditions, in-cluding Friedreich ataxia, Leigh syndrome, Leopard syndrome, Noonan syndrome, familial myopathy, Duchenne and other non-myotonic dystrophies, the aniridia-Wilms tumor complex, and various metabolic disorders (see Table 11.3) (Fried *et al.*,

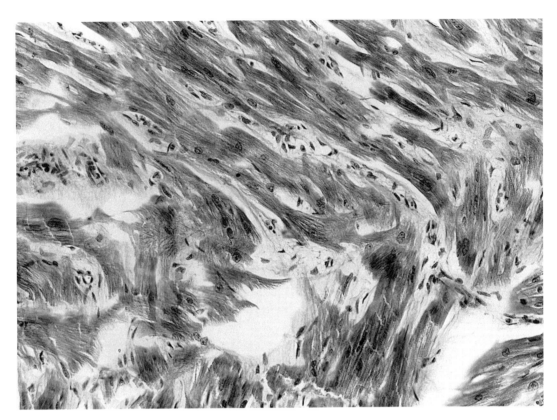

Figure 5.9 Disorganized cardiac myocytes in the lateral wall of the left ventricle in hypertrophic cardiomyopathy (hematoxylin and eosin, ×80).

1979; Gilgenkrantz *et al.*, 1982; Perloff, de Leon & O'Doherty, 1966; Senn, Hess & Krayenbuhl, 1984). In occasional families, both hypertrophic cardiomyopathy and Wolff–Parkinson–White syndrome may occur (MacRae *et al.*, 1995).

Dilated cardiomyopathy

This is another form of cardiomyopathy found in childhood in which there is massive enlargement of the heart due to ventricular dilation in the absence of valvular or congenital cardiac structural defects.

Clinical features

While the clinical course is usually chronic, complications such as atrial and ventricular arrhythmias, systemic embolization, and sudden unexpected death in childhood have been described (Friedman, Moak & Garson, 1991). Sudden death usually occurs only after the development of heart failure or arrhythmias (Davies & Popple, 1979).

Etiology

The etiology of dilated or congestive cardiomyopathy is heterogeneous, and the condition may result from a variety of toxins, metabolic abnormalities, and infectious or inflammatory diseases (Billingham & Tazelaar, 1986; Dec & Fuster, 1994). Inherited gene defects account for approximately 35% of cases, with reports of autosomal dominant, autosomal recessive, X-linked, and mitochondrial modes of inheritance (Berko & Swift 1987; Emanuel, Withers & O'Brien 1971; Gardner *et al.*, 1987; Schmidt *et al.*, 1988; Towbin & Bowles, 2001).

Autosomal dominant dilated cardiomyopathy has been linked to mutations on chromosomes 1q3, 1p1-q21, 1q11-21, 1q11-23, 1q32, 2q11-22, 2q31, 2q35, 3p22-25, 5q33, 6q23, 9q13-22, 10q21-23, 14q11, and 15q14, with defects occurring in both actin and desmin genes (Bowles *et al.*, 1996; Durand *et al.*, 1995; Krajinovic *et al.*, 1995; Li *et al.*, 1999; Olson & Keating, 1996; Olson *et al.*, 1998; Siu *et al.*, 1999; Towbin & Bowles, 2001). An autosomal recessive form is linked to 17q12-21.33 (Graham & Owens, 1999). Mutations in the dystrophin gene on chromosome Xp21 may cause structural protein defects, resulting in X-linked dilated cardiomyopathy and the dilated cardiomyopathies of Duchenne and Becker muscular dystrophies (Strauss & Johnson, 1996; Towbin, 1999). Barth syndrome is another X-linked cardiomyopathy, in which there is endocardial fibroelastosis and dilation and hypertrophy of the left ventricle (Towbin & Bowles, 2001).

The finding of a dilated cardiomyopathy at autopsy in a child should also raise the possibility of an underlying metabolic abnormality, such as a disorder of fatty acid oxidation or carnitine deficiency (Kelly & Strauss, 1994; Rocchiccioli *et al.*, 1990) (see Table 11.3). There is an association with neuromuscular disorders, such as Friedreich ataxia, Duchenne muscular dystrophy, myotonic dystrophy, facioscapulohumeral muscular dystrophy, and Erb limb-girdle dystrophy (Dec & Fuster, 1994).

Pathological features

Macroscopically, affected hearts show marked enlargement, with dilation of the ventricles (Figure 5.10), which may contain mural thrombi. Cardiac valves and vessels are usually normal. Microscopically, the changes present are non-specific, with focal hypertrophy and interstitial fibrosis being present in the majority of, but not all, cases (Roberts, 1978).

Restrictive cardiomyopathy

Restrictive cardiomyopathy is uncommon in children, accounting for 5% of all cardiomyopathies. The annual mortality rate for children with restrictive cardiomyopathy and sudden death has been

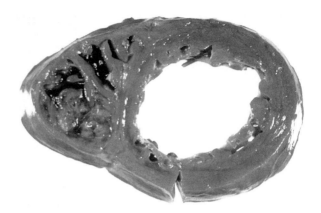

Figure 5.10 Dilation of the left ventricle in dilated cardiomyopathy.

reported as 7%, with affected children often having histories of chest pain or syncope (Rivenes *et al.*, 2000). Although rare in children from Western countries, so-called eosinophilic endomyocardial disease is found in children from tropical areas, where death may result from arrhythmias or thromboembolism (Edwards, 1991). Unexpected death has also been reported in a child with a restrictive cardiomyopathy, who was undergoing a pyruvate loading test as part of a metabolic work-up for a possible mitochondrial enzyme deficiency (Matthys, Van Coster & Verhaaren, 1991). Restrictive cardiomyopathy has been reported in Noonan syndrome (Cooke, Chambers & Curry, 1994), and may rarely be inherited autosomal dominantly (Fitzpatrick *et al.*, 1990).

Arrhythmogenic right ventricular cardiomyopathy

Arrhythmogenic right ventricular cardiomyopathy refers to a condition that is characterized by fibrofatty replacement of the right ventricular wall. It has a broad spectrum of clinical and pathological manifestations (Shrapnel, Gilbert & Byard, 2001). The term has been used to refer to Uhl anomaly, where replacement of the right ventricular wall by fibrous tissue results in a "parchment-like" effect, and also to right ventricular dysplasia, where the ventricular wall is

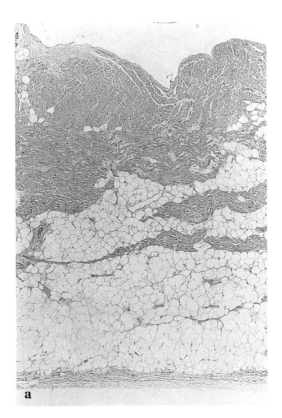 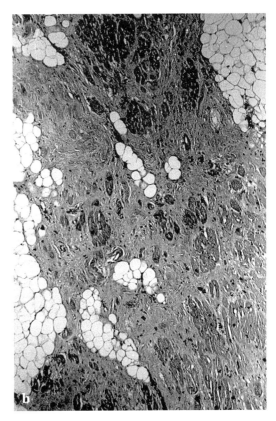

Figure 5.11 Fatty replacement of the wall of the right ventricle (a) (hematoxylin and eosin, ×60), with adjacent fibrous scarring (b) in an 18-year-old female who died unexpectedly from arrhythmogenic right ventricular cardiomyopathy. Her mother had died unexpectedly at the age of 24 years (hematoxylin and eosin, ×80).

replaced by fatty tissue but is of approximately normal width (Figure 5.11) (Maron, 1988).

While some authors suggest that Uhl anomaly and fibrolipomatous transformation ("dysplasia") are different manifestations of the same disease process, the underlying feature of which is right ventricular dysfunction, others would regard them as discrete disorders (Farb, Burke & Virmani, 1992; Goodin *et al.*, 1991; Marcus *et al.*, 1982; Maron, 1988; Nava *et al.*, 1988a; Nava *et al.*, 1988b; Smeeton & Smith, 1987; Sutter & Gujer, 1996; Virmani *et al.*, 1982). The occurrence of both entities within the same kindred may support an occasional association in some cases (Thiene *et al.*, 1988); however, it appears likely that ventricular dysplasia is a separate entity to Uhl

anomaly. Both are associated with sudden childhood death.

Clinical features

Clinical manifestations of arrhythmogenic right ventricular cardiomyopathy, including unexpected death, usually occur in adolescence and early adulthood, although the diagnosis has been made as early as 10 days of age (Kearney *et al.*, 1995). Congestive cardiac failure, complete heart block, and ventricular arrhythmias are characteristic. Deaths may occur during athletic activity due to sensitivity of the heart to elevated levels of exercise-induced catecholamines (Gemayel, Pelliccia & Thompson, 2001).

Etiology

A variety of causes have been proposed, including infectious and degenerative; however, many cases are inherited in an autosomal dominant manner, with variable expression and penetrance (Ibsen, Baandrup & Simonsen, 1985; Ruder *et al.*, 1985). Mutations have been identified on chromosomes 1q42-q43, 2q32.1-q32.2, 3p23, 10p12-p14, 14q12-q22, 14q23-q24, and 17q21 (Naxos disease) (Gemayel, Pelliccia & Thompson, 2001; Towbin, 2001; Towbin & Bowles, 2001). Mutations in the cardiac ryanodine receptor gene also identified in families affected by arrhythmogenic right ventricular cardiomyopathy may explain the tendency to exercise-induced arrhythmias, as the ryanodine receptor is responsible for catecholamine-induced ventricular tachycardia (Gemayel, Pelliccia & Thompson, 2001).

Pathological features

The diagnosis at autopsy is based upon demonstration of fibrolipomatous replacement of the right ventricular myocardium in the absence of any valvular, coronary artery, or congenital cardiac defects. Young adults may also have a background inflammatory infiltrate, which should not be mistaken for myocarditis. It is thought to be a secondary phenomenon as it has not been described in affected infants (Bharati *et al.*, 1983b) and is not invariably present in adults (Horiguchi *et al.*, 1990), although a light infiltrate of lymphocytes is not uncommon (Figure 5.12). The right atrium and left ventricle may show similar pathological changes (Marcus *et al.*, 1982), and on occasion only the left ventricle is involved. Whether the latter is a variant of arrhythmogenic right ventricular cardiomyopathy or a separate entity is yet to be determined (Shrapnel, Gilbert & Byard, 2001).

Occurrence of sudden death

In the USA, arrhythmogenic right ventricular cardiomyopathy has been responsible for 3–4% of sudden deaths in young athletes. A much higher incidence has been reported from other countries, possibly reflecting variation in the incidence of underlying gene mutations (Corrado *et al.*, 1990). Where

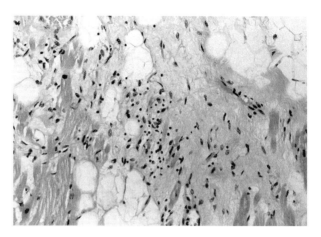

Figure 5.12 Fibrosis with a mild background lymphocytic infiltrate in arrhythmogenic right ventricular cardiomyopathy (hematoxylin and eosin, ×150).

documented, cardiac arrest has been associated with ventricular fibrillation (Gemayel, Pelliccia & Thompson, 2001). Sudden death is believed to result from arrhythmias generated at the junction of the normal and abnormal myocardium and has occurred in childhood (Bharati & Lev, 1985; Dungan, Garson & Gillette, 1981; Pawel *et al.*, 1994).

Histiocytoid cardiomyopathy

This rare entity, also known as foamy transformation of the myocardium or oncocytic cardiomyopathy, is characterized by cardiac hypertrophy with aggregated enlarged myocytes located particularly in the subendocardium of the left ventricle (Stahl, Couper & Byard, 1997).

Clinical features

Most affected children are girls under the age of two years (range three days to four years, mean 12.5 months) (Malhotra, Ferrans & Virmani, 1994). The clinical presentation usually involves a variety of cardiac rhythm disturbances, including ventricular, supraventricular, and junctional tachycardias, Lown–Ganong–Levine or Wolff–Parkinson–White syndromes, conduction disturbances, and atrial fibrillation or flutter (Boissy *et al.*, 1997).

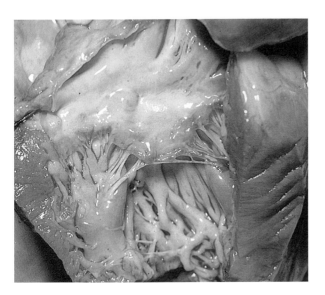

Figure 5.13 Nodular distortion of the papillary muscle and mitral valve leaflets with thickening of chordae tendinae in a 15-month-old girl with histiocytoid cardiomyopathy.

Affected children may also present with cyanotic episodes or congestive cardiac failure, and occasional cases have had seizures related to cardiac arrhythmias (Kearney *et al*, 1987; Stahl, Couper & Byard, 1997).

Etiology

The etiology of the foamy transformation is not understood; however, oncocytic change has also been demonstrated in other organs (Silver *et al.*, 1980). Although a viral etiology has been suggested, familial cases occur, with autosomal recessive rather than X-linked inheritance being proposed (Suarez *et al.*, 1987). Other postulated etiologies include a response to myocarditis, ischemia, or toxins, a variant of granular cell myoblastoma, and an occult metabolic disorder (Cunningham & Stewart, 1985). Deficiency in cytochrome c in cardiac mitochondria may suggest that defects in respiratory chain enzymes due to mutations in the mitochondrial genome may be responsible for some of the manifestations (Stahl, Couper & Byard, 1997).

Pathological features

At autopsy, there may be cardiomegaly with tan-white nodules apparent beneath the endocardium or epicardium on sectioning. Valves may be thickened (Figure 5.13). Histologically, the nodules are composed of aggregates of round to polygonal cells with granular cytoplasm (Figure 5.14). Occasional cells are multinucleate. Origin from myocytes is confirmed by positive immunohistochemical staining for actin, myoglobin, and desmin, with negative staining for lysozyme and CD 68. Electron microscopy has shown that the cytomegaly is due to increased numbers of abnormally formed mitochondria (Shehata *et al.*, 1998). Variable amounts of fibrous stroma and lymphocytic infiltrate are present (Boissy *et al.*, 1997; Ruszkiewicz & Vernon-Roberts, 1995).

A high rate of cardiac and extracardiac abnormalities has also been reported in affected children. These include cardiac septal defects, left ventricular hypoplasia and valve stenoses, hydrocephalus, agenesis of the corpus callosum, cerebellar, basal ganglia, and intracerebral vascular abnormalities, micropthalmia, corneal opacities, renal cysts, ovarian hypoplasia, laryngeal web, and cleft palate (Malhotra, Ferrans & Virmani, 1994).

Occurrence of sudden death

Sudden and unexpected death is also a possible presentation, occurring in 20% of cases, including some cases that mimic SIDS (Cunningham & Stewart, 1985; Grech, Ellul & Montalto, 2000).

Non-compaction of the left ventricle

This is a rare congenital cardiomyopathy in which there is a problem with left ventricular development, resulting in failure of compaction of loose fetal myocardial fibers. The left ventricle has a spongy appearance, with prominent trabeculation and deep recesses. Also known as "spongy myocardium," the condition leads to left ventricular hypertrophy, cardiac failure, fibroelastosis, mural thrombus formation with embolization, and lethal arrhythmias (Michel, Carpenter & Lovell, 1998; Valdés-Dapena &

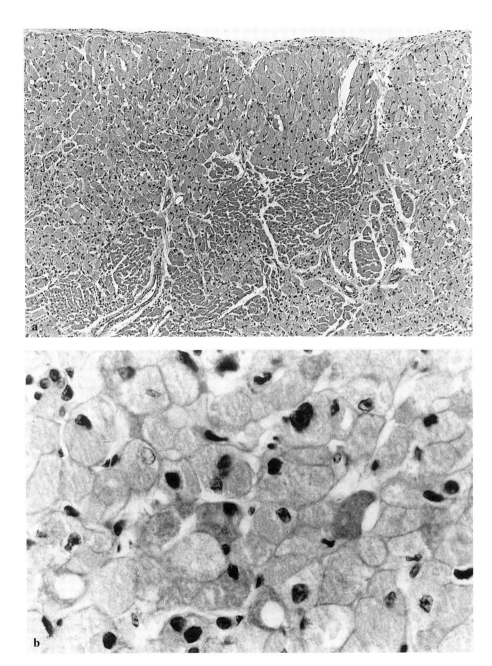

Figure 5.14 Subendocardial nodules in the case of histiocytoid cardiomyopathy shown in Figure 5.13, demonstrating well-defined aggregates of cells (a) (hematoxylin and eosin, ×120), which at higher power have granular cytoplasm and eccentrically placed nuclei (b) (hematoxylin and eosin, ×410).

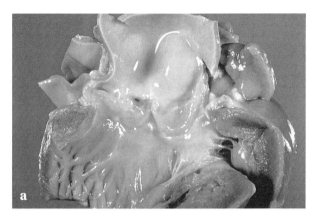

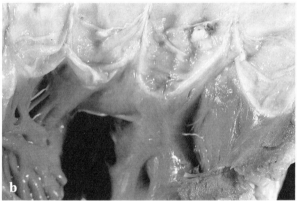

Figure 5.15 Congenital anomalies of the aortic valve, showing two cusps (a), and of the pulmonary valve, showing four cusps (b).

Gilbert-Barness, 2002). Typical features may occur in isolation, or there may be ventricular outflow obstruction, aortic stenosis, or atresia (Halbertsma, van't Hek & Daniels 2001). Familial cases have been reported, and there has been association with conduction tract disorders, Roifman syndrome, Melnick-needles syndrome, and Xq28-linked cardiomyopathy (Mandel, Grunebaum & Benson, 2001; Neudorf *et al.*, 2001).

Valvular abnormalities

Congenital valvular abnormalities with more or less than the usual number of cusps (Figure 5.15) will not usually cause clinical manifestations unless blood flow is compromised or coronary artery ostia are obstructed.

Aortic stenosis

Frequency
Congenital aortic stenosis is a common abnormality found in 3–6% of children with congenital heart disease and is a well known cause of sudden and unexpected death in the young, particularly during exercise (Denfield & Garson, 1990). It has been estimated that sudden death occurs in 1% of children with aortic stenosis per year, and that valvular stenosis has been responsible for sudden death in a total of 6–19% of children with this congenital cardiac defect (Glew *et al.*, 1969).

Clinical features
Most children with this anomaly are asymptomatic, even if significant obstruction is present. While sudden death usually occurs in symptomatic patients, reflecting the severity of the stenosis (Doyle *et al.*, 1974), occasionally completely asymptomatic individuals may die unexpectedly (Hossack *et al.*, 1980).

Etiology
The etiology of most cases is multifactorial; however, rare familial cases have occurred, with an autosomal dominant mode of inheritance (Emanuel *et al.*, 1978).

Pathological features
Examination of the unopened aortic valve from above is the best method of determining the morphology of the stenosis. The most common abnormality found in children under 15 years of age is a congenitally unicuspid valve (Roberts, 1980), of which two varieties occur: an acommissural type, in which there is central perforation of a dome-shaped valve, and a unicommissural type, in which the valve orifice has the shape of an exclamation mark (Figure 5.16) (Cohle *et al.*, 1988). In later adolescence, the valve is most commonly bicuspid and not stenotic unless it is also dysplastic (Figure 5.17) (Becker & Anderson, 1981). Calcification is a

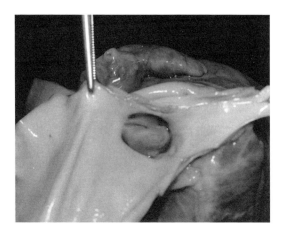

Figure 5.16 Unicommissural aortic valve with stenosis and associated cardiac hypertrophy found at autopsy in an asymptomatic four-month-old boy who suddenly screamed, collapsed, and died while out with his mother shopping.

significant cause of valvular stenosis in later life but is present only rarely in those under 30 years of age (Roberts, 1970).

Pathophysiology

Myocardial ischemia due to inadequate coronary artery perfusion occurs in children who have outflow obstruction (Figure 5.18). Coronary artery perfusion diminishes secondary to reduced cardiac output, and tissue hypoxia is exacerbated further by the presence of secondary left ventricular hypertrophy (Denfield & Garson, 1990; Vetter, 1985). Ischemia then predisposes to arrhythmia and sudden death. The occurrence of sudden death in children with mild stenosis, however, also raises the possibility of an associated abnormality in atrioventricular conduction. This occurred in a 16-year-old boy with mild subaortic stenosis who died suddenly and was found at autopsy to have fibrous replacement of the bundle of His and adjacent bundle branches (James *et al.*, 1988). Thus, surgical correction of the valvular stenosis, either by valve replacement or valvulotomy, reduces but does not eliminate the increased risk of sudden death. Other contributing factors may be permanent left ventricular damage from previous chronic pressure and volume overload, and failure to completely relieve the outflow obstruction at

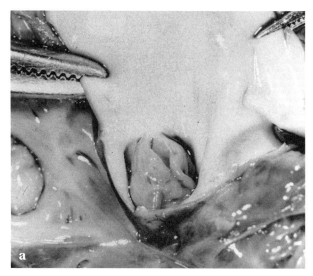

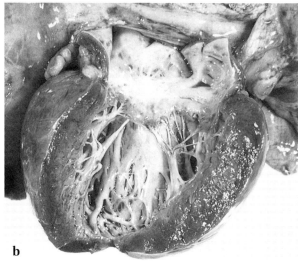

Figure 5.17 Bicuspid aortic valve with dysplasia (a) and marked cardiac hypertrophy (b) causing sudden death of an infant.

operation. Children with aortic stenosis are also at increased risk of developing infective endocarditis and aortic dissection.

Mitral valve prolapse syndrome

Frequency

Prolapse of the mitral valve is present in about 5% of the population, more often in young women than men (Virmani & Roberts, 1991).

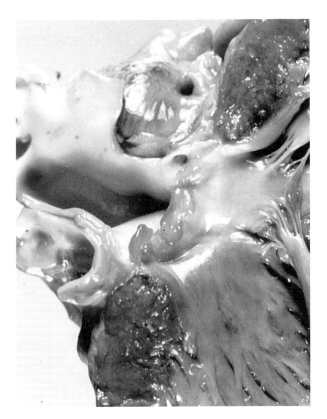

Figure 5.18 Marked aortic valve stenosis associated with dysplasia and compromise of coronary artery flow in a seven-week-old boy.

Etiology

There is considerable variability in underlying etiological mechanisms, with a number of cases being caused by alterations to the supporting valve annulus due to congenital cardiac anomalies or connective tissue disorders (Barlow & Pocock, 1979). Occasional cases may be inherited as an autosomal dominant condition linked to chromosome 16p11.2-p12.1 (Disse *et al.*, 1999; McKusick, 1990).

Pathological features

In cases of primary valvular abnormality, the underlying defect most often involves the posterior leaflet, and quite detailed descriptions are available of the pathological changes present (Edwards, 1988). The

Table 5.3. Grades of severity of mitral valve prolapse

Grade	Changes present
I	One leaflet involved: interchordal hooding of more than two-thirds of posterior leaflet, or more than half of anterior leaflet.
II	Two leaflets involved: interchordal hooding of more than two-thirds of posterior leaflet, and more than half of anterior leaflet.
III	Most of valve involved.

Adapted from Lucas & Edwards (1982).

essential features are increased leaflet tissue and/or increased length of the chordae tendinae, resulting in interchordal hooding and elongation of the involved leaflet, with hooding of the leaflets toward the left atrium and dilation of the valve annulus (Edwards, 1988; Virmani *et al.*, 1987). There is considerable variability in the extent of the changes present, and a grading system has been developed based on the amount of hooding that occurs (Lucas & Edwards, 1982) (Table 5.3).

In a series of 46 adults with mitral valve prolapse, those who died suddenly had larger mitral valve annuli, larger endocardial plaques, and thicker and longer posterior valve leaflets (Darcy *et al.*, 1988). Valve thickening, perivalvular thrombosis, and adjacent focal endocardial fibrosis represent secondary phenomena.

Microscopically, affected valves show thickening of the spongiosa, the centrally situated loose connective tissue that is a component of normal valves (Edwards, 1988), with increased deposition of acid mucopolysaccharides. The fibrosa is disrupted by the proliferating spongiosa, with loss of fibrous tissue and fragmentation of collagen (Davies, Moore & Braimbridge, 1978). The mucopolysaccharide within the spongiosa stains positively with colloidal iron and alcian blue (pH 2.5), as well as being periodic acid-Schiff positive, diastase resistant, and testicular hyaluronidase sensitive (Virmani *et al.*, 1987). Myxomatous mitral valves may indicate a more generalized derangement of the heart, as myxoid change has been demonstrated in extravalvular cardiac tissue in

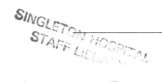

patients who have died from mitral valve prolapse (Morales *et al.*, 1992).

Occurrence of sudden death

Although mitral valve prolapse is almost invariably benign and rarely causes sudden death (Greenwood, 1984), it was held responsible for nearly a quarter of the cases of sudden cardiac death in the series of Topaz & Edwards (1985). This contrasts with another series, where only one case out of 101 children who died suddenly had a myxomatous mitral valve (Garson & McNamara, 1985). The latter study would accord with the author's experience. Sudden death is more likely to occur in females who have an associated chest wall deformity, ECG abnormality, or a positive family history of similar events (Anderson, 1980; Cooper & Abinader, 1981; Jeresaty, 1976; Shappell *et al.*, 1973; Topaz & Edwards, 1985; Virmani & Roberts, 1991). Occasional cases of sudden death have been reported in children as young as 13 and 14 years of age (Chesler, King & Edwards, 1983; Gillette & Garson, 1992), although there is always a possibility of mitral valve prolapse being coincidental to another cause of death. There is an increased risk of cerebrovascular accident in affected children (Rice *et al.*, 1980).

Pathophysiology

While the cause of sudden death in patients with significant mitral valve prolapse has been the subject of considerable debate, individuals with this anomaly are known to be at increased risk of developing arrhythmias (Swartz, Teichholz & Donoso, 1977). Electrocardiographic studies in affected individuals have demonstrated atrial fibrillation, paroxysmal atrial tachycardia, ventricular premature complexes, ventricular tachycardia and fibrillation, and prolonged QT intervals (Jeresaty, 1976; Nishimura *et al.*, 1985; Virmani & Roberts, 1991; Winkle *et al.*, 1975). Potentially serious arrhythmias have also been documented during exercise in a significant number of children with mitral prolapse (McNamara, 1982). Although the reasons for the increase in abnormal rhythms are uncertain, it has been proposed that papillary muscle ischemia, abnormal tension

on papillary muscles, or abnormal contact of chordae tendinae with the ventricle wall may stimulate premature myocyte contraction. Edwards (1988) has confirmed that patients at particular risk of sudden death are those with previously demonstrated electrocardiographic abnormalities.

Other complications that may lead to significant findings at autopsy are infective endocarditis, the reported incidence of which is between 6 and 9% (Allen, Harris & Leatham, 1974; Corrigall *et al.*, 1977; Mills *et al.*, 1977), cerebral embolism (Barnett *et al.*, 1980; Nishimura *et al.*, 1985), and cardiac failure. Endocarditis is generally only of significance in children who have had a murmur (McNamara, 1982).

Associated features

Mitral valve prolapse is associated with several connective tissue disorders and should be looked for in patients with pseudoxanthoma elasticum and Marfan or Ehlers–Danlos syndromes (Malcolm, 1985; Roberts & Honig, 1982). Floppy mitral valve might be a *forme fruste* of Marfan syndrome (Edwards, 1988). It also occurs more frequently in patients with other cardiac lesions, such as ventricular and atrial septal defects, supravalvular aortic stenosis, tetralogy of Fallot, Eisenmenger syndrome, pulmonary stenosis, Ebstein anomaly, and patent ductus arteriosus (Becker, Becker & Edwards, 1972; Malcolm, 1985; McDonald *et al.*, 1971), and it may be associated with other floppy valves (Lucas & Edwards, 1982). There is also an increased incidence of valve prolapse in hyperthyroidism and von Willebrand disease (Pickering, Brody & Barrett, 1981; Virmani *et al.*, 1987) (Table 5.4).

Tricuspid valve prolapse

Sudden and unexpected death is a well recognized complication of tricuspid incompetence when it occurs as part of the Ebstein anomaly (Bauer, 1945; Tuzcu *et al.*, 1989). In this malformation, the tricuspid valve leaflet attachment points are displaced from the atrioventricular junction into the body of the right ventricle. This may result in valvular

Table 5.4. Associations of mitral valve prolapse in childhood

Congenital cardiac disease
  Atrial septal defect
  Ventricular septal defect
  Supravalvular aortic stenosis
  Pulmonary stenosis
  Ebstein anomaly
  Transposition of the great vessels
  Tetralogy of Fallot
Connective tissue disorders
  Marfan disease
  Ehlers–Danlos syndrome
  Pseudoxanthoma elasticum
  Osteogenesis imperfecta
Hypertrophic cardiomyopathy
Inflammatory conditions
  Kawasaki disease
  Rheumatic fever
Metabolic conditions
  Mucopolysaccharidoses
  Sphingolipidoses
  Homocystinuria
Miscellaneous conditions
  Wolff–Parkinson–White syndrome
  Hyperthyroidism
  Von Willebrand disease

incompetence and also in obstruction of the right ventricular outflow tract in more severe forms. Tricuspid valve leaflets are usually dysplastic, and there may be associated pulmonary stenosis or atresia.

It is hypothesized that sudden death in Ebstein anomaly results from arrhythmias; however, there is no correlation between the likelihood of sudden death and anatomic or functional severity (Nihoyannopoulos et al., 1986). Sudden death has been reported in an 11-year-old girl with Ebstein anomaly associated with a septoseptal accessory conduction pathway (Corrado et al., 1990).

Much less commonly, sudden death has been reported in previously asymptomatic individuals who have tricuspid insufficiency in isolation, with normally positioned valve leaflets (Urban, 1964).

Miscellaneous

A wide variety of other valvular lesions may be found in congenital heart disease with dysplastic, stenotic, or atretic valves, resulting in a spectrum of clinical presentations (Figures 5.19 and 5.20 and Color Plate 11).

Subaortic stenosis

Although hypertrophic cardiomyopathy is a more common cause of subaortic stenosis, other entities and malformations may produce a similar effect. These include membranous and tunnel subtypes of subaortic stenosis that have been responsible for 8–20% of congenital left ventricular outflow obstruction (Edwards, 1965; Katz, Buckley & Liberthson, 1977; Maron et al., 1976; Newfeld et al., 1976; Petsas et al., 1998; Tentolouris et al., 1999).

Etiology
Autosomal dominant inheritance has been suggested in some cases (Petsas et al., 1998).

Pathological features
Discrete membranous subaortic stenosis consists of a cresent-shaped fibroelastic membrane located a variable distance beneath the aortic valve and attached to the ventricular septum and the anterior mitral valve leaflet (Katz, Buckley & Liberthson, 1977). Tunnel subaortic stenosis is caused by a more diffuse narrowing of the left ventricular outflow tract by fibromusuclar tissue. A third variant, the so-called fibromuscular collar, has a muscular base and a collar-like outflow obstruction and is intermediate between the other two entities (Newfeld et al., 1976).

Occurrence of sudden death

Sudden death may occur at any age from early childhood to adolescence. It may be precipitated by exercise, but it may also occur during sleep (Doyle et al.,1974).

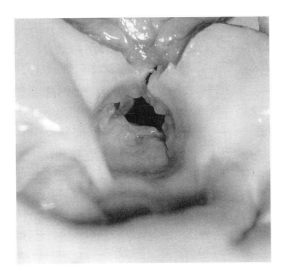

Figure 5.19 Dysplasia with fusing of mitral valve leaflets causing severe stenosis.

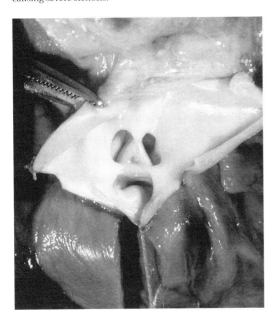

Figure 5.20 Pulmonary valve atresia.

Pathophysiology

As with other forms of cardiac outflow obstruction, lethal arrhythmias may be caused by myocardial hypertrophy or by left ventricular baroreceptor activation resulting in bradycardias. Myocardial ischemia may be a compounding factor arising from compression of intramural arteries from increased muscle bulk and increased end-diastolic pressures (Cohle *et al.*, 1988).

Associated features

There may also be associated congenital cardiac defects in one-half to two-thirds of patients, including valvular aortic stenosis, aortic coarctation, bicuspid aortic valve, aortopulmonary window, incomplete atrioventricular canal, double-outlet right ventricle, patent ductus arteriosus, infundibular pulmonary stenosis, ventricular septal defect, and persistent left superior vena cava (Cohle *et al.*, 1988). There may be overlap with hypertrophic cardiomyopathy in some cases. Patients may also have evidence of infective endocarditis or aortic incompetence, with thickening of the valve cusps due to high-pressure flow. Occasional patients have manifested specific rhythm disturbances such as Wolff–Parkinson–White syndrome (Newfeld *et al.*, 1976).

Tumors

Rhabdomyomas, fibromas, and myxomas constitute the three most common forms of primary tumors of the heart in children. Although it has been stated that the cardiac prognosis for most patients with these tumors is excellent (Abushaban, Denham & Duff, 1993), all have been associated with sudden and unexpected death (McAllister & Fenoglio, 1978). Intrapericardial teratomas may also be associated with sudden death, but this usually occurs around the time of birth or within the early neonatal period (Byard, Jimenez & Moore, 1992). Atrioventricular node tumors and fibroelastomas are rare in the pediatric age range (Thorgeirsson & Liebman, 1983; Topaz & Edwards, 1985).

Rhabdomyomas

Cardiac rhabdomyomas, the most common primary pediatric cardiac "tumor," are an integral part of the

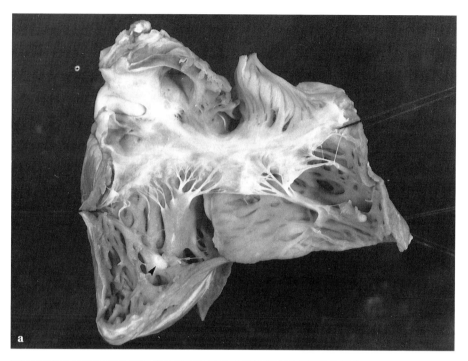

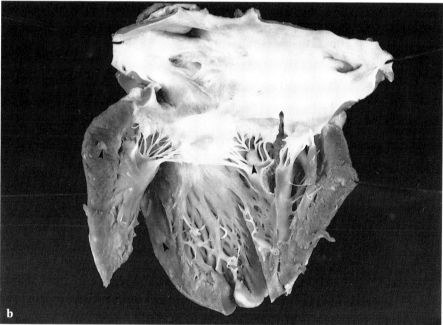

Figure 5.21 Opened right (a) and left (b) ventricles in a three-year-old girl who died suddenly, revealing unsuspected multiple small rhabdomyomas (arrowheads). There were no other stigmata of tuberous sclerosis.

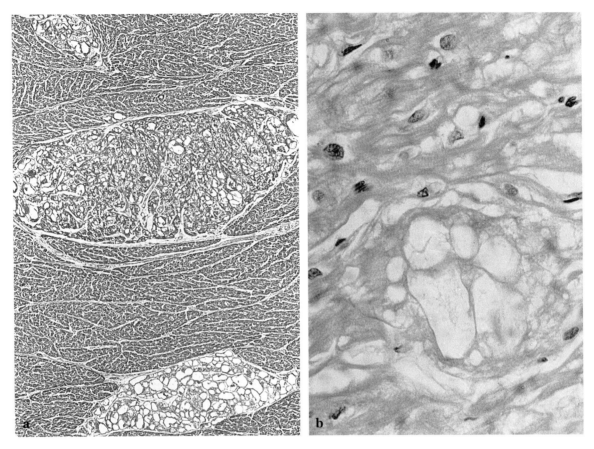

Figure 5.22 Low-power (×80) (a) and high-power (×440) (b) photomicrographs from the case shown in Figure 5.21, showing discrete aggregates of "spider" cells representing distorted glycogenated cardiac myocytes (hematoxylin and eosin).

tuberous sclerosis complex, an autosomal dominant condition described in detail in Chapter 8. However, rhabdomyomas may also occur as an isolated phenomenon (Figure 5.21). Sudden death in childhood occurs most often due to compromise of conduction pathways, obstruction to outflow, or distortion of valvular integrity (Couper *et al.*, 1991; Dubois, Neill & Hutchins, 1983; Rigle, Dexter & McGee, 1989; Violette, Hardin & McQuillen, 1981). A variant form has also been reported in which multifocal rhabdomyomas are found scattered throughout the myocardium, including the atria. This is termed "rhabdomyomatosis" and was associated with sudden death in a 13-year-old boy (Shrivastava *et al.*, 1977).

A case has also been reported of sudden death occurring in a 12-year-old boy with occult rhabdomyomas following the ingestion of a cold drink. It was considered that a temperature-related vasovagal reflex initiated the terminal arrhythmia (Burke *et al.*, 1999).

Rhabdomyomas are composed of vacuolated "spider" cells with thin cytoplasmic strands running between aggregates of glycogen (Figure 5.22). Debate over the precise nature of rhabdomyomas continues, with most authors favoring a hamartomatous malformation rather than a true neoplasm. Electron microscopy has confirmed their myogenic origin (Figure 5.23). These lesions may undergo

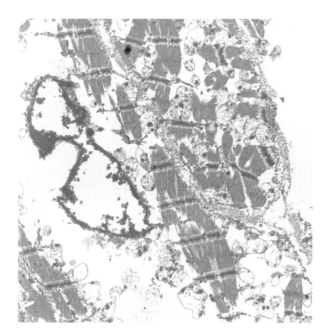

Figure 5.23 Electron micrograph from the case shown in Figure 5.22, showing disorganization of Z bands with numerous adjacent mitochondria.

spontaneous regression as children grow older (Shaher *et al.*, 1972). It is important to assess other autopsy findings and the history and circumstances of death, as rhabdomyomas may represent an incidental postmortem finding completely unrelated to the mechanisms responsible for the lethal episode (Byard, 1997).

Fibromas

Cardiac fibromas, the second most common primary pediatric cardiac tumor, usually form large solitary masses (Figure 5.24) composed of non-encapsulated bland spindled fibroblasts within the interventricular septum. Although these tumors appear to be well circumscribed, microscopic examination demonstrates extension of fibroblasts into the surrounding myocardium (Figure 5.25). As with rhabdomyomas, these neoplasms are predominantly a tumor of childhood and may result in sudden and unexpected death (Jokl & McClellan, 1970; Meissner *et al.*, 2000;

Rajs, Råsten-Almqvist & Nennesmo, 1997). Twenty-three percent of cases of cardiac fibromas in reviewed series have presented as sudden death, usually due to outflow obstruction or arrhythmia from involvement of conduction tracts (McAllister & Fenoglio, 1978).

Myxomas

Cardiac myxomas are a less common primary pediatric cardiac tumor that may be associated with mitral valve disturbance, systemic embolization, and sudden death (Vassiliades, Vassiliades & Karkavelos 1997). Myxomas are usually polypoidal lesions arising within the atria. They are gelatinous on sectioning, and composed of stellate mesenchymal cells embedded in a myxoid background of acid mucopolysaccharide (McAllister, 1979) (Figure 5.26).

Cerebral embolism arising from myxomas may occur in childhood (Pellegrino, Zanesco & Battistella, 1992) and may be lethal (Corrado *et al.*, 1990). One of the youngest cases of sudden death attributed to a cardiac myxoma was a six-week-old girl (Rabson, 1949). Becker & Anderson (1981) have described a case of a 17-year-old boy with a left ventricular myxoma who died suddenly while engaging in mild exercise, and Hals, Ek & Sandnes (1990) reported sudden and unexpected death in a 3.5-month-old infant due to occlusion of the tricuspid valve ring by a massive myxoma of the right atrium.

Cystic tumor of the atrioventricular node

These tumors occur within the inferior portion of the atrial septum in the region of the atrioventricular node. Replacement of the node may result in heart block and sudden and unexpected death (Becker & Anderson, 1981; Bharati & Lev, 1985; Ross, 1977).

The tumors consist of poorly circumscribed nests of uniform polygonal epithelial cells that surround cystic spaces and are embedded in dense fibrous stroma (Figure 5.27). The origin of these tumors is debated, but an endodermal rather than mesothelial origin is favored (Bharati *et al.*, 1976).

Although atrioventricular node tumors are found more commonly in adults, an 11-month-old boy has been reported with such a tumor and a lesion from a six-year-old girl is shown in Figure 5.27. Isolated Stokes–Adams attacks and sudden unexpected death (sometimes during cardiac catheterization) have also been described in children with these tumors (Bharati *et al.* 1976; McAllister & Fenoglio, 1978). Stokes–Adams attacks may precede the terminal event by many years (Lewman, Demany & Zimmerman, 1972).

Teratoma

Teratomas of the heart arise within the pericardial sac, usually adjacent to the root of the major vessels. In an Armed Forces Institute of Pathology (AFIP) series of 14 cases, there were 11 children. Two patients in this series died suddenly and unexpectedly (McAllister & Fenoglio, 1978). Intrapericardial teratomas can reach an extremely large size and on sectioning reveal a characteristic cystic parenchyma (Color Plate 12) composed of tissues derived from three germ cell layers (Figure 5.28) (Byard, Jimenez & Moore, 1992).

Fibroelastoma

Fibroelastomas are papillary tumors that occur very rarely in children, originating from the endocardium in the vicinity of the cardiac valves (McAllister & Fenoglio, 1978). Although fibroelastomas are usually an incidental finding at autopsy, sudden deaths in a 19-year-old woman and in a 21-year-old man have been reported secondary to coronary ostial occlusion and to coronary artery embolism, respectively (Amr & Abu al Ragheb, 1991).

Associated features

Very occasionally, cardiac tumors (e.g. rhabdomyomas, myxoma, and fibroma) have been found with significant congenital cardiac defects (Russell *et al.*, 1989). There is also an association of cardiac fibroma with the nevoid basal-cell carcinoma syndrome in a minority of children (Coffin, 1992). Myxomas may be associated with pigmented skin lesions, including lentiginoses and blue nevi, and with neural tumors in the so-called syndrome myxoma,

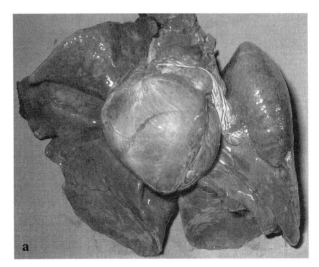

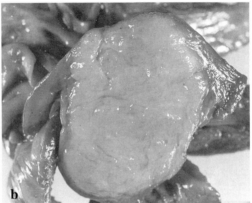

Figure 5.24 Cardiomegaly in a two-month-old infant who died suddenly (a). Sectioning of the heart revealed an unsuspected interventricular fibroma (b).

NAME (nevi, atrial myxoma, myxoid neurofibromata, and ephiledes), or LAMB (lentigenes, atrial myxoma, mucocutaneous myxoma, and blue nevi) syndromes (Atherton *et al.*, 1980; Rhodes *et al.*, 1984; Vidaillet *et al.*, 1987b).

Conduction defects

Conduction disturbances associated with sudden death in childhood can be classified on an anatomical basis into lesions involving the (i) sinoatrial

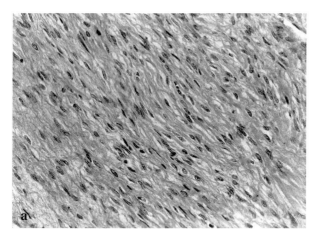

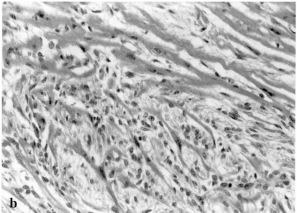

Figure 5.25 Bland fibroblasts within the cardiac fibroma shown in Figure 5.24 (a), with interdigitation with myocytes at the periphery of the tumor (b) (hematoxylin and eosin, ×440).

node, (ii) the atrioventricular node, (iii) the atrioventricular bundle and bundle branches, and (iv) the myocardium. Additionally, there is a group that includes occasional rare familial conditions, and a final miscellaneous group that includes accessory pathways, mitral valve prolapse, and postsurgical cases.

At autopsy, it may be difficult to determine whether a finding was functionally significant during life or is merely a variant of normal (Cohle & Lie, 1998), and it has been stated that the significance of histological findings in the absence of a clinical history must remain "speculative" (Basso *et al.*, 1995). The report

by Bharati & Lev (1985) may be of assistance in describing in detail the pathologic findings in a variety of conditions that resulted in sudden childhood death due to conduction tract disturbances. The paper emphasizes meticulous examination of the conduction pathways in cases of sudden death in children with histories of arrhythmias. The technical details of conduction pathway dissection may be found elsewhere (Anderson *et al.*, 1981b; Charlton & Williams, 1990).

Not all conduction disturbances and arrhythmias are associated with sudden childhood death. For example, supraventricular tachycardias are rarely associated with sudden death, except in children with pre-excitation syndrome or with multifocal atrial tachycardias (Gillette & Garson, 1992; Yeager, Hougen & Levy, 1984). On the other hand, both ventricular arrhythmias and complete heart block have a well known association with sudden death, even in the absence of symptomatic cardiac disease (Rowland & Schweiger, 1984). Conduction tract abnormalities may also predispose to accidental death, such as drowning if an arrhythmia occurs when the child is in water (Stumpp, Schneider & Bär, 1997).

The possibility of an underlying electrolyte imbalance such as hyper- or hypokalemia should also be considered in cases of lethal arrhythmia (Davies & Popple, 1979; Gettes, 1992), particularly in malnourished or anorexic children, and in children who have received intravenous fluids.

Iatrogenic exacerbation of an underlying rhythm disturbance due to medication may also be a possibility, as was suggested in a five-year-old boy with paroxysmal supraventricular tachycardia who suddenly collapsed and died while taking flecainide (Till & Herxheimer, 1992). It is, therefore, important to investigate serum drug levels at autopsy in similar cases.

Environmental factors may also have a profound influence on cardiac conduction. For example, sudden death following immersion in cold water, or consuming a cold drink, has been documented, possibly caused by vagally mediated asystole or ventricular fibrillation (Burke *et al.*, 1999; Keatinge & Hayward, 1981).

Sinoatrial nodal lesions

Interference with the function of the sinoatrial node and its connecting pathways may result in potentially lethal arrhythmias. Although the "sick sinus" syndrome is not common in children, a 16-year-old boy with a history of cardiac rhythm disturbances who died suddenly has been reported (Bharati *et al.*, 1980). At autopsy, extensive fibrosis around both the sinoatrial and atrioventricular nodes was found. Sick sinus syndrome is a very unusual cause of sudden pediatric death, but it is more likely to cause sudden death if it occurs after surgery (Gillette & Garson, 1992) or with myocarditis (Vetter, 1985). The syndrome may also occur in a heritable form (Barak *et al.*, 1987).

Thickening of the wall of the sinoatrial node artery ranging from intimal proliferation to fibromuscular hyperplasia has also been associated with sudden death at all ages, from infancy through childhood to later adolescence (James, Froggatt & Marshall, 1967; James & Marshall, 1976a).

Atrioventricular nodal lesions

Any lesion that interferes with conduction around the atrioventricular node may result in lethal arrhythmia. This includes fibrous scarring of uncertain etiology and atrioventricular node tumor (Topaz & Edwards, 1985). Fibromuscular hyperplasia of the atrioventricular nodal artery (Figure 5.29) has also been associated with sudden death in adolescence (Anderson *et al.*, 1981a; James, Hackel & Marshall, 1974).

Atrioventricular bundle and bundle branch lesions

"Fragmentation" of the bundle of His with surrounding fibrosis has been found in a 13-year-old boy with a past history of recurrent ventricular tachycardia who died suddenly, and in an 11-year-old boy who collapsed after exercise (Bharati *et al.*, 1979a; James & Marshall, 1976b). Although this pattern of dispersed fibers involving both the atrioventricular

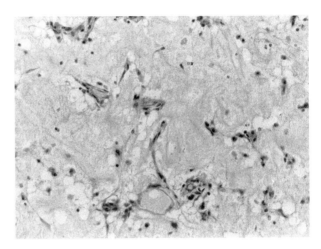

Figure 5.26 Typical loose stroma of a cardiac myxoma (hematoxylin and eosin, ×440).

node (Figure 5.30) and conduction tracts is more characteristic of the fetus, it may persist for years; some authors, however, consider it to be a feature of normal development and to be of little significance (Cohle & Lie, 1991; Cohle & Lie, 1998; Suárez-Mier & Aguilera, 1998). Sudden death has occurred in both children and young adults, associated with vascular malformations of the cardiac conduction system (Bell & Tate, 1994; Krous, Chapman & Altshuler, 1978).

Lesions of the myocardium

A variety of myocardial diseases described elsewhere in this chapter may result in sudden death due to involvement of the conduction pathways. These include myocarditis, right ventricular cardiomyopathy, fibrosis, tumors, and hypertrophic cardiomyopathy. Myocardial tumors, may cause incessant ventricular tachycardias despite apparently normal echocardiograms and angiocardiograms (Garson *et al.*, 1987).

Familial conditions

A range of lethal familial conduction disturbances, with variable inheritance patterns, may result in

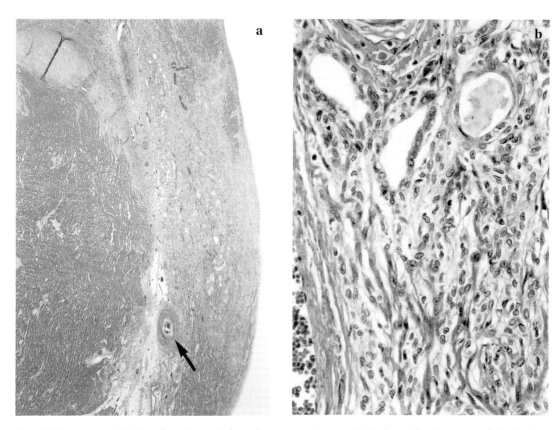

Figure 5.27 Low-power (×20) view of an atrioventricular node tumor in a six-year-old girl who was found unexpectedly dead in bed. The tumor abuts the atrioventricular node artery (arrow) (a). At higher power (×280), the tumor consisted of cystic spaces lined by flattened to cuboidal epithelium within a cellular fibrous stroma (b) (hematoxylin and eosin).

sudden childhood death. One of the better known conditions is prolongation of the QT interval (Moss & Robinson, 1992).

Prolonged QT interval syndromes

Two well recognized syndromes, the Romano–Ward syndrome and Jervell and Lange-Nielsen syndrome, have prolonged QT interval on electrocardiography and are associated with arrhythmias and sudden death.

Vigorous debate has occurred as to whether this conduction anomaly plays a significant role in the pathophysiology of SIDS (Byard & Krous, 2003). While not all studies have shown prolongation of the QT interval in SIDS infants (Southall *et al.*, 1986),

other studies have demonstrated an association in some cases (Schwartz *et al.*, 1998; Schwartz *et al.*, 2000; Schwartz, 2001; Ackerman *et al.*, 2001). However, there is certainly no doubt that individuals with this conduction disturbance have a significantly increased risk of sudden death in childhood and adolescence as well as in later adult life (Ackerman, Tester & Driscoll, 2001; Algra *et al.*, 1991; Weintraub, Gow & Wilkinson, 1990).

Children with prolonged QT syndrome may have 2:1 atrioventricular block, *torsade de pointes* (alternating positive and negative QRS complexes), and multiform premature ventricular contractions, with 9% of children in one study presenting with unexpected cardiac arrest. Children with QT intervals

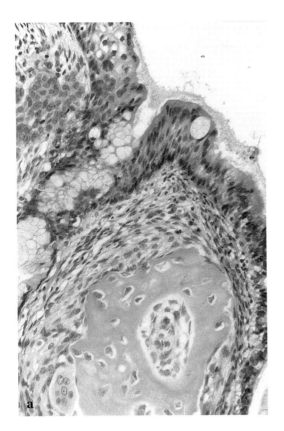 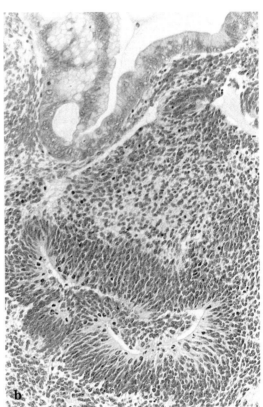

Figure 5.28 Typical tissues derived from an intrapericardial teratoma showing ciliated respiratory-type and mucinous epithelium overlying stroma containing aggregates of cartilage (a) and immature neural tissue (b) (hematoxylin and eosin, ×220).

greater than 0.60 are considered to be at particular risk for sudden death (Garson *et al.*, 1993).

Romano–Ward syndrome

This autosomal dominant condition is characterized by a prolonged QT interval, resting bradycardia, episodic ventricular fibrillation, tachycardia, and *torsade de pointes* (Bhandari *et al.*, 1985; Flugelman *et al.*, 1982; Vincent, 1986). These rhythm disturbances result in syncopal attacks and sudden death (Itoh, Munemura & Satoh, 1982). Abnormalities of the right or left ventricular myocardium have been suggested as a basis for the disturbance (Cross *et al.*, 1993).

The rhythm disturbance is caused by mutations in genes on chromosomes 3p21-24 (LQT3), 4q25-27

(LQT4), 7q35-36 (LQT2), and 11p15.5 (LQT1) (Curran *et al.*, 1995; Schott *et al.*, 1995; Splawski *et al.*, 1997a; Vincent *et al.*, 1992; Wang *et al.*, 1996). Specific mutations involve *KVLQT1(KCNQ1)*, *HERG*, and *SCN5A* genes, which are involved in potassium and sodium channels (Abbott *et al.*, 1999; Sanguinetti *et al.*, 1996; Splawski *et al.*, 1997a; Towbin, 1995; Wang, Bowles & Towbin, 1998; Wang *et al.*, 1995; Wang *et al.*, 1996).

Jervell and Lange-Nielson syndrome

This autosomal recessive condition is also characterized by prolongation of the QT interval, *torsade de pointes*, episodic ventricular fibrillation, syncope, and sudden death, with the added feature of congenital sensorineural deafness (Fraser, Froggatt & James, 1964; Jervell & Lange-Nielsen, 1957; Levine &

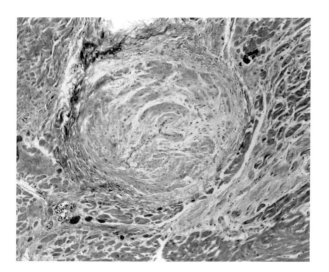

Figure 5.29 Marked fibromuscular hyperplasia of the atrioventricular node artery, causing lumenal narrowing in a 21-year-old male (elastic trichrome, ×200).

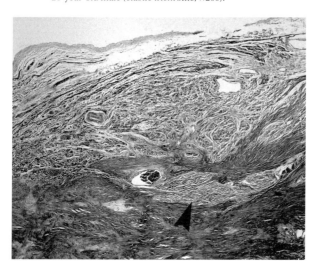

Figure 5.30 Persistent fetal dispersion of the atrioventricular node in a 17-year-old male with an island of conducting tissue (arrowhead) located beneath the main node surrounded by dense collagen of the central fibrous body (elastic trichrome, ×100).

Woodworth, 1958; Till *et al.*, 1988). Sudden death may be precipitated by strenuous exercise, an auditory startle, or a strong emotional stimulus (Moss *et al.*, 1985). Occasionally, the patient may also suffer

seizures, presumably secondary to reduced cardiac output with cerebral hypoperfusion (Bricker, Garson & Gillette, 1984). The genetic basis is mutation in the *KVLQT1* and *minK (KCNE1)* loci on chromosomes 11p15.5 and 21q22, which code for cardiac potassium channels (Neyroud *et al.*, 1997; Splawski *et al.*, 1997b; Wang, Bowles & Towbin, 1998).

As there are no pathognomonic features of these syndromes to be found at autopsy, determination of the cause of death and the likelihood of one of these syndromes being present must depend on appropriate clinicopathologic correlation with follow-up molecular and clinical studies. This includes a detailed family history and possible cardiological assessment of close relatives. Acquired causes of prolongation of the QT interval, such as hypokalemia, drugs, and anorexia nervosa, must be excluded (Isner *et al.*, 1985; Manning, 1977).

Other familial syndromes

Other families have been described where sudden and unexpected death occurred in children due to arrhythmias or conduction defects not associated with prolongation of the QT interval (Bharati & Lev, 1985; McRae *et al.*, 1974). For example, Gault and colleagues (1972) reported two sisters aged 16 and 18 years who both manifested intermittent tachycardia, without prolonged QT interval; sudden death occurred in the elder girl. Green and colleagues (1969) described another family with sudden death occurring in children, the youngest being four years of age. A family has also been described with congenital bundle branch disease, in which the conduction tracts were found to be absent or atrophic (Husson *et al.*, 1973). Other types of heritable conduction defects include bundle branch block, first-, second-, and third-degree heart block, and Wolff–Parkinson–White syndrome (Gillette, Freed & McNamara, 1978; Lynch *et al.*, 1973).

Miscellaneous syndromes

A number of other rare heritable syndromes are associated with cardiac conduction defects. One example is the Kearns–Sayre syndrome in which children exhibit external ophthalmoplegia, pigmentary retinopathy, short stature, and sudden death associated with heart block (Roberts, Perloff & Kark, 1979). Congenital complete heart block has been reported in a patient with a variant of Kartagener syndrome, who had sinusitis, bronchiectasis, and corrected transposition with normal visceral situs (Solomon *et al.*, 1976). Certain X-linked myopathies have also been associated with arrhythmias, heart block, and sudden death (Patterson, Donnelly & Dehner, 1992).

Isolated congenital heart block without associated congenital heart disease is rare, occurring in approximately one in 20,000 infants. While bradycardia is usually well tolerated, sudden death may occur due to bradycardia-related QT prolongation and *torsade de pointes* (Berger, Dhala & Friedberg, 1999), with up to 2–3% of patients dying suddenly (Vetter, 1985). An association between congenital heart block and maternal systemic lupus erythematosis has been noted, with immunoglobulin deposition being demonstrated around the sinoatrial node in affected infants (Patterson, Donnelly & Dehner, 1992). Congenital complete heart block has also been reported in a significant number of infants whose mothers have primary Sjögren syndrome (Manthorpe & Manthorpe, 1992).

An overlap between conduction pathway abnormalities and cardiomyopathies has been noted in some families (Massumi, 1967). For example, a 15.5-year-old adolescent in one kindred marked by a history of sudden death demonstrated right ventricular septal hypertrophy, with abnormalities of the penetrating bundle (Brookfield *et al.*, 1988). Graber and colleagues (1986) have reported a family with progressive cardiac failure due to myocardial dysfunction associated with lethal arrhythmias.

As a variety of polymorphic ventricular tachyarrhythmias may occur in the absence of structural heart disease, the autopsy may be of only limited value in establishing the diagnosis, except to exclude other entities. For example, certain children with apparently normal hearts may suffer from catecholamine-sensitive polymorphic ventricular tachycardia, in which atrial and ventricular arrhythmias are provoked by exercise (Viskin &

Belhassen, 1998), or from the Brugada syndrome. The latter is caused by mutations in the cardiac sodium channel gene *SCN5A* and is characterized by right bundle branch block and ST segment elevation in the right chest leads on electrocardiography in the presence of a normal heart. Ventricular fibrillation and sudden death may result (Brugada, Brugada & Brugada, 2000; Naccarelli *et al.*, 2002; Priori *et al.*, 2000). It has been proposed that cases of sudden nocturnal death occurring in young males in South East Asia (Laitai in Thailand, Bangungut in the Phillipines, and Pokkuri in Japan) are due to Brugada syndrome (Tatsanavivat *et al.*, 1992; Vatta *et al.*, 2002). As similar electrocardiographic features may occur with right ventricular cardiomyopathy and tricyclic drug toxicity, it is important to exclude these possibilities before the diagnosis is made (Virmani *et al.*, 2001).

Miscellaneous lesions

Bharati and colleagues (1983a) have described three cases of sudden death in adolescents in which conduction pathway abnormalities were associated with changes interpreted as being due to premature cardiac aging. Mitral valve prolapse was present in two of the patients, one of whom also had thrombosis of the sinoatrial node artery.

Sudden death may also occur due to accessory conduction pathways, which cause ventricular pre-excitation and re-entry, leading to fatal arrhythmias. There are three types of accessory pathways (Cohle & Lie, 1991):

1 Kent fibers (atrioventricular fibers), which are twigs of normal atrio-atrial fibers that run between the atrial and ventricular free walls.

2 Mahaim fibers (nodoventricular or fasciculoventricular tracts), which run between the ventricular septum and atrioventricular node, bundle of His, or left bundle branch (Figure 5.31).

3 James fibers, which run from the atrium to the bundle of His.

Examples of syndromes associated with accessory pathways are the pre-excitation (Wolff–Parkinson–White) and Lown–Ganong–Levine syndromes.

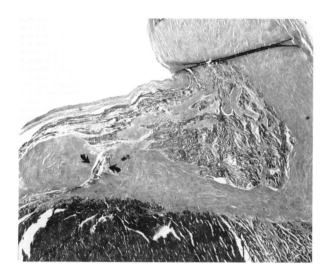

Figure 5.31 Mahaim fiber (arrows) extending from the junction of the bundle of His and left bundle branch through the central fibrous body to connect with the myocardium of the interventricular septum in a 20-year-old male (elastic trichrome, ×40).

However, there may be multiple anomalies present, for example a five-week-old infant has been reported with Mahaim fibers present as well as persistent fetal dispersion of conduction fibers (Buja *et al.*, 1986); a four-month-old infant has been described with Kent, Mahaim, and James fibers (Sturner *et al.*, 1980); and a previously well 17-year-old girl who was found dead in bed one morning had loop connections between different parts of the atrioventricular node, detached groups of nodal cells connecting with the interventricular septum, and Mahaim fibers (James, Marilley & Marriott, 1975). Multiple conduction tract anomalies may also be associated with other abnormalities. For example, Ebstein anomaly was associated with Kent and Mahaim fibers in an 11-year-old girl who collapsed and died while running (Rossi & Thiene, 1984). These complex cases demonstrate clearly the need for meticulous dissection and careful analysis of possible lethal mechanisms.

Wolff–Parkinson–White syndrome is characterized by the development of paroxysmal supraventricular tachycardia, cardiac arrest, and the possibility of sudden death during childhood and adolescence (Chia *et al.*, 1982; Rosenberg *et al.*, 1991; Vidaillet *et al.*, 1987a; Wiedermann *et al.*, 1987). Typical electrocardiographic abnormalities may have been present only intermittently.

James (1979) has reported inflammation of ganglia near the sinoatrial node in a series of individuals who died suddenly and unexpectedly, one of whom was in late adolescence. The exact relationship of this finding to sudden death is, however, unclear.

Miscellaneous conditions

Endocardial fibroelastosis

Endocardial fibroelastosis is characterized by diffuse thickening of the endocardium due to an increase in fibroelastotic tissue. It occurs most often within the left ventricle.

Etiology
The etiology is understood poorly, with most cases being idiopathic or representing a common end point for a number of diverse conditions. These include congenital cardiac defects, such as aortic stenosis and hypoplastic left heart syndrome, and myocarditis (Schryer & Karnauchow, 1974). An association with pre-excitation syndrome, anomalous conduction pathways, and complete heart block has been demonstrated (Bharati *et al.*, 1981). Rarely, familial cases have been reported, with variable inheritance patterns (Jennings, Hall & Kukolich, 1980; Rafinski *et al.*, 1967). In familial cases, the possibility of an underlying metabolic defect such as mucopolysaccharidosis or carnitine deficiency should also be considered (De Letter & Piette, 1999; Tripp *et al.*, 1981).

Clinical features
The usual clinical presentation in infants and children who do not have an associated congenital cardiac defect is with cardiac failure or arrhythmia. Occasionally, sudden death may occur (Lambert *et al.*, 1974), and endocardial fibroelastosis has been found

in cases mimicking SIDS (Williams & Emery, 1978). Cerebral embolism from detached mural thrombi may result in stroke.

Pathological features

Affected hearts may be markedly enlarged, with shortening of the chordae tendinae, flattening of the trabeculae carnae, and diffuse thickening of the endocardium (Figure 5.32). On microscopy, this consists of dense collagenized fibroelastic tissue (Figure 5.33) (Ino *et al.*, 1988). Specific staining of elastic fibers with van Giesson or orcein stains will enable endocardial fibroelastosis to be differentiated from pure endocardial fibrosis.

Pathophysiology

The mechanism by which endocardial fibroelastosis causes death is uncertain. It has been hypothesized that symptoms result from interference with contraction and relaxation of the heart, from interference with normal electrical conduction, or from interference with oxygenation of the subendocardial myocytes (Thomas *et al.*, 1954).

Myocardial infarction

Acute myocardial infarction may complicate congenital heart disease, as detailed above, or may be found in a variety of other situations. Table 5.5 lists a

Table 5.5. Causes of myocardial infarction in infants and children

Kawasaki disease
Congenital heart disease
Coronary artery anomalies
Coronary artery embolism
Infective endocarditis
Myocarditis
Chest trauma
Salmonella sepsis
Syphilis
Arterial calcinosis
William syndrome

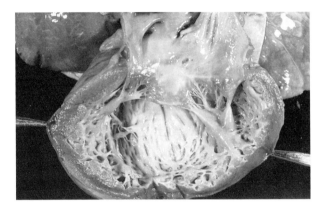

Figure 5.32 Glistening white endocardium within the left ventricle, typical of endocardial fibroelastosis.

number of different entities that should be checked for at autopsy if myocardial infarction is suspected.

Cardiac tamponade

The usual cause of cardiac tamponade in childhood is trauma, including problems related to medical procedures such as catheterization. Occasional cases arise from coronary artery dissection or aneurysm rupture.

Emotional stress

Although the most likely cause of sudden death following emotional stress is cardiac rhythm disturbance, this often has to be deduced from circumstantial rather than clinical or autopsy evidence (DeSilva & Lown, 1978; Dimsdale, 1977; Goodfriend & Wolpert, 1976).

A number of examples of sudden death in childhood following emotional stress can be found in the literature. For example, Engel (1971) described an 18-year-old girl who dropped dead when told of her grandfather's death, and a 14-year-old girl who suffered a fatal collapse on being informed of her 17-year-old brother's death. The occurrence of sudden collapse and death in another 14-year-old girl on being given the news of her 15-year-old brother's sudden death also suggests an underlying familial

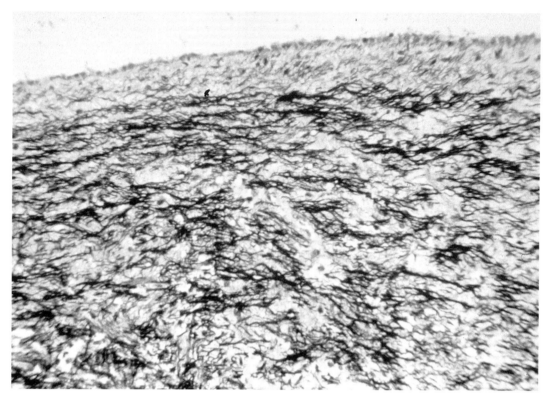

Figure 5.33 Histologic section of endocardial fibroelastosis, showing thickened layers of fibroelastic tissue (elastin stain, ×180).

conduction problem (Green *et al.*, 1969). The sudden death when stressed of children resident in institutions for the deaf raises the possibility of prolonged QT syndrome (Jervell, 1985).

It has been proposed that coronary artery spasm may also be induced by emotion (Comfort, 1981), and some researchers have found focal myocardial necrosis and myofibrillar degeneration in assault victims who die unexpectedly with no apparent lethal injuries discernible (Cebelin & Hirsch, 1980).

A stressful event for a child may also exacerbate an underlying pathological condition that may be demonstrated at autopsy. An example of this was a 10-year-old boy with severe aortic stenosis who died suddenly after being frightened and running during a thunder storm (Doyle *et al.*, 1974). The sudden death of a young woman with mitral valve prolapse

syndrome during a stressful argument provides another example (Shappell *et al.*, 1973).

REFERENCES

Abbott, G. W., Sesti, F., Splawski, I., *et al.* (1999). MiRP1 forms I_{Kr} potassium channels with HERG and is associated with cardiac arrhythmia. *Cell*, **97**, 175–87.

Abushaban, L., Denham, B. & Duff, D. (1993). 10 year review of cardiac tumours in childhood. *British Heart Journal*, **70**, 166–9.

Ackerman, M. J., Siu, B. L., Sturner, W. Q., *et al.* (2001). Postmortem molecular analysis of SCN5A defects in sudden infant death syndrome. *Journal of the American Medical Association*, **286**, 2264–9.

Ackerman, M. J., Tester, D. J. & Driscoll, D. J. (2001). Molecular autopsy of sudden unexplained death in the young.

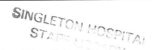

American Journal of Forensic Medicine and Pathology, **22**, 105–11.

Algra, A., Tijssen, J. G. P., Roelandt, J. R. T. C., Pool, J. & Lubsen, J. (1991). QTc prolongation measured by standard 12-lead electrocardiography is an independent risk factor for sudden death due to cardiac arrest. *Circulation*, **83**, 1888–94.

Allen, H., Harris, A. & Leatham, A. (1974). Significance and prognosis of an isolated late systolic murmur: a 9- to 22-year follow-up. *British Heart Journal*, **36**, 525–32.

Amr, S. S. & Abu al Ragheb, S. Y. (1991). Sudden unexpected death due to papillary fibroma of the aortic valve. Report of a case and review of the literature. *American Journal of Forensic Medicine and Pathology*, **12**, 143–8.

Anderson, R. C. (1980). Idiopathic mitral valve prolapse and sudden death. *American Heart Journal*, **100**, 941–2.

Anderson, P. A. W. (1995). The molecular genetics of cardiovascular disease. *Current Opinion in Cardiology*, **10**, 33–43.

Anderson, K. R., Bowie, J., Dempster, A. G. & Gwynne, J. F. (1981a). Sudden death from occlusive disease of the atrioventricular node artery. *Pathology*, **13**, 417–21.

Anderson, R. H., Ho, S. Y., Smith, A., Wilkinson, J. L. & Becker, A. E. (1981b). Study of the cardiac conduction tissues in the paediatric age group. *Diagnostic Histopathology*, **4**, 3–15.

Anderson, D. W., Virmani, R., Reilly, J. M., *et al.* (1988). Prevalent myocarditis at necropsy in the acquired immunodeficiency syndrome. *Journal of the American College of Cardiology*, **11**, 792–9.

Anonymous. (1975). Sudden infant death in children with heart disease. *British Medical Journal*, **1**, 1–2.

Arey, J. B. & Sotos, J. (1956). Unexpected death in early life. *Journal of Pediatrics*, **49**, 523–39.

Atherton, D. J., Pitcher, D. W., Wells, R. S. & MacDonald, D. M. (1980). A syndrome of various cutaneous pigmented lesions, myxoid neurofibromata and atrial myxoma: the NAME syndrome. *British Journal of Dermatology*, **103**, 421–9.

Barak, M., Herschkowitz, S., Shapiro, I. & Roguin, N. (1987). Familial combined sinus node and atrioventricular conduction dysfunctions. *International Journal of Cardiology*, **15**, 231–9.

Barlow, J. B. & Pocock, W. A. (1979). Mitral valve prolapse, the specific billowing mitral leaflet syndrome, or an insignificant non-ejection systolic click. *American Heart Journal*, **97**, 277–85.

Barnett, H. J. M., Boughner, D. R., Taylor, W., *et al.* (1980). Further evidence relating mitral-valve prolapse to cerebral ischemic heart events. *New England Journal of Medicine*, **302**, 139–44.

Basso, C., Frescura, C., Corrado, D., *et al.* (1995). Congenital heart disease and sudden death in the young. *Human Pathology*, **26**, 1065–72.

Bauer, D. (1945). Ebstein type of tricuspid insufficiency. Roentgen studies in a case with sudden death at the age of twenty-seven. *American Journal of Roentgenology*, **54**, 136–44.

Becker, A. E. & Anderson, R. H. (1981). *Pathology of Congenital Heart Disease*. London: Butterworth.

Becker, A. E., Becker, M. J. & Edwards, J. E. (1972). Mitral valvular abnormalities associated with supravalvular aortic stenosis. Observations in 3 cases. *American Journal of Cardiology*, **29**, 90–94.

Bell, M. D. & Tate, L. G. (1994). Vascular anomaly of the bundle of His associated with sudden death in a young man. *American Journal of Forensic Medicine and Pathology*, **15**, 151–5.

Berger, S., Dhala, A. & Friedberg, D. Z. (1999). Sudden cardiac death in infants, children and adolescents. *Pediatric Clinics of North America*, **46**, 221–34.

Berko, B. A. & Swift, M. (1987). X-linked dilated cardiomyopathy. *New England Journal of Medicine*, **316**, 1186–91.

Bhandari, A. K., Shapiro, W. A., Morady, F., *et al.* (1985). Electrophysiologic testing in patients with long QT syndrome. *Circulation*, **71**, 63–71.

Bharati, S. & Lev, M. (1983). The myocardium, the conduction system, and general sequelae after surgery for congenital heart disease. In *Congenital Heart Disease After Surgery*, ed. M. A. Engle & J. K. Perloff. New York: Yorke Medical Books, pp. 247–60.

Bharati, S. & Lev, M. (1985). The pathology of sudden death. In *Sudden Cardiac Death*, ed. M. E. Josephson & A. N. Brest. Philadelphia: F. A. Davis, pp. 1–27.

Bharati, S., Bauerfeind, R., Miller, L. B., Strasberg, B. & Lev, M. (1983a). Sudden death in three teenagers: conduction system studies. *Journal of the American College of Cardiology*, **1**, 879–86.

Bharati, S., Bauerfeind, R., Scheinman, M., *et al.* (1979a). Congenital abnormalities of the conduction system in two patients with tachyarrhythmias. *Circulation*, **59**, 593–606.

Bharati, S., Bicoff, J. P., Fridman, J. L., Lev, M. & Rosen, K. M. (1976). Sudden death caused by benign tumor of the atrioventricular node. *Archives of Internal Medicine*, **136**, 224–8.

Bharati, S., Feld, A. W., Bauerfeind, R., Kattus, A. A. & Lev, M. (1983b). Hypoplasia of the right ventricular myocardium with ventricular tachycardia. *Archives of Pathology and Laboratory Medicine*, **107**, 249–53.

Bharati, S., Molthan, M. E., Veasy, L. G. & Lev, M. (1979b). Conduction system in two cases of sudden death two years after the Mustard procedure. *Journal of Thoracic and Cardiovascular Surgery*, **77**, 101–8.

Bharati, S., Nordenberg, A., Bauerfiend, R., *et al.* (1980). The anatomic substrate for the sick sinus syndrome in adolescence. *American Journal of Cardiology*, **46**, 163–72.

Bharati, S., Strasberg, B., Bilitch, M., *et al.* (1981). Anatomic substrate for preexcitation in idiopathic myocardial hypertrophy with fibroelastosis of the left ventricle. *American Journal of Cardiology*, **48**, 47–58.

Bhavsar, P. K., Brand, N. J., Yacoub, M. H. & Barton, P. J. R. (1996). Isolation and characterization of the human cardiac troponin I gene (TNN13). *Genomics*, **35**, 11–23.

Billingham, M. E. & Tazelaar, H. D. (1986). The morphological progression of viral myocarditis. *Postgraduate Medical Journal*, **62**, 581–4.

Bloomfield, D. K. (1964). The natural history of ventricular septal defect in patients surviving infancy. *Circulation*, **29**, 914–55.

Boissy, C., Chevallier, A., Michiels, J.-F., *et al.* (1997). Histiocytoid cardiomyopathy: a cause of sudden death in infancy. *Pathology Research and Practice*, **193**, 589–93.

Bonadio, W. A. & Losek, J. D. (1987). Infants with myocarditis presenting with severe respiratory distress and shock. *Pediatric Emergency Care*, **3**, 110–13.

Bower, C. & Ramsay, J. M. (1994). Congenital heart disease: a 10 year cohort. *Journal of Paediatrics and Child Health*, **30**, 414–18.

Bowles, K. R., Gajarski, R., Porter, P., *et al.* (1996). Gene mapping of familial autosomal dominant familial dilated cardiomyopathy to chromosome 10q21–23. *Journal of Clinical Investigation*, **98**, 1355–60.

Branzi, A., Romeo, G., Specchia, S., *et al.* (1985). Genetic heterogeneity of hypertrophic cardiomyopathy. *International Journal of Cardiology*, **7**, 129–33.

Bricker, J. T., Garson, A. Jr & Gillette, P. C. (1984). A family history of seizures associated with sudden cardiac deaths. *American Journal of Diseases of Children*, **138**, 866–8.

Brookfield, L., Bharati, S., Denes, P., Halstead, R. D. & Lev, M. (1988). Familial sudden death. Report of a case and review of the literature. *Chest*, **94**, 989–93.

Brugada, P., Brugada, R. & Brugada, J. (2000). The Brugada syndrome. *Current Cardiology Report*, **2**, 507–14.

Bryant, R. M. (1999). Hypertrophic cardiomyopathy in children. *Cardiology in Review*, **7**, 92–100.

Buja, G. F., Corrado, D., Pellegrino, P. A., Nava, A. & Thiene, G. (1986). Fatal paroxysmal supraventricular tachycardia in an infant. *Chest*, **90**, 145–6.

Burke, A. P., Afzal, M. N., Barnett, D. S. & Virmani, R. (1999). Sudden death after a cold drink. Case report. *American Journal of Forensic Medicine and Pathology*, **20**, 37–9.

Byard, R. W. (1994). Ventricular septal defect and sudden death in early childhood. *Journal of Paediatrics and Child Health*, **30**, 439–40.

Byard, R. W. (1997). Significant coincidental findings at autopsy in accidental childhood death. *Medicine, Science and the Law*, **37**, 259–62.

Byard, R. W. (2002). Unexpected infant death: occult cardiac disease and sudden infant death syndrome – how much of an overlap is there? *Journal of Pediatrics*, **141**, 303–5.

Byard, R. W. & Krous, H. F. (2003). Sudden infant death syndrome: overview and update. *Pediatric and Developmental Pathology*, **6**, 112–27.

Byard, R. W., Bourne, A. J. & Adams, P. S. (1990). Subarterial ventricular septal defect in an infant with sudden unexpected death: cause or coincidence? *American Journal of Cardiovascular Pathology*, **3**, 333–6.

Byard, R. W., James, R. A. & Gilbert, J. D. (2002). Childhood sporting deaths. *American Journal of Forensic Medicine and Pathology*, **23**, 364–7.

Byard, R. W., Jimenez, C. L. & Moore, L. (1992). Mechanisms of sudden death in patients with congenital teratoma. *Pediatric Surgery International*, **7**, 464–7.

Carrier, L., Hengstenberg, C, Beckmann, J. S., *et al.* (1993). Mapping of a novel gene for familial hypertrophic cardiomyopathy to chromosome 11. *Nature Genetics*, **4**, 311–13.

Cebelin, M. S. & Hirsch, C. S. (1980). Human stress cardiomyopathy. Myocardial lesions in victims of homicidal assaults without internal injuries. *Human Pathology*, **11**, 123–32.

Chambers, J. (1995). Left ventricular hypertrophy. An underappreciated coronary risk factor. *British Medical Journal*, **311**, 273–4.

Charlton, I. & Williams, R. (1990). Cardiac conducting tissue. A simplified technique for examination of the SA and AV nodes. *American Journal of Forensic Medicine and Pathology*, **11**, 213–18.

Chesler, E., King, R. A. & Edwards, J. E. (1983). The myxomatous mitral valve and sudden death. *Circulation*, **67**, 632–9.

Chia, B. L., Yew, F. C., Chay, S. O. & Tan, A. T. H. (1982). Familial Wolff-Parkinson-White syndrome. *Journal of Electrocardiology*, **15**, 195–8.

Ciró, E., Nichols, P. F., III & Maron, B. J. (1983). Heterogeneous morphologic expression of genetically transmitted hypertrophic cardiomyopathy. Two-dimensional echocardiographic analysis. *Circulation*, **67**, 1227–33.

Coffin, C. M. (1992). Congenital cardiac fibroma associated with Gorlin syndrome. *Pediatric Pathology*, **12**, 255–62.

Cohle, S. D. & Lie, J. T. (1991). Pathologic changes of the cardiac conduction tissue in sudden unexpected death. A review. *Pathology Annual*, **26** (part 2), 33–57.

Cohle, S. D. & Lie, J. T. (1998). Histopathologic spectrum of the cardiac conducting tissue in traumatic and noncardiac sudden death patients under 30 years of age: an analysis of

100 cases. In *Anatomic Pathology*, vol. 3, ed. R. E. Fechner & P. P. Rosen. Chicago: American Society of Clinical Pathologists, pp. 53–76.

Cohle, S. D., Balraj, E. & Bell, M. (1999). Sudden death due to ventricular septal defect. *Pediatric and Developmental Pathology*, **2**, 327–32.

Cohle, S. D., Graham, M. A., Dowling, G. & Pounder, D. J. (1988). Sudden death and left ventricular outflow disease. *Pathology Annual*, **23** (part 2), 98–124.

Cohle, S. D., Graham, M. A., Sperry, K. L. & Dowling, G. (1989). Unexpected death as a result of infective endocarditis. *Journal of Forensic Sciences*, **34**, 1374–86.

Colman, J. M., Sermer, M., Seaward, P. G. R. & Siu, S. C. (2000). Congenital heart disease in pregnancy. *Cardiology in Review*, **8**, 166–73.

Comfort, A. (1981). Sorcery and sudden death. *Journal of the Royal Society of Medicine*, **74**, 332–3.

Cooke, R. A., Chambers, J. B. & Curry, P. V. L. (1994). Noonan's cardiomyopathy: a non-hypertrophic variant. *British Heart Journal*, **71**, 561–5.

Cooper, M. J. & Abinader, E. G. (1981). Family history in assessing the risk for progression of mitral valve prolapse. Report of a kindred. *American Journal of Diseases of Children*, **135**, 647–9.

Corrado, D., Thiene, G., Nava, A., Rossi, L. & Pennelli, N. (1990). Sudden death in young competitive athletes: clinicopathologic correlations in 22 cases. *American Journal of Medicine*, **89**, 588–96.

Corrigall, D., Bolen, J., Hancock, E. W. & Popp, R. L. (1977). Mitral valve prolapse and infective endocarditis. *American Journal of Medicine*, **63**, 215–22.

Cottrill, C. M. & Kaplan, S. (1973). Cerebral vascular accidents in cyanotic congenital heart disease. *American Journal of Diseases of Children*, **125**, 484–7.

Couper, R. T. L., Byard, R. W., Cutz, E., Stringer, D. A. & Durie, P. R. (1991). Cardiac rhabdomyomata and megacystis-microcolon-intestinal hypoperistalsis syndrome. *Journal of Medical Genetics*, **28**, 274–6.

Cross, S. J., Dean, J. C. S., Lee, H. S., *et al.* (1993). Study of left and right ventricular function in Romano-Ward syndrome. *British Heart Journal*, **70**, 266–71.

Cunningham, N. E. & Stewart, J. (1985). A rare cause of cot death – infantile xanthomatous cardiomyopathy. *Medicine, Science and the Law*, **25**, 149–52.

Curfman, G. D. (1992). Molecular insights into hypertrophic cardiomyopathy. *New England Journal of Medicine*, **326**, 1149–51.

Curran, M. E., Splawski, I., Timothy, K. W., *et al.* (1995). A molecular basis for cardiac arrhythmia: *HERG* mutations cause long QT syndrome. *Cell*, **80**, 795–803.

Darcy, T. P., Virmani, R., Cohen, I. S. & Robinowitz, M. (1988). Mitral valve prolapse associated with sudden death: morphologic spectrum and distinguishing features. *Journal of the American College of Cardiology*, **11**, 125A.

Davies, M. J. (1992). Anatomic features in victims of sudden coronary death. Coronary artery pathology. *Circulation*, **85** (suppl 1), I-19–24.

Davies, M. J. & Popple, A. (1979). Sudden unexpected cardiac death – a practical approach to the forensic problem. *Histopathology*, **3**, 255–77.

Davies, M. J., Moore, B. P. & Braimbridge, M. V. (1978). The floppy mitral valve. Study of incidence, pathology, and complications in surgical necropsy, and forensic material. *British Heart Journal*, **40**, 468–81.

Deanfield, J. E., McKenna, W. J. & Hallidie-Smith, K. A. (1980). Detection of late arrhythmia and conduction disturbance after correction of tetralogy of Fallot. *British Heart Journal*, **44**, 248–53.

Deanfield, J., McKenna, W. & Rowland, E. (1985). Local abnormalities of right ventricular depolarization after repair of tetralogy of Fallot: a basis for ventricular arrhythmia. *American Journal of Cardiology*, **55**, 522–5.

Dec, G. W. & Fuster, V. (1994). Idiopathic dilated cardiomyopathy. *New England Journal of Medicine*, **331**, 1564–75.

De Letter, E. A. & Piette, M. H. A. (1999). Endocardial fibroelastosis as a cause of sudden unexpected death. *American Journal of Forensic Medicine and Pathology*, **20**, 357–63.

Denfield, S. W. & Garson, A., Jr (1990). Sudden death in children and young adults. *Pediatric Clinics of North America*, **37**, 215–31.

DeSilva, R. A. & Lown, B. (1978). Ventricular premature beats, stress, and sudden death. *Psychosomatics*, **19**, 649–61.

Devine, W. A., Debich, D. E. & Anderson, R. H. (1991). Dissection of congenitally malformed hearts, with comments on the value of sequential segmental analysis. *Pediatric Pathology*, **11**, 235–59.

Dimsdale, J. E. (1977). Emotional causes of sudden death. *American Journal of Psychiatry*, **134**, 1361–6.

Disse, S., Abergel, E., Berrebi, A., *et al.* (1999). Mapping of a first locus for autosomal dominant myxomatous mitral-valve prolapse to chromosome 16p11. 2-p12. 1. *American Journal of Human Genetics*, **65**, 1242–51.

Doyle, E. F., Arumugham, P., Lara, E., Rutkowski, M. R. & Kiely, B. (1974). Sudden death in young patients with congenital aortic stenosis. *Pediatrics*, **53**, 481–9.

Dubois, R. W., Neill, C. A. & Hutchins, G. M. (1983). Rhabdomyoma of the heart producing right bundle branch block. *Pediatric Pathology*, **1**, 435–42.

Dungan, W. T., Garson, A., Jr & Gillette, P. C. (1981). Arrhythmogenic right ventricular dysplasia: a cause of ventricular tachycardia in children with apparently normal hearts. *American Heart Journal*, **102**, 745–50.

Dunn, F. G., Burns, J. M. A. & Hornung, R. S. (1991). Left ventricular hypertrophy in hypertension. *American Heart Journal*, **122**, 312–15.

Dunnigan, A., Pritzker, M. R., Benditt, D. G. & Benson, D. W., Jr (1984). Life threatening ventricular tachycardias in late survivors of surgically corrected tetralogy of Fallot. *British Heart Journal*, **52**, 198–206.

Durand, J.-B., Bachinski, L. L., Bieling, L. C., *et al.* (1995). Localization of a gene responsible for familial dilated cardiomyopathy to chromosome 1q32. *Circulation*, **92**, 3387–9.

Edwards, J. E. (1965). Pathology of left ventricular outflow tract obstruction. *Circulation*, **31**, 586–99.

Edwards, J. E. (1988). Floppy mitral valve syndrome. In *Contemporary Issues in Cardiovascular Pathology*, ed. B. F. Waller. Philadelphia: F. A. Davis, pp. 249–71.

Edwards, W. D. (1991). Cardiomyopathies. In *Cardiovascular Pathology, Major Problems in Pathology*, vol. 23, ed. R. Virmani, J. B. Atkinson & J. J. Fenoglio. Philadelphia: W. B. Saunders, pp. 257–309.

Emanuel, R., Withers, R. & O'Brien, K. (1971). Dominant and recessive modes of inheritance in idiopathic cardiomyopathy. *Lancet*, **ii**, 1065–7.

Emanuel, R., Withers, R., O'Brien, K., Ross, P. & Feizi, O. (1978). Congenitally bicuspid aortic valves. Clinicogenetic study of 41 families. *British Heart Journal*, **40**, 1402–7.

Engel, G. L. (1971). Sudden and rapid death during psychological stress. Folklore or folk wisdom? *Annals of Internal Medicine*, **74**, 771–82.

Epstein, N. D., Cohn, G. M., Cyran, F. & Fananapazir, L. (1992). Differences in clinical expression of hypertrophic cardiomyopathy associated with two distinct mutations in the β-myosin heavy chain gene A 908$^{\text{Leu}\to\text{Val}}$ mutation and a 403$^{\text{Arg}\to\text{Gln}}$ mutation. *Circulation*, **86**, 345–52.

Farb, A., Burke, A. P. & Virmani, R. (1992). Anatomy and pathology of the right ventricle (including acquired tricuspid and pulmonic valve disease). *Cardiology Clinics*, **10**, 1–21.

Fitzpatrick, A. P., Shapiro, L. M., Rickards, A. F. & Poole-Wilson, P. A. (1990). Familial restrictive cardiomyopathy with atrioventricular block and skeletal myopathy. *British Heart Journal*, **63**, 114–18.

Flugelman, M. Y., Pollack, S., Hammerman, H., Riss, E. & Barzilai, D. (1982). Congenital prolongation of Q-T interval: a family study of three generations. *Cardiology*, **69**, 170–74.

Franciosi, R. A. & Blanc, W. A. (1968). Myocardial infarcts in infants and children. I. A necropsy study in congenital heart disease. *Journal of Pediatrics*, **73**, 309–19.

Fraser, G. R., Froggatt, P. & James, T. N. (1964). Congenital deafness associated with electrocardiographic abnormalities, fainting attacks and sudden death. A recessive syndrome. *Quarterly Journal of Medicine*, **33**, 361–85.

Fried, K., Beer, S., Vure, E., Algom, M. & Shapira, Y. (1979). Autosomal recessive sudden unexpected death in children probably caused by a cardiomyopathy associated with myopathy. *Journal of Medical Genetics*, **16**, 341–6.

Friedman, R. A., Moak, J. P. & Garson, A., Jr (1991). Clinical course of idiopathic dilated cardiomyopathy in children. *Journal of the American College of Cardiology*, **18**, 152–6.

Gardner, R. J. M., Hanson, J. W., Ionasescu, V. V., *et al.* (1987). Dominantly inherited dilated cardiomyopathy. *American Journal of Medical Genetics*, **27**, 61–73.

Garson, A., Jr (1991). Sudden death in the young. *Hospital Practice*, **26**, 51–60.

Garson, A., Jr & McNamara, D. G. (1985). Sudden death in a pediatric cardiology population, 1958 to 1983: relation to prior arrhythmias. *Journal of the American College of Cardiology*, **5**, 134B–7B.

Garson, A., Jr, Dick, M., II, Fournier, A., *et al.* (1993). The long QT syndrome in children. An international study of 287 patients. *Circulation*, **87**, 1866–72.

Garson A., Jr, Smith, R. T., Moak, J. P., *et al.* (1987). Incessant ventricular tachycardia in infants: myocardial hamartomas and surgical care. *Journal of the American College of Cardiologists*, **10**, 619–26.

Gault, J. H., Cantwell, J., Lev, M. & Braunwald, E. (1972). Fatal familial cardiac arrhythmias. Histologic observations on the cardiac conduction system. *American Journal of Cardiology*, **29**, 548–53.

Gemayel, C., Pelliccia, A. & Thompson, P. D. (2001). Arrhythmogenic right ventricular cardiomyopathy. *Journal of the American College of Cardiology*, **38**, 1773–81.

Gettes, L. S. (1992). Electrolyte abnormalities underlying lethal and ventricular arrhythmias. *Circulation*, **85**, I-70–76.

Gheissari, A., Malm, J. R., Bowman, F. O., Jr & Bierman, F. Z. (1992). Cor triatriatum sinistrum: one institution's 28-year experience. *Pediatric Cardiology*, **13**, 85–8.

Gilgenkrantz, S., Vigneron, C., Gregoire, M. J., Pernot, C. & Raspiller, A. (1982). Association of del(11)(p15. 1p12), aniridia, catalase deficiency and cardiomyopathy. *American Journal of Medical Genetics*, **13**, 39–49.

Gillette, P. C., Freed, D. & McNamara, D. G. (1978). A proposed autosomal dominant method of inheritance of the

Wolff-Parkinson-White syndrome and supraventricular tachycardia. *Journal of Pediatrics*, **93**, 257–8.

Gillette, P. C. & Garson, A., Jr (1992). Sudden cardiac death in the pediatric population. *Circulation*, **85**, I-64–9.

Glew, R. H., Varghese, P. J., Krovetz, L. J., Dorst, J. P. & Rowe, R. D. (1969). Sudden death in congenital aortic stenosis. A review of eight cases with an evaluation of premonitory clinical features. *American Heart Journal*, **78**, 615–25.

Goodfriend, M. & Wolpert, E. A. (1976). Death from fright: report of a case and literature review. *Psychosomatic Medicine*, **38**, 348–56.

Goodin, J. C., Farb, A., Smialek, J. E., Field, F. & Virmani, R. (1991). Right ventricular dysplasia associated with sudden death in young adults. *Modern Pathology*, **4**, 702–6.

Gourdie, A. L., Robertson, C. E. & Busuttil, A. (1989). Sudden death in young people due to hypertrophic cardiomyopathy. *Archives of Emergency Medicine*, **6**, 220–24.

Gow, R. M. (1996). Sudden cardiac death in the young. *Canadian Journal of Cardiology*, **12**, 1157–60.

Graber, H. L., Unverferth, D. V., Baker, P. B., *et al.* (1986). Evolution of a hereditary cardiac conduction and muscle disorder: a study involving a family with six generations affected. *Circulation*, **74**, 21–35.

Graham, R. M. & Owens, W. A. (1999). Pathogenesis of inherited forms of dilated cardiomyopathy. *New England Journal of Medicine*, **341**, 1759–62.

Grech, V., Ellul, B. & Montalto, S. A. (2000). Sudden cardiac death in infancy due to histiocytoid cardiomyopathy. *Cardiology in the Young*, **10**, 49–51.

Green, J. R., Jr, Korovetz, M. J., Shanklin, D. R., Devito, J. J. & Taylor, W. J. (1969). Sudden unexpected death in three generations. *Archives of Internal Medicine*, **124**, 359–63.

Greenwood. R. D. (1984). Mitral valve prolapse. Incidence and clinical course in a pediatric population. *Clinical Pediatrics*, **23**, 318–20.

Guertl, B., Noehammer, C. & Hoefler, G. (2000). Metabolic cardiomyopathies. *International Journal of Experimental Pathology*, **81**, 349–72.

Halbertsma, F. J. J., van't Hek L. G. F. M. & Daniels, O. (2001). Spongy cardiomyopathy in a neonate. *Cardiology in the Young*, **11**, 458–60.

Hals, J., Ek, J. & Sandnes, K. (1990). Cardiac myxoma as the cause of death in an infant. *Acta Paediatrica Scandinavica*, **79**, 999–1000.

Hammon, J. W. & Bender, H. W. (1990). Major anomalies of pulmonary and thoracic systemic veins. In *Surgery of the Chest*, 5th edn, ed. D. C. Sabiston & F. C. Spencer. Philadelphia: W. B. Saunders, pp. 1274–97.

Hohn, A. R. & Stanton, R. E. (1987). Myocarditis in children. *Pediatrics in Review*, **9**, 83–8.

Horiguchi, H., Misawa, S., Ogata, T. & Doy, M. (1990). Sudden death due to right ventricular cardiomyopathy. *American Journal of Forensic Medicine and Pathology*, **11**, 261–4.

Hossack, K. F., Neutze, J. M., Lowe, J. B. & Barratt-Boyes, B. G. (1980). Congenital valvar aortic stenosis. Natural history and assessment of operation. *British Heart Journal*, **43**, 561–73.

Husson, G. S., Blackman, M. S., Rogers, M. C., Bharati, S. & Lev, M. (1973). Familial congenital bundle branch system disease. *American Journal of Cardiology*, **32**, 365–9.

Ibsen, H. H. W., Baandrup, U. & Simonsen, E. E. (1985). Familial right ventricular dilated cardiomyopathy. *British Heart Journal*, **54**, 156–9.

Ino, T., Benson, L. N., Freedom, R. M. & Rowe, R. D. (1988). Natural history and prognostic risk factors in endocardial fibroelastosis. *American Journal of Cardiology*, **62**, 431–4.

Isner, J. M., Roberts, W. C., Heymsfield, S. B. & Yager, J. (1985). Anorexia nervosa and sudden death. *Annals of Internal Medicine*, **102**, 49–52.

Itoh, S., Munemura, S. & Satoh, H. (1982). A study of the inheritance pattern of Romano-Ward syndrome. Prolonged Q-T interval, syncope and sudden death. *Clinical Pediatrics*, **21**, 20–24.

James, F. W., Kaplan, S. & Chou, T.-C. (1975). Unexpected cardiac arrest in patients after surgical correction of tetralogy of Fallot. *Circulation*, **52**, 691–5.

James, T. N. (1979). Intercardiac ganglionitis and sudden death. Herpes of the heart? *Transactions of the American Clinical and Climatological Association*, **91**, 177–90.

James, T. N. & Marshall, T. K. (1976a). De Subitaneis Mortibus. XVII. Multifocal stenoses due to fibromuscular dysplasia of the sinus node artery. *Circulation*, **53**, 736–42.

James, T. N. & Marshall, T. K. (1976b). De Subitaneis Mortibus. XVIII. Persistent fetal dispersion of the atrioventricular node and His bundle within the central fibrous body. *Circulation*, **53**, 1026–34.

James, T. N., Froggatt, P. & Marshall, T. K. (1967). Sudden death in young athletes. *Annals of Internal Medicine*, **67**, 1013–21.

James, T. N., Hackel, D. B. & Marshall, T. K. (1974). De Subitaneis Mortibus. V. Occluded A-V node artery. *Circulation*, **49**, 772–7.

James, T. N., Jordan, J. D., Riddick, L. & Bargeron, L. M. (1988). Subaortic stenosis and sudden death. *Journal of Thoracic Cardiovascular Surgery*, **95**, 247–54.

James, T. N., Marilley, R. J., Jr & Marriott, H. J. L. (1975). De Subitaneis Mortibus. XI. Young Girl with palpitations. *Circulation*, **51**, 743–8.

Jarcho, J. A., McKenna, W., Pare, J. A. P., (1989). Mapping a gene for familial hypertrophic cardiomyopathy to chromosome 14q1. *New England Journal of Medicine*, **321**, 1372–8.

Jennings, M. T., Hall, J. G. & Kukolich, M. (1980). Endocardial fibroelastosis, neurologic dysfunction and unusual facial appearance in two brothers, coincidentally associated with dominantly inherited macrocephaly. *American Journal of Medical Genetics*, **5**, 271–6.

Jeresaty, R. M. (1976). Sudden death in mitral valve prolapse-click syndrome. *American Journal of Cardiology*, **37**, 317–18.

Jervell, A. (1985). The surdo-cardiac syndrome. *European Heart Journal*, **6** (suppl D), 97–102.

Jervell, A. & Lange-Nielsen, F. (1957). Congenital deaf-mutism, functional heart disease with prolongation of the QT interval, and sudden death. *American Heart Journal*, **54**, 59–67.

Jokl, E. & McClellan, J. T. (1970). Exercise and cardiac death. *Journal of the American Medical Association*, **213**, 1489–91.

Katz, N. M., Buckley, M. J. & Liberthson, R. R. (1977). Discrete membranous subaortic stenosis. Report of 31 patients, review of the literature, and delineation of management. *Circulation*, **56**, 1034–8.

Kearney, D. L., Titus, J. L., Hawkins, E. P., Ott, D. A. & Garson, A. (1987). Pathologic features of myocardial hamartomas causing childhood tachyarrhythmias. *Circulation*, **75**, 705–10.

Kearney, D. L., Towbin, J. A., Bricker, J. T., Radovancevic, B. & Frazier, O. H. (1995). Case 5. Familial right ventricular dysplasia (cardiomyopathy). *Pediatric Pathology and Laboratory Medicine*, **15**, 181–9.

Keatinge, W. R. & Hayward, M. G. (1981). Sudden death in cold water and ventricular arrhythmia. *Journal of Forensic Sciences*, **26**, 459–61.

Kelly, D. P. & Strauss, A. W. (1994). Inherited cardiomyopathies. *New England Journal of Medicine*, **330**, 913–19.

Kiuchi, M., Kawachi, Y. & Kimura, Y. (1988). Sudden infant death due to asplenia syndrome. *American Journal of Forensic Medicine and Pathology*, **9**, 102–4.

Kojima, H., Ohgimi, Y., Mizutani, K. & Nishimura, Y. (1969). Hypoplastic-left-heart syndrome in siblings. *Lancet*, **ii**, 701.

Krajinovic, M., Pinamonti, B., Sinagra, G., *et al.* (1995). Linkage of familial dilated cardiomyopathy to chromosome 9. *American Journal of Human Genetics*, **57**, 846–52.

Krous, H. F., Chapman, A. J. & Altshuler, G. (1978). Cardiac hemangioma: a rare (or possible) cause of sudden death in children. *Journal of Forensic Sciences*, **23**, 375–8.

Kulbertus, H. E., Coyne, J. J. & Hallidie-Smith, K. A. (1969). Conduction disturbances before and after surgical closure of ventricular septal defect. *American Heart Journal*, **77**, 123–31.

Lambert, E. C., Menon, V. A., Wagner, H. R. & Vlad, P. (1974). Sudden unexpected death from cardiovascular disease in children. A cooperative international study. *American Journal of Cardiology*, **34**, 89–96.

Landing, B. H., Recalde, A. L., Lawrence, T. Y. K. & Shankle, W. R. (1994). Cardiomyopathy in childhood and adult life, with emphasis on hypertrophic cardiomyopathy. *Pathology Research and Practice*, **190**, 737–49.

Lecomte, D., Fornes, P., Fouret, P. & Nicolas, G. (1993). Isolated myocardial fibrosis as a cause of sudden cardiac death and its possible relation to myocarditis. *Journal of Forensic Sciences*, **38**, 617–21.

Levine, S. A. & Woodworth, C. R. (1958). Congenital deaf-mutism, prolonged QT interval, syncopal attacks and sudden death. *New England Journal of Medicine*, **259**, 412–17.

Lewman, L. V., Demany, M. A. & Zimmerman, H. A. (1972). Congenital tumor of atrioventricular node with complete heart block and sudden death. Mesothelioma or lymphangioendothelioma of atrioventricular node. *American Journal of Cardiology*, **29**, 554–7.

Li, D., Tapscoft, T., Gonzalez, O., *et al.* (1999). Desmin mutation responsible for idiopathic dilated cardiomyopathy. *Circulation*, **100**, 461–4.

Liberthson, R. R. (1996). Sudden death from cardiac causes in children and young adults. *New England Journal of Medicine*, **334**, 1039–44.

Lucas, R. V., Jr & Edwards, J. E. (1982). The floppy mitral valve. *Current Problems in Cardiology*, **7**, 1–48.

Lynch, H. T., Mohiuddin, S., Sketch, M. H., *et al.* (1973). Hereditary progressive atrioventricular conduction defect. A new syndrome? *Journal of the American Medical Association*, **225**, 1465–70.

MacRae, C. A., Ghaisas, N., Kass, S., *et al.* (1995). Familial hypertrophic cardiomyopathy with Wolff-Parkinson-White syndrome maps to locus on chromosome 7q3. *Journal of Clinical Investigation*, **96**, 1216–20.

Malcolm, A. D. (1985). Mitral valve prolapse associated with other disorders. Casual coincidence, common link, or fundamental genetic disturbance? *British Heart Journal*, **53**, 353–62.

Malhotra, V., Ferrans, V. J. & Virmani, R. (1994). Infantile histiocytoid cardiomyopathy: three cases and literature review. *American Heart Journal*, **128**, 1009–21.

Mandel, K., Grunebaum, E. & Benson, L. (2001). Noncompaction of the myocardium associated with Roifman syndrome. *Cardiology in the Young*, **11**, 240–43.

Manning, J. A. (1977). Sudden, unexpected death in children. *American Journal of Diseases of Children*, **131**, 1201–2.

Manthorpe, T. & Manthorpe, R. (1992). Congenital complete heart block in children of mothers with primary Sjogren's syndrome. *Lancet*, **340**, 1359–60.

Marcus, F. I., Fontaine, G. H., Guiraudon, G., *et al.* (1982). Right ventricular dysplasia: a report of 24 adult cases. *Circulation*, **65**, 384–98.

Markus, C. K., Chow, L. H., Wycoff, D. M. & McManus, B. M. (1989). Pet food-derived penicillin residue as a potential cause of hypersensitivity myocarditis and sudden death. *American Journal of Cardiology*, **63**, 1154–6.

Maron, B. J. (1988). Right ventricular cardiomyopathy: another cause of sudden death in the young. *New England Journal of Medicine*, **318**, 178–80.

Maron, B. J. & Fananapazir, L. (1992). Sudden cardiac death in hypertrophic cardiomyopathy. *Circulation*, **85** (suppl 1), I-57–63.

Maron, B. J., Bonow, R. O., Cannon, R. O., III, Leon, M. B. & Epstein, S. E. (1987a). Hypertrophic cardiomyopathy. Inter-relations of clinical manifestations, pathophysiology, and therapy (first of two parts). *New England Journal of Medicine*, **316**, 780–89.

Maron, B. J., Bonow, R. O., Cannon, R. O., III, Leon, M. B. & Epstein, S. E. (1987b). Hypertrophic cardiomyopathy. Interrelations of clinical manifestations, pathophysiology, and therapy (second of two parts). *New England Journal of Medicine*, **316**, 844–52.

Maron, B. J., Bonow, R. O., Seshagiri, T. N. R., Roberts, W. C. & Epstein, S. E. (1982). Hypertrophic cardiomyopathy with ventricular septal hypertrophy localized to the apical region of the left ventricle (apical hypertrophic cardiomyopathy). *American Journal of Cardiology*, **49**, 1838–48.

Maron, B. J., Edwards, J. E., Henry, W. L., *et al.* (1974). Asymmetric septal hypertrophy (ASH) in infancy. *Circulation*, **50**, 809–20.

Maron, B. J., Redwood, D. R., Roberts, W. C., *et al.* (1976). Tunnel subaortic stenosis. Left ventricular outflow tract obstruction produced by fibromuscular tubular narrowing. *Circulation*, **54**, 404–16.

Maron, B. J., Roberts, W. C. & Epstein, S. E. (1982). Sudden death in hypertrophic cardiomyopathy: a profile of 78 patients. *Circulation*, **65**, 1388–94.

Maron, B. J., Roberts, W. C., McAllister, H. A., Rosing, D. R. & Epstein, S. E. (1980). Sudden death in young athletes. *Circulation*, **62**, 218–29.

Maron, B. J., Wolfson, J. K., Epstein, S. E. & Roberts, W. C. (1989). Structural basis for myocardial ischemia in hypertrophic cardiomyopathy. In *Nonatherosclerotic Ischemic Heart Disease*, ed. R. Virmani & M. B. Forman. New York: Raven Press, pp. 305–24.

Massumi, R. A. (1967). Familial Wolff-Parkinson-White syndrome with cardiomyopathy. *American Journal of Medicine*, **43**, 951–5.

Matthys, D., Van Coster, R. & Verhaaren, H. (1991). Fatal outcome of pyruvate loading test in child with restrictive cardiomyopathy. *Lancet*, **338**, 1020–21.

McAllister, H. A., Jr (1979). Primary tumors and cysts of the heart and pericardium. *Current Problems in Cardiology*, **4**, 1–51.

McAllister, H. A., Jr & Fenoglio, J. J., Jr (1978). *Tumors of the Cardiovascular System*, fascicle 15. Washington, DC: Armed Forces Institute of Pathology.

McDonald, A., Harris, A., Jefferson, K., Marshall, J. & McDonald, L. (1971). Association of prolapse of posterior cusp of mitral valve and atrial septal defect. *British Heart Journal*, **33**, 383–7.

McKenna, W. J. & Deanfield, J. E. (1984). Hypertrophic cardiomyopathy: an important cause of sudden death. *Archives of Disease in Childhood*, **59**, 971–5.

McKusick, V. A. (1990). *Mendelian Inheritance in Man. Catalogs of Autosomal Dominant, Autosomal Recessive, and X-linked Phenotypes*, 9th edn. Baltimore: Johns Hopkins University Press.

McNamara, D. G. (1982). Idiopathic benign mitral leaflet prolapse. The pediatrician's view. *American Journal of Diseases of Children*, **136**, 152–6.

McRae, J. R., Wagner, G. S., Rogers, M. C. & Canent, R. V. (1974). Paroxysmal familial ventricular fibrillation. *Journal of Pediatrics*, **84**, 515–18.

Meijboom, F., Szatmari, A., Utens, E., *et al.* (1994). Long-term follow-up after surgical closure of ventricular septal defect in infancy and childhood. *Journal of the American College of Cardiologists*, **24**, 1358–64.

Meissner, C., Minnasch, P., Gafumbegete, E., *et al.* (2000). Sudden unexpected infant death due to fibroma of the heart. *Journal of Forensic Sciences*, **45**, 731–3.

Messerli, F. H. (1990). Left ventricular hypertrophy, arterial hypertension and sudden death. *Journal of Hypertension*, **8** (suppl 7), S181–5.

Michel, R. S., Carpenter, M. A. & Lovell, M. A. (1998). Pathological case of the month (non-compaction of the left ventricular myocardium). *Archives of Pediatric and Adolescent Medicine*, **152**, 709–10.

Mills, P., Rose, J., Hollingsworth, J., Amara, I. & Craige, E. (1977). Long-term prognosis of mitral-valve prolapse. *New England Journal of Medicine*, **297**, 13–18.

Mogensen, J., Klausen, I. C., Pedersen, A. K., *et al.* (1999). α-cardiac actin is a novel disease gene in familial hypertrophic cardiomyopathy. *Journal of Clinical Investigation*, **103**, R39–43.

Morales, A. R., Romanelli, R., Boucek, R. J., *et al.* (1992). Myxoid heart disease: an assessment of extravalvular cardiac pathology in severe mitral valve prolapse. *Human Pathology*, **23**, 129–37.

Moss, A. J. & Robinson, J. (1992). Clinical features of the idiopathic long QT syndrome. *Circulation*, **85** (Suppl 1), I-140–44.

Moss, A. J., Schwartz, P. J., Crampton, R. S., Locati, E. & Carleen, E. (1985). The long QT syndrome: a prospective international study. *Circulation*, **71**, 17–21.

Murphy, J. C., Gersh, B. J., Mair, D. D., *et al.* (1993). Long-term outcome in patients undergoing surgical repair of tetralogy of Fallot. *New England Journal of Medicine*, **329**, 593–9.

Naccarelli, G. V., Antzelevitch, C., Wolbrette, D. L. & Luck, J. C. (2002). The Brugada syndrome. *Current Opinion in Cardiology*, **17**, 19–23.

Nava, A., Canciani, B., Daliento, L., *et al.* (1988a). Juvenile sudden death and effort ventricular tachycardias in a family with right ventricular cardiomyopathy. *International Journal of Cardiology*, **21**, 111–23.

Nava, A., Thiene, G., Canciani, B., *et al.* (1988b). Familial occurrence of right ventricular dysplasia: a study involving nine families. *Journal of the American College of Cardiology*, **12**, 1222–8.

Neudorf, U. E., Hussein, A., Trowitzsch, E. & Schmaltz, A. A. (2001). Clinical features of isolated noncompaction of the myocardium in children. *Cardiology in the Young*, **11**, 439–42.

Neyroud, N., Tesson, F., Denjoy, I., *et al.* (1997). A novel mutation in the potassium channel gene *KVLQT1* causes the Jervell and Lange-Nielsen cardioauditory syndrome. *Nature Genetics*, **15**, 186–9.

Newfeld, E. A., Muster, A. J., Paul, M. H., Idriss, F. S. & Riker, W. L. (1976). Discrete subvalvular aortic stenosis in childhood. Study of 51 patients. *American Journal of Cardiology*, **38**, 53–61.

Nihoyannopoulos, P., McKenna, W. J., Smith, G. & Foale, R. (1986). Echocardiographic assessment of the right ventricle in Ebstein's anomaly: relation to clinical outcome. *Journal of the American College of Cardiology*, **8**, 627–35.

Nishimura, R. A., McGoon, M. D., Shub, C., *et al.* (1985). Echocardiographically documented mitral-valve prolapse. Long-term followup of 237 patients. *New England Journal of Medicine*, **313**, 1305–9.

Norwood, W. I. (1989). Hypoplastic left heart syndrome. *Cardiology Clinics*, **7**, 377–85.

Okoye, M. I., Congdon, D. E. & Mueller, W. F., Jr (1985). Asymmetric septal hypertrophy of the heart. New findings concerning the possible etiology of sudden deaths in five males.

American Journal of Forensic Medicine and Pathology, **6**, 105–24.

Olson, T. M. & Keating, M. T. (1996). Mapping a cardiomyopathy locus to chromosome 3p22-p25. *Journal of Clinical Investigation*, **97**, 528–32.

Olson, T. M., Michels, V. V., Thibodeau, S. N., Tai, Y.-S. & Keating, M. T. (1998). Actin mutations in dilated cardiomyopathy, a heritable form of heart failure. *Science*, **280**, 751–2.

Patterson, K., Donnelly, W. H. & Dehner, L. P. (1992). The cardiovascular system. In *Pediatric Pathology*, vol. 1, ed. J. T. Stocker & L. P. Dehner. Philadelphia: J. B. Lippincott, pp. 575–651.

Pawel, B. R., de Chadarévian, J.-P., Wolk, J. H., *et al.* (1994). Sudden death in childhood due to right ventricular dysplasia: report of two cases. *Pediatric Pathology*, **14**, 987–95.

Pellegrino, P. A., Zanesco, L. & Battistella, P. A. (1992). Coagulopathies and vasculopathies. In *Cerebrovascular Diseases in Children*, ed. A. J. Raimondi, M. Choux & C. Di Rocco. New York: Springer-Verlag, pp. 189–204.

Perloff, J. K., De Leon, A. C., Jr & O'Doherty, D. (1966). The cardiomyopathy of progressive muscular dystrophy. *Circulation*, **33**, 625–48.

Pesonen, E. (1974). Myocardial damage in children and its relation to coronary artery lesions. *Acta Pathologica Microbiologica Scandinavica*, **82**, 648–54.

Petsas, A. A., Anastassiades, L. C., Constantinou, E. C. & Antonopoulos, A. G. (1998). Familial discrete subaortic stenosis. *Clinics in Cardiology*, **21**, 63–5.

Phornphutkul, C., Rosenthal, A., Nadas, A. S. & Berenberg, W. (1973). Cerebrovascular accidents in infants and children with cyanotic congenital heart disease. *American Journal of Cardiology*, **32**, 329–34.

Pickering, N. J., Brody, J. I. & Barrett, M. J. (1981). Von Willebrand syndromes and mitral-valve prolapse. Linked mesenchymal dysplasias. *New England Journal of Medicine*, **305**, 131–4.

Poetter, K., Jiang, H., Hassanzadeh, S., *et al.* (1996). Mutations in either the essential or regulatory light chains of myosin are associated with a rare myopathy in human heart and skeletal muscle. *Nature Genetics*, **13**, 63–9.

Pringle, S. D., Dunn, F. G., Tweddel, A. C., *et al.* (1992). Symptomatic and silent myocardial ischaemia in hypertensive patients with left ventricular hypertrophy. *British Heart Journal*, **67**, 377–82.

Priori, S. G., Napolitano, C., Giordano, U., Collisani, G. & Memmi, M. (2000). Brugada syndrome and sudden cardiac death in children. *Lancet*, **355**, 808–9.

Quattlebaum, T. G., Varghese, P. J., Neill, C. A. & Donahoo, J. S. (1976). Sudden death among postoperative patients with tetralogy of Fallot. A follow-up study of 243 patients for an average of twelve years. *Circulation*, **54**, 289–93.

Rabson, S. M. (1949). Sudden and unexpected natural death. IV. Sudden and unexpected natural death in infants and young children. *Journal of Pediatrics*, **34**, 166–73.

Rafinski, T., Golenia, A., Wozniewicz, B. & Wlad, S. (1967). Familial endocardial fibroelastosis. *Journal of Pediatrics*, **70**, 574–6.

Rajs, J., Råsten-Almqvist, P. & Nennesmo, I. (1997). Unexpected death in two young infants mimics SIDS. Autopsies demonstrate tumors of medulla and heart. *American Journal of Forensic Medicine and Pathology*, **18**, 384–90.

Rhodes, A. R., Silverman, R. A., Harrist, T. J. & Perez-Atayde, A. R. (1984). Mucocutaneous lentigines, cardiomucocutaneous myxomas, and multiple blue nevi: the 'Lamb' syndrome. *Journal of the American Academy of Dermatology*, **10**, 72–82.

Rice, G. P. A., Boughner, D. R., Stiller, C. & Ebers, G. C. (1980). Familial stroke syndrome associated with mitral valve prolapse. *Annals of Neurology*, **7**, 130–34.

Rigle, D. A., Dexter, R. D. & McGee, M. B. (1989). Cardiac rhabdomyoma presenting as sudden infant death syndrome. *Journal of Forensic Sciences*, **34**, 694–8.

Rivenes, S. M., Kearney, D. L., Smith, E. O., Towbin, J. A. & Denfield, S. W. (2000). Sudden death and cardiovascular collapse in children with restrictive cardiomyopathy. *Circulation*, **102**, 876–82.

Roberts, W. C. (1970). The congenitally bicuspid aortic valve. A study of 85 autopsy cases. *American Journal of Cardiology*, **26**, 72–83.

Roberts, W. C. (1978). Cardiomyopathy and myocarditis: morphologic features. *Advanced Cardiology*, **22**, 184–98.

Roberts, W. C. (1980). Congenital cardiovascular abnormalities usually "silent" until adulthood: morphologic features of the floppy mitral valve, valvular aortic stenosis, discrete subvalvular aortic stenosis, hypertrophic cardiomyopathy, sinus of valsalva aneurysm, and the Marfan syndrome. In *Congenital Heart Disease in Adults*, ed. W. C. Roberts. Philadelphia: F. A. Davis, pp. 407–53.

Roberts, W. C. & Honig, H. S. (1982). The spectrum of cardiovascular disease in the Marfan syndrome: a clinico-morphologic study of 18 necropsy patients and comparison to 151 previously reported necropsy patients. *American Heart Journal*, **104**, 115–35.

Roberts, N. K., Perloff, J. K. & Kark, R. A. P. (1979). Cardiac conduction in the Kearns-Sayre syndrome (a neuromuscular disorder associated with progressive external ophthalmoplegia and pigmentary retinopathy). Report of 2 cases and review of 17 published cases. *American Journal of Cardiology*, **44**, 1396–400.

Rocchiccioli, F., Wanders, R. J. A, Aubourg, P., *et al.* (1990). Deficiency of long-chain 3-hydroxyacyl-CoA dehydrogenase: a cause of lethal myopathy and cardiomyopathy in early childhood. *Pediatric Research*, **28**, 657–62.

Rosenberg, H. C., Yee, R., Sharma, A. D., *et al.* (1991). Near miss sudden death in an infant with Wolff-Parkinson-White syndrome. *Journal of Paediatrics and Child Health*, **27**, 62–3.

Rosenthal, A. (1993). Adults with tetralogy of Fallot – repaired, yes; cured, no. *New England Journal of Medicine*, **329**, 655–6.

Ross, J. S. (1977). Heart block, sudden death, and atrioventricular node mesothelioma. *American Journal of Diseases of Children*, **131**, 1209–11.

Rossi, L. & Thiene, G. (1984). Mild Ebstein's anomaly associated with supraventricular tachycardia and sudden death: clinicomorphologic features in 3 patients. *American Journal of Cardiology*, **53**, 332–4.

Rowland, T. W. & Schweiger, M. J. (1984). Repetitive paroxysmal ventricular tachycardia and sudden death in a child. *American Journal of Cardiology*, **53**, 1729.

Ruder, M. A., Winston, S. A., Davis, J. C., *et al.* (1985). Arrhythmogenic right ventricular dysplasia in a family. *American Journal of Cardiology*, **56**, 799–800.

Russell, G. A. (1992). Congenital heart disease. In *Recent Advances in Histopathology*, no. 15, ed. P. P. Anthony & R. N. M. MacSween. Edinburgh: Churchill Livingstone, pp. 219–39.

Russell, G. A. & Berry, P. J. (1989). Postmortem audit in a paediatric cardiology unit. *Journal of Clinical Pathology*, **42**, 912–18.

Russell, G. A., Dhasmana, J. P., Berry, P. J. & Gilbert-Barness, E. F. (1989). Coexistent cardiac tumours and malformations of the heart. *International Journal of Cardiology*, **22**, 89–98.

Ruszkiewicz, A. R. & Vernon-Roberts, E. (1995). Sudden death in an infant due to histiocytoid cardiomyopathy. A light microscopic, ultrastructural and immunohistochemical study. *American Journal of Forensic Medicine and Pathology*, **16**, 74–80.

Rutledge, J. M. & Boor, P. J. (1989). Eisenmenger's: a case study and review of the syndrome and complex. *American Journal of Cardiovascular Pathology*, **2**, 285–94.

Samanek, M., Goetzova, J. & Benesova, D. (1985). Distribution of congenital heart malformations in an autopsied child population. *International Journal of Cardiology*, **8**, 235–48.

Sanguinetti, M. C., Curran, M. E., Spector, P. S. & Keating, M. T. (1996). Spectrum of HERG K^+ channel dysfunction in an inherited cardiac arrhythmia. *Proceedings of the National Academy of Science USA*, **93**, 2208–12.

Schmidt, M. A., Michels, V. V., Edwards, W. D. & Miller, F. A. (1988). Familial dilated cardiomyopathy. *American Journal of Medical Genetics*, **31**, 135–43.

Schott, J.-J., Benson, D. W., Basson, C. T., *et al.* (1998). Congenital heart disease caused by mutations in the transcription factor NKX2-5. *Science*, **281**, 108–11.

Schott, J.-J., Charpentier, F., Peltier, S., *et al.* (1995). Mapping a gene for long QT syndrome to chromosome 4q25-27. *American Journal of Human Genetics*, **57**, 1114–22.

Schryer, M. J. P. & Karnauchow, P. N. (1974). Endocardial fibroelastosis. Etiologic and pathogenetic considerations in children. *American Heart Journal*, **88**, 557–65.

Schwartz, M. L., Cox, G. F., Lin, A. E., *et al.* (1996). Clinical approach to genetic cardiomyopathy in children. *Circulation*, **94**, 2021–38.

Schwartz, P. J. (2001). QT prolongation and SIDS – from theory to evidence. In *Sudden Infant Death Syndrome. Problems, Progress and Possibilities*, ed. R. W. Byard & H. F. Krous. London: Arnold, pp. 83–95.

Schwartz, P. J., Priori, S. G., Dumaine, R., *et al.* (2000). A molecular link between the sudden infant death syndrome and the long QT syndrome. *New England Journal of Medicine*, **343**, 262–7.

Schwartz, P. J., Stramba-Badiale, M., Segantini, A., *et al.* (1998). Prolongation of the QT interval and the sudden infant death syndrome. *New England Journal of Medicine*, **338**, 1709–14.

Senn, M., Hess, O. M. & Krayenbuhl, H. P. (1984). Hypertrophe kardiomyopathie und lentiginose. *Schweizerische Medizinische Wochenschrift*, **114**, 838–41.

Shaher, R. M., Farina, M., Alley, R., Hansen, P. & Bishop, M. (1972). Congenital subaortic stenosis in infancy caused by rhabdomyoma of the left ventricle. *Journal of Thoracic and Cardiovascular Surgery*, **63**, 157–63.

Shappell, S. D., Marshall, C. E., Brown, R. E. & Bruce, T. A. (1973). Sudden death and the familial occurrence of midsystolic click, late systolic murmur syndrome. *Circulation*, **48**, 1128–34.

Shehata, B. M., Patterson, K., Thomas, J. E., *et al.* (1998). Histiocytoid cardiomyopathy: three new cases and a review of the literature. *Pediatric and Developmental Pathology*, **1**, 56–69.

Shrapnel, M., Gilbert, J. D. and Byard, R. W. (2001). 'Arrhythmogenic left ventricular dysplasia' and sudden death. *Medicine, Science and the Law*, **41**, 159–62.

Shrivastava, S., Jacks, J. J., White, R. S. & Edwards, J. E. (1977). Diffuse rhabdomyomatosis of the heart. *Archives of Pathology and Laboratory Medicine*, **101**, 78–80.

Silka, M. J., Hardy, B. G., Menashe, V. D. & Morris, C. D. (1998). A population-based prospective evaluation of risk of sudden cardiac death after operation for common congenital heart defects. *Journal of the American College of Cardiology*, **32**, 245–51.

Silka, M. J., Kron, J. & McAnulty, J. (1992). Supraventricular tachyarrhythmias, congenital heart disease, and sudden cardiac death. *Pediatric Cardiology*, **13**, 116–18.

Silka, M. J., Kron, J., Walance, C. G., Cutler, J. E. & McAnulty, J. H. (1990). Assessment and follow up of pediatric survivors of sudden cardiac death. *Circulation*, **82**, 341–9.

Silver, M. M., Burns, J. E., Sethi, R. K. & Rowe, R. D. (1980). Oncocytic cardiomyopathy in an infant with oncocytosis in exocrine and endocrine glands. *Human Pathology*, **11**, 598–605.

Siu, S. C. & Colman, J. M. (2001). Heart disease and pregnancy. *Heart*, **85**, 710–15.

Siu, B. L., Niimura, H., Osbourne, J. A., *et al.* (1999). Familial dilated cardiomyopathy locus maps to chromosome 2q31. *Circulation*, **99**, 1022–6.

Smeeton, W. M. I. & Smith, W. M. (1987). Sudden death due to a cardiomyopathy predominantly affecting the right ventricle – right ventricular dysplasia. *Medicine, Science and the Law*, **27**, 207–12.

Smith, N. M. & Ho, S. Y. (1994). Heart block and sudden death associated with fibrosis of the conduction system at the margin of a ventricular septal defect. *Pediatric Cardiology*, **15**, 139–42.

Solomon, M. H., Winn, K. J., White, R. D., *et al.* (1976). Kartagener's syndrome with corrected transposition. Conducting system studies and coronary arterial occlusion complicating valvular replacement. *Chest*, **69**, 677–80.

Southall, D. P., Arrowsmith, W. A., Stebbens, V. & Alexander, J. R. (1986). QT interval measurements before sudden infant death syndrome. *Archives of Disease in Childhood*, **61**, 327–33.

Splawski, I., Timothy, K. W., Vincent, G. M., Atkinson, D. L. & Keating, M. T. (1997a). Molecular basis of the long QT syndrome associated with deafness. *New England Journal of Medicine*, **336**, 1562–7.

Splawski, I., Tristani-Firouzi, M., Lehmann, M. H., Sanguinetti, M. C. & Keating, M. T. (1997b). Mutations in the hminK gene cause long QT syndrome and suppress I_{Ks} function. *Nature Genetics*, **17**, 338–40.

Stahl, J., Couper, R. T. L. & Byard, R. W. (1997). Oncocytic cardiomyopathy: a rare cause of unexpected early childhood death associated with fitting. *Medicine, Science and the Law*, **37**, 84–7.

Strauss, A. W. & Johnson, M. C. (1996). The genetic basis of pediatric cardiovascular disease. *Seminars in Perinatology*, **20**, 564–76.

Stumpp, J. W. H., Schneider, J. & Bär, W. (1997). Drowning of a girl with anomaly of the bundle of His and the right bundle branch. *American Journal of Forensic Medicine and Pathology*, **18**, 208–10.

Sturner, W. Q., Lipsitt, L. P., Oh, W., Barrett, J. & Truex, R. C. (1980). Abnormal heart rate response during newborn sucking behaviour study: subsequent sudden infant death syndrome with cardiac conduction abnormality. *Forensic Science International*, **16**, 201–12.

Suarez, V., Fuggle, W. J., Cameron, A. H., French, T. A. & Hollingsworth, T. (1987). Foamy myocardial transformation of infancy: an inherited disease. *Journal of Clinical Pathology*, **40**, 329–34.

Suárez-Mier, M. P. & Aguilera, B. (1998). Histopathology of the conduction system in sudden infant death. *Forensic Science International*, **93**, 143–54.

Sutter, A. & Gujer, H-R. (1996). Left and right ventricular dysplasia and Uhl's anomaly. *American Journal of Forensic Medicine and Pathology*, **17**, 141–5.

Swartz, M. H., Teichholz, L. E. & Donoso, E. (1977). Mitral valve prolapse. A review of associated arrhythmias. *American Journal of Medicine*, **62**, 377–89.

Tatsanavivat, P., Chiravatkul, A., Klungboonkrong, V., *et al.* (1992). Sudden and unexplained deaths in sleep (Laitai) of young men in rural northeastern Thailand. *International Journal of Epidemiology*, **21**, 904–10.

Tentolouris, K., Kontozoglou, T., Trikas, A., *et al.* (1999). Fixed subaortic stenosis revisited. Congenital abnormalities in 72 new cases and review of the literature. *Cardiology*, **92**, 4–10.

Terplan, K. L. (1973). Patterns of brain damage in infants and children with congenital heart disease. Association with catheterization and surgical procedures. *American Journal of Diseases of Children*, **125**, 175–85.

Thiene, G., Nava, A., Corrado, D., Rossi, L. & Pennelli, N. (1988). Right ventricular cardiomyopathy and sudden death in young people. *New England Journal of Medicine*, **318**, 129–33.

Thierfelder, L., MacRae, C., Watkins, H., *et al.* (1993). A familial hypertrophic cardiomyopathy locus maps to chromosome 15q2. *Proceedings of the National Academy of Science USA*, **90**, 6270–74.

Thomas, W. A., Randall, R. V., Bland, E. F. & Castleman, B. (1954). Endocardial fibroelastosis: a factor in heart disease of obscure etiology. A study of 20 autopsied cases in children and adults. *New England Journal of Medicine*, **251**, 327–38.

Thorgeirsson, G. & Liebman, J. (1983). Mesothelioma of the AV node. *Pediatric Cardiology*, **4**, 219–24.

Till, J. & Herxheimer, A. (1992). Death of a child with supraventricular tachycardia. *Lancet*, **339**, 1597–8.

Till, J. A., Shinebourne, E. A., Pepper, J., Camm, A. J. & Ward, D. E. (1988). Complete denervation of the heart in a child with congenital long QT and deafness. *American Journal of Cardiology*, **62**, 1319–21.

Topaz, O. & Edwards, J. E. (1985). Pathologic features of sudden death in children, adolescents, and young adults. *Chest*, **87**, 476–82.

Towbin, J. A. (1995). New revelations about the long-QT syndrome. *New England Journal of Medicine*, **333**, 384–5.

Towbin, J. A. (1999). Pediatric myocardial disease. *Pediatric Clinics of North America*, **46**, 289–312.

Towbin, J. A. (2001). Molecular genetic basis of sudden cardiac death. *Cardiovascular Pathology*, **10**, 283–95.

Towbin, J. A. & Bowles, N. E. (2001). Arrhythmogenic inherited heart muscle diseases in children. *Journal of Electrocardiology*, **34** (suppl), 151–65.

Tripp, M. E., Katcher, M. L., Peters, H. A., *et al.* (1981). Systemic carnitine deficiency presenting as familial endocardial fibroelastosis. A treatable cardiomyopathy. *New England Journal of Medicine*, **305**, 385–90.

Tuzcu, E. M., Moodie, D. S., Ghazi, F., *et al.* (1989). Ebstein's anomaly: natural and unnatural history. *Cleveland Clinic Journal of Medicine*, **56**, 614–18.

Urban, C. H. (1964). Congenital tricuspid insufficiency. Report of an asymptomatic case with sudden death. *Journal of Forensic Sciences*, **9**, 396–402.

Valdés-Dapena, M. & Gilbert-Barness, E. (2002). Cardiovascular causes for sudden infant death. *Pediatric Pathology and Molecular Medicine*, **21**, 195–211.

Vassiliades, N., Vassiliades, K. & Karkavelas, G. (1997). Sudden death due to cardiac myxoma. *Medicine, Science and the Law*, **37**, 76–7.

Vatta, M., Dumaine, R., Varghese, G., *et al.* (2002). Genetic and biophysical basis of sudden unexplained nocturnal death syndrome (SUNDS), a disease allelic to Brugada syndrome. *Human and Molecular Genetics*, **11**, 337–45.

Vetter, V. L. (1985). Sudden death in infants, children and adolescents. *Cardiovascular Clinics*, **15**, 301–13.

Vidaillet, H. J., Jr, Pressley, J. C., Henke, E., Harrell, F. E. & German, L. D. (1987b). Familial occurrence of accessory atrioventricular pathways (preexcitation syndrome). *New England Journal of Medicine*, **317**, 65–9.

Vidaillet, H. J., Jr, Seward, J. B., Fyke, F. E., III, Su, W. P. D. & Tajik, A. J. (1987a). "Syndrome myxoma": a subset of patients with cardiac myxoma associated with pigmented skin lesions and peripheral and endocrine neoplasms. *British Heart Journal*, **57**, 247–55.

Vincent, G. M. (1986). The heart rate of Romano-Ward syndrome. *American Heart Journal*, **112**, 61–4.

Vincent, G. M., Timothy, K. W., Leppert, M. & Keating, M. (1992). The spectrum of symptoms and QT intervals in carriers of the gene for the long-QT syndrome. *New England Journal of Medicine*, **327**, 846–52.

Violette, E. J., Hardin, N. J. & McQuillen, E. N. (1981). Sudden unexpected death due to asymptomatic cardiac rhabdomyoma. *Journal of Forensic Sciences*, **26**, 599–604.

Virmani, R. & Roberts, W. C. (1991). Sudden cardiac death. In *Cardiovascular Pathology, Major Problems in Pathology*, vol. 23, ed. R. Virmani, J. B. Atkinson & J. J. Fenoglio. Philadelphia: W. B. Saunders, pp. 134–51.

Virmani, R., Atkinson, J. B., Forman, M. B. & Robinowitz, M. (1987). Mitral valve prolapse. *Human Pathology*, **18**, 596–602.

Virmani, R., Burke, A., Farb, A. & Atkinson, J. B. (2001). In *Cardiovascular Pathology*, 2nd edn. Philadelphia: W. B. Saunders, p. 373.

Virmani, R., Robinowitz, M., Clark, M. A. & McAllister, H. A., Jr (1982). Sudden death and partial absence of the right ventricular myocardium. *Archives of Pathology and Laboratory Medicine*, **106**, 163–7.

Virmani, R., Ursell, P. C. & Fenoglio, J. J. (1987). Examination of the heart. *Human Pathology*, **18**, 432–40.

Viskin, S. & Belhassen, B. (1998). Polymorphic ventricular tachyarrhythmias in the absence of organic heart disease: classification, differential diagnosis, and implications for therapy. *Progress in Cardiovascular Disease*, **41**, 17–34.

Wang, Q., Bowles, N. E. & Towbin, J. A. (1998). The molecular basis of long QT syndrome and prospects for therapy. *Molecular Medicine Today*, **4**, 382–8.

Wang, Q., Curran, M. E., Splawski, I., *et al.* (1996). Positional cloning of a novel potassium channel gene: KVLQT1 mutations cause cardiac arrhythmias. *Nature Genetics*, **12**, 17–23.

Wang, Q., Shen, J., Splawski, I., *et al.* (1995). *SCN5A* mutations associated with an inherited cardiac arrhythmia, long QT syndrome. *Cell*, **80**, 805–11.

Watkins, H., MacRae, C., Thierfelder, L., *et al.* (1993). A disease locus for familial hypertrophic cardiomyopathy maps to chromosome 1q3. *Nature Genetics*, **3**, 333–7.

Watkins, H., Rosenzweig, A., Hwang, D.-S., (1992). Characteristics and prognostic implications of myosin missense mutations in familial hypertrophic cardiomyopathy. *New England Journal of Medicine*, **326**, 1108–14.

Weintraub, R. G., Gow, R. M. & Wilkinson, J. L. (1990). The congenital long QT syndromes in childhood. *Journal of the American College of Cardiology*, **16**, 674–80.

Wiedermann, C. J., Becker, A. E., Hopferwieser, T., Mühlberger, V. & Knapp, E. (1987). Sudden death in a young competitive athlete with Wolff-Parkinson-White syndrome. *European Heart Journal*, **8**, 651–5.

Wilkinson, J. L. (1994). Sudden cardiac death in childhood and adolescence. *Journal of Paediatrics and Child Health*, **30**, 384–5.

Williams, R. B. & Emery, J. L. (1978). Endocardial fibrosis in apparently normal infant hearts. *Histopathology*, **2**, 283–90.

Winkle, R. A., Lopes, M. G., Fitzgerald, J. W., *et al.* (1975). Arrhythmias in patients with mitral valve prolapse. *Circulation*, **52**, 73–81.

Yeager, S. B., Hougen, T. J. & Levy, A. M. (1984). Sudden death in infants with chaotic atrial rhythm. *American Journal of Diseases of Children*, **138**, 689–92.

Yetman, A. T., Hamilton, R. M., Benson, L. N. & McCrindle, B. W. (1998). Long-term outcome and prognostic determinants in children with hypertrophic cardiomyopathy. *Journal of the American College of Cardiology*, **32**, 1943–50.

6

Vascular conditions

Introduction

A number of unique vascular disorders of childhood that may cause sudden death should always be sought assiduously at the time of autopsy, even in the absence of a suggestive clinical history (Byard, 1996a). Disorders may be hereditary or acquired and may be manifest by increased bruising, hemorrhage, or thromboembolic phenomena (Bick, 2001). A list of possible vascular causes of sudden pediatric death can be found in Table 6.1.

Aortic abnormalities

Overview

Obstructive lesions of the left ventricular outflow tract are well-known causes of sudden and unexpected death in children (Anonymous, 1975; Cohle *et al.*, 1988; Doyle *et al.*, 1974; Lambert *et al.*, 1974). Obstruction to the outflow tract may involve the aortic valve or the proximal aorta, with lesions such as supravalvular stenosis and tubular hypoplasia leading to rapid clinical deterioration and death (Byard, 1996a).

Occurrence of sudden death

The frequency of sudden death in one study of 916 patients under 21 years of age with left ventricular outflow obstruction was 1% (Thornback & Fowler, 1975). Sudden death in children with obstructive lesions sometimes may also be associated with a medical procedure such as cardiac catheterization (Noonan, Cottrill & O'Connor, 1982).

Pathophysiology

Sudden death in obstructive aortic disease usually results from a complex series of interactions involving myocardial ischemia and arrhythmias. An increase in myocardial mass without an increase in the number of nutrient vessels results in relative reduction in blood flow, unless a compensatory increase in vessel cross-sectional area occurs (Lewis & Gotsman, 1973). There may also be actual reduction in blood flow due to systolic compression of intramural coronary arteries from the hypertrophied myocardium, or reduction in subendocardial coronary perfusion pressures from increased end-diastolic pressures. Ischemia has been exacerbated in patients with aortic stenosis from reflex bradycardia and peripheral vasodilation, thought to be initiated by left ventricular baroreceptors (Johnson, 1971).

In all types of supravalvular stenosis, the coronary arteries are subjected to elevated systolic pressures that may cause narrowing of the vessels from medial smooth muscle hypertrophy (Edwards, 1965). Significant intimal and medial hyperplasia of the coronary arteries, resulting in luminal narrowing and myocardial infarction, have been reported as early as the second year of life, and atherosclerosis has occurred in later childhood (Edwards, 1965; Neufeld & Blieden,

Table 6.1. Vascular causes of sudden pediatric death

Aortic abnormalities	Coronary artery abnormalities	Venous abnormalities	Vascular malformations	Abnormalities of pulmonary vessels	Miscellaneous vascular abnormalities
Supravalvular stenosis	Idiopathic arterial calcinosis	Total anomalous pulmonary venous drainage	Kasabach–Merritt syndrome	Pulmonary hypertension (primary and secondary)	Arterial dissection/rupture
Coarctation	Anomalous coronary arteries		Diffuse infantile hemangiomatosis	Persistent pulmonary hypertension of the newborn	Arterial fibromuscular dysplasia
William syndrome	Coronary artery aplasia/hypoplasia		Sturge–Weber syndrome		Atherosclerosis
Aortic cystic medial necrosis	Coronary arteritis (Kawasaki disease)		Osler–Weber–Rendu syndrome	Pulmonary veno-occlusive disease	Cerebral sinus thrombosis
Persistent ductus arteriosus					Acquired immunodeficiency syndrome (AIDS)
Vascular rings					Connective tissue disorders
DiGeorge syndrome					Budd-Chiari syndrome
Aortitis					Hypertension
					Embolic phenomena
					Behçet disease

1975; Terhune, Buchino & Rees, 1985). It is likely that these changes either are caused by the same ill-understood factors responsible for the supravalvular stenosis itself (Noonan, Cottrill & O'Connor, 1982) or are exacerbated by the higher-than-normal systolic pressures within the arteries (Neufeld *et al.*, 1962).

Left ventricular hypertrophy on its own, in the absence of mechanical obstruction, may be arrhythmogenic due to lowering of the electrical threshold and increase in the irritability of individual hypertrophic myocytes (Myerburg, Kessler & Castellanos, 1992). All of these factors may combine to produce precipitate clinical deterioration, sometimes in children who were thought to be completely well prior to their sudden death.

Supravalvular stenosis

Etiology
Congenital supravalvular aortic stenosis has an incidence of one in 20,000 births with an autosomal dominant inheritance linked to mutation or loss of the elastin gene on chromosome 7q11.23 (Stamm *et al.*, 2001; Towbin, Casey & Belmont, 1999).

Pathological features
There are several different anatomical subtypes, including a membranous form, in which a discrete fibrous membrane is found distal to the coronary artery ostia, and an "hourglass" form, in which thickening of the aortic media with intimal proliferation results in luminal narrowing distal to the aortic valve (Morrow *et al.*, 1959; Neufeld *et al.*, 1962; Peterson, Todd & Edwards, 1965). In either type of supravalvular stenosis, the aorta distal to the obstruction may be dilated due to a Venturi effect on blood flow (Cohle *et al.*, 1988). The final type of supravalvular aortic obstruction is represented by tubular hypoplasia (Neufeld *et al.*, 1962), in which there is segmental uniform narrowing of the aortic isthmus without distal dilation (Logan *et al.*, 1965) (Figure 6.1).

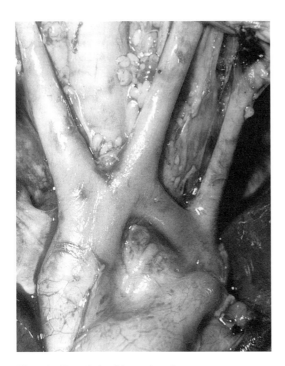

Figure 6.1 Hypoplasia of the aortic arch.

Histologically, there is disorganization of elastic and smooth muscle fibers of the media in all of the above entities, with smooth muscle hypertrophy, intimal proliferation, and loss of glycosaminoglycans. In the membranous form, the constriction occasionally may be composed of loose fibroconnective tissue without medial tissue (O'Connor *et al.*, 1985). Accelerated coronary artery atherosclerosis may occur, resulting in myocardial infarction at an early age (Neufeld & Blieden, 1975).

Associated features
Supravalvular stenosis may be isolated or associated with other congenital vascular defects, such as aortic coarctation, aortic and pulmonary valve dysplasia, fusion of the coronary cusps to the aortic ridge, mitral valve prolapse, aortic arch branch stenoses, and proximal and peripheral pulmonary artery stenoses (Becker, Becker & Edwards, 1972; Sun, Jacot & Brenner, 1992). It may also be associated with Marfan syndrome (Peterson, Todd &

Edwards, 1965), form part of William syndrome (Logan *et al.*, 1965) (*vide infra*), or be inherited as an autosomal dominant trait with variable penetrance (Cohle *et al.*, 1988). There is an association with both congenital rubella syndrome and generalized arterial fibromuscular dysplasia (Schmidt *et al.*, 1969). The genetic aspects of this condition emphasize the need for accurate identification at autopsy so that appropriate family investigation and counselling can be undertaken.

Coarctation

Coarctation of the aorta consists of a well-defined narrowing or "shelf-like" constriction. Although it may be present at any point along the aorta, the usual site is adjacent to the ductus arteriosus or ligamentum arteriosum (Figure 6.2) (Rosenberg, 1973). An association with bicuspid aortic valve and cystic medial necrosis suggests that it may sometimes represent one element of a more generalized connective tissue defect (Lindsay, 1988). Familial occurrence of coarctation of the abdominal aorta may also occur (Hallidie-Smith & Olsen, 1968).

Although the ridge of medial tissue in coarctation is often continuous with the ductus and may appear to be composed of similar tissue, the ductus is usually readily distinguishable histologically (Ho & Anderson, 1979).

Pathophysiology
Coarctation has caused rapid clinical deterioration and death from cardiac decompensation even in very early infancy (Bahn, Edwards & DuShane, 1951). Aortic rupture, with and without superadded infection, has also been documented in childhood (Nikaidoh, Idriss & Riker, 1973). Death may be caused occasionally by associated intracranial aneurysm rupture (Reifenstein, Levine & Gross, 1947; Shearer *et al.*, 1970) or may follow surgical repair.

Associated features
When the ductus is patent, there may be a range of outlet obstructions present, such as tubular hypoplasia, and a variety of associated congenital cardiac

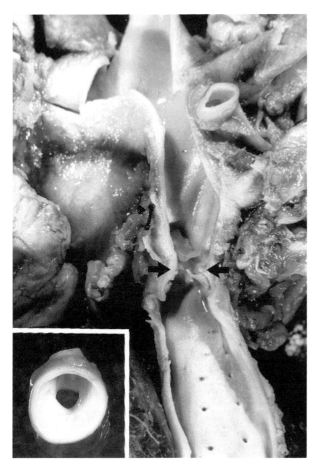

Figure 6.2 Discrete area of narrowing in aortic coarctation (arrows). Inset demonstrates marked luminal stenosis in a surgically resected specimen.

lesions, such as transposition of the great vessels. If the anomaly occurs with a closed ductus, then there is an increased association with bicuspid aortic valve (Becker & Anderson, 1981).

William syndrome

Clinical features

William syndrome is an autosomal dominant condition characterized by mental and physical retardation with supravalvular aortic stenosis, peripheral pulmonary arterial stenoses, dental abnormalities, elfin facies, infantile hypercalcemia, and a predisposition to sudden and unexpected death. While the mechanism of sudden death is not always obvious, it may result from aortic outflow obstruction, associated coronary artery stenoses, or acute myocardial ischemia (Noonan, Cottrill & O'Connor, 1982; Terhune, Buchino & Rees, 1985).

Due to the variability in clinical presentations of William syndrome (Jones & Smith, 1975; White *et al.*, 1977), there is confusion in early reports regarding the relationship between supravalvular aortic stenosis and idiopathic infantile hypercalcemia (Fanconi *et al.*, 1952; Sissman *et al.*, 1959). However, it now appears that both represent different manifestations of the same syndrome (Beuren, 1972), with hypercalcemia occurring before cardiovascular anomalies are detected (Martin & Moseley, 1973). Thus, although sporadic and familial supravalvular aortic stenosis may still occur in isolation (O'Connor *et al.*, 1985), the stigmata of William syndrome should always be looked for carefully at autopsy before this possibility is accepted. A history of irritability and vomiting may be a clue to the presence of antemortem hypercalcemia in an affected infant (Folger, 1977).

Etiology

Although it was suggested historically that William syndrome was related to exposure to excessive amounts of vitamin D, an in-born error of vitamin D metabolism, or *in utero* rubella exposure (Fellers & Schwartz, 1958; Friedman & Roberts, 1966; Varghese, Izukawa & Rowe, 1969), it is now known that William syndrome is due to mutation or deletion of the elastin gene on chromosome 7q11.23 (Donnai & Karmiloff-Smith, 2000; Morris & Mervis, 2000; Strauss & Johnson, 1996).

Pathological features

Typical microscopic changes in the aorta are disorganization of the media with randomly arranged thickened elastic fibers (Figure 6.3), hypertrophic smooth muscle cells, and increased collagen deposition with fibrous thickening of the intima (O'Connor *et al.*,

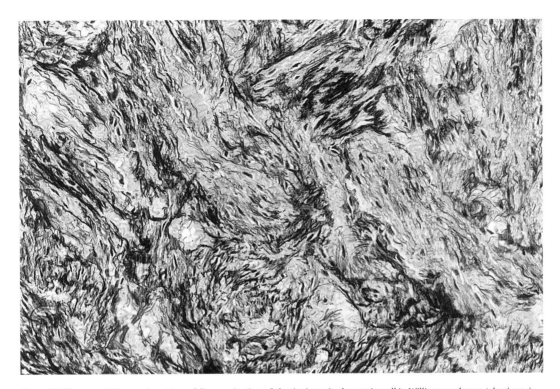

Figure 6.3 Characteristic mosaic pattern of disorganization of elastic tissue in the aortic wall in William syndrome (elastin stain, ×150).

1985). Stenosis of the coronary arteries occurs either as part of the syndrome complex or secondary to elevated arterial pressures proximal to the aortic obstruction (Neufeld *et al.*, 1962).

Associated features

Other cardiovascular anomalies described in patients with William syndrome include atrial and ventricular septal defects, tetralogy of Fallot, aortic coarctation, aortic hypoplasia, tortuosity of the coronary arteries, mitral valve prolapse, and bicuspid aortic valve (Folger, 1977; Hallidie-Smith & Karas, 1988; Maisuls, Alday & Thüer, 1987). Systemic hypertension is a common complication (Morris *et al.*, 1988). Children with William syndrome are also at increased risk of sudden death following cardiac catheterization (Conway *et al.*, 1990).

Aortic cystic medial necrosis

Although cystic medial necrosis is characteristic of Marfan syndrome, sudden death from aortic dissection associated with cystic medial necrosis may occur in non-Marfanoid children (Nicod *et al.*, 1989). However, while familial cases occur, with inheritance in some instances being autosomal dominant, the term is primarily descriptive and does not generally refer to a specific disease entity (Fann, Dalman & Harris, 1993; Hanley & Jones, 1967; Toyama, Amano & Kameda, 1989). Further details of cystic medial necrosis and Marfan syndrome may be found in Chapter 12.

Persistent ductus arteriosus

Children with uncorrected persistent ductus arteriosus have a higher mortality rate than age-matched controls due to infective endocarditis and cardiac failure. The occurrence of sudden death is, however, not well documented in the literature. Nevertheless, this is a possibility if left ventricular hypertrophy, endocarditis, or pulmonary hypertension develops (Campbell, 1968).

Vascular rings

Vascular rings occur when an anomalous vessel encircles and compresses the esophagus and trachea (Hewitt, Brewer & Drapanas, 1970).

Clinical features

As a large number of anatomical variations are possible with vascular rings, a spectrum of clinical presentations occurs. This ranges from an incidental finding with no symptoms or signs, to acute respiratory obstruction (Lincoln *et al.*, 1969) with the possibility of death (Filston, Ferguson & Oldham, 1987). Most symptomatic patients present early in life with stridor, cyanotic episodes, respiratory and feeding difficulties, recurrent respiratory infections, or failure to thrive (Smith *et al.*, 1984). Acute episodes in which death occurs are rare, and some infants become less symptomatic over time without intervention.

Pathological features

The most common vascular anomalies that form rings around the trachea and esophagus are double aortic arch and right-sided aortic arch with a left-sided ligamentum arteriosum (Backer *et al.*, 1989). Other anomalies include retro-esophageal aortic arch, retro-esophageal left and right subclavian arteries (Figure 6.4), anomalous subclavian arteries passing anterior to the trachea, anomalous innominate artery origin, and pulmonary vascular ring (Fearon & Shortreed, 1963; Strife, Baumel & Dunbar, 1981).

Pathophysiology

Most vascular rings are not associated with sudden and unexpected death, and even where death has occurred from airway obstruction it is seldom sudden. When there is sudden death, the mechanisms

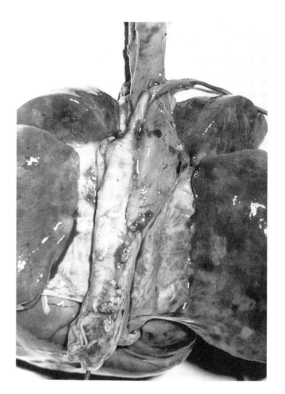

Figure 6.4 Compression of the esophagus by a retro-esophageal right subclavian artery (containing a probe).

are variable and include reflex apnea and respiratory arrest, for example, in infants with an innominate artery origin that is more distal than usual (Lima *et al.*, 1983; Mustard *et al.*, 1969). Airway blockage may also occur when a bolus of food within the esophagus compresses the membranous part of the trachea (Backer *et al.*, 1989); the trachea is prevented from moving anteriorly by the unusual position of the aberrant vessel, resulting in obstructive symptoms (Binet & Langlois, 1977). Rarely, airway obstruction can occur from a persistent truncus arteriosus due to compression of the bronchi between the aortic arch and pulmonary artery (Habbema, Losekoot & Becker, 1980).

Associated features

Other anomalies that may be present with vascular rings, such as bronchomalacia and congenital long-segment tracheal stenosis, may also predispose an infant to airway obstruction (Berdon *et al.*, 1984; Koopot, Nikaidoh & Idriss, 1975). Careful examination of the trachea should, therefore, always be performed, as this may reveal hypoplasia with complete cartilagenous rings or absent pars membranacea (Hickey & Wood, 1987). Given the spectrum of abnormalities that may be present at autopsy, each case should be assessed thoroughly before death is attributed to a vascular ring.

DiGeorge syndrome

DiGeorge syndrome refers to a complex congenital malformation of tissues derived from the third and fourth pharyngeal pouches. Specific features are thymic and parathyroid aplasia or hypoplasia, with 95% of cases demonstrating conotruncal cardiac defects, with anomalies of the aortic arch, truncus arteriosus, or tetralogy of Fallot (Cuneo, 2001; Levy-Mozziconacci *et al.*, 1994). Some authors reserve the term "DiGeorge syndrome" for cases in which there is complete absence of the thymus, referring to other complex malformations of the third, fourth, and fifth aortic arches as partial DiGeorge or III–IV pharyngeal pouch syndromes (Lischner, 1972). Given the possibility that small ectopic thymic rests may not be found during autopsy dissection, this separation may be of more theoretical than practical significance.

Clinical features

The spectrum of clinical presentations in infancy is wide, ranging from neonatal hypocalcemia to cardiac failure. Affected children have characteristic dysmorphic facies, with low-set ears, short philtrum, hypertelorism, micrognathia, and retrognathia (Moerman *et al.*, 1980). Older infants and children manifest infective problems due to defective thymus-dependent cell-mediated immunity (Conley *et al.*, 1979).

Rarely, the condition causes sudden death, as in a 2.5-week-old girl who exhibited no external dysmorphic features and whose only clinical abnormality was a loud systolic murmur. She was found unexpectedly dead in bed before formal cardiological review could be undertaken. The diagnosis of DiGeorge syndrome was made at autopsy, when thymic hypoplasia was observed in association with persistence of the right ductus arteriosus, an anomalous origin and course of the right subclavian artery, and absence of the parathyroid glands.

Etiology

The genetic basis for DiGeorge syndrome is microdeletion of chromosome 22q11.2, which can be inherited autosomal dominantly or can arise as a de novo translocation or deletion (Cuneo, 2001; Lammer & Opitz, 1986; Sullivan, 2001; Wilson *et al.*, 1992). Other associated chromosomal abnormalities include 10p13, 10p14, and 17p13 deletions (Punnett & Zakai, 1990). Microdeletion of chromosome 22q11.2 is also found in the majority of patients with velocardiofacial or Shprintzen syndrome and conotruncal anomaly face syndrome, suggesting an overlap between these conditions (Cuneo, 2001; Scambler *et al.*, 1992; Shprintzen *et al.*, 1981). It is likely that the ubiquitin-fusion-degradation-1-like gene is involved in the pathogenesis of these syndromes, given its expression in both embryonic branchial arch tissues and the conotruncus (Cuneo, 2001).

While it has been proposed that conotruncal anomalies may initiate vascular compromise of the left fourth aortic arch and its dependent tissues, this is unconfirmed (Robinson, 1975). Other authors have suggested that there may be defective migration of, or injury to, neural crest tissue in early embryonic life (Bockman & Kirby, 1984; Kirby & Bockman, 1984), supported by the demonstration of thyroid C-cell deficiency in affected patients (Burke *et al.*, 1987). An unconfirmed relationship with fetal alcohol syndrome has also been proposed, based on the overlap of morphologic features (Ammann *et al.*, 1982).

Pathological features

At autopsy, the neck and anterior mediastinal structures must be carefully dissected, as both thymus and parathyroid glands may be situated ectopically. Soft tissues of the neck from the thoracic inlet to above the inlet of the larynx may need to be blocked in toto if glandular aplasia is to be confirmed histologically.

The most common cardiovascular anomalies include aortic arch abnormalities, such as a right-sided arch with an anomalous subclavian artery, and conotruncal abnormalities, such as truncus arteriosus or tetralogy of Fallot (Freedom, Rosen & Nadas, 1972). As other anomalies such as choanal atresia (Dische, 1968) have been reported, careful examination of the upper aerodigestive tract is required. An important aspect in correctly establishing or confirming the diagnosis at autopsy is the heritable nature of some cases (Driscoll, Budarf & Emanuel, 1992).

Aortitis

Inflammation of the aorta in children may be due to microbiological infection, to Takayasu aortitis, or to familial granulomatous aortitis.

Bacterial aortitis
Bacterial aortitis may be associated with a congenital malformation, such as coarctation, and may cause sudden death due to weakening of the vessel wall with rupture.

Takayasu arteritis
Takayasu arteritis (aortitis syndrome) is an inflammatory condition of uncertain etiology that affects the aorta, proximal portions of its major branches, the pulmonary artery, and rarely the coronary arteries (Cohle, Graham & Pounder, 1986; Haas & Stiehm, 1986; Hall *et al.*, 1985). The syndrome involves mainly young women, but it may also be found in childhood (Ishikawa, 1981; Lee *et al.*, 1967; Sánchez-Torres *et al.*, 1983), where a characteristic granulomatous arteritis can be demonstrated within the walls of involved arteries. The youngest patient in the series of Lupi-Herrera and colleagues (1977) was four years of age.

Although the inflammatory response generally resolves without sequelae, sudden and unexpected death has been described occasionally in adult patients due to arterial rupture, dissection, and cerebral embolism (Ishikawa, 1978; Lie, 1987b; Subramanyan, Joy & Balakrishnan, 1989). Stroke is a complication that may occur in infants. Resultant ostial stenosis is also a potential cause of sudden death in children (Seguchi *et al.*, 1990).

Familial granulomatous arteritis
A familial granulomatous arteritis involving both the aorta and coronary arteries has been reported associated with polyarthritis, hypertension (Rotenstein *et al.*, 1982), and sudden death during early childhood (Di Liberti, 1982). An apparently sporadic giant cell arteritis with aneurysm formation may also occur in children (Wagenvoort *et al.*, 1963).

Coronary artery abnormalities

Idiopathic arterial calcinosis

Idiopathic arterial calcinosis is a rare entity characterized by widespread intimal hyperplasia with calcium deposition along the internal elastic lamina and media of arteries throughout the body, usually excluding the central nervous system (Byard, 1996b; Lipman, Rosenthal & Lowenberg, 1951; Moran & Steiner, 1962; Van Dyck *et al.*, 1989). Although it is a generalized condition, the lethal consequences result from coronary artery occlusion.

Clinical features
Presenting symptoms and signs are extremely variable, reflecting the widespread distribution of arterial lesions. Infants may present dead on arrival with no preceeding history, or they may have relatively non-specific histories of respiratory distress, vomiting, diarrhea, irritability, anorexia, listlessness, or fever (Hunt & Leys, 1957; Hussain *et al.*, 1991; Meurman, Somersalo & Tuuteri, 1965; Paine & Grafton, 1970). Intestinal obstruction and subarachnoid hemorrhage have both been described.

Previous clinical examinations may have documented signs of congestive cardiac failure with tachycardia, cyanosis, and lethargy, hypertension, or signs of apparent respiratory infection (Milner *et al.*, 1984). These may lead to mistaken diagnoses of myocarditis or pneumonia. As cases are often not identified before death, the onus may be on the pathologist to establish the diagnosis correctly.

In a review of 62 cases of idiopathic arterial calcification, Moran (1975) noted that 85% of patients died under six months of age, and that death generally occurred between the ages of three days and 28 months. Rare patients have survived into adult life (Marrott *et al.*, 1984), and spontaneous regression of the calcification has been documented (Sholler *et al.*, 1984). The male-to-female ratio in Moran's review was 1:1, with Caucasian infants forming the majority of cases.

Etiology

The etiology of the changes in idiopathic arterial calcinosis is not known, although an autosomal recessive mode of inheritance is considered likely (Carles *et al.*, 1992; Juul *et al.*, 1990; Meradji *et al.*, 1978; Moran & Becker, 1959). While an identical pattern of arterial calcification may be found in patients with hypercalcemia from chronic renal failure, hyperparathyroidism, or hypervitaminosis D, no metabolic abnormalities have been detected in infants with idiopathic arterial calcinosis. Specifically, renal function is not deranged, and lipid, amino acid, and mucopolysaccharide metabolism are not defective; serum calcium, phosphate, and electrolyte levels are all within the normal ranges (Juul *et al.*, 1990).

Similar arterial calcification has also been documented in infants with congenital heart defects, presumably secondary to abnormal hemodynamics or ischemia and degeneration of elastin fibers. Thus, it is important to exclude local structural abnormalities before labeling arterial calcification as idiopathic.

The role of elastin fibers in the pathogenesis of the calcification is uncertain, with suggestions made that elastin fibers are unusually sensitive to toxic insult in predisposed infants (Bird, 1974). This contrasts with assertions that calcification occurs primarily in the media of involved arteries and is resisted by the adjacent elastica interna, which prevents the intima becoming similarly calcified (Gower & Pinkerton, 1963). As noted by Morton (1978), other authors have suggested that the primary event is intimal thickening and that changes in elastin fibers represent a secondary phenomenon. It is also possible that several mechanisms may cause a similar morphological outcome.

Radiological features

Radiological examination shows calcification of larger elastic arteries, such as the thoracic and abdominal aorta, carotid, axillary, and femoral arteries (Parker, Smith & Stoneman, 1971), as well as smaller muscular arteries in the hands and feet (Moran & Erickson, 1974). An unusual pattern of periarticular stippled calcification has been noted (Maayan *et al.*, 1984; Moran & Erickson, 1974), similar to that seen in chondrodysplasia punctata. However, the latter disorder is quite different from idiopathic arterial calcinosis, being characterized by dysmorphic features and shortened long bones, with no evidence of arterial calification (Tasker, Mastri & Gold, 1970). Postmortem radiological examination of tissues may provide a clearer definition of the pattern of vascular calcification than is possible during life.

Pathological features

Vascular changes usually affect large elastic to smaller muscular arteries in all organs, except the brain and spinal cord. Visceral changes observed at autopsy are often limited to the heart, which may show left or biventricular enlargement, endocardial fibroelastosis, thickened coronary arteries, and evidence of recent infarction (Byard, 1996b; Thomas *et al.*, 1956; Weens & Marin, 1956). The aorta may feel slightly firmer than usual, or it may show no gross abnormalities. Parathyroid glands are normal in size.

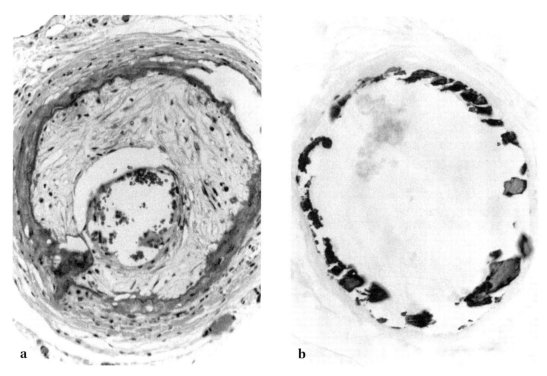

Figure 6.5 Cross-section of small arteries, showing fibrointimal proliferation and medial calcification in idiopathic arterial calcification (a, hematoxylin and eosin, ×110; B, Von Kossa, ×110).

Involved arteries show microscopic calcification and fragmentation of the internal elastic lamina, with mild to marked fibrointimal hyperplasia (Menten & Fetterman, 1948; Stryker, 1946) (Figures 6.5–6.7). The lesions stain positively with Alazarin red, von Kossa, and Perls stains, indicating the presence of calcium, phosphate, and iron. They do not contain lipid and thus they are readily distinguishable from atherosclerotic plaques. They also differ from the diffuse medial calcific lesions found in older patients with Monckeberg medial calcific sclerosis (Cochrane & Bowden, 1954). Similar changes of uncertain significance have been described within both the iliac arteries and the carotid siphon of normal infants in the absence of calcification elsewhere (Meyer & Lind, 1972a; Meyer & Lind, 1972b).

Inflammation is not generally a feature of idiopathic arterial calcification in infancy, although a focal foreign-body giant-cell reaction may develop around mineralized aggregates (Bird, 1974). However, the presence of an occasional aggregate of adventitial or subintimal lymphocytes and neutrophils suggests the possibility of an inflammatory etiology in some cases (Anderson *et al.*, 1985; Paine & Grafton, 1970). Involved arteries may be occluded by thrombi.

The myocardium shows a range of pathological changes with variable degrees of hypertrophy and interstitial fibrosis (Figure 6.8), reflecting chronic ischemic damage. There may be evidence of more recent ischemia in the form of acute myocardial infarction with focal myocyte necrosis (Traisman, Limperis & Traisman, 1956). Occasionally, dystrophic calcification will be found within the myocardium along with prominent subendocardial fibrosis.

Although arteries supplying a number of other organs, such as the lungs, kidneys, adrenal glands, pancreas, and thyroid gland, may be affected, these organs do not usually demonstrate ischemic changes.

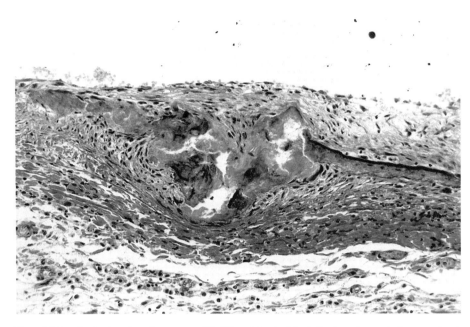

Figure 6.6 Longitudinal section of an artery wall in idiopathic arterial calcification, demonstrating prominent focal calcification (hematoxylin and eosin, ×110).

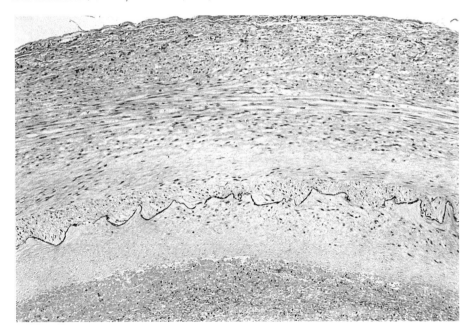

Figure 6.7 Fine calcification of the internal elastic lamina of the aorta with fibrointimal proliferation in a two-week-old girl with idiopathic arterial calcification (Von Kossa, ×60).

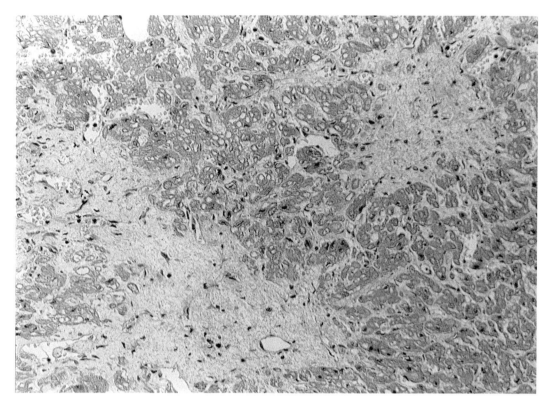

Figure 6.8 Fibrous scarring of the wall of the left ventricle in a three-month-old boy with idiopathic arterial calcification and resultant coronary artery narrowing (hematoxylin and eosin, ×160).

Pulmonary hypertensive changes with right heart failure may occur secondary to obliteration of the pulmonary vasculature (Morton, 1978). The kidneys may show focal glomerular calcification (Hunt & Leys, 1957), but no bone lesions have been described and there is no evidence of visceral calcification of the type seen in hypercalcemic disorders. There is also no evidence of abnormal storage of lipid or mucopolysaccharide.

Differential diagnosis

The arteriopathy decribed in children with AIDS is characterized by similar calcific lesions. However, variations in the clinical presentation enable separation of the two entities (Joshi *et al.*, 1987). Aneurysms and a different pattern of vascular obliteration are present in lesions of Kawasaki disease.

Anomalous coronary arteries

Normal anatomy

The normal heart is supplied by two extramural muscular coronary arteries that arise from ostia within the left and right sinuses of Valsalva. The right coronary artery runs in a subepicardial location along the sulcus between the right atrium and ventricle. The left coronary artery divides into the circumflex artery, which courses between the left atrium and ventricle, and the left anterior descending artery, which descends in the anterior interventricular groove.

Considerable normal variation in this pattern occurs; for example, in 50% of individuals, the first branch of the right coronary artery arises separately from the right sinus of Valsalva as the conus artery (Lauridson, 1988). Three major patterns of arterial distribution are recognized. In type I (77% of cases), the posterior descending artery arises from the right coronary artery; in type II (8%), it arises from the circumflex branch of the left coronary artery; and in type III (15%), two posterior descending arteries are present, arising from each of the major coronary arteries (Baroldi, 1991).

Anomalous anatomy

Coronary arteries are regarded as anomalous if they arise from an unusual site in the aorta, such as the opposite sinus of Valsalva, the ascending portion of the aortic arch, the opposite coronary artery, or from the pulmonary trunk (Table 6.2) (Figure 6.9). Variable courses may result, with arteries running behind the aorta, between the aorta and pulmonary trunk, within the myocardium of the crista supraventricularis and ventricular septum, or anterior to the pulmonary trunk (Angelini, 1989; Byard, 1996a). Sudden and unexpected death has been described in children with each of these anomalies.

Frequency

The occurrence of anomalous coronary arteries varies in different studies and age groups. While Hobbs and colleagues (1981) found that 1.55% of patients undergoing angiography at the Cleveland Clinic Foundation had aberrant coronary arteries, Samanek, Goetzova & Benesova (1985) found only 0.6% of children in an autopsy series with similar

Table 6.2. Classification of coronary artery anomalies

Anomalous origin from aorta
  Anomalous origin and course
  High origin
Anomalous origin from pulmonary artery
Anomalous origin from other vessels
Aplasia/hypoplasia
Fistula
Aneurysm
Vascular malformation
Bridging
Intussusception
Vasospasm

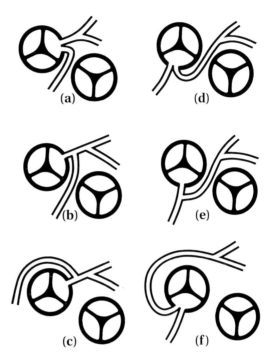

Figure 6.9 Patterns of anomalous coronary arteries arising from the aorta: (a–c) aberrant right coronary arteries; (d–f) aberrant left coronary arteries.

anomalies. This compares with a study of sudden unexpected cardiac death under 21 years of age, where 50% of the 20 infants and 24% of the 50 older individuals had anomalous coronary arteries (Steinberger *et al.*, 1996).

Associated features

Aberrant coronary arteries may be associated with other congenital heart defects, such as bicuspid aortic valve, mitral valve prolapse, tetralogy of Fallot, and transposition of the great vessels (Topaz *et al.*, 1992; Werner *et al.*, 2001). In these cases, the anomalous coronary arteries may have been diagnosed prior to autopsy, given the extensive cardiological work-up that occurs in such children. On the other hand, anomalous coronary arteries in isolation may be clinically occult until the patient suffers sudden death (McClellan & Jokl, 1968). Sudden death was found in 45% of cases in an autopsy series of

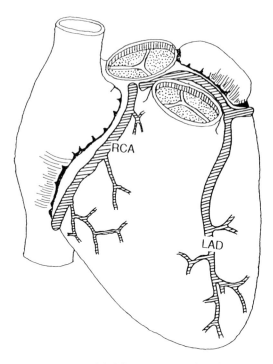

Figure 6.10 Origin of the left coronary artery from the right sinus of Valsalva, with a course between the great vessels. (RCA, right coronary artery; LAD, left anterior descending artery.)

35 infants and children with congenital coronary anomalies (Lipsett *et al.*, 1994).

Anomalous origin from the aorta

There are many variations in the patterns of distribution of anomalous coronary arteries that arise from the aorta involving both left and right coronary arterial systems (Figures 6.10 and 6.11). While the majority of anomalous arteries arise from either the left or right sinuses of Valsalva, in occasional cases the anomalous artery may arise from the posterior non-coronary sinus. These, too, may be associated with sudden and unexpected death in childhood (Ishikawa, Otsuka & Suzuki, 1990).

Frequency

The specific frequency of anomalous coronary arteries with an aortic origin is difficult to determine in children, as most large angiographic studies have

been performed in symptomatic adults. Kimbiris and colleagues (1978) studied 7000 symptomatic patients and found that 0.64% had an anomalous aortic coronary artery origin, the most common being an anomalous circumflex artery. Other studies have shown a range of 0.6–0.83% (Chaitman *et al.*, 1976; Liberthson *et al.*, 1974). Depending on the series and whether the circumflex artery is included, right coronary artery anomalies have been equal in frequency to (Liberthson, Dinsmore & Fallon, 1979), more common than (Hobbs *et al.*, 1981; Kimbiris *et al.*, 1978; Topaz *et al.*, 1992), or less common than (Engel, Torres & Page, 1975) left coronary anomalies. All of these reviews were based on angiographic data, except for the study of Liberthson, Dinsmore & Fallon (1979), which combined angiographic and autopsy data.

In a retrospective pediatric autopsy study, Lipsett and colleagues (1991) described three cases of

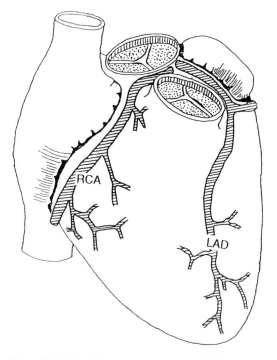

Figure 6.11 Origin of the right coronary artery (RCA) from the left sinus of Valsalva. (LAD, left anterior descending artery.)

sudden and unexpected death in infants and young children under two years of age, with anomalous coronary arteries, out of a total autopsy population of 812 (giving a frequency of 0.4%). However, as the authors point out, this rate may be falsely low due to variable interpretation of the significance of anomalous vessels and to the possibility that not every anomaly was documented.

Pathological features

At autopsy, the coronary arteries should be examined for anomalies in any infant or child who has died suddenly. This should include careful tracing of the epicardial courses of the vessels, ideally with coronary angiography if an anomaly is detected (Virmani, Ursell & Fenoglio, 1987). Examination of the sinuses alone may lead to some confusion, as an artery may be thought to be absent merely because the aortic valve has been opened through an ostium, or if an ostium is off centre, "hidden" by the point of attachment of the valve cusp. Opening the aortic valve between cusps and carefully inspecting the sinuses and epicardial courses of the arteries should prevent this error.

Particular abnormalities that may be overlooked in patients with normally sited ostia are ostial stenoses and acute angles of arterial take-off. When an anomalous artery has been identified, the presence of ostial hypoplasia and luminal ridges should be assessed. The vessel should then be dissected from the epicardial fat, and its course plotted accurately, although this may be technically difficult in very young infants. Cross-sectioning of the vessel and major branches at 2–3-mm intervals will provide important information about possible occlusive lesions and relative vessel caliber (Byard, Smith & Bourne, 1991).

The extent of histologic changes found at autopsy will be influenced to some degree by the nature of the aberrant vessel. Whereas chronic ischemia may be tolerated in a small area of myocardium supplied by an anomalous minor artery, a lesser degree of compromise in a more significant vessel may result in sudden death. This produces the histologic paradox that a less significant coronary artery anomaly may

show chronic ischemic change with fibrous scarring, whereas the pathophysiologically more important coronary artery anomaly may have only minimal histologic findings. Given the time that it takes for microscopically detectable ischemic myocardial damage to develop, it is perhaps not surprising that children dying rapidly often have hearts that are apparently normal histologically. Nevertheless, contraction band necrosis does develop rapidly, and its presence in the myocardium supplied by an anomalous vessel may be significant. In addition, lethal arrhythmias may develop in the absence of permanent ischemic damage.

A major problem may also exist in trying to determine whether an aberrant coronary artery was the cause of sudden death or was merely a coincidental finding entirely unrelated to the terminal episode. Occasionally in the older child, there may be a history that is suggestive of angina or an arrhythmia, but this cannot always be relied upon. Similarly, not all patients will have evidence of acute or chronic myocardial damage (Figure 6.12). In these cases, the cause of death may remain conjectural, although the demonstration of a congenital vascular abnormality that is associated with an increased risk of sudden

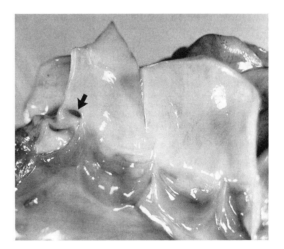

Figure 6.12 Right coronary artery ostium (arrow) situated above the left coronary ostium in the left sinus of Valsalva in a three-month-old boy found dead in bed. Microscopically, there was no evidence of myocardial ischemia.

death at all stages of childhood (and even in utero) (Muus & McManus, 1984), in the absence of other findings at autopsy, must place it at the top of the list of possibilities. It is likely in such cases that lethal arrhythmias have occurred in the absence of detectable ischemic damage.

Occurrence of sudden death

As noted above, the likelihood of sudden death depends to a certain extent on the amount of myocardium supplied by the anomalous artery. For example, the effects of occluding an artery that supplies a large muscle mass are far more profound than occlusion of a minor branch. Liberthson (1989) noted chest pain or sudden death in at least 75% of adults with aberrant left main coronary arteries, compared with less than 25% of cases of anomalous right coronary arteries in which ventricular fibrillation or sudden death occurred.

It was originally considered that only anomalous coronary arteries arising from the pulmonary trunk (Ogden, 1970), or left coronary arteries running between the aortic and pulmonary trunks, were of clinical importance (Benson & Lack, 1968); i.e. anomalous right coronary arteries were thought to be relatively harmless. However, reports have subsequently demonstrated myocardial infarction and sudden death in victims at all ages with aberrant right coronary arteries (Barth, Bray & Roberts, 1986; Benge, Martins and Funk, 1980; Byard, 1996a; Liberthson, Gang & Custer, 1983; McManus *et al.*, 1990; Ness & McManus, 1988).

The frequency of sudden death in two series of adults with coronary anomalies was 18% (9/51) and 30% (3/10), respectively (Cheitlin, DeCastro & McAllister, 1974; Roberts, Siegel & Zipes, 1982).

While infants with coronary artery anomalies who have died suddenly may have minimal or nonspecific symptoms and signs (Byard *et al.*, 1991c; Herrmann, Dousa & Edwards, 1992; Lipsett *et al.*, 1991), this is not always the case, and careful review of the presenting history may reveal significant features. For example, children may develop preterminal chest pain if they have myocardial ischemia (Cohen & Shaw, 1967). Liberthson (1989) has described a nine-month-old infant with an aberrant right coronary artery who, on waking, "screamed, clutched his chest, and became limp." Histologic evidence of acute myocardial ischemia was subsequently demonstrated. It is interesting to note that both this infant and two from the series of Lipsett and colleagues (1991) died in the absence of exertion, during or soon after sleep. This suggests that young children with this anomaly may become compromised without exerting themselves excessively, and that a history of exercise is not, therefore, necessary to support this as a cause of death in early childhood.

While an anomalous left anterior descending coronary artery has also been regarded as a benign phenomenon in the past, sudden death has occurred, and children with this anomaly have developed symptoms (Liberthson, 1989).

Pathophysiology

The pathological effects of aberrant coronary arteries arising from the aorta derive from reduction in blood flow causing myocardial ischemia, arrhythmia, and sudden death (Lipsett, *et al.*, 1991).

Reduction in blood flow through an abnormally placed vessel is caused by a variety of mechanisms (Table 6.3). The ostium and initial portion of the artery may be stenotic (Jokl *et al.*, 1966) and are often slit-like when there is a tangential take-off (Mahowald *et al.*, 1986). Virmani and colleagues (1984a) have estimated that the critical angle between the aorta and the proximal portion of an aberrant artery is 45 degrees. They also noted that a

Table 6.3. Factors associated with reduced blood flow in aberrant coronary arteries

Ostial stenosis
Ostial ridges
Acute angle of arterial take-off
Arterial hypoplasia
External compression
Intra-arterial compression
Intramyocardial compression
Intrinsic obliterative lesions

normally situated coronary artery may also have an acute angle of take-off and that this too may have an association with sudden death. This may be an important factor in coronary ostia that are found above the valve sinuses.

Further narrowing of the ostia may occur during exercise as the aortic root dilates and undergoes torsion (Barth & Roberts, 1986), with the unusual ostial shape and tangential vessel angle interfering with blood flow during diastole. Arteries that run posteriorly around the aorta may also be narrowed due to stretching (Figures 6.13 and 6.14).

Membranous occlusion of a coronary ostium may occur with aortic valvular stenosis (Josa *et al.*, 1981), and a 16-year-old boy has been reported who died following obstruction of the left coronary ostium by an anomalous cusp of a quadricuspid aortic valve (Kurosawa, Wagenaar & Becker, 1981).

Virmani and colleagues (1984a) discuss the significance of ridges within the ostia that function as valves and cause occlusion of the arterial lumen as the aortic root dilates. These "valve-like" ridges were regarded as a contributor to sudden death if they occupied more than half of the ostial area.

The role of compression of an aberrant coronary artery between the aortic and pulmonary roots has been debated as a causal factor in reducing blood supply. While some authors point out that normal coronary artery pressure is greater than pulmonary pressure, thus preventing coronary arterial collapse (Baltaxe & Wixson, 1977), this does not take into account the possibility of reduced pressures in the abnormal vessel from ostial stenoses or valve-like ridges. Compression of an abnormal vessel may also occur if the vessel has an oblique course through the wall of the aorta or, less commonly, through the conal or interventricular septum (Cheitlin, De Castro & McAllister, 1974; Liberthson, 1989).

Aberrant coronary arteries may develop atherosclerosis prematurely, leading to luminal stenosis, with further reduction in blood flow and increasing myocardial hypoxia. For example, a 17-year-old boy has been reported with focal obstructive atherosclerosis in an aberrant coronary at the point where it passed between the aorta and

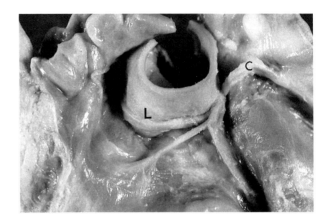

Figure 6.13 External view demonstrating an acute angle of take-off of an aberrant left coronary artery (L), with attenuation as it passes behind the aorta. A separate conus artery (C) was also present.

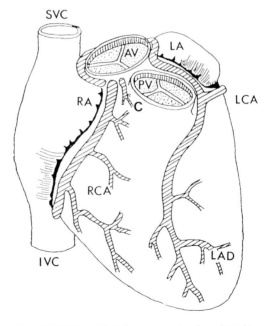

Figure 6.14 Origin of the left coronary artery from the right sinus of Valsalva with a course behind the aorta. (RA, right atrium; LA, left atrium; AV, aortic valve; PV, pulmonary valve; RCA, right coronary artery; LCA, left coronary artery; LAD, left anterior descending artery; C, conus artery; SVC, superior vena cava; IVC, inferior vena cava.)

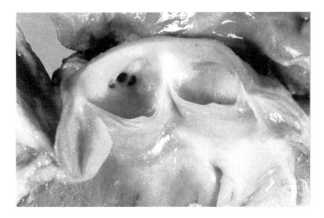

Figure 6.15 Three coronary ostia in the right sinus of Valsalva, including a separate conus artery ostium, in a 19-month-old girl who died in her sleep.

right ventricular infundibulum (Liberthson *et al.*, 1974).

Although the most common angiographically demonstrated anomalies involve the circumflex artery (Engel, Torres & Page, 1975), these anomalies are usually of minimal significance and are associated only rarely with sudden death (Cohle, Graham & Pounder, 1986; Page *et al.*, 1974). Arterial transection or ligation may, however, be a problem during cardiac surgery for other congenital heart defects if an anomalous coronary artery is unsuspected (Anderson, McGoon & Lie,1978; Landolt *et al.*, 1986; Nagao *et al.*, 1967).

An important point with all of these anomalies is that unless a pathological lesion or anatomic arrangement can be demonstrated that could convincingly lead to a marked reduction in blood flow along an aberrant vessel, then there is no reason to believe that an abnormality, per se, has clinical significance. For example, the finding of a separate ostium for the conus artery in the right sinus of Valsalva represents a normal variant rather than an anomaly with possible pathological consequences (Figure 6.15).

High aortic origin
There is debate as to whether aberrantly placed coronary ostia located in the aortic wall distal to the valve sinuses are of clinical significance (Virmani, Rogan &

Cheitlin, 1989). However, the positioning of ostia more than 1 cm above the sinotubular junction may be significant if this results in ostial narrowing, an acute angle of take-off, or reduction in coronary artery filling pressure (Cohle, Graham & Pounder, 1986).

Anomalous origin from the pulmonary artery

A variety of anomalies have been described involving origin of one or both coronary arteries from the pulmonary trunk. The most common anomaly is origin of the left coronary artery from the pulmonary artery, with the right coronary artery arising from the aorta (Bland, White & Garland; 1933; Wesselhoeft, Fawcett & Johnson, 1968) (Figure 6.16). This is followed in frequency by the much less common origin of the right coronary from the pulmonary artery, with the left anterior descending (Schwartz & Robicsek, 1971) and the circumflex arteries arising from the pulmonary

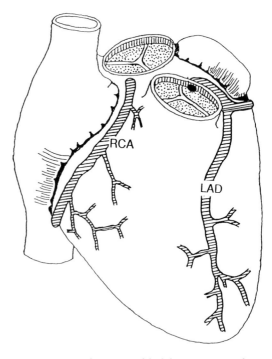

Figure 6.16 Anomalous origin of the left coronary artery from the pulmonary trunk. (RCA, right coronary artery; LAD, left anterior descending artery.)

artery even less frequently. Rarely, a single coronary artery will arise from the pulmonary trunk (Hoganson *et al.*, 1983).

Frequency

In studies of congenital cardiac disease, anomalous origin of the coronary arteries from the pulmonary artery occurred in 0.24% of cases, compared with a frequency in angiographic studies of less than 0.1% (Liberthson, 1989). The estimated frequency of the Bland–White–Garland syndrome in the general population is one in 300,000 children (Cohle, Graham & Pounder, 1986).

Clinical features

The clinical presentation of an anomalous coronary artery arising from the pulmonary trunk has been classified as "infantile" when symptoms and signs occur early, with death before one year of age; as "adult" when symptoms occur in later life; and as "intermediate" when symptoms that are present in infancy resolve by the age of three to four years due to improvement in collateral circulation (Neufeld & Blieden, 1975).

Symptoms and signs are often of heart failure (Driscoll *et al.*, 1981; Menahem & Venables, 1987), although affected infants may present as an apparent SIDS death or with rapid clinical deterioration (Lalu, Karhunen & Rautiainen, 1992). Older children may also die very suddenly and unexpectedly, with minimal antemortem symptoms (Bunton *et al.*, 1987; Perper, Rozin & Williams, 1985).

Anomalous coronary arteries may arise from both the aorta and the pulmonary trunk in the same patient (Chaitman *et al.*, 1975), and occasionally both coronary arteries arise from the pulmonary trunk. Usually, patients with both coronary arteries arising from the pulmonary trunk die at an early age (Heifetz *et al.*, 1986), although sometimes there has been surprisingly long survival (Feldt, Ongley & Titus, 1965). In children with prolonged survival, other congenital cardiac defects are usually present that cause elevation of pulmonary arterial pressure and prevent arterial shunting (Cheitlin, 1989; Keeton, Keenan & Monro, 1983).

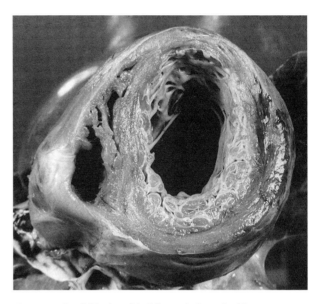

Figure 6.17 Focal thinning of the left ventricular wall, with fibrous scarring and endocardial fibroelastosis caused by an anomalous left coronary artery arising from the pulmonary trunk.

Pathological features

On gross examination of the heart in the most common variant, the anomalous left coronary artery may be thin-walled and vein-like (Virmani, Rogan & Cheitlin, 1989), perfusing a thinned and dilated left ventricle. The corresponding normally placed right coronary artery, on the other hand, is often quite large, with a number of intercoronary collateral channels demonstrable on injection studies. The left ventricle may show evidence of acute infarction in evolution or may show interstitial fibrosis, calcification, and endocardial fibroelastosis (Figure 6.17), with atrophy of the anterior papillary muscle. There may be dilation of the mitral valve ring.

Occurrence of sudden death

Sudden and unexpected death has been reported in patients with anomalous left or right coronary arteries arising from the pulmonary trunk (Bunton *et al.*, 1987; Lerberg *et al.*, 1979; Mintz *et al.*, 1983; Wilson, Dlabal & McGuire, 1979). Patients having anomalous origin of the right coronary artery tend to present at a later age (Bregman *et al.*, 1976; Roberts & Robinowitz, 1984).

Pathophysiology

The unique position of aberrant vessels arising from the pulmonary artery results in a different pathophysiological sequence of events to that found with anomalous arteries arising from the aorta. However, reduction in blood flow is caused by similar mechanisms to those described for anomalous coronary arteries with an aortic origin.

Due to the high pulmonary vascular resistance that is present in fetal life, similar blood flow occurs in coronary arteries arising either from the pulmonary artery or from the aorta. As the lungs expand after birth, pulmonary vascular resistance begins to fall and blood flow along the aberrant vessel arising from the pulmonary trunk reduces (Liberthson, 1989). At the same time, blood oxygenation levels in the anomalous artery also decline. These changes result in ischemia of the dependent myocardium and may lead to infarction and death at that stage. In infants who survive, blood flow along the aberrant vessel eventually reverses, with flow being maintained through intercoronary collaterals from the other normally positioned coronary artery. The extent of the left-to-right shunting is not significant in terms of overall volume, but the resulting "myocardial steal" phenomenon exacerbates myocardial hypoxia and may also predispose to sudden death (Mintz *et al.*, 1983).

Left ventricular rupture with fatal cardiac tamponade has occasionally been documented in infancy associated with an anomalous left coronary artery arising from the pulmonary trunk (McKinley, Andrews & Neill, 1951).

Anomalous origin from other vessels

Aberrant coronary arteries may arise from the proximal portion of another coronary artery (Figure 6.18). In these cases, comparable mechanisms causing luminal narrowing with blood flow reduction apply. Rarely, anomalous origin of a coronary artery from a carotid artery has been reported (Knop & Bennett, 1944; Smith, 1950).

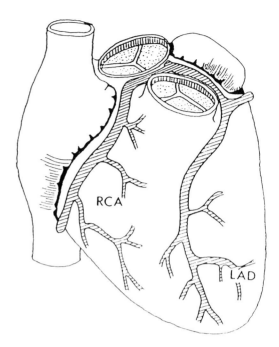

Figure 6.18 Origin of the right coronary artery (RCA) from the left coronary artery. (LAD, left anterior descending artery.)

Coronary artery aplasia/hypoplasia

Aplasia

A variety of patterns may be found in the distribution of epicardial vessels when one artery is absent. A common feature is a single coronary ostium from which arises an artery that provides the entire cardiac blood supply (Smith, 1950) (Figure 6.19).

Frequency

Complete absence of a coronary artery has an estimated frequency of 0.02% within the general population (Lipton *et al.*, 1979), increasing to around 0.4% in the highly selected population of adults undergoing angiography. It has been reported in 4.5% of patients with anomalies of the coronary arteries (Kelley, Wolfson & Marshall, 1977).

Occurrence Of sudden death

The clinical significance of a single coronary artery is extremely variable; some individuals remain completely asymptomatic until well into adult life, while others die suddenly and unexpectedly in infancy or childhood (Okuni & Sumitomo, 1987; Vestermark, 1965; Virmani, Rogan & Cheitlin, 1989). Before death is ascribed to this anomaly, additional causes of coronary vascular obstruction should be looked for carefully.

Pathophysiology

A solitary coronary artery becomes significant only when there is a critical reduction in blood supply along the vessel, resulting in myocardial hypoxia. If obstructive lesions are not present, then there may be no cardiac problems or reduction in life expectancy (Dent & Fisher, 1955).

Blood flow may be compromised in a single coronary artery if it has an anomalous course or if the solitary ostium is narrowed. Dye injection or postmortem angiography may demonstrate a functional problem if there is kinking. For example, a two-month-old boy who died suddenly and unexpectedly was found at autopsy to have a single left coronary artery of apparently normal caliber with a normal ostium (Moore & Byard, 1992b). Further dissection and injection studies revealed obstruction to flow due to kinking near the origin of the posterior descending branch (Figure 6.20).

Associated features

Single coronary arteries may occur independently in approximately 60% of patients, or they may be associated with congenital heart defects, such as bicuspid aortic valve, truncus arteriosus, transposition of the great vessels, coronary fistula, pulmonary or aortic valvular atresia, or tetralogy of Fallot in the remainder (Ogden & Goodyer, 1970; Sharbaugh & White, 1974). One case of absent circumflex artery in a 12-year-old girl was associated with dilated cardiomyopathy (Bestetti *et al.*, 1985).

Hypoplasia

A hypoplastic coronary artery is one that is situated normally but that has a markedly reduced caliber. However, relating hypoplasia to functional

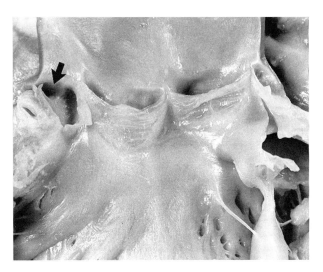

Figure 6.19 Single coronary ostium in the left sinus of Valsalva (arrow).

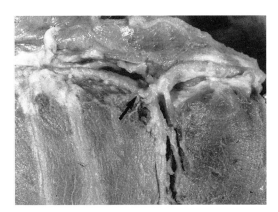

Figure 6.20 Single left coronary artery with obstruction to flow due to kinking at a point of arterial branching (arrow). Opening of the vessels demonstrated no intrinsic obstructive lesions.

significance may be extremely difficult if there are no signs of acute or chronic myocardial ischemia in the distribution of the hypoplastic vessel. An 11-year-old boy who died suddenly while swimming demonstrates the difficulties that may occur in trying to determine correctly the cause of death in such patients (Byard, Smith & Bourne, 1991). However, a history of exercise-induced collapse on several occasions enabled clinicopathological correlation with

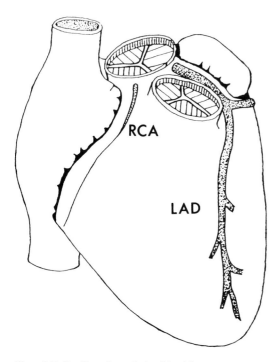

Figure 6.21 Significant hypoplasia of the right coronary artery (RCA) in an 11-year-old boy with a history of exercise-induced collapse. (LAD, left anterior descending artery.)

the findings at autopsy (Figures 6.21 and 6.22). Other cases of sudden death in adolescence due to coronary artery hypoplasia have been reported (Jokl & McClellan, 1970; Virmani, Rogan & Cheitlin, 1989).

As arteries with an anomalous course may show a degree of hypoplasia, the contribution of a reduced luminal diameter to the fatal outcome must also be assessed. An additional problem is the subjective nature of these assessments and the absence of published normal ranges for coronary artery diameters.

Coronary arteritis

Kawasaki disease

This acute febrile illness of childhood was first described in 1967 by Kawasaki as "acute febrile muco-cutaneous lymph node syndrome." Also known as infantile polyarteritis nodosa (Landing & Larson, 1977; Lie, 1987a), it is now recognized as a relatively common illness in childhood. Unfortunately, it is also one that may have serious sequelae due to inflammation of the coronary arteries (Byard, 1996a). In North America and Japan, it is now the major cause of acquired heart disease in children under five years of age, following the decline in cases of rheumatic fever (Byard *et al.*, 1991b; Freeman & Shulman, 2001; Gedalia, 2002). Because of its importance in terms of sudden childhood death, this section includes additional epidemiological and clinical information.

Epidemiology
Kawasaki disease generally affects children aged between six months and five years, with the highest rate noted between nine and 11 months (Levin, Tizard & Dillon, 1991). It is rare over ten years of age, and it has a male predilection, with a male-to-female ratio of approximately 3:2 (Wreford *et al.*, 1991), a difference that is even more exaggerated in fatal cases, where the ratio is 3:1. There appears to be a racial bias, with oriental children being the most, and Caucasian children the least, susceptible (Melish, 1982). Cases tend to cluster.

Clinical features
The clinical presentation of Kawasaki disease is usually quite sudden, with fever followed by features that are summarized in Table 6.4 (Centers for Disease Control, 1980; Koike & Freedom, 1989). Certain atypical cases may not have all of the features, particularly in infants under the age of six months (Burns *et al.*, 1986; Rowley & Shulman, 1999). Other clinical and pathological features are abdominal pain, diarrhea, arthritis, urethritis, aseptic meningitis, acute hydrops of the gallbladder, hepatitis, cholangitis, and proliferative lesions of the bile ducts (Bader-Meunier *et al.*, 1992). Cardiac manifestations include mitral and aortic valve insufficiency.

There are four stages in the evolution of Kawasaki disease: (i) an "acute febrile" stage, which lasts 1–11 days; (ii) a "subacute" stage, where there is non-specific but persistent irritability and anorexia lasting 11–21 days associated with thrombocytosis; (iii) a "convalescent" stage, lasting from 21 to 60 days;

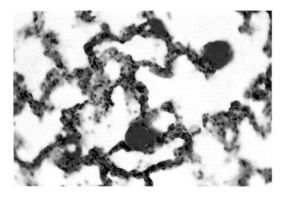

Color Plate 1 Fat emboli present within the lungs of the nine-year-old cyclist illustrated in Figure 2.8 (hematoxylin and eosin, ×200).

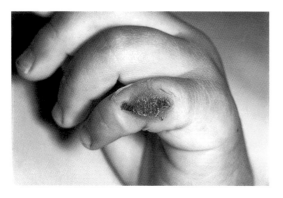

Color Plate 3 Classical electrical burns in a case of childhood electrocution, showing targetoid appearances with peripheral blanching and hyperemic borders.

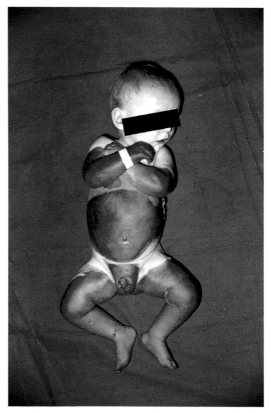

Color Plate 2 Extensive scalding of an infant in the bath with sparing of flexural creases.

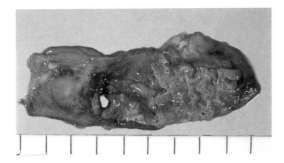

Color Plate 4 Minimal external signs of injury were present in a three-year-old boy who died following perforation of the small intestine due to inflicted abdominal trauma, with peritonitis and fatal sepsis.

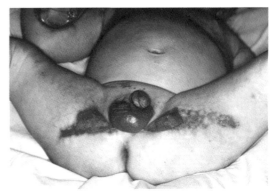

Color Plate 5 An unusual pattern of upper thigh and scrotal scalds in the case shown in Figure 3.58, with a sharp line of demarcation, suggesting that the perineum had been pushed firmly against the bath, with the legs out of the water.

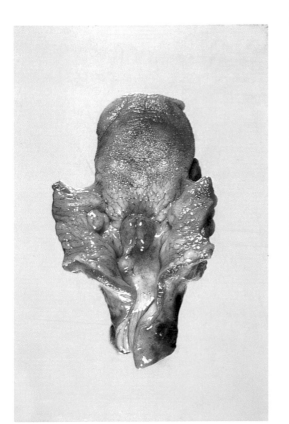

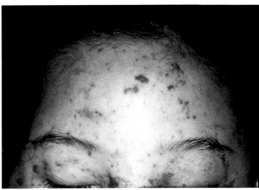

Color Plate 7 Diffuse rash over the forehead in a young girl dying from fulminant meningococcemia.

Color Plate 6 Marked swelling of the epiglottis with occlusion of the airway due to *Hemophilus influenzae* type B infection. The eight-month-old boy had "croup-like" symptoms for only a short time before his terminal respiratory arrest.

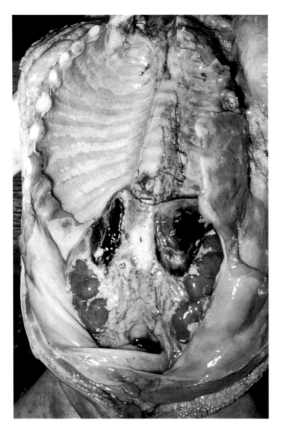

Color Plate 8 Bilateral adrenal hemorrhages (Waterhouse–Friderichson syndrome) in a two-month-old infant with meningococcal meningitis and septicemia.

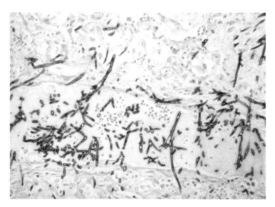

Color Plate 9 Hyphae of *Aspergillus* sp. infiltrating a blood vessel (hematoxylin and eosin, ×110).

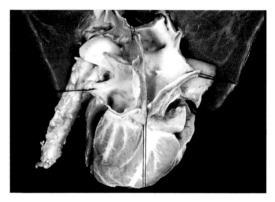

Color Plate 10 Cor triatriatum in a 2.5-month-old boy, showing complete separation of the pulmonary venous return from the left atrial cavity by a muscular septum.

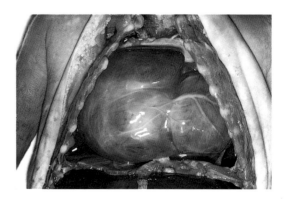

Color Plate 11 Marked right atrial dilation due to pulmonary valve atresia.

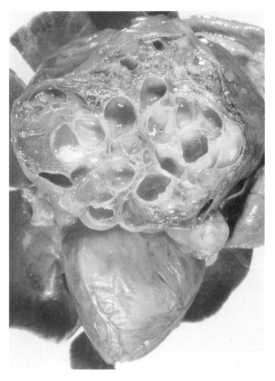

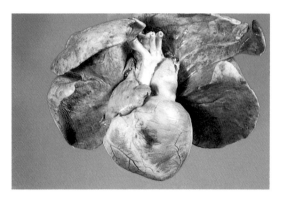

Color Plate 13 Markedly dilated right atrial appendage, right atrium, ventricle, and pulmonary outflow tract in a 14-year-old boy with primary pulmonary hypertension.

Color Plate 12 Cross-section of an intrapericardial teratoma, revealing multiple cystic spaces. In this case, death occurred soon after birth.

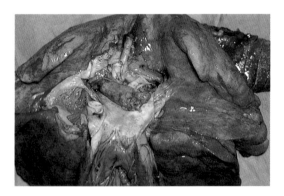

Color Plate 14 Large saddle thromboembolus causing sudden and unexpected death in a nine-year-old girl with unsuspected primary pulmonary hypertension.

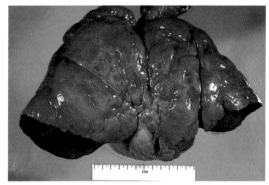

Color Plate 15 Hyperinflated lungs in a case of sudden death of a five-year-old asthmatic boy. Air-trapping caused the bulky lungs to obscure the anterior surface of the heart almost completely.

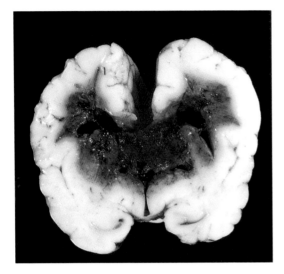

Color Plate 16 Venous thrombosis with symmetric cerebral infarction in a two-week-old girl with sepsis and dehydration.

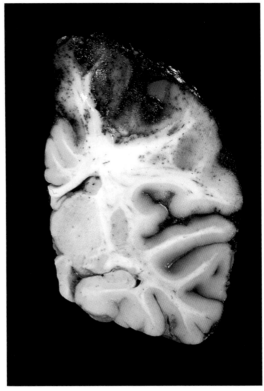

Color Plate 17 Intracerebral and subarachnoid hemorrhage in a 10-month-old girl with scurvy.

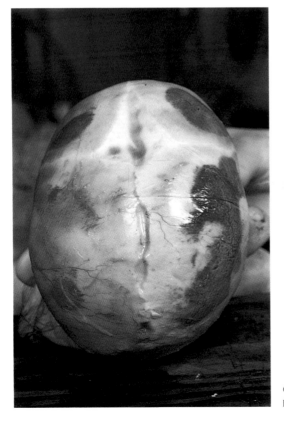

Color Plate 18 Bossing of the skull in an infant with marrow hyperplasia.

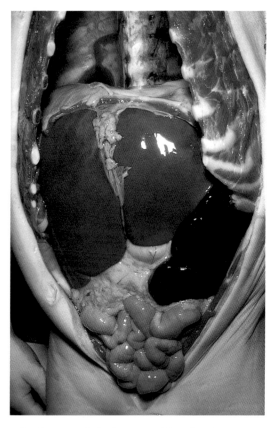

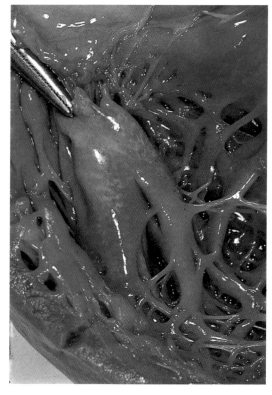

Color Plate 21 "Thrush breast" dappling of the heart due to marked fatty change in an anemic nine-year-old boy with acute lymphoblastic leukemia in relapse.

Color Plate 19 Marked enlargement of the spleen due to acute splenic sequestration in an eight-year-old boy with a southern European background and combined sickle cell disease–β thalassemia.

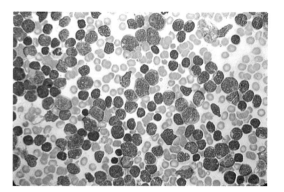

Color Plate 20 Peripheral blood smear from the three-year-old girl illustrated in Figure 9.7, demonstrating numerous blast cells (Giemsa, ×1100).

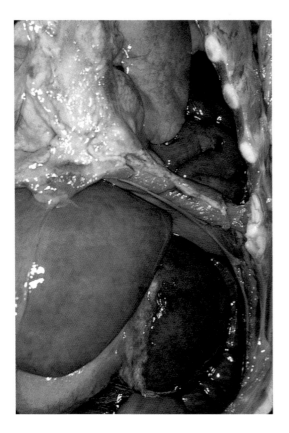

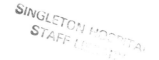

Color Plate 22 Herniation of the abdominal contents through a small left-sided diaphragmatic hernia in a four-month-old boy resulted in sudden death.

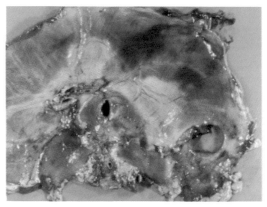

Color Plate 24 The relatively small size of the diaphragmatic defect in a late-presenting case can be appreciated when the diaphragm has been removed, as in Case 2 in Table 10.2.

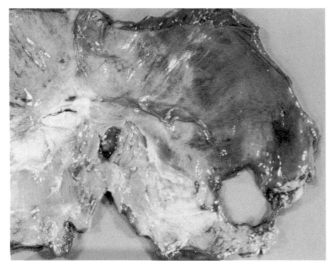

Color Plate 23 The relatively small size of the diaphragmatic defect in a late-presenting case can be appreciated when the diaphragm has been removed, as in Case 1 in Table 10.2.

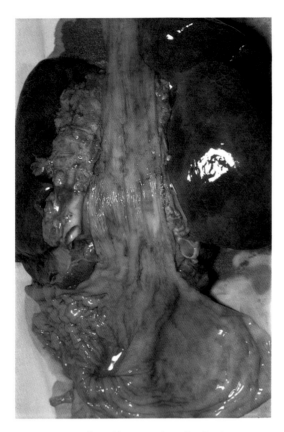

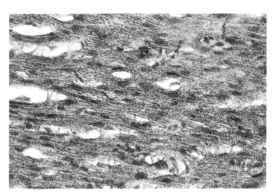

Color Plate 26 Oil-red O staining of a frozen section of the heart, demonstrating extensive lipid deposition (×440).

Color Plate 25 Collapsed lower-esophageal varices in a 9.5-year-old boy with congenital biliary atresia and biliary cirrhosis, who died following massive upper-gastrointestinal hemorrhage.

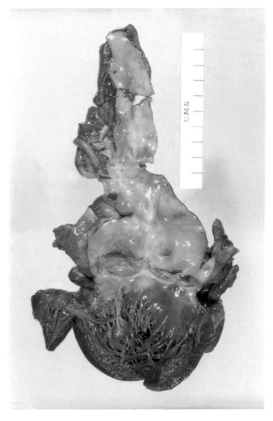

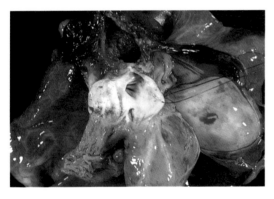

Color Plate 28 Massive intrathoracic hemorrhage from dissection and rupture of a patent ductus arteriosus as the presenting feature of Marfan syndrome resulted in sudden and unexpected death of a four-month-old girl.

Color Plate 27 Marked dilation of the aortic root, with microscopic features of cystic medial necrosis, in a six-year-old boy with Marfan syndrome, who collapsed and died while bathing.

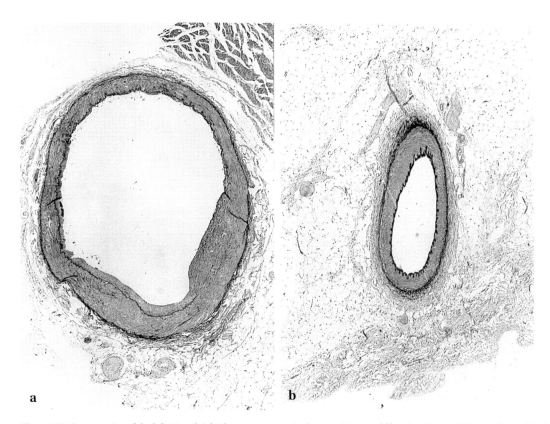

Figure 6.22 Cross-section of the left (a) and right (b) coronary arteries from an 11-year-old boy (see Figure 6.21) who died suddenly and unexpectedly, demonstrating marked disparity in their luminal diameters (Movat pentachrome, ×20).

Table 6.4. Criteria for diagnosis of Kawasaki disease*

Fever for at least five days
Bilateral conjunctival injection
Changes in the oropharynx:
   Erythema and cracking of the lips, or
   Oropharyngeal edema, or
   Strawberry tongue
Changes in extremities:
   Edema of hands and feet, or
   Erythema of palms or soles, or
   Desquamation of fingertips and toe tips
Erythematous rash
Lymphadenopathy (>15 mm diameter)

*Diagnosis requires fever plus four of the remaining five criteria.

and (iv) a "healed" stage after this (Hicks & Melish, 1986).

Kawasaki disease once had a mortality rate of 1–2% (Wreford *et al.*, 1991); however, a striking decrease has followed the use of intravenous immunoglobulin therapy (Barron *et al.*, 1990; Nakamura *et al.*, 1991). Included in the group with a fatal outcome are infants and children who die suddenly, sometimes without having an established antemortem diagnosis of Kawasaki disease. On careful review of the history, there may, however, be evidence of a febrile illness that was not considered particularly severe at the time but that in retrospect had typical features (McCowen & Henderson, 1988).

Less than 5% of deaths occur in the acute stage of the disease, with most (70%) lethal cases being found in the subacute and healing stages (Melish, 1982).

Death usually occurs within six months of the onset of symptoms (Wreford *et al.*, 1991), although sudden and unexpected death may occur at any stage, sometimes many years after symptoms have subsided (Kegel *et al.*, 1977; Kohr, 1986; Quam *et al.*, 1986). Fatal myocardial infarction is not necessarily precipitated by exertion and may occur during sleep or at rest (Kato, Ichinose & Kawasaki, 1986).

Kawasaki disease and infantile polyarteritis nodosa are now considered to be the same disease and are quite distinct from classical polyarteritis nodosa, which tends to be more chronic, with a different pattern of vessel involvement and a higher rate of renal and pulmonary complications (Landing & Larson, 1977; Melish, 1982).

Etiology

Clustering of cases of Kawasaki disease suggests an infectious etiology complicated by an immune complex vasculitis (Freeman & Shulman, 2001; Gedalia, 2002; Levin *et al.*, 1985; Yanagawa *et al.*, 1986). However, no specific agent has been identified. Staphylococci, streptococci, *Propionobacterium acnes*, retrovirus, Epstein–Barr virus, parvovirus B19, parainfluenza virus, herpes simplex virus, adenovirus, echovirus, rotavirus, leptospira, rickettsia, *Coxiella burnetti*, yersinia, and house dust mite have all been implicated as possible etiological agents (Hicks & Melish, 1986; Kato *et al.*, 1983; Nigro *et al.*, 1994), but none has been found consistently (Glode *et al.*, 1986; Klein *et al.*, 1986; Rowley, Gonzalez-Crussi & Shulman, 1988). Furthermore, the lack of response to antibiotic therapy implies that acute bacterial sepsis is unlikely. Repeatedly negative viral cultures and serological examinations reduce the likelihood of a standard viral infection being present.

While a possible association between outbreaks of Kawasaki disease and recent carpet cleaning has been reported (Fatica *et al.*, 1989; Ichida *et al.*, 1989; Patriarca *et al.*, 1982), with the suggestion that cleaning may liberate an infectious or toxic agent (Rauch *et al.*, 1991), this connection has not been confirmed (Lin *et al.*, 1985; Rogers *et al.*, 1985). The possibility of an animal reservoir/arthropod vector has been proposed, based on the finding that children with

Table 6.5. Immunological features of Kawasaki disease

Polyclonal B-cell stimulation
Antineutrophil antibodies
Antiendothelial cell antibodies
Circulating immune complexes
Increased T4 helper cells
Decreased T8 suppressor cells
Elevated serum cytokine levels
Variable interferon levels
Increased numbers of CD14+ macrophages/monocytes
Increased lymphocyte interleukin-2 surface receptors

Kawasaki disease tend to live closer than controls to water (Rauch *et al.*, 1988).

The similarity in clinical presentation to conditions caused by known enterotoxins, such as staphylococcal scalded skin syndrome, staphylococcal toxic shock syndrome, and scarlet fever, and the similarity in immunological alterations to toxin-induced disorders, supports the possibility of an unidentified toxin being responsible for Kawasaki disease. The toxin may be derived from organisms that are either commensals or of only very low virulence (Levin, Tizard & Dillon, 1991), thus affecting only a small number of predisposed individuals.

Immunological studies have demonstrated a wide variety of abnormalities in patients with acute phase Kawasaki disease, summarized in Table 6.5 (Furukawa, Matsubara & Yabuta, 1992; Lang *et al.*, 1990; Leung *et al.*, 1983; Leung *et al.*, 1989; Mason *et al.*, 1985; Ogle *et al.*, 1991; Savage *et al.*, 1989; Tizard *et al.*, 1991). These findings suggest that a variety of inflammatory pathways are involved in the pathogenesis of the disease.

Although there is a higher incidence in siblings of affected children, particularly in those under two years of age, where 8–9% develop the disease, person-to-person transmission has not been proven. This, together with the lack of major outbreaks in schools or specific districts where cases have occurred, argues against an infectious etiology. In examining the higher incidence in siblings of affected children, it is also apparent that the disease usually begins at around the same time in both children, implying that exposure to a common etiological agent would be a more likely event than secondary transmission (Fujita *et al.*, 1989; Levin, Tizard & Dillon, 1991). If an as yet unidentified infectious agent is responsible for Kawasaki disease, then it must either have a very low infectivity or be more widespread than thought previously, with a large number of subclinical cases.

The higher incidence in children of oriental families resident in the USA (Ichida *et al.*, 1989) has suggested a genetic basis to the disorder, with the possibility of an aberrant response to a common infectious agent being considered (Levin, Tizard & Dillon, 1991). However, studies of Japanese twins have not supported this, with no difference in concordance being shown between monozygotic and dizygotic twins (Sasazuki, Harada & Kawasaki, 1987).

Pathological features

On external examination of the heart, there may be thickening of the coronary arteries or aneurysm formation (Figures 6.23 and 6.24). The aneurysms that form tend to be saccular and involve the proximal portions of the major coronary arteries (Takahashi, Mason & Lewis, 1987) and can be demonstrated on postmortem coronary angiography (Figure 6.25). Giant aneurysms may occur very early in the course of the disease, although not every involved artery develops them (Figure 6.26) (Avner, Shaw & Chin, 1989; Fujiwara, Fujiwara & Nakano, 1988; Fujiwara & Hamashima, 1978). There may also be valvular involvement (Figure 6.27).

The microscopic features of involved arteries are summarized in Table 6.6. They range from an early acute vasculitis with fibrointimal proliferation to aneurysmal dilation and thrombosis (Figures 6.28–6.30).

Coronary artery aneurysms may appear to regress on angiography (Akagi *et al.*, 1992), but the process is one of luminal remodeling due to intimal proliferation, thrombus recanalization, and contractive scarring of the damaged arterial wall (Zuccollo & Byard, 2001). The damaged arteries do not, therefore, return to normal (Landing & Larson, 1987) but will always

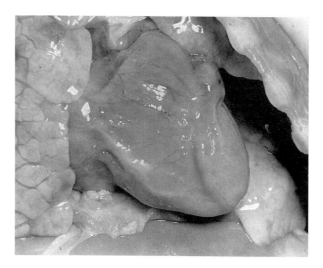

Figure 6.23 External view of the heart, showing thickening of the coronary arteries in a four-month-old girl who died suddenly due to Kawasaki disease.

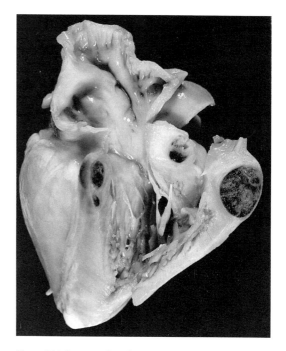

Figure 6.24 Cross-section of a coronary artery aneurysm (maximum diameter 1 cm), with a superimposed occluding thrombus in a 5.5-month-old girl with healed Kawasaki disease who died suddenly.

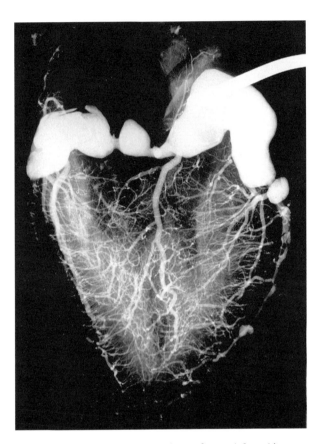

Figure 6.25 Postmortem angiogram from an infant with Kawasaki disease, showing marked aneurysmal dilation of the proximal coronary arteries.

Table 6.6. Pathological changes within the heart and coronary arteries in Kawasaki disease

Stage	Pathological changes
I	Acute inflammation of extramural arterial adventitia and intima
	Acute endocarditis, myocarditis, and pericarditis
II	Acute panvasculitis of extramural coronary arteries, with aneurysm formation and thrombosis
	Acute endocarditis, myocarditis, and pericarditis
III	Arterial intimal hyperplasia
	Resolving myocardial and pericardial inflammation
IV	Arterial stenosis with intimal fibrosis, calcification, and recanalization
	Myocardial fibrosis

show evidence of a healed vasculitis with fibrous scarring, disruption of elastic lamina, intimal thickening, and dystrophic calcification. This may predispose survivors to coronary artery atherosclerosis in early adult life (Kato *et al.*, 1992).

If myocardial ischemia following vessel thrombosis is non-fatal, then the organized luminal thrombus may recanalize (Fujiwara *et al.*, 1986), thus predisposing to sudden and unexpected death, possibly many years later due to marginal adequacy of the subsequent blood flow (Fineschi, Paglicci Reatelli & Baroldi, 1999; Kegel *et al.*, 1977; Pounder, 1985). This occurred in a two-year-old boy who collapsed and died of an acute myocardial infarct. Histological

examination of the heart revealed extensive scarring in addition to more recent ischemic changes and an occluded right main coronary artery (Figure 6.31) (Byard *et al.*, 1991c).

As well as damaging coronary arteries, Kawasaki disease may cause a generalized vasculitis, which affects small to medium-sized muscular arteries throughout the body (Amano *et al.*, 1980) (Figure 6.32). Similar inflammation and necrosis are found in the arteries of the mesentery, spleen, adrenal glands, and kidneys, all of which should be sampled at autopsy. The involved segments of vessel wall tend to be extraparenchymal and may occasionally involve medium-sized and large veins (Melish, 1982). Reticulin or trichrome stains may be useful in delineating obliterated, thrombosed vessels.

Histologic similarities, including the presence of arterial aneurysms, are also found in childhood AIDS, which may sometimes be included in the differential diagnosis (Joshi *et al.*, 1987). Usually, however, the central nervous system is spared in Kawasaki disease (Terasawa *et al.*, 1983).

Most fatal cases of Kawasaki disease seen by pathologists no longer demonstrate an erythematous skin rash. Even if this is present, it is of little diagnostic help, since histologic examination merely shows non-specific dilation of superficial dermal capillaries, with mild edema and a

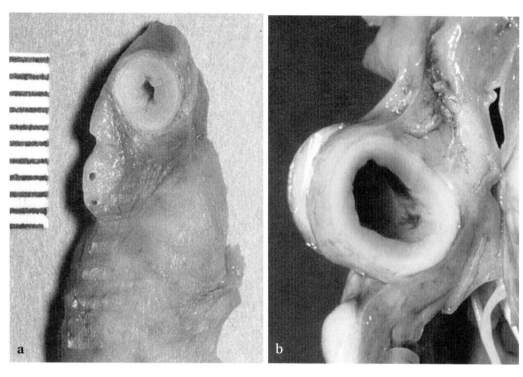

Figure 6.26 Features of Kawasaki disease were found at autopsy in a 10-month-old boy with no significant history, who died suddenly one night. Variable changes have occurred in different sections of the same coronary artery: (a) marked fibrointimal proliferation; (b) aneurysmal dilation.

perivascular chronic inflammatory infiltrate. Lymph node changes are similarly non-diagnostic, with follicular hyperplasia and a non-specific interfollicular infiltrate of immunoblasts and atypical mononuclear cells (Melish, 1982).

Occurrence of sudden death

The mechanism of sudden death in Kawasaki disease is variable, with death resulting from ischemically induced arrhythmia, inflammation of cardiac conduction tracts, acute myocardial infarction, or, less commonly, acute cardiac tamponade due to rupture of an aneurysmally dilated artery. Fujiwara and colleagues (1986) documented the cause of death at autopsy in 69 cases as myocardial ischemia in 56 (81%), aneurysm rupture 6 (9%), myocarditis 5 (7%), and miscellaneous 2 (3%). Patients who die of

myocarditis are more likely to do so at an earlier stage than patients who die of myocardial infarction.

Critical compromise of arterial blood flow may occur due to aneurysm thrombosis or reduction of the caliber of the vessel lumen because of the profound intimal hyperplasia that characterizes the middle stages of the disease. Diffuse obliterative vasculitis may also result in vessel occlusion and sudden death months after the disease (McConnell *et al.*, 1998). In the past, 20% of cases have manifested panvasculitis of the coronary arteries, with aneurysm formation and subsequent scarring (Fujiwara, Fujiwara & Hamashima, 1987; Koike & Freedom, 1989), with resultant lethal sequelae involving only a minority of patients (1–2%).

Given that early treatment with gamma globulin and aspirin appears to have reduced the incidence of cardiac complications from 20% to around 5% (Byard

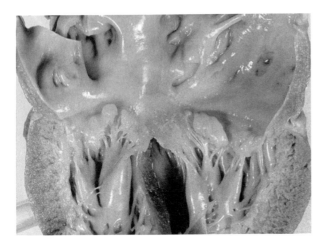

Figure 6.27 Ballooning and dysplasia of the mitral valve in a three-month-old boy due to Kawasaki disease.

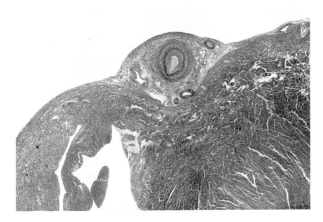

Figure 6.28 Marked intimal thickening in the healing phase of Kawasaki disease (Movat pentachrome, ×20).

et al., 1991b), it is to be hoped that pathologists will see even less of this disorder on the autopsy table in the future.

Miscellaneous coronary vasculitis

Less commonly, coronary arteritis may be associated with rheumatic fever or found in transplanted hearts.

Rheumatic fever

Vascular involvement is unusual in rheumatic fever. However, occasionally there may be evidence of an acute coronary arteritis, with fibrinoid necrosis, lymphocytic infiltration, and mural thrombi. More chronic vascular changes involve intimal fibrosis and medial elastification (Virmani, Robinowitz & Darcy, 1991).

Post-cardiac transplantation

Following cardiac transplantation in children, acute rejection may also result in fibrinoid medial necrosis of coronary arteries, with resultant thrombosis. More chronic changes of concentric fibrointimal proliferation may result in luminal narrowing (Virmani, Robinowitz & Darcy, 1991).

Miscellaneous conditions

Other conditions that affect the coronary arteries are included here because of their potential for unexpected lethal consequences.

Coronary artery fistulas

Direct communication between a major coronary artery and a heart chamber, major vein, coronary sinus, or pulmonary artery is reported as one of the most common hemodynamically important abnormalities of the coronary circulation (Cheitlin, 1989). These coronary-cardiac, coronary-venous, and coronary-arterial fistulas are distinct from fistulas that develop as a result of an anomalous coronary artery arising from the pulmonary trunk. They were present in 0.2% of patients undergoing coronary angiography in one series (Lowe & Sabiston, 1990) and in 13% of cases in another series of congenital coronary artery anomalies (Hobbs *et al.*, 1981). Most coronary artery fistulas drain into the right side of the heart (Cheng, 1982).

Almost 50% of patients with coronary artery fistulas are symptomatic, with heart failure, exertional dyspnea, or angina pectoris (Hallman, Cooley and Singer, 1966). Potentially lethal complications include acute myocardial infarction, ventricular rupture, and embolization (Lowe & Sabiston, 1990). Bacterial endocarditis has been reported in 10% of cases (Neufeld & Blieden, 1975). Three percent of patients with coronary artery fistulas have an associated single coronary artery (Levin, Fellows and Abrams, 1978; Morgan *et al.*, 1972); however, sudden

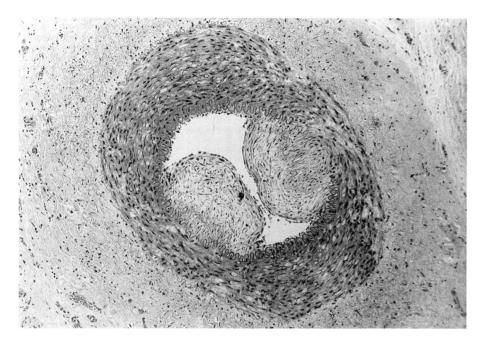

Figure 6.29 Symmetrical focal fibrointimal proliferation in a mesenteric vessel of a three-month-old boy with Kawasaki disease (hematoxylin and eosin, ×145).

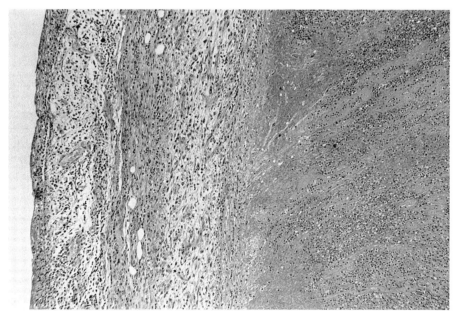

Figure 6.30 A portion of recent thrombus in an aneurysmally dilated coronary artery from a six-month-old infant with Kawasaki disease (hematoxylin and eosin, ×110).

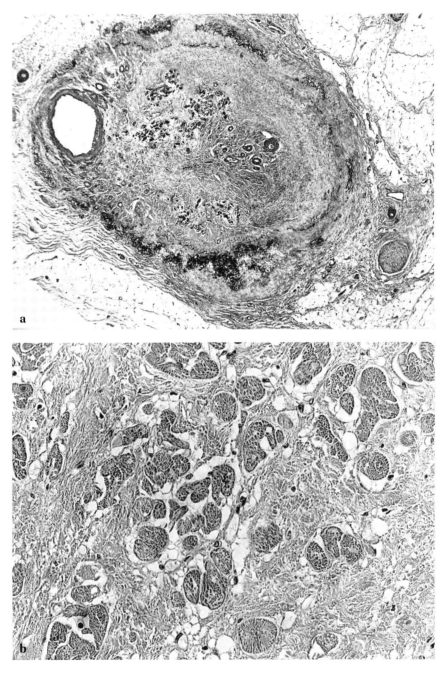

Figure 6.31 A previously thrombosed right coronary artery with organization and recanalization in a two-year-old boy who collapsed and died unexpectedly at home (a). There had been no clear history of Kawasaki disease (Movat pentachrome, ×45). Section of the left ventricle in this case showing extensive fibrous scarring (b) from a previous healed infarct (Masson trichrome stain, ×280).

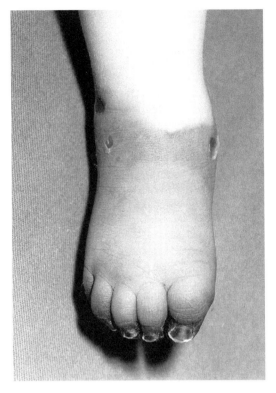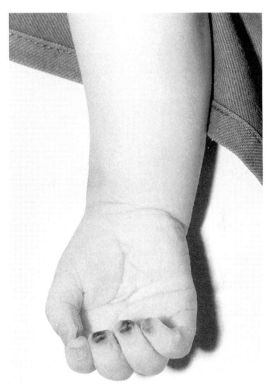

Figure 6.32 Ischemic changes of the feet and fingers in a three-month-old boy with widespread arterial disease and who died of Kawasaki disease.

death in childhood in these cases is not usual (Daniel, Graham & Sabiston, 1970).

Congenital coronary artery aneurysm

The majority of coronary artery aneurysms in children are acquired either as a result of Kawasaki disease or from localized infection following mycotic embolism. They may also occur in AIDS. However, a small number of apparent congenital aneurysms may occur in isolation or in association with fistulas (Robinowitz, Forman & Virmani, 1989). Determining the etiology of coronary aneurysms may be difficult in cases of sudden death in childhood (Trillo, Scharyj & Prichard, 1980), as the occurrence of complications such as thrombotic occlusion, peripheral embolization, or rupture of an aneurysm (Lowe & Sabiston, 1990) is independent of pathogenesis. Other cases in which multiple multifocal arterial aneurysms are

present (Short, 1978) must raise the possibility of a generalized connective tissue disorder, such as Ehlers–Danlos syndrome. In such cases, it is essential to perform collagen and molecular analyses.

Congenital coronary artery arteriovenous malformation

Rarely, cases of sudden infant death are due to rupture of a coronary artery arteriovenous malformation, with resultant hemopericardium and tamponade (Dancea *et al.*, 2002).

Intramural coronary arteries: coronary artery bridging

The presence of an intramural coronary artery and the occurrence of sudden death may be a purely co-incidental association (Roberts *et al.*, 1982), as such vessels have been observed in up to 86% of autopsied

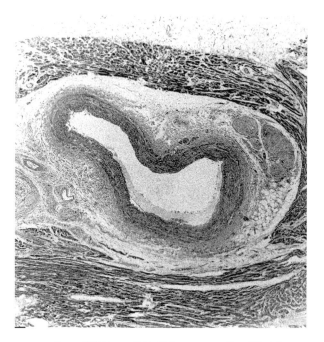

Figure 6.33 Myocardial bridging over a portion of the left anterior descending coronary artery in a 12-year-old girl who died suddenly while swimming. No other abnormality was found at autopsy (hematoxylin and eosin, ×45).

hearts (Cheitlin, 1980). However, the demonstration at autopsy of an acute myocardial infarct in a 17-year-old girl who died suddenly while swimming, in association with a long segment of intramural left anterior descending artery, and sudden death in another 17-year-old athelete with coronary artery hypoplasia and tunnelling of the distal circumflex artery, may suggest a causal relationship in at least some cases (McManus *et al.*, 1981; Morales, Romanelli & Boucek, 1980). Coronary artery bridging (Figure 6.33) has certainly been associated with the development of arrhythmias, such as ventricular fibrillation and paroxysmal supraventricular tachycardia in the adult population, as well as scarring of the myocardium (Basso *et al.*, 1995; Faruqui *et al.*, 1978).

Coronary artery intussusception

Roberts, Silver & Sapala (1986) described a 19-year-old male footballer who died suddenly during exercise and who had coronary artery occlusion caused by distal prolapse of portions of the intima and media.

Coronary artery vasospasm

Vasospasm in the presence of angiographically normal coronary arteries was considered responsible for episodic angina in an 11-year-old boy (Wilkes *et al.*, 1985). Whether vasospasm could be of sufficient intensity to provoke a fatal arrhythmia or infarction in childhood is arguable, as no cases of exercise-related sudden death from coronary spasm were found in the review by McManus and colleagues (1981). As coronary artery spasm is a physiological event, certain criteria have been proposed to assist in evaluating it as a cause of death. These include a complete clinical history with electrocardiographic evidence of ischemia in the absence of significant fixed arterial obstruction. In an ideal world, clinical evidence of previous spasm would be available before autopsy (Cohle, Graham & Pounder, 1986).

Venous abnormalities

With the exception of anomalous pulmonary venous drainage described below, abnormalities in the origin and courses of veins are generally of minimal clinical significance. There is, however, an association between persistent left superior vena cava and fatal cardiac arrhythmias in adolescence, which appears to relate to concomitant conduction tract abnormalities (James, Marshall & Edwards, 1976).

Total anomalous pulmonary venous drainage

Anomalous drainage of the pulmonary veins into the systemic venous system rather than into the left atrium is the main structural venous abnormality associated with sudden and unexpected death. This occurs when there is persistence of the fetal connection between intrapulmonary veins and the splanchnic venous plexus, with failure to form the common pulmonary vein (Rammos, Gittenberger-de Groot & Oppenheimer-Dekker, 1990; Wilson, 1798).

Anomalous drainage of blood into the right side of the heart may be total, involving both lungs, or only

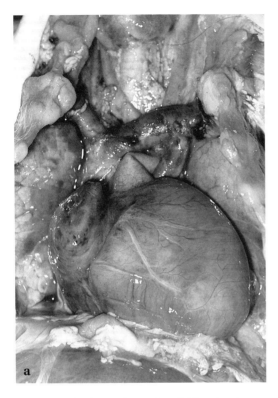 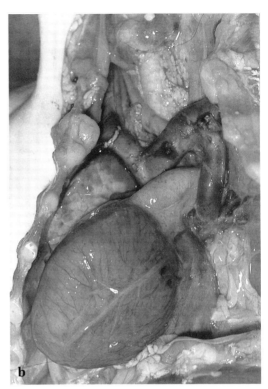

Figure 6.34 Dilated innominate vein and right atrium in a case of total anomalous pulmonary venous drainage and left ventricular hypoplasia with passage of pulmonary venous blood via a common vein into the innominate vein (a). Reflection of the heart to the right, demonstrating the lack of normal connection of the pulmonary veins to the left atrium (b).

partial, involving all or only a portion of one lung. The point of entry of oxygenated pulmonary blood into the systemic venous circulation may be either above or below the diaphragm (Lamb *et al.*, 1988).

The type of drainage has been classified into four groups: (i) supracardiac, (ii) cardiac, (iii) infracardiac, and (iv) mixed (Darling, Rothney & Craig, 1957). The most common connection is to the left innominate vein (Figure 6.34) followed by the coronary sinus (Figure 6.35), right superior vena cava, portal vein and right atrium, in descending order of occurrence (Carter, Capriles & Noe, 1969). Very uncommonly, drainage will be into the azygous vein or into a persistent left superior vena cava (Delisle *et al.*, 1976).

Clinical features

Total anomalous pulmonary venous drainage (TAPVD) accounts for 1–2% of all congenital cardiovascular malformations. In untreated infants it has a mortality rate of 80% within the first year of life (Hawkins, Clark & Doty, 1983; Turley *et al.*, 1980), although survival to adult life is possible (Gomes *et al.*, 1970; Hammon & Bender, 1990). Continued postnatal survival is possible only when an alternative mechanism exists for diverting blood into the left side of the heart, such as through a patent foramen ovale or ductus arteriosus. Male infants are affected more often than females (Hammon & Bender, 1990), and rare familial cases have been documented (Paz & Castilla, 1971; Solymar, Sabel & Zetterqvist, 1987).

Most patients present with respiratory symptoms and cardiac failure in early infancy (Behrendt *et al.*, 1972; Hammon *et al.*, 1980). However, in spite of the presence of a major vascular malformation, clinical symptoms in the immediate postnatal period may be

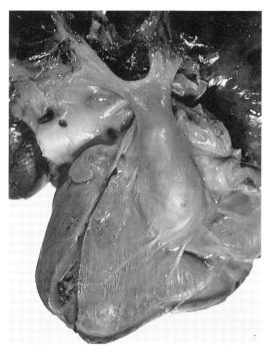

Figure 6.35 Posterior view of a heart with total anomalous pulmonary venous drainage into a markedly dilated coronary sinus.

either absent or quite non-specific, and so of no help in arriving at the diagnosis prior to autopsy (Byard & Moore, 1991). For example, 12 (23%) cases in an autopsy series of 52 infants presented as sudden and unexpected death with no significant antemortem symptoms (James *et al.*, 1994).

Pathological features

In otherwise normally formed hearts, the first indication of TAPVD at autopsy may be dilation and hypertrophy of the right atrium and ventricle, with engorgement of the major veins (see Figure 6.34). Once the pericardium has been removed completely, the heart will often be unusually mobile due to loss of the tethering effect normally provided by the pulmonary veins.

The marked variability in the arrangement of venous connections, coupled with great difficulties that occur in trying to reconstruct venous pathways

after evisceration of organs, makes careful *in situ* dissection particularly important in this entity (Devine, Debich & Anderson, 1991). It is also important to check for luminal narrowing at autopsy. In particular, postmortem angiography complements careful dissection and may be the only way to adequately demonstrate the site and degree of obstruction in cases of extrinsic compression. Silicone rubber casting is an alternative method for demonstrating luminal stenosis (Seo *et al.*, 1991).

Persistent obstruction may result in pulmonary hypertension due to increased venous pressure (Haworth & Reid, 1977), and so all lobes of the lung should be sampled adequately at autopsy to enable subsequent careful microscopic assessment of the morphology of the intrapulmonary vessels. Pulmonary hypertension has also been documented in scimitar syndrome, where there is partial anomalous pulmonary venous drainage from a hypoplastic right lung that receives a systemic arterial supply.

Pathophysiology

A major problem in children with TAPVD is blood flow obstruction within the common draining vein (Sano, Brawn & Mee, 1989). This is particularly so in cases where drainage is infradiaphragmatic, caused by extrinsic compression at the diaphragmatic hiatus (Figure 6.36), exacerbated by the greater length of the draining vein. Obstruction has also been reported in as many as 50% of cases where drainage occurs above the diaphragm due to segmental hypoplasia of the draining vein or to compression between the bronchi and pulmonary arteries. The importance of this phenomenon lies in the predisposition to death at an earlier age in children who have significant obstruction (Delisle *et al.*, 1976).

Associated features

Anomalous pulmonary venous drainage may be associated with the asplenia/polysplenia complex (Petersen & Edwards, 1983). It may also be found with other congenital heart defects, such as tetralogy of Fallot, double-outlet right ventricle, common atrioventricular canal, transposition of the great vessels, other venous anomalies, and pulmonary

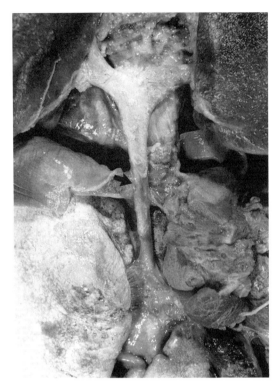

Figure 6.36 Infradiaphragmatic drainage in an infant with total anomalous pulmonary venous drainage with obstruction of the common vein at the level of the diaphragm (arrow).

stenosis/atresia (DeLeon *et al.*, 1987; Muster, Paul & Nikaidoh, 1973; Redington *et al.*, 1990). Anomalous pulmonary venous drainage has also been found in 8% of patients with hypoplastic left heart syndrome (Byard & Moore, 1991; Murphy, 1991). The presence of coexisting skeletal abnormalities should raise the possibility of Holt–Oram or Ellis–van Creveld syndromes (Husson & Parkman, 1961; Sahn *et al.*, 1981).

Vascular malformations

Vascular malformations may be responsible for rapid clinical deterioration and sudden death if there is significant spontaneous hemorrhage, particularly if this is intracranial (Figure 6.37) (Demick, 1991). While most affected children have symptoms and signs of raised intracranial pressure, subarachnoid hemorrhage, or convulsions for some time, death may occur within hours of sudden collapse (Byard, Bourne & Hanieh, 1991–2). This is dealt with in greater detail in Chapter 8.

Congenital arteriovenous malformations have also been documented as sites of origin of fatal pulmonary thromboemboli in the pediatric age group and should always be examined carefully at autopsy with this in mind (Byard & Cutz, 1990; Machin & Kent, 1989).

Aneurysms of major intracranial vessels may produce catastrophic hemorrhage in childhood (Meldgaard, Vesterby & Østergaard, 1997; Plunkett, 1999; Prahlow, Rushing & Barnard, 1998). In these cases, cystic renal disease or a positive family history may provide clues to the presence of cerebral vessel aneurysms as some cases appear to be inherited in an autosomal dominant fashion (McKusick, 1990). Vascular malformations of the coronary arteries may hemorrhage and cause fatal tamponade (Dancea *et al.*, 2002).

Kasabach-Merritt syndrome

Kasabach–Merritt syndrome is characterized by the appearance of large hemangiomas soon after birth associated with thrombocytopenia due to platelet entrapment and destruction. Further details may be found in Chapter 9.

Diffuse infantile hemangiomatosis

Diffuse infantile hemangiomatosis is a rare condition characterized by multiple hemangiomas of the skin and internal organs. It is associated with considerable morbidity and a relatively chronic course, with death usually resulting from high-output cardiac failure. Occasionally, death may occur with hemorrhage from vascular lesions, associated with thrombocytopenia, or from obstruction of the upper airway (Byard *et al.*, 1991a) (Figures 6.38 and 6.39).

Sturge-Weber syndrome

Sturge–Weber syndrome is one of the neurocutaneous syndromes, or phakomatoses, characterized

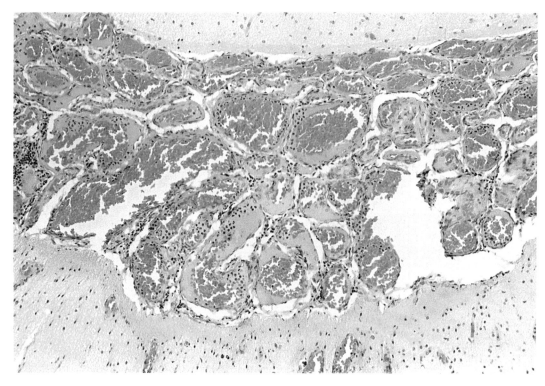

Figure 6.37 Abnormal and dilated vessels within the meninges of a seven-year-old girl who died from an intracranial hemorrhage (hematoxylin and eosin, ×60).

by unilateral hemangiomas of the face, neck, mucous membranes, and meninges. Although not usually considered a cause of sudden death, individuals with this syndrome suffer from epilepsy and sub-arachnoid hemorrhage associated with meningeal involvement.

Osler–Weber–Rendu syndrome

Osler–Weber–Rendu syndrome, or hereditary hem-orrhagic telangiectasia, is an autosomal dominant condition characterized by the presence of vascular malformations in a variety of organ systems (Byard, Schliebs & Koszyca, 2001).

Clinical features
Diagnostic criteria for Osler–Weber–Rendu syn-drome are slightly variable, with the diagnosis being

made when two of three criteria – mucocuta-neous telangiectasia, spontaneous epistaxis more than three times per month, and an affected parent (Sharma & Howden, 1998), or three of four criteria – telangiectasias at typical sites, recurrent sponta-neous epistaxis, a visceral manifestation, and an af-fected first-degree relative (Shovlin & Letarte, 1999) – are met. The incidence varies among communi-ties from two to 19 per 100,000 of the population (Kjeldsen, Vase & Green, 1999).

Studies have shown that 20% of affected individ-uals have lesions within the lungs, with the risk of pulmonary hemorrhage being present at any age, in-cluding early childhoood (Reyes-Mújica *et al.*, 1988). Pulmonary lesions may also be responsible for high-output cardiac failure due to shunting and may lead to paradoxical embolism to the brain, causing strokes or brain abscesses (Haitjema *et al.*, 1996). Pulmonary

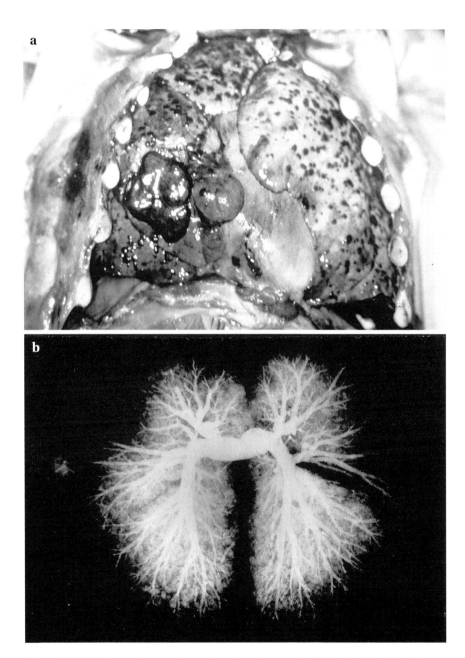

Figure 6.38 Multiple intrapulmonary hemangiomas in a four-month-old girl with diffuse infantile hemangiomatosis (a). Postmortem pulmonary angiography demonstrated multiple lesions throughout the lung parenchyma (b).

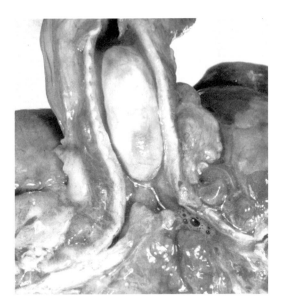

Figure 6.39 Obstruction of the lower trachea in an infant by a large intraluminal hemangioma.

hypertension may also develop. Intracerebral vascular malformations occur in 5–10% of cases and may cause epilepsy, hemorrhage, or ischemia from a vascular steal phenomenon (Shovlin & Letarte, 1999). Gastrointestinal hemorrhage is not usually a problem in children. Hepatic telangiectasia may be associated with fibrosis producing a "pseudocirrhosis" picture (Weik & Greiner, 1999).

Etiology

At least two gene loci have been implicated in the etiology of Osler–Weber–Rendu syndrome. A mutation on chromosome 9q3, which encodes for the protein endoglin, is responsible for Osler–Weber–Rendu 1, and a mutation on chromosome 12q causing defects in the activin receptor-like kinase 1 gene is responsible for Osler–Weber–Rendu 2 (Sharma & Howden, 1998; Shovlin, 1997). Both of these are highly expressed in endothelial cells and are involved in the regulation of endothelial cell migration, adhesion, and proliferation through transforming growth factor beta (Guttmacher, Marchuk & White, 1995).

Pathological features

Vascular lesions are caused by defects in vessel walls, resulting in dilation of postcapillary venules. These ectatic vessels arise in any tissues, particularly the skin, mucus membranes, lung, brain, and gastrointestinal tract, and may connect directly to dilated arterioles, resulting in arteriovenous shunting (Guttmacher, Marchuk & White, 1995).

While examination of the brain may reveal telangiectasias with evidence of previous hemorrhage, ischemia, or gliosis (Figure 6.40), symptomatic spinal cord lesions are rare (Mandzia *et al.*, 1999). Typical vascular malformations may also be found in the lungs (Figures 6.41 and 6.42), liver, skin, mucous membranes, kidneys, and bone (Shovlin, 1997).

Occurrence of sudden death

Despite assertions that individuals with Osler–Weber–Rendu syndrome usually have a normal life expectancy (Robbins, Cotran & Kumar, 1984), there is no doubt that the syndrome is associated with an increased mortality risk, particularly in those with manifestations in childhood (Byard, Schliebs & Koszyca, 2001; Kjeldsen, Vase & Green, 1999). Sudden death is rare but may be caused by a variety of mechanisms, as detailed in Table 6.7.

Malignant hemangioendothelioma

This exceedingly rare tumor of childhood has been associated with thrombocytopenia, high-output cardiac failure, cyanotic episodes, and death from massive exsanguination (Perrot, 1997).

Abnormalities of pulmonary vessels

Pulmonary hypertension

A sustained increase in blood pressure within the pulmonary arterial system from any cause will result in a series of characteristic microscopic changes (Edwards & Edwards, 1978b).

Clinical features

Symptoms in children with pulmonary hypertension vary depending partly on the etiology, but they

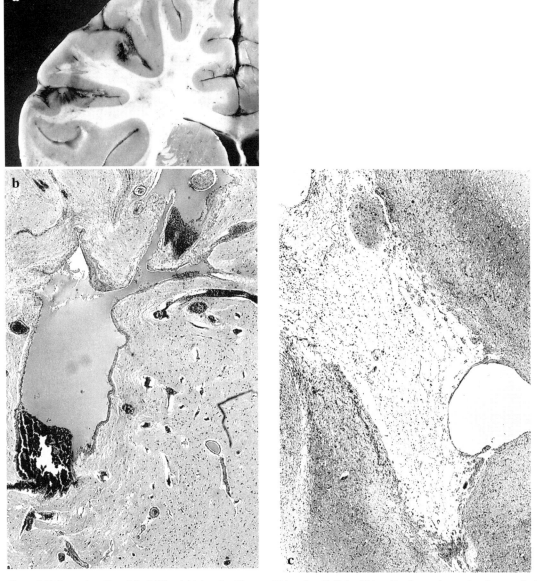

Figure 6.40 Coronal section of the left frontal lobe of an 18-year-old female with Osler–Weber–Rendu, syndrome showing a cortical vascular malformation (a). Irregularly dilated vascular spaces were found within the brain (b). Extensive areas of gliosis and cystic necrosis were also present (c) (hematoxylin and eosin, ×60).

often include syncope, dizziness, and dyspnea. In some cases, however, no warning symptoms or signs occur, and the first indication of pulmonary vascular pathology is the occurrence of sudden death (Ackermann & Edwards, 1987; Brown, Wetli & Davis, 1981; Robertson, 1971). This may occur at all ages from early infancy to later adult life. Thornback & Fowler (1975) documented sudden death in seven

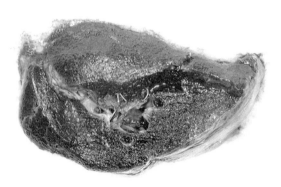

Figure 6.41 Section of the upper lobe of the left lung from the case shown in Figure 6.40, demonstrating a coiled embolizing wire within an arteriovenous malformation.

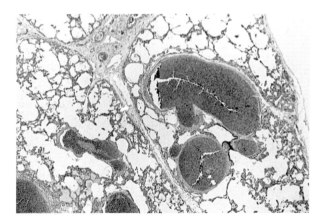

Figure 6.42 Histologic section of the lung of a six-year-old boy with Osler–Weber–Rendu syndrome, showing characteristic large dilated vascular spaces (hematoxylin and eosin, ×60).

(7.5%) of 93 patients with pulmonary hypertension, all of whom were under the age of 21 years. Cardiac catheterization and pregnancy are exacerbating factors that may precipitate unexpected death in these patients (Fuster *et al.*, 1984; Loyd, Primm & Newman, 1984).

Etiology

The etiology of some cases of pulmonary hypertension is poorly understood, resulting in an

Table 6.7. Causes of unexpected death in Osler–Weber–Rendu syndrome

Cerebral
Hemorrhage
Infection/abscess
Epilepsy
Pulmonary
Hemorrhage
Gastrointestinal
Hemorrhage

"idiopathic" group. Even in those cases with a known cause, the underlying pathophysiology may not be known completely. Generally, chronic pulmonary hypertension can be divided into six broad categories:

1 Primary idiopathic pulmonary hypertension, in which, by definition, the etiology is not known.
2 Hyperkinetic pulmonary hypertension, in which there is an increased pulmonary blood flow due to congenital cardiac defects, with left-to-right shunting.
3 Pulmonary hypertension associated with postcapillary obstruction.
4 Pulmonary hypertension associated with mechanical obstruction from embolic material.
5 Pulmonary hypertension associated with chronic hypoxia from disorders that interfere with normal oxygen exchange.
6 Miscellaneous.

(A more complete listing of these entities is given in Table 6.8.)

Pathological features

In longstanding cases of pulmonary hypertension, there is right ventricular hypertrophy with prominence of the infundibulum (Edwards, 1974) (Color Plate 13). Histologically, several classification systems have been proposed for the changes observed in the small pulmonary vessels. The widely used Heath–Edwards system (Heath & Edwards, 1958), based largely on observations of pulmonary hypertension due to shunting through septal defects, divides the pathological changes into six major groups:

Table 6.8. Causes of chronic pulmonary hypertension

Primary idiopathic pulmonary hypertension (plexogenic arteriopathy), persistent pulmonary hypertension of the newborn
Hyperkinetic pulmonary hypertension associated with congenital cardiac defects with left-to-right shunting, such as:
    ventricular septal defect (without pulmonary stenosis), transposition of the great vessels, patent ductus arteriosus, TAPVD, rarely atrial septal defect, and other more complex anomalies with shunts
Postcapillary obstruction due to:
    lesions such as cor triatriatum, mitral stenosis, aortic stenosis, aortic coarctation, sub- and supravalvular aortic stenosis, and hypertrophic or restrictive cardiomyopathy
    veno-occlusive disease
    other phenomena resulting in increased venous pressure, such as chronic left ventricular failure, mitral incompetence, aortic incompetence, TAPVD with obstruction, constrictive pericarditis, and mediastinal fibrosis or neoplasia
Mechanical arterial obstruction from:
    pulmonary thromboemboli, sickle cell disease, or foreign body material in intravenous drug abusers
Chronic hypoxia associated with:
    upper airway obstruction due to congenital webs, tracheomalacia, and tonsillar enlargement
    impaired chest expansion due to muscular dystrophy, poliomyelitis, and severe kyphoscoliosis
    reduced central respiratory drive
    high altitude
    destructive interstitial lung conditions, such as bronchopulmonary dysplasia, mucoviscidosis, and bronchiectasis, asthma, interstitial pneumonitis, Langerhan cell granulomatosis, post-irradiation change, meconium aspiration, cholesterol ester storage disease, and idiopathic pulmonary hemosiderosis
Miscellaneous conditions, such as:
    pulmonary vasculitis in cases of Wegener's granulomatosis, congenital pulmonary vascular anomalies, capillary hemangiomatosis, or in association with portal hypertension due to cirrhosis

Grade I: Medial hypertrophy of small, muscular pulmonary arteries (width of the media >7% of the artery's external diameter) (Wagenvoort & Wagenvoort, 1977). Smooth muscle also extends into the walls of the more peripheral arterioles.

Grade II: Intimal proliferation in small pulmonary arteries, with accumulation of subendothelial myofibroblasts.

Grade III: Marked concentric lamellar intimal fibrosis in addition to smooth muscle hypertrophy and intimal proliferation (Figure 6.43).

Grade IV: Dilation of small pulmonary arteries and arterioles, with plexiform lesions. These changes are found most often at a point just distal to the origin of smaller from larger arteries, and consist of aggregates of vascular channels within dilated muscular arteries that later become separated by fibrous tissue.

Grade V: Dilated vein-like branches from hypertrophied muscular arteries, with loss of media, which causes a resemblance to pulmonary veins. This results in the so-called "angiomatoid" lesion, which consists of a well-defined aggregate of thin-walled, vein-like vessels adjacent to a muscular artery (Figure 6.44). Prominent hemosiderin-containing macrophages within the alveoli at this stage result from rupture of these distended thin-walled vascular lesions.

Grade VI: Necrotizing vasculitis with prominent fibrinoid degeneration of muscular arteries and a transmural infiltrate of neutrophils. Eosinophils are occasionally seen in the inflammatory infiltrate, which progresses to granulation tissue formation.

Adequate sampling of the lung at autopsy should include portions from each lobe, as the extent of the pathological changes varies depending on the site from where the tissue was taken, and to some extent on the underlying etiological condition (Haworth & Reid, 1978).

The clinicopathological significance of the different Heath–Edwards grades in young children with cardiac shunts has been questioned, as muscularization of distal arterioles appears to be a more reliable indicator of severe pulmonary hypertension than the higher Heath–Edwards grades (Rabinovitch & Reid, 1981). An alternative grading system has therefore been proposed (Rabinovitch *et al.*, 1980) consisting of:

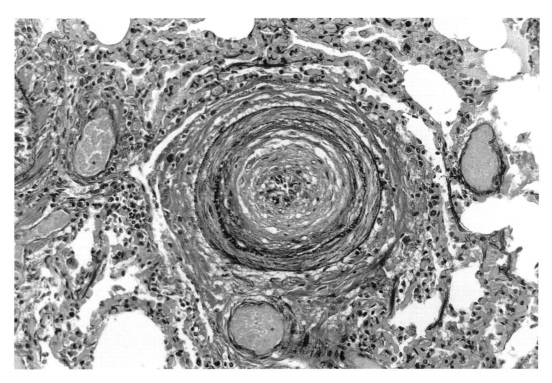

Figure 6.43 Pulmonary artery showing marked hypertensive changes with concentric intimal fibroplasia and smooth muscle hypertrophy within the media (elastin stain, ×110).

Grade A: Abnormal extension of smooth muscle into peripheral arteries.

Grade B: Increased medial thickness of muscular arteries.

Grade C: Increased medial thickness of muscular arteries plus reduction in the number of small peripheral arteries.

Occurrence of sudden death

While various theories have been proposed to explain the occurrence of sudden death in pulmonary hypertension, it is most likely that arrhythmias secondary to myocardial ischemia occur with increasing right ventricular strain. James (1962) proposed that similar changes to those present in the pulmonary arteries may be found in the atrioventricular nodal artery in the heart, resulting in nodal ischemia. An unusual case of death due to pulmonary artery dissection in a 17-year-old with complex congenital heart disease and pulmonary hypertension has also been reported (Walley, Virmani & Silver, 1990).

Idiopathic (plexogenic) pulmonary hypertension

Primary pulmonary hypertension (plexogenic pulmonary angiopathy) is a diagnosis of exclusion once congenital heart disease and other possible causes have been ruled out.

Clinical features

Although the clinical presentation is often of effort-related dyspnea, syncope, or fatiguability, with a steadily downhill course culminating in death after several years (Michael & Summer, 1985), sudden and unexpected death may occur in the pediatric age group (Brown, Wetli & Davis, 1981). The typical age range of presentation is from 16 to 40 years, but some patients are much younger than this. A female predominance noted in adults is not found in children (Wagenvoort & Wagenvoort, 1970).

Etiology
The etiology of primary pulmonary hypertension is unknown. The underlying pathophysiology may involve sustained vasoconstriction (Anderson, Simon & Reid, 1973; Haworth, 1983a; Haworth, 1983b) however, it is also possible that this represents a secondary phenomenon. Familial cases occur (Loyd, Primm & Newman, 1984).

Pathological features and differential diagnosis
Histologic changes including all of the Heath–Edwards grades may develop quite rapidly in childhood (Juaneda, Watson & Haworth, 1985), although advanced changes tend to be more common in adults (Yamaki & Wagenvoort, 1985). Absence of widespread fibrotic occlusion of pulmonary venules helps to distinguish primary from postcapillary obstructive causes of pulmonary hypertension, such as pulmonary veno-occlusive disease.

The presence of recent pulmonary thromboemboli is more suggestive of a thromboembolic etiology, which may be supported by a lack of true plexiform lesions. The presence of occasional focal areas of eccentric intimal fibroplasia and mural thrombi in cases of primary pulmonary hypertension may, however, make this distinction less easy. It has been suggested that this apparent overlap occurs because the pathogenesis of both entities is similar (Loyd *et al.*, 1988).

Hyperkinetic pulmonary hypertension
The majority of cases in this category result from shunting of blood from the left side of the heart to the right in congenital heart disease, with increased pulmonary vascular blood flow and intravascular pressures (Haworth, 1983c; Haworth *et al.*, 1977; Hoffman, Rudolph & Heymann, 1981). An example of this occurs when intrapulmonary pressures increase in transposition of the great vessels (Newfeld *et al.*, 1974; Viles, Ongley & Titus, 1969). The fact that pulmonary vascular changes may develop in infants with transposition and an intact ventricular septum

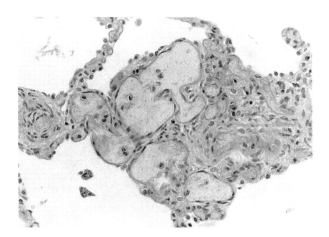

Figure 6.44 Angiomatoid lesion with numerous dilated thin-walled vessels adjacent to a muscular artery (hematoxylin and eosin, ×280).

prior to a significant increase in pulmonary arterial pressure implies that additional mechanisms may be involved in the generation of pulmonary hypertension in this malformation (Edwards & Edwards, 1978a; Newfeld *et al.*, 1979).

Pathological features
All grades of the Heath–Edwards classification may be found in cases of hyperkinetic pulmonary hypertension. However, while there are similarities with idiopathic pulmonary hypertension, the level at which shunting occurs and the age of the child may influence the type of morphological changes that develop (Haworth, 1984). Young children may not show the typical changes of the higher grades, despite having significantly elevated arterial pressures (Rabinovitch *et al.*, 1978). Although plexiform lesions have been documented in an eight-week-old girl with a patent ductus arteriosus and atrial and ventricular septal defects (Wagenvoort, 1973), most children under three years of age with septal defects do not show marked histologic changes (Bessinger, Blieden & Edwards, 1975). In particular, severe hypertensive changes are not usual in pretricuspid lesions, and marked medial hypertrophy is found most often in young children with ventricular (Haworth, 1984;

Haworth, 1987) rather than atrial septal defects (Wagenvoort *et al.*, 1961).

Pulmonary hypertension due to postcapillary obstruction

Pulmonary hypertension occurs in this group of diverse disorders due to obstruction of venous return. Lesions may be present within the heart (e.g. valve stenoses or cor triatriatum), within the pulmonary veins (e.g. TAPVD with obstruction), or within the smaller intrapulmonary veins (e.g. pulmonary veno-occlusive disease, *vide infra*) (Lucas *et al.*, 1962; Tandon & Kasturi, 1975). Hypertensive pulmonary changes may be found in very young infants who present with obstructive TAPVD (Haworth & Reid, 1977; Newfeld *et al.*, 1980) or with pulmonary vein stenosis (Presbitero, Bull & Macartney, 1983). Rarely, fibrosing mediastinitis may also result in pulmonary vein obstruction in childhood (Katzenstein & Mazur, 1980).

Pathological features

Histologic changes begin within the intrapulmonary veins, with intimal fibroelastosis, medial hypertrophy, and arterialization. However, cellular intimal proliferation is not found within the altered veins (Hutchins & Ostrow, 1976). There is geographic variability in the distribution of vascular lesions present in venous obstruction, with medial hypertrophy occurring in lower-lobe arteries and intimal fibrosis occurring in upper-lobe arteries (Wagenvoort, 1975). Intra-alveolar hemosiderin-containing macrophages are markers of longstanding chronic venous congestion, and alveolar septa may contain dilated lymphatics and increased fibrous tissue. Changes within the arteries and arterioles are generally grade III or lower.

Embolic causes of pulmonary hypertension

Recurrent thromboemboli, pulmonary hypertension, and sudden death may occur at quite young ages in children with ventriculoatrial shunts for hydrocephalus. Talc or mycotic emboli may be found in intravenous drug abusers, although their role in the causation of death has been questioned (Siegel, 1972), and reported cases have involved adults rather than children (Arnett *et al.*, 1976; Navarro *et al.*, 1984; Pare, Cote & Fraser, 1989). Foreign body granulomas of uncertain etiology, possibly related to intravenous infusions (Bowen *et al.*, 1981) or to surgical procedures (Favara & Moores, 1991), have been described in the lungs in children, although again their functional significance is far from clear. Recurrent emboli may also be associated with parasitic infestation in areas where schistosomiasis is endemic (Naeye, 1960). Hemoglobinopathies, such as sickle cell disease, may result in intravascular thrombosis within the lungs, with subsequent obstruction. Pulmonary vascular changes of sickle cell disease are illustrated in Figure 9.5.

Clinical features

A typical clinical history of recurrent pulmonary embolism with progressive dyspnea may not be obtained (Rich, Levitsky & Brundage, 1988), as recurrent thromboemboli may remain subclinical until established pulmonary hypertension produces sudden death. Such was the case of a three-year-old girl who had a ventriculoatrial shunt for hydrocephalus secondary to Arnold Chiari malformation and who died suddenly after apparently only one day of right heart failure. On the other hand, symptoms of episodic dyspnea that may have been noted prior to death may have been overlooked or ascribed to some other cause, such as asthma (Byard, 1996c).

Pathological features

The histological features of pulmonary thromboemboli vary depending on the age of the lesion. In the acute stage, recent thromboemboli will show laminated fibrin, platelet, and red blood cell bands (Figure 6.45). Later, organized lesions demonstrate fibrous obliteration of the lumina of small muscular arteries with recanalization (Figure 6.46). Eccentrically placed fibrous tissue and intimal aggregates are also characteristic of organized thromboemboli, although it has been noted that patients with idiopathic ("plexogenic") pulmonary hypertension may also have evidence of thromboemboli, with

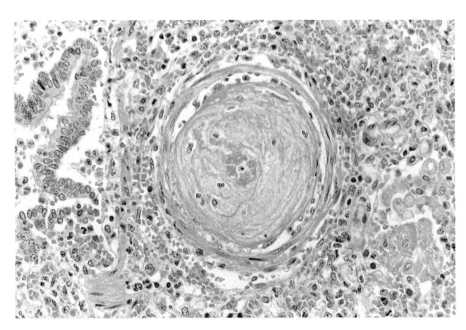

Figure 6.45 Recent pulmonary thromboembolus with surrounding intra-alveolar hemorrhage (hematoxylin and eosin, ×180).

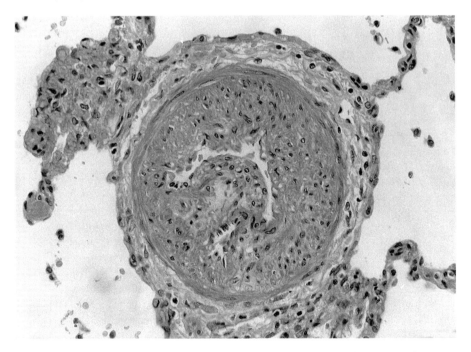

Figure 6.46 Recanalized pulmonary thromboembolus in an infant with pulmonary hypertension due to recurrent thromboembolism from a ventriculoatrial shunt inserted for hydrocephalus (hematoxylin and eosin, ×280).

occasional areas of focal eccentric intimal fibrosis (Wagenvoort, 1980).

Reactive arterial changes away from sites of thromboembolic occlusion usually consist of medial smooth muscle hypertrophy of the type seen in Heath–Edwards grades I and II. Concentric intimal fibroplasia and the plexiform and angiomatoid lesions of higher grades are not usually seen, although it may on occasion be difficult to distinguish a plexiform lesion from a recanalized thrombus.

Hypoxic causes of pulmonary hypertension

A wide variety of conditions in childhood associated with chronic hypoxia may cause pulmonary hypertension. These include bronchopulmonary dysplasia, idiopathic pulmonary hemosiderosis, and chronic destructive lung diseases such as cystic fibrosis, cholesterol ester storage disease, and Langerhan cell granulomatosis. Pulmonary hypertension in these cases is caused partly by destruction and fibrous obliteration of portions of the pulmonary capillary bed, as well as by sustained vasoconstriction (Wagenvoort & Wagenvoort, 1976). Restrictive lung disease in cases of severe scoliosis may also be associated with pulmonary arterial medial hypertrophy (Haworth, 1983a), and similar changes may be found within the pulmonary vasculature in high-altitude dwellers. The reasons for hypoxic pulmonary vasoconstriction, rather than vasodilation, are poorly understood (Kay, 1997).

Significant pulmonary hypertension with cor pulmonale may result from chronic upper-airway obstruction due to enlarged tonsils and adenoids (Bland, Edwards & Brinsfield, 1969; Levy *et al.*, 1967). Recurrent sleep apnea in children with Down syndrome has been proposed as a possible cause of pulmonary hypertension, particularly in cases where underlying cardiac defects are not severe (Loughlin, Wynne & Victorica, 1981).

Pathological features

Histologic changes found in pulmonary vessels consist primarily of medial hypertrophy of smaller pulmonary arteries, with muscularization of arterioles, sometimes also with a degree of medial hypertrophy of the pulmonary veins.

Miscellaneous causes of pulmonary hypertension

A variety of unrelated conditions, including Wegener granulomatosis, non-granulomatous arteritis, capillary hemangiomatosis, congenital alveolar dysplasia, Osler–Weber–Rendu syndrome, schistosomiasis, hydatid disease, collagen vascular disease, hemophilia, and portal hypertension associated with cirrhosis or portal vein thrombosis, may be found in conjunction with pulmonary hypertension, although several of these entities tend to effect mainly older individuals (Bjornsson & Edwards, 1985; Faber *et al.*, 1989; Gilsanz *et al.*, 1977; Heath & Reid, 1985; Katzenstein & Askin, 1990; Rich & Brundage, 1984; Silver *et al.*, 1992; Tron *et al.*, 1986).

Etiology

The etiology of pulmonary hypertension in many of these conditions is obscure. Destruction of the pulmonary capillary bed may be the basis of pulmonary hypertension in the vasculitides, while space-occupying aggregates of capillaries in hemangiomatosis may act as postcapillary obstructive lesions. Arteriovenous fistulae in Osler–Weber–Rendu syndrome may rarely cause pulmonary hypertension due to increased intrapulmonary blood flow and hypoxia.

The cause of pulmonary hypertension in patients with established portal hypertension (Moscoso *et al.*, 1991) and portal vein thrombosis or obstruction (Cohen *et al.*, 1983) is uncertain. It may be related to an as-yet-unidentified toxin that either is produced by or bypasses the liver, causing pulmonary vasoconstriction (Haworth, 1974; Kibria *et al.*, 1980). The condition is rare, with Rossi and colleagues (1992) finding only six other pediatric cases in the literature in addition to their own. Sudden death is, however, a possible outcome in children with portal hypertension who develop secondary pulmonary hypertension (Levine *et al.*, 1973).

A number of drugs, such as mitomycin, aminorex, carmustine, zinostatin, and bleomycin, and toxins, such as rapeseed oil, have been shown to cause pulmonary hypertension (Garcia-Dorado *et al.*, 1983).

Persistent pulmonary hypertension of the newborn

This entity represents persistence of fetal circulation in neonatal life and is thought to be a separate entity from primary idiopathic pulmonary hypertension. The morphology of the pulmonary arterial bed varies, with marked muscularization of distal pulmonary arterioles being found in only some cases. The remainder of cases have either underdeveloped or normal pulmonary arteries (Patterson, Kapur & Chandra, 1988). The condition is believed to be a response to sustained hypoxia and acidosis resulting from a number of diverse entities, including congenital diaphragmatic hernia, birth asphyxia, maternal drug ingestion, hyaline membrane disease, sepsis, congenital heart disease, meconium aspiration, and cystic adenomatoid malformation (Atkinson *et al.*, 1992; Graves, Redmond & Arensman, 1988; Meyrick & Reid, 1983; Tiefenbrunn & Riemenschneider, 1986). As right ventricular strain may develop in infants with this condition, there is a potential for sudden death due to arrhythmia.

Pulmonary veno-occlusive disease

Pulmonary veno-occlusive disease is a postcapillary cause of secondary pulmonary hypertension whose unique pathological features and association with sudden and unexpected death in both infancy and later childhood (Hasleton *et al.*, 1986) warrant separate description.

Clinical features

A significant number of patients with pulmonary veno-occlusive disease are under 16 years of age, although all ages are susceptible (Dail *et al.*, 1978). The sexes are affected equally. While the classical presentation is with increasing dyspnea, sometimes with a preceding flu-like illness and fever (Wagenvoort & Wagenvoort, 1977), cases have occurred in which the first manifestation is sudden and unexpected death

(Bolster, Hogan & Bredin, 1990; Cagle & Langston, 1984). In those cases investigated prior to autopsy, there may have been considerable difficulty in excluding primary idiopathic pulmonary hypertension or recurrent thromboembolic disease (Thadani *et al.*, 1975).

Etiology

The etiology of pulmonary veno-occlusive disease is not known, although infection and autoimmune disease have been suggested as causative agents. Familial cases have been reported (Hasleton *et al.*, 1986; Voordes, Kuipers & Elema, 1977), and lesions found at very early ages suggest that changes may begin during intrauterine life (Wagenvoort, Losekoot & Mulder, 1971). The presence of recognizable organizing mural thrombi with a preceding history of a mild febrile illness led to the hypothesis that the initial insult consisted of viral damage to pulmonary venular endothelium followed by thrombosis (Bolster, Hogan & Bredin, 1990), but not all cases demonstrate evidence of new and organizing thrombi (Stoler, Anderson & Stuard, 1982).

The possibility of damage due to circulating toxin has also been considered, based on cases of veno-occlusive disease of the liver associated with ingestion of *Crotalaria* alkaloids (Hughes & Rubin, 1986). These alkaloids have caused similar changes in the pulmonary veins of rats.

The possibility of several diverse etiologies has, therefore, led to the suggestion that pulmonary veno-occlusive disease is not a pure entity but represents a common end point for a variety of causative agents (Justo *et al*, 1993; Wagenvoort, 1976).

Pathological features and differential diagnosis

The most obvious changes occur within small intrapulmonary veins and venules, where there is marked intimal proliferation and fibrosis with occlusion of vessel lumina by loose edematous connective tissue. Residual occluded pulmonary veins may be obvious only if an elastin stain is used. The histologic changes are widespread, with involvement of up to 95% of venules and small veins. Prominent aggregates of intra-alveolar hemosiderin-containing macrophages may be present, as in idiopathic pulmonary hemosiderosis. In the latter entity, however, fibrous obliteration of pulmonary veins and hypertensive changes within pulmonary arteries are not seen.

In pulmonary veno-occlusive disease, pulmonary arteries do not show striking changes, with medial hypertrophy and some degree of intimal fibrosis occurring as secondary phenomena. A notable feature resulting from repeated hemorrhage is the presence of degenerating, iron-encrusted, basophilic elastic fibers within the walls of fibrotic veins, and within the interstitium, which may be associated with a foreign-body granulomatous inflammatory response. Perls stain for hemosiderin may be used to outline the wall of an affected vein in such cases. Other features that may be present are small paraseptal infarcts and dilation of the interstitial lymphatics.

The finding of widespread fibrotic obliteration of pulmonary venules helps to differentiate pulmonary veno-occlusive disease from other causes of postcapillary obstruction that may have induced pulmonary hypertension. Other possible diagnoses, such as primary idiopathic pulmonary hypertension and recurrent thromboembolic disease, will not show the profound venular fibrosis of pulmonary veno-occlusive disease.

Miscellaneous vascular conditions

Arterial dissection/rupture

The aorta and branches, including the ductus arteriosus, may dissect in childhood, with catastrophic results (Byard *et al.*, 1991c; Cooper, Lucke & Moseson, 1986; Nakashima *et al.*, 1990). In these cases, an underlying connective tissue disorder, such as Ehlers–Danlos or Marfan syndromes (Serry, Agomuoh & Goldin, 1988; Virmani & Forman, 1989), should always be considered, although the children may appear unremarkable on external examination (Coleman, 1955; Panja *et al.*, 1990). Sudden death may also occur in children with Ehlers–Danlos syndrome due to rupture of other large arteries such as the popliteal and subclavian (McFarland & Fuller, 1964). Pregnancy may predispose to dissection (Colman *et al.*, 2000), as in the case of a 20-year-old pregnant woman who dissected her peripheral pulmonary arteries (Figure 6.47). While no predisposing cause for dissection will be discovered in occasional cases even after careful investigation (York & Dimon, 1988), the possibility of an unknown defect in connective tissue remains (Nicod *et al.*, 1989).

Aortic dissection

Aortic dissection may occur in children with Turner syndrome, Marfan syndrome, Ehlers–Danlos syndrome, familial cystic medial necrosis (Cooper, Lucke & Moseson, 1986), and congenital cardiovascular malformations, such as coarctation (2% of cases) and bicuspid aortic valve (1% of cases) (Huntington & Hirst, 1967; Roberts & Roberts, 1991; Virmani & Forman, 1989). Other conditions predisposing to aortic dissection in children are cystinosis, rheumatic fever, Takayasu aortitis, and trauma (Fikar *et al.*, 1981). There is an association with cocaine usage and weightlifting (Fikar & Koch, 2000).

Carotid artery dissection

Spontaneous dissection of the carotid artery siphon has resulted in fatal stroke at an early age (Bergevin *et al.*, 1991). Postulated causes of intracranial artery dissection include trauma, intense physical exertion, fibromuscular dysplasia, congenital medial defects, homocystinuria (Jackson *et al.*, 1983; Manz, Vester & Lavenstein, 1979), and Moyamoya disease, a craniocentric arteriopathy that causes death through the development of multiple dissecting aneurysms (Pilz & Hartjes, 1976) (see Chapter 8). Usually, death in childhood cases of spontaneous carotid dissection is not sudden but occurs days to weeks after the onset of stroke (Hochberg *et al.*, 1975).

Coronary artery dissection

Spontaneous dissection of the coronary arteries is usually limited to young adult females, with one of the youngest reported cases involving a 17-year-old

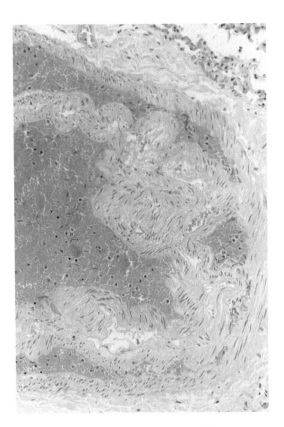 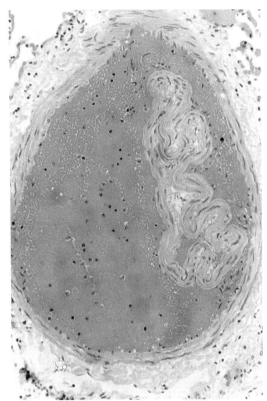

Figure 6.47 Spontaneous dissection of the peripheral pulmonary arteries in a young pregnant woman (hematoxylin and eosin, ×140).

girl (Cohle, Graham & Pounder, 1986; Glasgow, Tift & Alexander, 1984; Virmani *et al.*, 1984b). In adults, it may be associated with recent pregnancy or severe exercise (Ellis, Haywood & Monro, 1994).

Arterial fibromuscular dysplasia

This heterogeneous group of exceedingly rare and ill-understood entities demonstrates varying degrees of intimal and medial hyperplasia of the arteries, with luminal narrowing. Based on a study of renal artery dysplasia (Devaney *et al.*, 1991), the typical histologic changes consist of:
- intimal fibrous dysplasia
- medial fibrous dysplasia
- medial muscular dysplasia
- perimedial elastic dysplasia.

Fatal myocardial or cerebral infarction are frequent sequelae when coronary or cerebral vessels are involved. While it has been suggested that at least 85% luminal stenosis is necessary to cause sudden death in adults with ischemic atherosclerotic heart disease (Davies & Popple, 1979), it is uncertain whether this applies to children with stenoses due to fibromuscular dysplasia. Familial cases with sudden unexpected death in infancy may occur (Dominguez, Tate & Robinson, 1988).

Fibromuscular dysplasia may be idiopathic, associated with certain syndromes, or may occur secondary to known toxin exposure or metabolic defects. Although arterial fibrointimal proliferation represents a common end point for a wide variety of disease processes, pathologic effects usually derive from two basic mechanisms – arterial occlusion by the proliferating mural tissue (Arey & Segal, 1987) and spontaneous dissection (Lie & Berg, 1987).

Idiopathic fibromuscular dysplasia

Occlusive fibromuscular dysplasia most often occurs sporadically in middle-aged women involving the renal arteries, but it may be found in the coronary arteries and elsewhere in younger individuals (Price & Vawter, 1972; Siegal & Dunton, 1991). In infants and children, it may result in sudden and unexpected death (Arey & Segal, 1987; Siegal & Dunton, 1991; Strong *et al.*, 1970). Dominguez, Tate & Poppitti (1987) described a five-month-old girl who died suddenly while being fed and who had marked fibromuscular dysplasia of the coronary arteries associated with papillary muscle infarction. Fatal aortic dissection may also complicate generalized disease in later adolescence (Gatalica, Gibas & Martinez-Hernandez, 1992).

Pathological features
Large to medium-sized arteries in affected children have variable degrees of intimal proliferation (Figure 6.48) and medial hyperplasia. Arterial inflammation and calcification are not generally features of the proliferative mural tissue, which may be focal

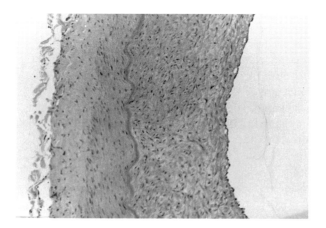

Figure 6.48 Idiopathic fibromuscular dysplasia in an adolescent, showing intimal thickening (hematoxylin and eosin, ×150).

and eccentric, or multifocal and circumferential in nature (Lüscher *et al.*, 1987).

Differential diagnosis
The histologic features of fibromuscular dysplasia are not specific. Similar changes have been reported in the coronary arteries in early infancy in association with congenital cardiac defects (MacMahon & Dickinson, 1967). Moyamoya disease also has similar arterial lesions (Yamashita *et al.*, 1984), as does progressive arterial occlusive (Kohlmeier–Degos) disease, which may affect the arteries of the gastrointestinal tract, eyes, central nervous system, and heart, in association with skin lesions (Sotrel, Lacson & Huff, 1983; Strole, Clark & Isselbacher, 1967). Fibrointimal proliferation may occur in vessels affected by Henoch–Schönlein purpura (Figure 6.49), resulting in tissue ischemia (Lipsett & Byard, 1995), or may represent a reactive response to adjacent infection (Figure 6.50).

Fibromuscular dysplasia associated with syndromes

Arterial fibrointimal proliferative lesions have been documented in a wide range of other inherited and genetically based syndromes, including tuberous sclerosis, neurofibromatosis, Alport syndrome, Down syndrome, progeria, and Friedreich ataxia (Fleisher, Buck & Cornfeld, 1978; Greene, Fitzwater & Burgess, 1974; Levin, Fellows & Abrams, 1978; Lüscher *et al.*, 1987; Nadas, Alimurung & Sieracki, 1951; Rolfes, Towbin & Bove, 1985). Patients with congenital rubella syndrome may also have similar arterial changes (Fortuin, Morrow & Roberts, 1971). Involvement of the renal arteries in these conditions may result in hypertension (Wallis, Deutsch & Azizi, 1970).

Fibromuscular dysplasia associated with metabolic conditions or toxin exposure

Metabolic disorders such as Hurler syndrome and homocystinuria may have associated proliferative arterial lesions (Schimke *et al.*, 1965) (see Figure 11.6). Similar changes occur from toxic exposure to arsenic (Rosenberg, 1974). Radiation may

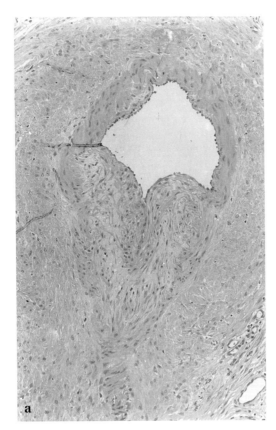 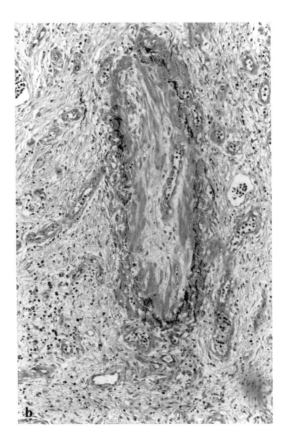

Figure 6.49 Eccentric fibrointimal proliferation of the intestinal vessels (a) of a five-year-old boy with Henoch–Schönlein purpura and bowel obstruction. Thrombotic obstruction with recanalization was also seen (b) (hematoxylin and eosin, ×140).

cause coronary arterial narrowing from intimal proliferation with medial and adventitial fibrosis and from accelerated atherosclerosis (Angelini, Benciolini & Thiene, 1985; Applefeld & Wiernik, 1983; Brosius, Waller & Roberts, 1981). De Sa (1979) reported proliferative intimal lesions in the coronary arteries of stillbirths and infants associated with ischemic myocardial damage, and suggested that the changes may have developed as a sequel to severe hypoxia.

Atherosclerosis

Although degenerative atherosclerotic vascular disease is generally a problem in older adults, patients with inherited disorders of lipid metabolism, such as hypercholesterolemia, and with diabetes mellitus may manifest atherosclerosis and its sequelae at quite early ages. Such sequelae include cerebral ischemic events in childhood (Daniels *et al.*, 1982; Glueck *et al.*, 1982). This is discussed further in Chapter 11.

Premature atherosclerosis with its attendant cardiovascular complications has also been described in Cockayne and Hutchinson–Gilford (progeria) syndromes (Gabr *et al.*, 1960). Children with progeria, a rare syndrome characterized by dwarfism and premature aging, have hyperlipidemia and die in childhood or early adolescence (Atkins, 1954; Makous *et al.*, 1962; Reichel & Garcia-Bunuel, 1970). Premature atherosclerosis may also be found in Werner syndrome, although cardiac changes may occur in

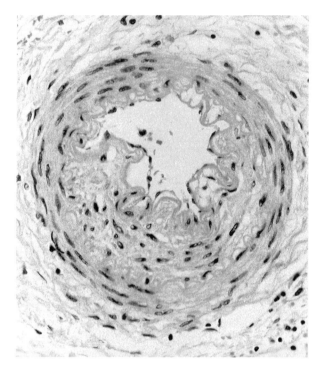

Figure 6.50 Fibrointimal proliferation within a meningeal arteriole in a case of chronic meningitis in a young boy (hematoxylin and eosin, ×280).

the absence of atherosclerosis in these children (Tri & Combs, 1978). Sudden death has been documented in children with all of these conditions (Lambert *et al.*, 1974). Sudden death during late adolescence may also occur rarely from ischemic heart disease due to atherosclerotic plaques in the absence of evidence of hyperlipidemia (Koskenvuo, Karvonen & Rissanen, 1978).

Cerebral sinus thrombosis

Thrombosis of the cerebral sinuses occurs as a secondary phenomenon and may result in death if the degree of thrombosis is substantial. Dehydration from fulminant gastroenteritis in infants may result in quite rapid demise from cerebral sinus thrombosis, with or without adjacent brain infarc-

tion. Other diverse disorders associated with thrombotic phenomena include cyanotic congenital heart disease and hematological conditions such as sickle cell disease and familial hypercoagulable syndromes (Abrantes *et al.*, 2002; Nuss, Hays & Manco-Johnson, 1995) (see Chapters 5 and 9).

Acquired immunodeficiency syndrome

Vascular involvement may occur in children with AIDS, resulting in death due to coronary artery occlusion or to intracerebral hemorrhage or ischemia. This is discussed further in Chapter 4.

Connective tissue disorders

Sudden death may occur in the pediatric age range from disorders of connective tissue such as Marfan or Ehlers–Danlos syndromes due to inherent weaknesses in the walls of arteries and arterioles resulting in spontaneous rupture and hemorrhage (Byard, Keeley & Smith, 1990). Death may occur before the condition has been diagnosed and may be due to subarachnoid hemorrhage from intracranial bleeding or from major arterial dissection. Marfan syndrome also has an association with bicuspid aortic valve (Emanuel *et al.*, 1978) and with left ventricular outflow disease in the form of supravalvular aortic stenosis (Peterson, Todd & Edwards, 1965).

Hepatic vein thrombosis/Budd-Chiari syndrome

Thrombosis of the hepatic vein (Budd–Chiari syndrome) is a rare disorder in early childhood that may be associated with trauma (Powell-Jackson *et al.*, 1982). Although the course is often chronic, rapid deterioration may occur over a period of days. Alternatively, it has been reported as a cause of sudden death in infancy with minimal preceding symptoms or signs (Carlson, Arya & Gilbert, 1985). The etiology of the venous thrombosis in the latter report is uncertain.

Hypertension

While hypertensive disorders are not common in childhood, there are a number of well-defined entities, some of which have already been described in detail, that are associated with significant systemic hypertension (Eden, Sills & Brown, 1977; Loggie, 1969; Loggie, New & Robson, 1979; Londe, 1978; Sumboonnanonda et al., 1992). These can be grouped into the categories listed in Table 6.9. The possibility of intracerebral hemorrhage in these cases warrants their consideration as potential causes of sudden death in children.

Embolic phenomena

Thromboembolism

Pulmonary thromboembolism
Massive pulmonary embolism is a well-recognized cause of sudden and unexpected death in adults due to sudden obstruction of the pulmonary outflow tract with acute right ventricular decompensation (Becker, Graor & Holloway, 1984). This is a less frequent phenomenon in children and infants (Champ & Byard, 1994; de la Grandmaison & Durigon, 2002; Evans & Wilmott, 1994; Freeman, 1999) and is often not considered in cases of sudden death even when known predisposing conditions are present.

Various autopsy studies have demonstrated that pulmonary thromboembolism is a relatively rare event in children, having a frequency of between 0.73% and 4.2% (Buck et al., 1981; Jones & Sabiston, 1966). The percentage of cases in which pulmonary thromboembolism has caused sudden death has varied considerably in different studies, with Emery (1962) reporting sudden collapse and death in more than 60% of children in a series of 25 cases with pulmonary thromboembolism, compared with Buck and colleagues (1981), who found embolism a causal factor in death in only 31% of their 116 cases accumulated over a 25-year period. In a series of 24,250 hospitalized patients aged between 12 and 21 years, only 10 patients aged 19 years or younger were found (Bernstein, Coupey & Schonberg, 1986).

In a study from Canada, Byard & Cutz (1990) found only eight cases of sudden unexpected death due to pulmonary thromboembolism in a total of 17,500 autopsies (0.05%) over a 50-year period.

The factors predisposing to thromboembolism in infants and children are similar to those causing thromboembolism in adults, and included in-dwelling central venous catheters, sepsis, inflammatory bowel disease, recent surgery, prolonged immobility, and occult metastatic carcinoma (Rubinstein, Murray & Hoffstein, 1988) (Table 6.10). Similarly, in three patients aged 16 years or younger in Bernstein, Coupey & Schonberg's study (1986), surgery, trauma, rheumatic heart disease, sepsis, and inflammatory bowel disease were predisposing factors. The mortality rate in this latter group was 33%. Parenteral alimentation, central venous catheterization, and ventriculoatrial shunts (Figure 6.51) have been associated with sudden death in a small number of infants and children due to pulmonary embolism (Firor, 1972; Müller & Blaeser, 1976; Nichols & Tyson, 1978). Ventriculoatrial shunts may also result in death from the more chronic effects of pulmonary hypertension (McMahon & Aterman, 1978). Color Plate 14 and Figures 6.52–6.54 demonstrate massive pulmonary thromboemboli causing sudden death in early infancy and childhood due to a variety of conditions.

It is worthwhile reviewing the clinical and family histories of young patients who die suddenly from massive pulmonary thromboemboli. For example, a 21-year-old man with spina bifida and a ventriculoatrial shunt for hydrocephalus who died suddenly from a large pulmonary thromboembolus was found at autopsy to have numerous old and organized pulmonary emboli with arterial recanalization. Previous episodes of shortness of breath during adolescence had been attributed to asthma; however, there was no evidence of asthma, grossly or microscopically, at autopsy (Byard, 1996c) (Figure 6.55). The possibility of an hereditary condition predisposing to thrombosis, such as lupus anticoagulant, deficiencies of protein C or S, or factor V Leiden or prothrombin gene mutations, should also be considered (Heller et al.,

Table 6.9. Causes of hypertension in childhood

Vascular	Renal	Metabolic	Endocrine	Neurologic	Hematologic	Infective	Miscellaneous
Takayasu aortitis	Acute and chronic renal disorders such as:	Several of the mucopolysaccharidoses	Congenital adrenal hyperplasia	Poliomyelitis	Anemia	Subacute bacterial endocarditis	Heavy metal poisoning
Middle aortic syndrome	Hemolytic-uremic syndrome	Hypercalcemia	Cushing disease	Neurofibromatosis	Polycythemia		Steroid ingestion
Aortic coarctation	Glomerulonephritis	Diabetes mellitus	Pheochromocytoma	Guillain–Barré syndrome	Leukemia		Following genitourinary surgery
Fibromuscular dysplasia	Pyelonephritis	Porphyria	Hyperthyroidism	Dysautonomia			Burns
Pseudoxanthoma elasticum	Henoch–Schönlein purpura		Hyperparathyroidism	Associated with disorders causing raised intracranial pressure			Pregnancy
Radiation aortitis	Obstructive uropathy		Neuroblastoma				Stevens–Johnson syndrome.
Patent ductus arteriosus	Congenital hypoplastic or polycystic kidneys		Primary hyperaldosteronism				
Arteriovenous fistula	Medullary cystic disease						
	Renal artery anomalies						
	Renal artery thrombosis						
	Tumors						
	Fabry disease						
	Alport disease						
	Systemic lupus erythematosis						
	Polyarteritis nodosa						
	Following transplantation						

Table 6.10. Clinicopathologic features of a series of infants and children dying of pulmonary thromboembolism

Age/Sex	Primary disease	Presentation	Origin of thromboembolus	Infarct	Cause of death	Additional features
1 month F	Epidermolysis bullosa	SUD in sleep	Innominate vein catheter	–	Massive recent bilateral PTE	Multifocal organized small thromboemboli, recent sepsis
15 months F	Restrictive cardiomyopathy	SUD	Right atrium	–	Massive recent bilateral PTE	–
18 months M	Tetralogy of Fallot	Several hours of respiratory distress, SUD	Right ventricle	–	Massive recent bilateral PTE	Surgical repair 12 days before death
4 years F	Bronchopneumonia	SUD	Not found	+	Multifocal recent PTE	Recent infarct of lower lobe, septicemia (*Escherichia coli*)
4 years M	Arteriovenous malformations in left leg and perineum	SUD	Arteriovenous malformations in leg and perineum	–	Massive recent bilateral PTE	Congenital hypothyroidism, surgical repair of leg lesion 5 days before death
10 years M	Poliomyelitis/paraplegia (1-year duration)	SUD	Right profunda femoris vein	–	Massive recent bilateral PTE	–
13 years F	Dystonia musculorum deformans	SUD	Not found	–	Multifocal bilateral recent PTE	–
13 years F	Crohn disease	SUD	Subclavian vein catheter	–	Massive recent left-sided PTE	Pelvic abscess, hyperalimentation, papillary carcinoma of thyroid

PTE, pulmonary thromboembolism; SUD, sudden unexpected death.

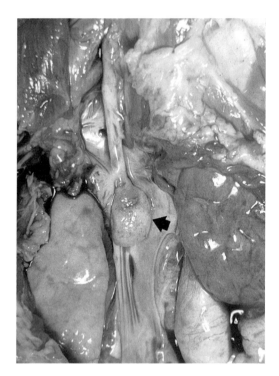

Figure 6.51 An organized thrombus (arrow) adherent to the tip of a ventriculoatrial catheter in a child with Arnold–Chiari malformation and obstructive hydrocephalus.

2000; Nuss, Hays & Manco-Johnson, 1995; Segel & Francis, 2000; Thomas, 2001).

Arteriovenous malformations and congenital cardiac anomalies are two conditions associated with thromboembolism that are more likely to be found in the pediatric age group than in adults. Children who have a communication from the right side to the left side of the heart may develop paradoxical embolism and sudden death due to cerebral infarction.

Coronary artery thromboembolism

Although coronary artery embolism appears to be a disease mainly of adult life, sudden death may occur rarely in childhood due to emboli associated with infective endocarditis (Bor, 1969). Two children aged 10 months and 12 years, respectively, have been reported who suffered infarcts attributed to

thromboemboli derived from left ventricular thrombi associated with underlying myocarditis (Celermajer *et al.*, 1991). Theoretically, any intracavity neoplasm or any of the causes of intracardiac mural thrombi (Roberts, 1978) could give rise to coronary embolism in younger age groups. An example of fatal coronary artery embolization in a six-year-old girl with acute rheumatic fever is illustrated in Figure 4.6. Underlying congenital heart disease may also act as a source of thromboemboli, as in the case of an 18-year-old adolescent with Down syndrome and a complete atrioventricular canal defect with associated Eisenmenger complex who died of a myocardial infarct following left anterior coronary artery embolization (Stahl, Santos & Byard, 1995) (Figure 6.56).

Spontaneous thrombosis of coronary arteries may occur in Kawasaki disease or in children with thrombocytosis (Spach, Howell & Harris, 1963). Paradoxical embolism with subsequent myocardial infarction has been reported in both childhood and very early infancy (Berry, 1970; Brown, 1974; Kilbride *et al.*, 1980).

Mycotic embolism

One of the most common causes of microbiological thromboembolism nowadays involves opportunistic fungi in immunocompromised children on chemotherapy for malignancy (Byard *et al.*, 1987). The likelihood of fungal thromboemboli is highest in febrile, neutropenic children with treated acute leukemia and who have recently received antibiotics. In spite of the extensive literature, however, cases still occur in which fungal thromboemboli are a "surprise" finding at autopsy. Postmortem blood cultures should include arterial blood, as it is possible that thread-like fungal hyphae may be filtered from venous blood by the capillary bed, thus rendering venous blood cultures inadequate for microbiological assessment (Byard, 1989).

Septic thromboemboli due to infection are also found occasionally in children with bacterial endocarditis (Schwöbel & Stauffer, 1983), often in association with congenital structural defects or prosthetic material.

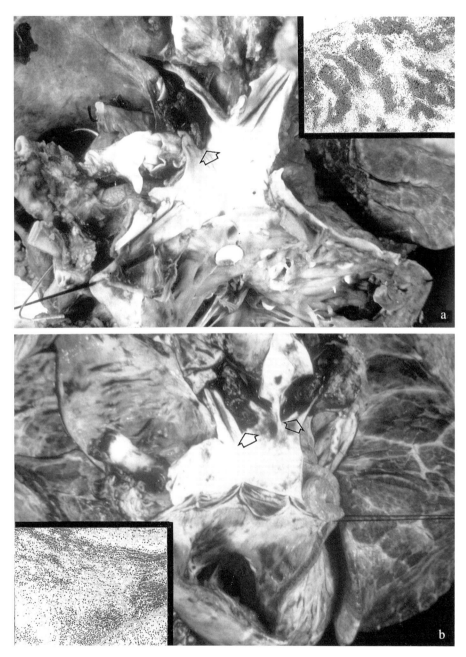

Figure 6.52 Large pulmonary thromboembolus (arrow) within the right main pulmonary artery of an 18-month-old boy with a recent surgical repair of a tetralogy of Fallot (a). Bilateral pulmonary thromboemboli (arrows) present in a four-year-old girl with bronchopneumonia (b).

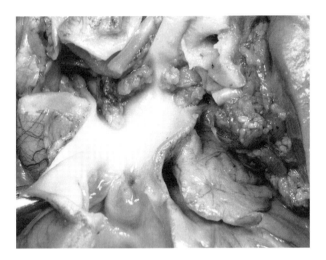

Figure 6.53 Fatal pulmonary thromboembolism in an infant following successful small-intestinal resection for necrotizing enterocolitis.

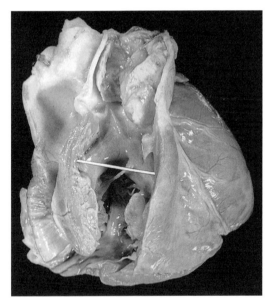

Figure 6.54 Fatal saddle pulmonary thromboembolism in an infant with undiagnosed idiopathic arterial calcification.

Parasitic thromboembolism is more prevalent in tropical regions, where children with schistosomiasis or cerebral malaria may develop occluded vessels. This possibility should be considered in ill children who have a history of recent travel to endemic areas.

An unusual case of sudden death due to rupture of a left ventricular hydatid cyst with embolization of material into both middle cerebral arteries has been reported in a previously well seven-year-old boy who lived in a rural Australian sheep-raising community (see Figure 4.31) (Byard & Bourne, 1991). Cardiac involvement in hydatid disease in childhood is quite rare, being present in less than 5% of cases (Auldist & Myers, 1974; Slim & Akel, 1982). Consequently, the likelihood of rupture causing fatal embolism is extremely unlikely, although embolism of hydatid debris to the brain, periphery, and lungs have all been documented in adults (Buris, Takacs & Varga, 1987).

Tumor embolism

The most common type of childhood tumor associated with embolic phenomenon is nephroblastoma/Wilms' tumor (Akyön & Arslan, 1981), although intraoperative embolization of hepatoblastoma has also been described (Dorman, Sumner & Spitz, 1985). Embolization in the case of Wilms' tumor is a direct result of the tumor's angio-invasive nature, with its propensity to grow into the renal vein and thence into the inferior vena cava. Cases have even been documented in which a tongue of tumor has extended as far as the right atrium (Anselmi *et al.*, 1970). In such an instance, it is not difficult to imagine a terminal portion of the tumor breaking off and embolizing to the pulmonary vessels. If the fragment is large, then saddle embolism may occur, with impaction of the tumor at the bifurcation of the pulmonary artery resulting in sudden death. Such a case is illustrated in Figure 10.24. Paradoxical tumor embolism may occur if there is a congenital communication between the right and left sides of the heart (see Figure 10.25) (Moore & Byard, 1992a). Cerebral embolism may also result from fragmentation of pulmonary metastases (Chan *et al.*, 1985). Fatal embolization of embryonal carcinoma of the testis and seminoma has been reported in young adults (Aronsohn & Nishiyama, 1974; Saukko & Lignitz, 1990).

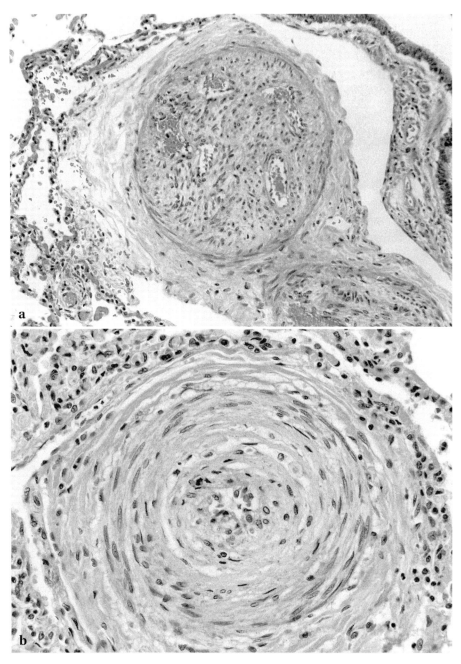

Figure 6.55 A recanalized pulmonary artery in a 21-year-old male with recurrent thromboembolism from a ventriculoatrial catheter (×180) (a). Marked fibrointimal proliferation in pulmonary vessels in a three-year-old girl with recurrent thromboembolism from a ventriculoatrial catheter (b) (hematoxylin and eosin, ×280).

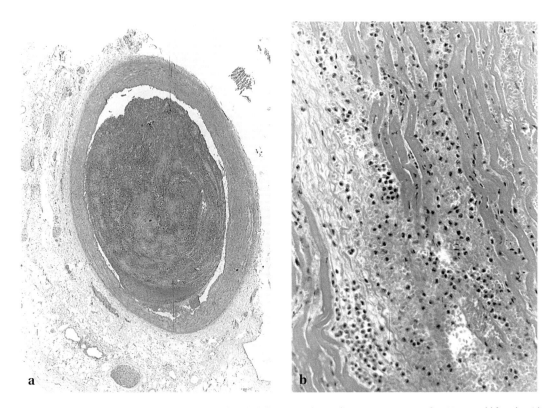

Figure 6.56 Coronary artery thromboembolism within the left anterior descending coronary artery of an 18-year-old female with congenital heart disease (×30) (a). The myocardium distal to the occlusion demonstrated changes of acute myocardial infarction (b) (hematoxylin and eosin, ×160).

Obstetrical embolism

Obstetrical sudden death must be considered a possibility in sexually mature adolescents, and a certain number of these include embolic deaths. Material such as amniotic fluid and trophoblast may embolize to the lungs, resulting in sudden collapse and death (Anonymous, 1979; Cohle & Petty, 1985) (see Chapter 10).

Fat embolism

Fat embolism occurs most often in children following trauma and may result in death (Weisz *et al.*, 1974) (see Chapter 2). It has also been reported in infants during prolonged intravenous lipid administration, and it may occur in children with hemoglobinopathies, sometimes associated with viral infection (Barson, Chiswick & Doig, 1978; Kolquist *et al.*, 1996).

Behçet disease

This systemic vasculitis is characterized by mucosal ulcers, arthralgia, uveitis, and thrombophlebitis. Although usually a disease of adults, 1–3% of cases occur in childhood. Pulmonary artery involvement may result in aneurysm formation, with lethal hemoptysis, as occurred in a 10-year-old boy illustrated in Figure 6.57. Other potentially lethal manifestations include aortitis with aneurysm formation and myocarditis (Cohle & Colby, 2002).

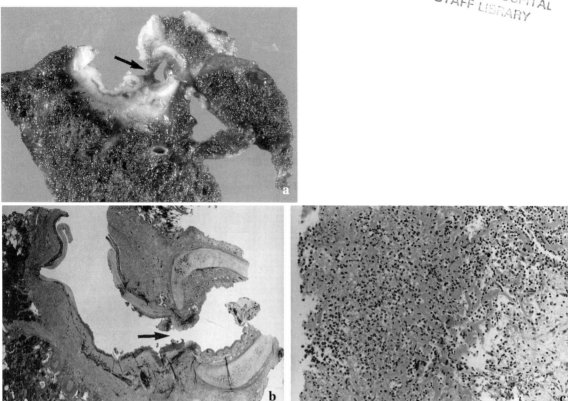

Figure 6.57 Section of lung from a 10-year-old boy with Behçet disease who died following massive hemoptysis. An inflammatory aneurysm of the pulmonary artery had eroded into an adjacent bronchus (arrow) (a). Wholemount section demonstrates the area of erosion (arrow) (b). Section of the wall of the aneurysm, demonstrating necrotic and inflammatory debris (c) (hematoxylin and eosin, ×110).

REFERENCES

Abrantes, M., Lacerda, A. F., Abreu, C. R., *et al.* (2002). Cerebral venous sinus thrombosis in a neonate due to factor V Leiden deficiency. *Acta Paediatrica*, **91**, 243–5.

Ackermann, D. M. & Edwards, W. D. (1987). Sudden death as the initial manifestation of primary pulmonary hypertension. Report of four cases. *American Journal of Forensic Medicine and Pathology*, **8**, 97–102.

Akagi, T., Rose, V., Benson, L. N., Newman, A. & Freedom, R. M. (1992). Outcome of coronary artery aneurysms after Kawasaki disease. *Journal of Pediatrics*, **121**, 689–94.

Akyön, M. G. & Arslan, G. (1981). Pulmonary embolism during surgery from a Wilms' tumour (nephroblastoma): case report. *British Journal of Anaesthesia*, **53**, 903–4.

Amano, S., Hazama, F., Kubagawa, H., *et al.* (1980). General pathology of Kawasaki disease: on the morphological alterations corresponding to the clinical manifestations. *Acta Pathologica Japanonica*, **30**, 681–94.

Ammann, A. J., Wara, D. W., Cowan, M. J., Barrett, D. J. & Stiehm, E. R. (1982). The DiGeorge syndrome and the fetal alcohol syndrome. *American Journal of Diseases of Children*, **136**, 906–8.

Anderson, E. G., Simon, G. & Reid, L. (1973). Primary and thrombo-embolic pulmonary hypertension: a quantitative pathological study. *Journal of Pathology*, **110**, 273–93.

Anderson, K. A., Burbach, J. A., Fenton, L. J., Jaqua, R. A. & Barlow, J. F. (1985). Idiopathic arterial calcification of infancy in newborn siblings with unusual light and electron microscopic manifestations. *Archives of Pathology and Laboratory Medicine*, **109**, 838–42.

Anderson, K. R., McGoon, D. C. & Lie, J. T. (1978). Vulnerability of coronary arteries in surgery for transposition of the great arteries. *Journal of Thoracic and Cardiovascular Surgery*, **76**, 135–9.

Angelini, A., Benciolini, P. & Thiene, G. (1985). Radiation induced coronary obstructive atherosclerosis and sudden death in a teenager. *International Journal of Cardiology*, **9**, 371–3.

Angelini, P. (1989). Normal and anomalous coronary arteries: definition and classification. *American Heart Journal*, **117**, 418–34.

Anonymous. (1975). Sudden death in children with heart disease. *British Medical Journal*, **i**, 1–2.

Anonymous. (1979). Amniotic fluid embolism. *Lancet*, **i**, 398–400.

Anselmi, G., Suarez, J. A., Machado, I., Moleiro, F. & Blanco, P. (1970). Wilms' tumour propagated through the inferior vena cava into the right heart cavities. *British Heart Journal*, **32**, 575–8.

Applefeld, M. M. & Wiernik, P. H. (1983). Cardiac disease after radiation therapy for Hodgkin's disease: analysis of 48 patients. *American Journal of Cardiology*, **51**, 1679–81.

Arey, J. B. & Segal, R. (1987). Case 4. Fibromuscular dysplasia of intramyocardial coronary arteries. *Pediatric Pathology*, **7**, 97–103.

Arnett, E. N., Battle, W. E., Russo, J. V. & Roberts, W. C. (1976). Intravenous injection of talc-containing drugs intended for oral use. A cause of pulmonary granulomatosis and pulmonary hypertension. *American Journal of Medicine*, **60**, 711–18.

Aronsohn, R. S. & Nishiyama, R. H. (1974). Embryonal carcinoma. An unexpected cause of sudden death in a young adult. *Journal of the American Medical Association*, **229**, 1093–4.

Atkins, L. (1954). Progeria. Report of a case with postmortem findings. *New England Journal of Medicine*, **250**, 1065–9.

Atkinson, J. B., Ford, E. G., Kitagawa, H., Lally, K. P. & Humphries, B. (1992). Persistent pulmonary hypertension complicating cystic adenomatoid malformation in neonates. *Journal of Pediatric Surgery*, **27**, 54–6.

Auldist, A. W. & Myers, N. A. (1974). Hydatid disease in children. *Australian and New Zealand Journal of Surgery*, **44**, 402–7.

Avner, J. R., Shaw, K. N. & Chin, A. J. (1989). Atypical presentation of Kawasaki disease with early development of giant coronary artery aneurysms. *Journal of Pediatrics*, **114**, 605–6.

Backer, C. L., Ilbawi, M. N., Idriss, F. S. & DeLeon, S. Y. (1989). Vascular anomalies causing tracheoesophageal compression. Review of experience in children. *Journal of Thoracic and Cardiovascular Surgery*, **97**, 725–31.

Bader-Meunier, B., Hadchouel, M., Fabre, M., Arnoud, M. D. & Dommergues, J. P. (1992). Intrahepatic bile duct damage in children with Kawasaki disease. *Journal of Pediatrics*, **120**, 750–52.

Bahn, R. C., Edwards, J. E. & DuShane, J. W. (1951). Coarctation of the aorta as a cause of death in early infancy. *Journal of Pediatrics*, **8**, 192–203.

Baltaxe, H. A. & Wixson, D. (1977). The incidence of congenital anomalies of the coronary arteries in the adult population. *Radiology*, **122**, 45–52.

Baroldi, G. (1991). Diseases of extramural coronary arteries. In *Cardiovascular Pathology*, 2nd edn, vol. 1, ed. M. D. Silver. New York: Churchill Livingstone, pp. 487–563.

Barron, K. S., Murphy, D. J., Jr, Silverman, E. D., *et al.* (1990). Treatment of Kawasaki syndrome: a comparison of two dosage regimens of intravenously administered immune globulin. *Journal of Pediatrics*, **117**, 638–44.

Barson, A. J., Chiswick, M. L. & Doig, C. M. (1978). Fat embolism in infancy after intravenous fat infusions. *Archives of Disease in Childhood*, **53**, 218–23.

Barth, C. W., III & Roberts, W. C. (1986). Left main coronary artery originating from the right sinus of Valsalva and coursing between the aorta and pulmonary trunk. *Journal of the American College of Cardiology*, **7**, 366–73.

Barth, C. W., III, Bray, M. & Roberts, W. C. (1986). Sudden death in infancy associated with origin of both left main and right coronary arteries from a common ostium above the left sinus of Valsalva. *American Journal of Cardiology*, **57**, 365–6.

Basso, C., Frescura, C., Corrado, D., *et al.* (1995). Congenital heart disease and sudden death in the young. *Human Pathology*, **26**, 1065–72.

Becker, A. E. & Anderson, R. H. (1981). Malformations of the aortic arch. In *Pathology of Congenital Heart Disease*. London: Butterworth, pp. 321–9.

Becker, A. E., Becker, M. J. & Edwards, J. E. (1972). Mitral valvular abnormalities associated with supravalvular aortic stenosis. Observations in 3 cases. *American Journal of Cardiology*, **29**, 90–94.

Becker, R. C., Graor, R. & Holloway, J. (1984). Pulmonary embolism: a review of 200 cases with emphasis on pathophysiology, diagnosis and treatment. *Cleveland Clinical Quarterly*, **51**, 519–29.

Behrendt, D. M., Aberdeen, E., Waterson, D. J. & Bonham-Carter, R. E. (1972). Total anomalous pulmonary venous drainage in infants. I. Clinical and hemodynamic findings, methods, and results of operation in 37 cases. *Circulation*, **46**, 347–56.

Benge, W., Martins, J. B. & Funk, D. C. (1980). Morbidity associated with anomalous origin of the right coronary artery from the left sinus of Valsalva. *American Heart Journal*, **99**, 96–100.

Benson, P. A. & Lack, A. R. (1968). Anomalous aortic origin of left coronary artery. Report of two cases. *Archives of Pathology*, **86**, 214–16.

Berdon, W. E., Baker, D. H., Wung, J. F., *et al.* (1984). Complete cartilage-ring tracheal stenosis associated with anomalous left pulmonary artery: the ring-sling complex. *Pediatric Radiology*, **152**, 57–64.

Bergevin, M. A., Daugherty, C. C., Bove, K. E. & McAdams, A. J. (1991). The internal carotid artery siphon in children and adolescents. *Human Pathology*, **22**, 603–6.

Bernstein, D., Coupey, S. & Schonberg, S. K. (1986). Pulmonary embolism in adolescents. *American Journal of Diseases of Children*, **140**, 667–71.

Berry, C. L. (1970). Myocardial infarction in a neonate. *British Heart Journal*, **32**, 412–15.

Bessinger, F. B., Jr, Blieden, L. C. & Edwards, J. E. (1975). Hypertensive pulmonary vascular disease associated with patent ductus arteriosus. Primary or secondary? *Circulation*, **52**, 157–61.

Bestetti, R. B., Costa, R. B., Oliveira, J. S. M., Rossi, M. A. & Correa de Araujo, R. (1985). Congenital absence of the circumflex coronary artery associated with dilated cardiomyopathy. *International Journal of Cardiology*, **8**, 331–5.

Beuren, A. J. (1972). Supravalvular aortic stenosis: a complex syndrome with and without mental retardation. *Birth Defects: Original Article Series*, **8**, 45–6.

Bick, R. (2001). Vascular thrombohemorrhagic disorders: hereditary and acquired. *Clinical and Applied Thrombosis/Hemostasis*, **7**, 178–94.

Binet, J. P. & Langlois, J. (1977). Aortic arch anomalies in children and infants. *Journal of Thoracic and Cardiovascular Surgery*, **73**, 248–52.

Bird, T. (1974). Idiopathic arterial calcification in infancy. *Archives of Disease in Childhood*, **49**, 82–9.

Bjornsson, J. & Edwards, W. D. (1985). Primary pulmonary hypertension: a histopathologic study of 80 cases. *Mayo Clinic Proceedings*, **60**, 16–25.

Bland, E. F., White, P. D. & Garland, J. (1933). Congenital anomalies of the coronary arteries: report of an unusual case associated with cardiac hypertrophy. *American Heart Journal*, **8**, 787–801.

Bland, J. W., Jr, Edwards, F. K. & Brinsfield, D. (1969). Pulmonary hypertension and congestive heart failure in children and chronic upper airway obstruction. New concepts of etiologic factors. *American Journal of Cardiology*, **23**, 830–37.

Bockman, D. E. & Kirby, M. L. (1984). Dependence of thymus development on derivatives of the neural crest. *Science*, **223**, 498–500.

Bolster, M. A., Hogan, J. & Bredin, C. P. (1990). Pulmonary vascular occlusive disease presenting as sudden death. *Medicine, Science and the Law*, **30**, 26–8.

Bor, I. (1969). Myocardial infarction and ischaemic heart disease in infants and children. Analysis of 29 cases and review of the literature. *Archives of Disease in Childhood*, **44**, 268–81.

Bowen, J. H., Woodard, B. H., Barton, T. K., Ingram, P. & Shelburne, J. D. (1981). Infantile pulmonary hypertension associated with foreign body vasculitis. *American Journal of Clinical Pathology*, **75**, 609–13.

Bregman, D., Brennan, F. J., Singer, A., *et al.* (1976). Anomalous origin of the right coronary artery from the pulmonary artery. *Journal of Thoracic and Cardiovascular Surgery*, **72**, 626–30.

Brosius, F. C., III, Waller, B. F. & Roberts, W. C. (1981). Radiation heart disease. Analysis of 16 young (aged 15 to 33 years) necropsy patients who received over 3500 rads to the heart. *American Journal of Medicine*, **70**, 519–30.

Brown, D. L., Wetli, C. V. & Davis, J. H. (1981). Sudden unexpected death from primary pulmonary hypertension. *Journal of Forensic Sciences*, **26**, 381–6.

Brown, N. J. (1974). Myocardial infarction in the newborn. *Archives of Disease in Childhood*, **49**, 494.

Buck, J. R., Connors, R. H., Coon, W. W., *et al.* (1981). Pulmonary embolism in children. *Journal of Pediatric Surgery*, **16**, 385–91.

Bunton, R., Jonas, R. A., Lang, P., Rein, A. J. J. T. & Castaneda, A. R. (1987). Anomalous origin of left coronary artery from pulmonary artery. Ligation versus establishment of a two coronary artery system. *Journal of Thoracic and Cardiovascular Surgery*, **93**, 103–8.

Buris, L., Takacs, P. & Varga, M. (1987). Sudden death caused by hydatid embolism. *Zeutschrift fur Rechtsmedizen*, **98**, 125–8.

Burke, B. A., Johnson, D., Gilbert, E. F., *et al.* (1987). Thyrocalcitonin-containing cells in the Di George anomaly. *Human Pathology*, **18**, 355–60.

Burns, J. C., Wiggins, J. W., Jr, Toews, W. H., *et al.* (1986). Clincial spectrum of Kawasaki disease in infants younger than 6 months of age. *Journal of Pediatrics*, **109**, 759–63.

Byard, R. W. (1989). Arterial blood cultures in disseminated fungal disease. *Pediatric Infectious Disease Journal*, **8**, 728–9.

Byard, R. W. (1996a). Vascular causes of sudden death in infancy, childhood and adolescence. *Cardiovascular Pathology*, **5**, 243–57.

Byard, R. W. (1996b). Idiopathic arterial calcification and unexpected infant death. *Pediatric Pathology and Laboratory Medicine*, **16**, 985–94.

Byard, R. W. (1996c). Mechanisms of sudden death and autopsy findings in patients with Arnold–Chiari malformation and ventriculoatrial catheters. *American Journal of Forensic Medicine and Pathology*, **17**, 260–63.

Byard, R. W. & Bourne, A. J. (1991). Cardiac echinococcosis with fatal intracerebral embolism. *Archives of Disease in Childhood*, **66**, 155–6.

Byard, R. W. & Cutz, E. (1990). Sudden and unexpected death in infancy and childhood due to pulmonary thromboembolism. *Archives of Pathology and Laboratory Medicine*, **114**, 142–4.

Byard, R. W. & Moore, L. (1991). Total anomalous pulmonary venous drainage and sudden death in infancy. *Forensic Science International*, **51**, 197–202.

Byard, R. W., Bourne, A. J. & Hanieh, A. (1991–2). Sudden and unexpected death due to hemorrhage from occult central nervous system lesions. A pediatric autopsy study. *Pediatric Neurosurgery*, **17**, 88–94.

Byard, R. W., Burrows, P. E., Izakawa, T. & Silver, M. M. (1991a) Diffuse infantile haemangiomatosis: clinicopathological features and management problems in five fatal cases. *European Journal of Pediatrics*, **150**, 224–7.

Byard, R. W., Edmonds, J. F., Silverman, E. & Silver, M. M. (1991b). Respiratory distress and fever in a two-month-old infant. *Journal of Pediatrics*, **118**, 306–13.

Byard, R. W., Jimenez, C. L., Carpenter, B. F., Cutz, E. & Smith, C. R. (1991c). Four unusual cases of sudden and unexpected cardiovascular death in infancy and childhood. *Medicine, Science and the Law*, **31**, 157–61.

Byard, R. W., Jimenez, C. L., Carpenter, B. F. & Hsu, E. (1987). Aspergillus-related aortic thrombosis. *Canadian Medical Association Journal*, **136**, 155–6.

Byard, R. W., Keeley, F. W. & Smith, C. R. (1990). Type IV Ehlers–Danlos syndrome presenting as sudden infant death. *American Journal of Clinical Pathology*, **93**, 579–82.

Byard, R. W., Schliebs, J. & Koszyca, B. A. (2001). Osler–Weber–Rendu syndrome – pathological manifestations and autopsy considerations. *Journal of Forensic Sciences*, **46**, 698–701.

Byard, R. W., Smith, N. M. & Bourne, A. J. (1991). Association of right coronary artery hypoplasia with sudden death in an eleven-year-old child. *Journal of Forensic Sciences*, **36**, 1234–9.

Cagle, P. & Langston, C. (1984). Pulmonary veno-occlusive disease as a cause of sudden infant death. *Archives of Pathology and Laboratory Medicine*, **108**, 338–40.

Campbell, M. (1968). Natural history of persistent ductus arteriosus. *British Heart Journal*, **30**, 4–13.

Carles, D., Serville, F., Dubecq, J.-P., *et al.* (1992). Idiopathic arterial calcification in a stillborn complicated by pleural hemorrhage and hydrops fetalis. *Archives of Pathology and Laboratory Medicine*, **116**, 293–5.

Carlson, R. A., Arya, S. & Gilbert, E. F. (1985). Budd–Chiari syndrome presenting as sudden infant death. *Archives of Pathology and Laboratory Medicine*, **109**, 379–80.

Carter, R. E. B., Capriles, M. & Noe, Y. (1969). Total anomalous pulmonary venous drainage. A clinical and anatomical study of 75 children. *British Heart Journal*, **31**, 45–51.

Celermajer, D. S., Sholler, G. F., Howman-Giles, R. & Celermajer, J. M. (1991). Myocardial infarction in childhood: clinical analysis of 17 cases and medium term follow up of survivors. *British Heart Journal*, **65**, 332–6.

Centers for Disease Control (1980). Kawasaki disease – New York. *Morbidity and Mortality Weekly Report*, **29**, 61–3.

Chaitman, B. R., Bourassa, M. G., Lesperance, J., Dominguez, J. L. D. & Saltiel, J. (1975). Aberrant course of the left anterior descending coronary artery associated with anomalous left circumflex origin from the pulmonary artery. *Circulation*, **52**, 955–8.

Chaitman, B. R., Lesperance, J., Saltiel, J. & Bourassa, M. G. (1976). Clinical, angiographic and hemodynamic findings in patients with anomalous origin of the coronary arteries. *Circulation*, **53**, 122–31.

Champ, C. & Byard, R. W. (1994). Pulmonary thromboembolism and unexpected death in infancy. *Journal of Paediatrics and Child Health*, **30**, 550–51.

Chan, K. W., Fryer, C. J. H., Fraser, G. C. & Dimmick, J. E. (1985). Sudden cerebral death in malignant presacral teratoma. *Medical and Pediatric Oncology*, **13**, 395–7.

Cheitlin, M. D. (1980). The intramural coronary artery: another cause for sudden death with exercise? *Circulation*, **62**, 238–9.

Cheitlin, M. D. (1989). Coronary arterial anomalies. Clinical and angiographic aspects. In *Nonatherosclerotic Ischemic Heart Disease*, ed. R. Virmani & M. B. Forman. New York: Raven Press, pp. 125–51.

Cheitlin, M. D., De Castro, C. M. & McAllister, H. A. (1974). Sudden death as a complication of anomalous left coronary origin from the anterior sinus of Valsalva. A not-so-minor congenital anomaly. *Circulation*, **50**, 780–87.

Cheng, T. O. (1982). Left coronary artery-to-left ventricular fistula: demonstration of coronary steal phenomenon. *American Heart Journal*, **104**, 870–72.

Cochrane, W. A. & Bowden, D. H. (1954). Calcification of the arteries in infancy and childhood. *Pediatrics*, **14**, 222–31.

Cohen, L. S. & Shaw, L. D. (1967). Fatal myocardial infarction in an 11 year old boy associated with a unique coronary artery anomaly. *American Journal of Cardiology*, **19**, 420–23.

Cohen, M. D., Rubin, L. J., Taylor, W. E. & Cuthbert, J. A. (1983). Primary pulmonary hypertension: an unusual case associated with extrahepatic portal hypertension. *Hepatology*, **3**, 588–92.

Cohle, S. D. & Colby, T. (2002). Fatal hemoptysis from Behcet's disease in a child. *Cardiovascular Pathology*, **11**, 296–9.

Cohle, S. D. & Petty, C. S. (1985). Sudden death caused by embolization of trophoblast from hydatidiform mole. *Journal of Forensic Sciences*, **30**, 1279–83.

Cohle, S. D., Graham, M. A., Dowling, G. & Pounder, D. J. (1988). Sudden death and left ventricular outflow disease. *Pathology Annual*, **23** (part 2), 97–124.

Cohle, S. D., Graham, M. A. & Pounder, D. J. (1986). Nonatherosclerotic sudden coronary death. *Pathology Annual*, **21** (part 2), 217–49.

Coleman, P. N. (1955). A case of dissecting aneurysm in a child. *Journal of Clinical Pathology*, **8**, 313–17.

Colman, J. M., Sermer, M., Seaward, P. G. R. & Siu, S. C. (2000). Congenital heart disease in pregnancy. *Cardiology in Review*, **8**, 166–73.

Conley, M. E., Beckwith, J. B., Mancer, J. F. K. & Tenckhoff, L. (1979). The spectrum of the DiGeorge syndrome. *Journal of Pediatrics*, **94**, 883–90.

Conway, E. E., Jr, Noonan, J., Marion, R. W. & Steeg, C. N. (1990). Myocardial infarction leading to sudden death in the Williams syndrome: report of three cases. *Journal of Pediatrics*, **117**, 593–5.

Cooper, D. R., Lucke, W. C. & Moseson, D. L. (1986). Aortic dissection in adolescence. *American Family Physican*, **34**, 137–42.

Cuneo, B. F. (2001). 22q11. 2 deletion syndrome: DiGeorge, velocardiofacial, and conotruncal anomaly face syndromes. *Current Opinion in Pediatrics*, **13**, 465–72.

Dail, D. H., Liebow, A. A., Gmelich, J., Carrington, C. B. & Churg, A. (1978). A study of 43 cases of pulmonary veno-occlusive (PVO) disease. *Laboratory Investigation*, **38**, 340–41.

Dancea, A., Côté, A., Rohlicek, C., Bernard, C. & Oligny, L. L. (2002). Cardiac pathology in sudden unexpected infant death. *Journal of Pediatrics*, **141**, 336–42.

Daniel, T. M., Graham, T. P. & Sabiston, D. C., Jr (1970). Coronary artery-right ventricular fistula with congestive heart failure: surgical correction in the neonatal period. *Surgery*, **67**, 985–94.

Daniels, S. R., Bates, S., Lukin, R. R., *et al.* (1982). Cerebrovascular arteriopathy (arteriosclerosis) and ischemic childhood stroke. *Stroke*, **13**, 360–65.

Darling, R. C., Rothney, W. B. & Craig, J. M. (1957). Total pulmonary venous drainage into the right side of the heart. Report of 17 autopsied cases not associated with other major cardiovascular anomalies. *Laboratory Investigation*, **6**, 44–64.

Davies, M. J. & Popple, A. (1979). Sudden unexpected cardiac death – a practical approach to the forensic problem. *Histopathology*, **3**, 255–77.

De la Grandmaison, G. L. & Durigon, M. (2002). Pulmonary embolism. A rare cause of sudden infant death. *American Journal of Forensic Medicine and Pathology*, **23**, 247–9.

DeLeon, S. Y., Gidding, S. S., Ilbawi, M. N., *et al.* (1987). Surgical management of infants with complex cardiac anomalies associated with reduced pulmonary blood flow and total anomalous pulmonary venous drainage. *Annals of Thoracic Surgery*, **43**, 207–11.

Delisle, G., Ando, M., Calder, A. L., *et al.* (1976). Total anomalous pulmonary venous connection: report of 93 autopsied cases with emphasis on diagnostic and surgical considerations. *American Heart Journal*, **91**, 99–122.

Demick, D. A. (1991). Cerebrovascular malformation causing sudden death. Analysis of three cases and review of the literature. *American Journal of Forensic Medicine and Pathology*, **12**, 45–9.

Dent, E. D., Jr & Fisher, R. S. (1955). Single coronary artery: report of two cases. *Annals of Internal Medicine*, **44**, 1024–30.

De Sa, D. J. (1979). Coronary arterial lesions and myocardial necrosis in stillbirths and infants. *Archives of Disease in Childhood*, **54**, 918–30.

Devaney, K., Kapur, S. P., Patterson, K. & Chandra, R. S. (1991). Pediatric renal artery dysplasia: a morphologic study. *Pediatric Pathology*, **11**, 609–21.

Devine, W. A., Debich, D. E. & Anderson, R. H. (1991). Dissection of congenitally malformed hearts, with comments on the value of sequential segmental analysis. *Pediatric Pathology*, **11**, 235–59.

Di Liberti, J. H. (1982). Granulomatous vasculitis. *New England Journal of Medicine*, **306**, 1365.

Dische, M. R. (1968). Lymphoid tissue and associated congenital malformations in thymic agenesis. Findings in one infant and two severely malformed stillborns. *Archives of Pathology*, **86**, 312–16.

Dominguez, F. E., Tate, L. G. & Poppitti, R. J. (1987). Sudden infant death from fibromuscular dysplasia. Paper presented to the American Academy of Forensic Sciences Annual Meeting, San Diego, February 1987.

Dominguez, F. E., Tate, L. G. & Robinson, M. J. (1988). Familial fibromuscular dysplasia presenting as sudden death. *American Journal of Cardiovascular Pathology*, **2**, 269–72.

Donnai, D. & Karmiloff-Smith, A. (2000). Williams syndrome: from genotype through to the cognitive phenotype. *American Journal of Medical Genetics*, **97**, 164–71.

Dorman, F., Sumner, E. & Spitz, L. (1985). Fatal intraoperative tumour embolism in a child with hepatoblastoma. *Anesthesiology*, **63**, 692–3.

Doyle, E. F., Arumugham, P., Lara, E., Rutkowski, M. R. & Kiely, B. (1974). Sudden death in young patients with congenital aortic stenosis. *Pediatrics*, **53**, 481–9.

Driscoll, D. A., Budarf, M. L. & Emanuel, B. S. (1992). A genetic etiology for DiGeorge syndrome: consistent deletions and microdeletions of 22q11. *American Journal of Human Genetics*, **50**, 924–33.

Driscoll, D. J., Nihill, M. R., Mullins, C. E., Cooley, D. A. & McNamara, D. G. (1981). Management of symptomatic infants with anomalous origin of the left coronary artery from the pulmonary artery. *American Journal of Cardiology*, **47**, 642–8.

Eden, O. B., Sills, J. A. & Brown, J. K. (1977). Hypertension in acute neurological diseases of childhood. *Developmental Medicine in Child Neurology*, **19**, 437–45.

Edwards, J. E. (1965). Pathology of left ventricular outflow tract obstruction. *Circulation*, **31**, 586–99.

Edwards, J. E. (1974). Pathology of chronic pulmonary hypertension. *Pathology Annual*, **9**, 1–25.

Edwards, W. D. & Edwards, J. E. (1978a). Hypertensive pulmonary vascular disease in d-transposition of the great arteries. *American Journal of Cardiology*, **41**, 921–4.

Edwards, W. D. & Edwards, J. E. (1978b). Recent advances in the pathology of the pulmonary vasculature. *Monographs in Pathology*, **19**, 235–61.

Ellis, C. J., Haywood, G. A. & Monro, J. L. (1994). Spontaneous coronary artery dissection in a young woman resulting from intense gymnasium "work-out". *International Journal of Cardiology*, **47**, 193–4.

Emanuel, R., Withers, R., O'Brien, K., Ross, P. & Feizi, D. (1978). Congenitally bicuspid aortic valves. Clinicogenetic study of 41 families. *British Heart Journal*, **40**, 1462–7.

Emery, J. L. (1962). Pulmonary embolism in children. *Archives of Disease in Childhood*, **37**, 591–5.

Engel, H. J., Torres, C. & Page, H. L., Jr (1975). Major variations in anatomical origin of the coronary arteries: angiographic observations in 4250 patients without associated congenital heart disease. *Catheterisation and Cardiovascular Diagnosis*, **1**, 157–69.

Evans, D. A. & Wilmott, R. W. (1994). Pulmonary embolism in children. *Pediatric Clinics of North America*, **41**, 569–84.

Faber, C. N., Yousem, S. A., Dauber, J. H., *et al.* (1989). Pulmonary capillary hemangiomatosis. A report of three cases and a review of the literature. *American Review of Respiratory Disease*, **140**, 808–13.

Fanconi, G., Giradet, P., Schlesinger, B., Butler, N. & Black, J. (1952). Chronische hypercalcämie, kombiniert mit osteosklerose, hyperazotämie, minderwuchs und kongenitalen mibbilungen. *Helvetica Paediatrica Acta*, **7**, 314–49.

Fann, J. I., Dalman, R. L. & Harris, E. J. (1993). Genetic and metabolic causes of arterial disease. *Annals of Vascular Surgery*, **7**, 594–604.

Faruqui, A. M. A., Maloy, W. C., Felner, J. M., *et al.* (1978). Symptomatic myocardial bridging of coronary artery. *American Journal of Cardiology*, **41**, 1305–10.

Fatica, N. S., Ichida, F., Engel, M. A. & Lesser, M. L. (1989). Rug shampoo and Kawasaki disease. *Pediatrics*, **84**, 231–4.

Favara, B. E. & Moores, H. K. (1991). Foreign-body pulmonary embolism. *Pediatric Pathology*, **11**, 371–9.

Fearon, B. & Shortreed, R. (1963). Tracheobronchial compression by congenital cardiovascular anomalies in children. Syndrome of apnea. *Annals of Otology, Rhinology and Larngology*, **72**, 949–69.

Feldt, R. H., Ongley, P. A. & Titus, J. L. (1965). Total coronary arterial circulation from pulmonary artery with survival to age seven: report of case. *Mayo Clinic Proceedings*, **40**, 539–43.

Fellers, F. X. & Schwartz, R. (1958). Etiology of the severe form of idiopathic hypercalcemia of infancy. A defect in Vitamin D metabolism. *New England Journal of Medicine*, **259**, 1050–58.

Fikar, C. R., Amrhein, J. A., Harris, P. & Lewis, E. R. (1981). Dissecting aortic aneurysm in childhood and adolescence. Case report and literature review. *Clinical Pediatrics*, **20**, 578–83.

Fikar, C. R., & Koch, S. (2000). Etiologic factors of acute aortic dissection in children and young adults. *Clinical Pediatrics*, **39**, 71–80.

Filston, H. C., Ferguson, T. B., Jr & Oldham, H. N. (1987). Airway obstruction by vascular anomalies: importance of telescopic bronchoscopy. *Annals of Surgery*, **205**, 541–9.

Fineschi, V., Paglicci Reatelli, L. & Baroldi, G. (1999). Coronary artery aneurysms in a young adult: a case of sudden death. A late sequelae to Kawasaki disease? *International Journal of Legal Medicine*, **112**, 120–23.

Firor, H. V. (1972). Pulmonary embolization complicating total intravenous alimentation. *Journal of Pediatric Surgery*, **7**, 81.

Fleisher, G. R., Buck, B. E. & Cornfeld, D. (1978). Primary intimal fibroplasia in a child with Down's syndrome. *American Journal of Diseases of Children*, **132**, 700–703.

Folger, G. M., Jr (1977). Further observations on the syndrome of idiopathic infantile hypercalcemia associated with supravalvular aortic stenosis. *American Heart Journal*, **93**, 455–62.

Fortuin, N. J., Morrow, A. G. & Roberts, W. C. (1971). Late vascular manifestations of the rubella syndrome. A roentgenographic-pathologic study. *American Journal of Medicine*, **51**, 134–40.

Freedom, R. M., Rosen, F. S. & Nadas, A. S. (1972). Congenital cardiovascular disease and anomalies of the third and fourth pharyngeal pouch. *Circulation*, **46**, 165–72.

Freeman, A. F. & Shulman, S. T. (2001). Recent developments in Kawasaki disease. *Current Opinion in Infectious Diseases*, **14**, 357–61.

Freeman, L. (1999). Pulmonary embolism in a 13-year-old boy. *Pediatric Emergency Care*, **15**, 422–4.

Friedman, W. F. & Roberts, W. C. (1966). Vitamin D and the supravalvular aortic stenosis syndrome. The transplacental effects of vitamin D on the aorta of the rabbit. *Circulation*, **34**, 77–86.

Fujita, Y., Nakamura, Y., Sakata, K., *et al.* (1989). Kawasaki disease in families. *Pediatrics*, **84**, 666–9.

Fujiwara, H., Fujiwara, T., Kao, T.-C., Ohshio, G. & Hamashima, Y. (1986). Pathology of Kawasaki disease in the healed stage: relationships between typical and atypical cases of Kawasaki disease. *Acta Pathologica Japonica*, **36**, 857–67.

Fujiwara, H. & Hamashima, Y. (1978). Pathology of the heart in Kawasaki disease. *Pediatrics*, **61**, 100–107.

Fujiwara, T., Fujiwara, H. & Hamashima, Y. (1987). Frequency and size of coronary arterial aneurysm at necropsy in Kawasaki disease. *American Journal of Cardiology*, **59**, 808–11.

Fujiwara, T., Fujiwara, H. & Nakano, H. (1988). Pathological features of coronary arteries in children with Kawasaki disease in which coronary arterial aneurysm was absent at autopsy. Quantitative analysis. *Circulation*, **78**, 345–50.

Furukawa, S., Matsubara, T. & Yabuta, K. (1992). Mononuclear cell subsets and coronary artery lesions in Kawasaki disease. *Archives of Disease in Childhood*, **67**, 706–8.

Fuster, V., Steele, P. M., Edwards, W. D., *et al.* (1984). Primary pulmonary hypertension: natural history and the importance of thrombosis. *Circulation*, **70**, 580–87.

Gabr, M., Hashem, N., Hashem, M., Fahmi, A. & Safouh, M. (1960). Progeria, a pathologic study. *Journal of Pediatrics*, **57**, 70–77.

Garcia-Dorado, D., Miller, D. D., Garcia, E. J., *et al.* (1983). An epidemic of pulmonary hypertension after toxic grapeseed oil ingestion in Spain. *Journal of the American College of Cardiology*, **1**, 1216–22.

Gatalica, Z., Gibas, Z. & Martinez-Hernandez, A. (1992). Dissecting aortic aneurysm as a complication of generalized fibromuscular dysplasia. *Human Pathology*, **23**, 586–8.

Gedalia, A. (2002). Kawasaki disease: an update. *Current Rheumatology Reports*, **4**, 25–9.

Gilsanz, V., Campo, C., Cue R., *et al.* (1977). Recurrent pulmonary embolism due to hydatid disease of heart. Study of 3 cases, one with intermittent tricuspid valve obstruction (atrial pseudomyxoma). *British Heart Journal*, **39**, 553–8.

Glasgow, B. J., Tift, J. P. & Alexander, C. B. (1984). Spontaneous primary dissecting coronary artery aneurysm. Report of two cases. *American Journal of Forensic Medicine and Pathology*, **5**, 155–9.

Glode, M., Brogden, R., Joffe, L., *et al.* (1986). Kawasaki syndrome and house dust mite exposure. *Pediatric Infectious Diseases Journal*, **5**, 644–8.

Glueck, C. J., Daniels, S. R., Bates, S., *et al.* (1982). Pediatric victims of unexplained stroke and their families: familial lipid and lipoprotein abnormalities. *Pediatrics*, **69**, 308–16.

Gomes, M. M. R., Feldt, R. H., McGoon, D. C & Danielson, G. K. (1970). Total anomalous pulmonary venous connection. Surgical considerations and results of operation. *Journal of Thoracic and Cardiovascular Surgery*, **60**, 116–22.

Gower, N. D. & Pinkerton, J. R. H. (1963). Idiopathic arterial calcification in infancy. *Archives of Disease in Childhood*, **38**, 408–11.

Graves, E. D., III, Redmond, C. R. & Arensman, R. M. (1988). Persistent pulmonary hypertension in the neonate. *Chest*, **93**, 638–41.

Greene, J. F., Jr, Fitzwater, J. E. & Burgess, J. (1974). Arterial lesions associated with neurofibromatosis. *American Journal of Clinical Pathology*, **62**, 481–7.

Guttmacher, A. E., Marchuk, D. A. & White, R. I., Jr (1995). Hereditary hemorrhagic telangiectasia. *New England Journal of Medicine*, **333**, 918–24.

Haas, A. & Stiehm, E. R. (1986). Takayasu's arteritis presenting as pulmonary hypertension. *American Journal of Diseases of Children*, **140**, 372–4.

Habbema, L., Losekoot, T. G. & Becker, A. E. (1980). Respiratory distress due to bronchial compression in persistent truncus arteriosus. *Chest*, **77**, 230–32.

Haitjema, T., Westerman, C. J. J., Overtoom, T. T. C., *et al.* (1996). Hereditary hemorrhagic telangiectasia (Osler–Weber–Rendu disease): new insights in pathogenesis, complications, and treatment. *Archives of Internal Medicine*, **156**, 714–19.

Hall, S., Barr, W., Lie, J. T., *et al.* (1985). Takayasu arteritis. A study of 32 North American patients. *Medicine*, **64**, 89–99.

Hallidie-Smith, K. A. & Karas, S. (1988). Cardiac anomalies in Williams–Beuren syndrome. *Archives of Disease in Childhood*, **63**, 809–13.

Hallidie-Smith, K. A. & Olsen, E. G. J. (1968). Endocardial fibroelastosis, mitral incompetence, and coarctation of abdominal aorta. A report of three cases. *British Heart Journal*, **30**, 850–58.

Hallman, G. L., Cooley, D. A. & Singer, D. B. (1966). Congenital anomalies of the coronary arteries: anatomy, pathology and surgical treatment. *Surgery*, **59**, 133–44.

Hammon, J. W., Jr & Bender, H. W., Jr (1990). Major anomalies of pulmonary and thoracic systemic veins. In *Surgery of the Chest*, 5th edn, vol. 2, ed. D. C. Sabiston & F. C. Spencer. Philadelphia: W. B. Saunders, pp. 1274–97.

Hammon, J. W., Jr, Bender, H. W., Jr, Graham, T. P., Jr, *et al.* (1980). Total anomalous pulmonary venous connection in infancy. Ten years experience including studies of postoperative ventricular function. *Journal of Thoracic Cardiovascular Surgery*, **80**, 544–51.

Hanley, W. B. & Jones, N. B. (1967). Familial dissecting aortic aneurysm. A report of three cases within two generations. *British Heart Journal*, **29**, 852–8.

Hasleton, P. S., Ironside, J. W., Whittaker, J. S., *et al.* (1986). Pulmonary veno-occlusive disease. A report of four cases. *Histopathology*, **10**, 933–44.

Hawkins, J. A., Clark, E. B. & Doty, D. B. (1983). Total anomalous pulmonary venous connection. *Annals of Thoracic Surgery*, **36**, 548–60.

Haworth, S. G. (1974). Progressive pulmonary hypertension in children with portal hypertension. *Journal of Pediatrics*, **84**, 783–5.

Haworth, S. G. (1983a). Primary and secondary pulmonary hypertension in childhood: a clinicopathological reappraisal. *Current Topics in Pathology*, **73**, 91–152.

Haworth, S. G. (1983b). Primary pulmonary hypertension. *British Heart Journal*, **49**, 517–21.

Haworth, S. G. (1983c). Pulmonary vascular disease in secundum atrial septal defect in childhood. *American Journal of Cardiology*, **51**, 265–72.

Haworth, S. G. (1984). Pulmonary vascular disease in different types of congenital heart disease. Implications for interpretation of lung biopsy findings in early childhood. *British Heart Journal*, **52**, 557–71.

Haworth, S. G. (1987). Pulmonary vascular disease in ventricular septal defect: structural and functional correlations in lung biopsies from 85 patients, with outcome of intracardiac repair. *Journal of Pathology*, **152**, 157–68.

Haworth, S. G. & Reid, L. (1977). Structural study of pulmonary circulation and of heart in total anomalous pulmonary venous return in early infancy. *British Heart Journal*, **39**, 80–92.

Haworth, S. G. & Reid, L. (1978). A morphometric study of regional variation in lung structure in infants with pulmonary hypertension and congenital cardiac defect. A justification of lung biopsy. *British Heart Journal*, **40**, 825–31.

Haworth, S. G., Sauer, U., Bühlmeyer, K. & Reid, L. (1977). Development of the pulmonary circulation in ventricular septal defect: a quantitative structural study. *American Journal of Cardiology*, **40**, 781–8.

Heath, D. & Edwards, J. E. (1958). The pathology of hypertensive pulmonary vascular disease. A description of six grades of structural changes in the pulmonary arteries with special reference to congenital cardiac septal defects. *Circulation*, **18**, 533–47.

Heath, D. & Reid, R. (1985). Invasive pulmonary haemangiomatosis. *British Journal of Diseases of the Chest*, **79**, 284–94.

Heifetz, S. A., Robinowitz, M., Mueller, K. H. & Virmani, R. (1986). Total anomalous origin of the coronary arteries from the pulmonary artery. *Pediatric Cardiology*, **7**, 11–18.

Heller, C., Schobess, R., Kurnik, K., *et al.* (2000). Abdominal venous thrombosis in neonates and infants: role of prothrombotic risk factors – a multicentre case–control study. *British Journal of Haematology*, **111**, 534–9.

Herrmann, M. A., Dousa, M. K., & Edwards, W. D. (1992). Sudden infant death with anomalous origin of the left coronary artery. *American Journal of Forensic Medicine and Pathology*, **13**, 191–5.

Hewitt, R. L., Brewer, P. L. & Drapanas, T. (1970). Aortic arch anomalies. *Journal of Thoracic and Cardiovascular Surgery*, **60**, 746–53.

Hickey, M. S. & Wood, A. E. (1987). Pulmonary artery sling with tracheal stenosis: one-stage repair. *Annals of Thoracic Surgery*, **44**, 416–17.

Hicks, R. V. & Melish, M. E. (1986). Kawasaki syndrome. *Pediatric Clinics of North America*, **33**, 1151–75.

Ho, S. Y. & Anderson, R. H. (1979). Coarctation, tubular hypoplasia and the ductus arteriosus: histological study of 35 specimens. *British Heart Journal*, **41**, 268–74.

Hobbs, R. E., Millit, D., Raghavan, P. V., Moodie, D. S. & Sheldon, W. C. (1981). Congenital coronary artery anomalies: clinical and therapeutic implications. *Cardiovascular Clinics*, **12**, 43–58.

Hochberg, F. H., Bean, C., Fisher, C. M. & Roberson, G. H. (1975). Stroke in a 15-year-old girl secondary to terminal carotid dissection. *Neurology*, **25**, 725–9.

Hoffman, J. I. E., Rudolph, A. M. & Heymann, M. A. (1981). Pulmonary vascular disease with congenital heart lesions: pathologic features and causes. *Circulation*, **64**, 873–7.

Hoganson, G., McPherson, E., Piper, P. & Gilbert, E. F. (1983). Single coronary artery arising anomalously from the pulmonary trunk. *Archives of Pathology and Laboratory Medicine*, **107**, 199–201.

Hughes, J. D. & Rubin, L. J. (1986). Primary pulmonary hypertension. An analysis of 28 cases and a review of the literature. *Medicine*, **65**, 56–72.

Hunt, A. C. & Leys, D. G. (1957). Generalised arterial calcification of infancy. *British Medical Journal*, **i**, 385–6.

Huntington, R. W., Jr & Hirst, A. E., Jr (1967). Dissecting aneurysm of the aorta in a 16-year-old girl. *American Journal of Clinical Pathology*, **48**, 44–8.

Hussain, T., Patrick, W. A., Gibson, A. A. & Fitzpatrick, D. R. (1991). Idiopathic arterial calcification: a further six cases. *Journal of Medical Genetics*, **28**, 554.

Husson, G. S. & Parkman, P. (1961). Chondroectodermal dysplasia (Ellis-van Creveld syndrome) with a complex cardiac malformation. *Pediatrics*, **28**, 285–92.

Hutchins, G. M. & Ostrow, P. T. (1976). The pathogenesis of the two forms of hypertensive pulmonary vascular disease. *American Heart Journal*, **92**, 797–803.

Ichida, F., Fatica, N. S., O'Loughlin, J. E., *et al.* (1989). Epidemiologic aspects of Kawasaki disease in a Manhattan hospital. *Pediatrics*, **84**, 235–41.

Ishikawa, K. (1978). Natural history and classification of occlusive thromboaortopathy (Takayasu's disease). *Circulation*, **57**, 27–35.

Ishikawa, K. (1981). Survival and morbidity after diagnosis of occlusive thromboaortopathy (Takayasu's disease). *American Journal of Cardiology*, **47**, 1026–32.

Ishikawa, T., Otsuka, T. & Suzuki, T. (1990). Anomalous origin of the left main coronary artery from the noncoronary sinus of Valsalva. *Pediatric Cardiology*, **11**, 173–4.

Jackson, M. A., Hughes, R. C., Ward, S. P. & McInnes, E. G. (1983). "Headbanging" and carotid dissection. *British Medical Journal*, **287**, 1262.

James, C. L., Keeling, J. W., Smith, N. M. & Byard, R. W. (1994). Total anomalous pulmonary venous drainage (TAPVD) associated with fatal outcome in infancy and early childhood – an autopsy study of 52 cases. *Pediatric Pathology*, **14**, 665–78.

James, T. N. (1962). On the cause of syncope and sudden death in primary pulmonary hypertension. *Annals of Internal Medicine*, **56**, 252–64.

James, T. N., Marshall, T. K. & Edwards, J. E. (1976). Cardiac electrical instability in the presence of a left superior vena cava. *Circulation*, **54**, 689–97.

Johnson, A. M. (1971). Aortic stenosis, sudden death and the left ventricular baroceptors. *British Heart Journal*, **33**, 1–5.

Jokl, E. & McClellan, J. T. (1970). Exercise and cardiac death. *Journal of the American Medical Association*, **213**, 1489–91.

Jokl, E., McClellan, J. T., Williams, W. C., Gouze, F. J. & Bartholomew, R. D. (1966). Congenital anomaly of left coronary artery in young athletes. *Cardiologia*, **49**, 253–8.

Jones, R. H. & Sabiston, D. C., Jr (1966). Pulmonary embolism in childhood. *Monographs in the Surgical Sciences*, **3**, 35–51.

Jones, K. L. & Smith, D. W. (1975). The Williams elfin facies syndrome. A new perspective. *Journal of Pediatrics*, **86**, 718–23.

Josa, M., Danielson, G. K., Weidman, W. H. & Edwards, W. D. (1981). Congenital ostial membrane of left main coronary artery. *Journal of Thoracic and Cardiovascular Surgery*, **81**, 338–46.

Joshi, V. V., Pawel, B., Connor, E., *et al.* (1987). Arteriopathy in children with acquired immune deficiency syndrome. *Pediatric Pathology*, **7**, 261–75.

Juaneda, E., Watson, H. & Haworth, S. G. (1985). An unusual case of rapidly progressive primary pulmonary hypertension in childhood. *International Journal of Cardiology*, **7**, 306–9.

Justo, R. N., Dare, A. J., Whight, C. M. & Radford, D. J. (1993). Pulmonary veno-occlusive disease: diagnosis during life in four patients. *Archives of Disease in Childhood*, **68**, 97–100.

Juul, S., Ledbetter, D., Wight, T. N. & Woodrum, D. (1990). New insights into idiopathic infantile arterial calcinosis. Three patient reports. *American Journal of Diseases of Children*, **144**, 229–33.

Kato, H., Ichinose, E. & Kawasaki, T. (1986). Myocardial infarction in Kawasaki disease: clinical analyses in 195 cases. *Journal of Pediatrics*, **108**, 923–7.

Kato, H., Inoue, O., Kawasaki, T., *et al.* (1992). Adult coronary artery disease probably due to childhood Kawasaki disease. *Lancet*, **340**, 1127–9.

Kato, H., Inoue, O., Koga, Y., *et al.* (1983). Variant strain of *Propionibacterium acnes*: a clue to the aetiology of Kawasaki disease. *Lancet*, **ii**, 1383–7.

Katzenstein, A.-L. A. & Askin, F. B. (1990). Pulmonary hypertension and other vasaular disorders. In *Surgical Pathology of Non-neoplastic Lung Disease*, 2nd edn. Philadelphia: W. B. Saunders, pp. 432–48.

Katzenstein, A.-L. A. & Mazur, M. T. (1980). Pulmonary infarct: an unusual manifestation of fibrosing mediastinitis. *Chest*, **77**, 521–4.

Kawasaki, T. (1967). Acute febrile mucotaneous lymph node syndrome [in Japanese]. *Allergy*, **16**, 178–222.

Kay, J. M. (1997). Hypoxia, obstructive sleep apnea syndrome, pulmonary hypertension. *Human Pathology*, **28**, 261–3.

Keeton, B. R., Keenan, D. J. M. & Monro, J. L. (1983). Anomalous origin of both coronary arteries from the pulmonary trunk. *British Heart Journal*, **49**, 397–9.

Kegel, S. M., Dorsey, T. J., Rowen, M. & Taylor, W. F. (1977). Cardiac death in mucocutaneous lymph node syndrome. *American Journal of Cardiology*, **40**, 282–6.

Kelley, M. J., Wolfson, S. & Marshall, R. (1977). Single coronary artery from the right sinus of Valsalva: angiography, anatomy and clinical significance. *American Journal of Roentgenology*, **128**, 257–62.

Kibria, G., Smith, P., Heath, D. & Sagar, S. (1980). Observations on the rare association between portal and pulmonary hypertension. *Thorax*, **35**, 945–9.

Kilbride, H., Way, G. L., Merenstein, G. B. & Winfield, J. M. (1980). Myocardial infarction in the neonate with normal heart and coronary arteries. *American Journal of Diseases of Children*, **134**, 759–62.

Kimbiris, D., Iskandrian, A. S., Segal, B. L. & Bemis, C. E. (1978). Anomalous aortic origin of coronary arteries. *Circulation*, **58**, 606–15.

Kirby, M. L. & Bockman, D. E. (1984). Neural crest and normal development: a new perspective. *Anatomical Record*, **209**, 1–6.

Kjeldsen, A. D., Vase, P. & Green, A. (1999). Hereditary haemorrhagic telangiectasia: a population-based study of prevelance and mortality in Danish patients. *Journal of Internal Medicine*, **245**, 31–9.

Klein, B. S., Rogers, M. F., Patrican, L. A., *et al.* (1986). Kawasaki syndrome: a controlled study of an outbreak in Wisconsin. *American Journal of Epidemiology*, **124**, 306–16.

Knop, C. Q. & Bennett, W. A. (1944). Sudden death from coronary insufficiency: report of case of an infant. *Mayo Clinic Proceedings*, **19**, 574–7.

Kohr, R. M. (1986). Progressive asymptomatic coronary artery disease as a late fatal sequela of Kawasaki disease. *Journal of Pediatrics*, **108**, 256–9.

Koike, K. & Freedom, R. M. (1989). Kawasaki disease, with a focus on cardiovascular manifestations. *Current Opinion in Pediatrics*, **1**, 135–41.

Kolquist, K. A., Vnencak-Jones, C. L., Swift, L., *et al.* (1996). Fatal fat embolism syndrome in a child with undiagnosed hemoglobin S/beta+ thalassemia: a complication of acute parvovirus B19 infection. *Pediatric Pathology and Laboratory Medicine*, **16**, 71–82.

Koopot, R., Nikaidoh, H. & Idriss, F. S. (1975). Surgical management of anomalous left pulmonary artery causing tracheobronchial obstruction. Pulmonary artery sling. *Journal of Thoracic and Cardiovascular Surgery*, **69**, 239–46.

Koskenvuo, K., Karvonen, M. J. & Rissanen, V. (1978). Death from ischemic heart disease in young Finns aged 15 to 24 years. *American Journal of Cardiology*, **42**, 114–18.

Kurosawa, H., Wagenaar, S. S. & Becker, A. E. (1981). Sudden death in a youth. A case of quadricuspid aortic valve with isolation of origin of left coronary artery. *British Heart Journal*, **46**, 211–15.

Lalu, K., Karhunen, P. J. & Rautiainen, P. (1992). Sudden and unexpected death of a 6-month-old baby with silent heart failure due to anomalous origin of the left coronary artery from the pulmonary artery. *American Journal of Forensic Medicine and Pathology*, **13**, 196–8.

Lamb, R. K., Qureshi, S. A., Wilkinson, J. L., *et al.* (1988). Total anomalous pulmonary venous drainage: seventeen-year surgical experience. *Journal of Thoracic and Cardiovascular Surgery*, **96**, 368–75.

Lambert, E. C., Menon, V. A., Wagner, H. R. & Vlad, P. (1974). Sudden unexpected death from cardiovascular disease in children. A cooperative international study. *American Journal of Cardiology*, **34**, 89–96.

Lammer, E. J. & Opitz, J. M. (1986). The Di George anomaly as a developmental field defect. *American Journal of Medical Genetics Supplement*, **2**, 113–27.

Landing, B. H. & Larson, E. J. (1977). Are infantile periarteritis nodosa with coronary artery involvement and fatal mucocutaneous lymph node syndrome the same? Comparison of 20 patients from North America with patients from Hawaii and Japan. *Pediatrics*, **59**, 651–62.

Landing, B. H. & Larson, E. J. (1987). Pathological features of Kawasaki disease (mucocutaneous lymph node syndrome). *American Journal of Cardiovascular Pathology*, **1**, 215–29.

Landolt, C. C., Anderson, J. E., Zorn-Chelton, S., *et al.* (1986). Importance of coronary artery anomalies in operations for congenital heart disease. *Annals of Thoracic Surgery*, **41**, 351–5.

Lang, B. A., Silverman, E. D., Laxer, R. M., *et al.* (1990). Serum-soluble interleukin-2 receptor levels in Kawasaki disease. *Journal of Pediatrics*, **116**, 592–6.

Lauridson, J. R. (1988). Sudden death and anomalous origin of the coronary arteries from the aorta. A case report and review. *American Journal of Forensic Medicine and Pathology*, **9**, 236–40.

Lee, K.-S., Sohn, K.-Y., Hong, C.-Y., Kang, S.-R. & Berg, K. (1967). Primary arteritis (pulseless disease) in Korean children. *Acta Paediatrica Scandinavica*, **56**, 526–36.

Lerberg, D. B., Ogden, J. A., Zuberbuhler, J. R. & Bahnson, H. T. (1979). Anomalous origin of the right coronary artery from the pulmonary artery. *Annals of Thoracic Surgery*, **27**, 87–94.

Leung, D. Y. M., Chu, E. T., Wood, N., *et al.* (1983). Immunoregulatory T cell abnormalities in mucocutaneous lymph node syndrome. *Journal of Immunology*, **130**, 2002–4.

Leung, D. Y. M., Kurt-Jones, E., Newburger, J. W., *et al.* (1989). Endothelial cell activation and high interleukin-1 secretion in the pathogenesis of acute Kawasaki disease. *Lancet*, **ii**, 1298–302.

Levin, D. C., Fellows, K. E. & Abrams, H. L. (1978). Hemodynamically significant primary anomalies of the coronary arteries. *Circulation*, **58**, 25–34.

Levin, M., Holland, P. C., Nokes, T. J. C., *et al.* (1985). Platelet immune complex interaction in pathogenesis of Kawasaki disease and childhood polyarteritis. *British Medical Journal*, **290**, 1456–60.

Levin, M., Tizard, E. J. & Dillon, M. J. (1991). Kawasaki disease: recent advances. *Archives of Disease in Childhood*, **66**, 1369–74.

Levine, O. R., Harris, R. C., Blanc, W. A. & Mellins, R. B. (1973). Progressive pulmonary hypertension in children with portal hypertension. *Journal of Pediatrics*, **83**, 964–72.

Levy, A. M., Tabakin, B. S., Hanson, J. S. & Narkewicz, R. M. (1967). Hypertrophied adenoids causing pulmonary hypertension and severe congestive heart failure. *New England Journal of Medicine*, **277**, 506–11.

Levy-Mozziconacci, A., Wernert, F., Scambler, P., *et al.* (1994). Clinical and molecular study of DiGeorge sequence. *European Journal of Pediatrics*, **153**, 813–20.

Lewis, B. S. & Gotsman, M. S. (1973). Relation between coronary artery size and left ventricular wall mass. *British Heart Journal*, **35**, 1150–53.

Liberthson, R. R. (1989a). Anomalous origins of a coronary artery from the pulmonary artery. In *Congenital Heart Disease. Diagnosis and Management in Children and Adults*. Boston: Little, Brown, pp. 201–8.

Liberthson, R. R. (1989b). Ectopic origin of a coronary artery from the aorta with aberrant proximal course. In *Congenital Heart Disease. Diagnosis and Management in Children and Adults*. Boston: Little, Brown, pp. 209–17.

Liberthson, R. R., Dinsmore, R. E., Bharati, S., *et al.* (1974). Aberrant coronary artery origin from the aorta. Diagnosis and clinical significance. *Circulation*, **50**, 774–9.

Liberthson, R. R., Dinsmore, R. E. & Fallon, J. T. (1979). Aberrant coronary artery origin from the aorta: report of 18 patients, review of the literature and delineation of natural history and management. *Circulation*, **59**, 748–54.

Liberthson, R. R., Gang, D. L. & Custer, J. (1983). Sudden death in an infant with aberrant origin of the right coronary artery from the left sinus of Valsalva of the aorta: case report and review of the literature. *Pediatric Cardiology*, **4**, 45–8.

Lie, J. T. (1987a). Coronary vasculitis: a review in the current scheme of classification of vasculitis. *Archives of Pathology and Laboratory Medicine*, **111**, 224–33.

Lie, J. T. (1987b). Segmental Takayasu (giant cell) aortitis with rupture and limited dissection. *Human Pathology*, **18**, 1183–5.

Lie, J. T. & Berg, K. K. (1987). Isolated fibromuscular dysplasia of the coronary arteries with spontaneous dissection and myocardial infarction. *Human Pathology*, **18**, 654–6.

Lima, J. A., Rosenblum, B. N., Reilly, J. S., Pennington, D. G. & Nouri-Moghaddam, S. (1983). Airway obstruction in aortic arch anomalies. *Otolaryngology, Head and Neck Surgery*, **91**, 605–9.

Lin, F.-Y. C., Bailowitz, A., Koslowe, P., Israel, E. & Kaslow, R. A. (1985). Kawasaki syndrome. A case control study during an outbreak in Maryland. *American Journal of Diseases of Children*, **139**, 277–9.

Lincoln, J. C. R., Deverall, P. B., Stark, J., Aberdeen, E. & Waterston, D. J. (1969). Vascular anomalies compressing the oesophagus and trachea. *Thorax*, **24**, 295–306.

Lindsay, J., Jr (1988). Coarctation of the aorta, bicuspid aortic valve and abnormal ascending aortic wall. *American Journal of Cardiology*, **61**, 182–4.

Lipman, B. L., Rosenthal, I. M. & Lowenburg, H., Jr (1951). Arteriosclerosis in infancy. *American Journal of Diseases of Children*, **82**, 561–6.

Lipsett, J. & Byard, R. W. (1995). Small bowel stricture due to vascular compromise: a late complication of Henoch–Schönlein purpura. *Pediatric Pathology and Laboratory Medicine*, **15**, 333–40.

Lipsett, J., Byard, R. W., Carpenter, B. F., Jimenez, C. L. & Bourne, A. J. (1991). Anomalous coronary arteries arising from the aorta associated with sudden death in infancy and early childhood. *Archives of Pathology and Laboratory Medicine*, **115**, 770–73.

Lipsett, J., Cohle, S. D., Russell, G., Berry, P. J. & Byard, R. W. (1994) Anomalous coronary arteries: a multicentre pediatric autopsy study. *Pediatric Pathology*, **14**, 287–300.

Lipton, M. J., Barry, W. H., Obrez, I. Silverman, J. F. & Wexler L. (1979). Isolated single coronary artery: diagnosis, angiographic classification and clinical significance. *Diagnostic Radiology*, **130**, 39–47.

Lischner, H. W. (1972). DiGeorge syndrome(s). *Journal of Pediatrics*, **81**, 1042–4.

Logan, W. F. W. E., Jones E. W., Walker, E., Coulshed, N. & Epstein, E. J. (1965). Familial supravalvar aortic stenosis. *British Heart Journal*, **27**, 547–59.

Loggie, J. M. H. (1969). Hypertension in children and adolescents. I. Causes and diagnostic studies. *Journal of Pediatrics*, **74**, 331–55.

Loggie, J. M. H., New, M. I. & Robson, A. M. (1979). Hypertension in the pediatric patient: a reappraisal. *Journal of Pediatrics*, **94**, 685–99.

Londe, S. (1978). Causes of hypertension in the young. *Pediatric Clinics of North America*, **25**, 55–65.

Loughlin, G. M., Wynne, J. W. & Victorica, B. E. (1981). Sleep apnea as a possible cause of pulmonary hypertension in Down syndrome. *Journal of Pediatrics*, **98**, 435–7.

Lowe, J. E. & Sabiston, D. C., Jr (1990). Congenital malformations of the coronary circulation. In *Surgery of the Chest*, 5th edn, vol. 2, ed. D. C. Sabiston & F. C. Spencer. Philadelphia: W. B. Saunders, pp. 1689–707.

Loyd, J. E., Atkinson, J. B., Pietra, G. G. Virmani, R. & Newman, J. H. (1988). Heterogeneity of pathologic lesions in familial primary pulmonary hypertension. *American Review of Respiratory Disease*, **138**, 952–7.

Loyd, J. E., Primm, R. K. & Newman, J. H. (1984). Familial primary pulmonary hypertension: clinical patterns. *American Review of Respiratory Disease*, **129**, 194–7.

Lucas, R. V., Jr, Anderson, R. C., Amplatz, K., Adams, P. & Edwards, J. E. (1962). Congenital causes of pulmonary venous obstruction. *Pediatric Clinics of North America*, **10**, 781–836.

Lupi-Herrera, E., Sanchez-Torres, G., Marcushamer, J., *et al.* (1977). Takayasu's arteritis. Clinical study of 107 cases. *American Heart Journal*, **93**, 94–103.

Lüscher, T. F., Lie, J. T., Stanson, A. W., *et al.* (1987). Arterial fibromuscular dysplasia. *Mayo Clinic Proceedings*, **62**, 931–2.

Maayan, C., Peleg, O., Eyal, F., *et al.* (1984). Idiopathic infantile arterial calcification: a case report and review of the literature. *European Journal of Pediatrics*, **142**, 211–15.

Machin, G. A. & Kent, S. (1989). Pulmonary thromboembolism from a large hemangioma in a 4-week-old infant. *Pediatric Pathology*, **9**, 73–8.

MacMahon, H. E. & Dickinson, P. C. T. (1967). Occlusive fibroelastosis of coronary arteries in the newborn. *Circulation*, **35**, 3–9.

Mahowald, J. M., Blieden, L. C., Coe, J. I. & Edwards, J. E. (1986). Ectopic origin of a coronary artery from the aorta: sudden death in 3 of 23 patients. *Chest*, **89**, 668–72.

Maisuls, H., Alday, L. E. & Thüer, O. (1987). Cardiovascular findings in the Williams–Beuren syndrome. *American Heart Journal*, **114**, 897–9.

Makous, N., Friedman, S., Yakovac, W. & Maris, E. P. (1962). Cardiovascular manifestations in progeria. Report of clinical and pathologic findings in a patient with severe arteriosclerotic heart disease and aortic stenosis. *American Heart Journal*, **64**, 334–46.

Mandzia, J. L., terBrugge, K. G., Faughnan, M. E. & Hyland, R. H. (1999). Spinal cord arteriovenous malformations in two patients with hereditary hemorrhagic telangiectasia. *Child's Nervous System*, **15**, 80–83.

Manz, H. J., Vester, J. & Lavenstein, B. (1979). Dissecting aneurysm of cerebral arteries in childhood and adolescence. *Virchows Archive (Pathological Anatomy and Histology)*, **384**, 325–35.

Marrott, P. K., Newcombe, K. D., Becroft, D. M. O. & Friedlander, D. H. (1984). Idiopathic infantile arterial calcification with survival to adult life. *Pediatric Cardiology*, **5**, 119–22.

Martin, E. C. & Moseley, I. F. (1973). Supravalvular aortic stenosis. *British Heart Journal*, **35**, 758–65.

Mason, W. H., Jordan, S. C., Sakai, R., Takashima, M. & Bernstein, B. (1985). Circulating immune complexes in Kawasaki syndrome. *Pediatric Infectious Disease*, **4**, 48–51.

McClellan, J. T. & Jokl, E. (1968). Congenital anomalies of coronary arteries as cause of sudden death associated with physical exertion. *American Journal of Clinical Pathology*, **50**, 229–33.

McConnell, M. E., Hannon, D. W., Steed, R. D. & Gilliland, M. G. F. (1998). Fatal obliterative coronary vasculitis in Kawasaki disease. *Journal of Pediatrics*, **133**, 259–61.

McCowen, C. & Henderson, D. C. (1988). Sudden death in incomplete Kawasaki's disease. *Archives of Disease in Childhood*, **63**, 1254–71.

McFarland, W. & Fuller, D. E. (1964). Mortality in Ehlers–Danlos syndrome due to spontaneous rupture of large arteries. *New England Journal of Medicine*, **271**, 1309–10.

McKinley, H. I., Andrews, J. & Neill, C. A. (1951). Left coronary artery from the pulmonary artery. Three cases, one with cardiac tamponade. *Pediatrics*, **8**, 828–40.

McKusick, V. A. (1990). *Mendelian Inheritance in Man. Catalogs of Autosomal Dominant, Autosomal Recessive, and X-linked Phenotypes*, 9th edn. Baltimore: Johns Hopkins University Press.

McMahon, D. P. & Aterman, K. (1978). Pulmonary hypertension due to multiple emboli. *Journal of Pediatrics*, **92**, 841–5.

McManus, B. M., Gries, L. A., Ness, M. J. & Galup, L. N. (1990). Anomalous origin of the right coronary artery from the left sinus of Valsalva. *Pediatric Pathology*, **10**, 987–91.

McManus, B. M., Waller, B. F., Graboys, T. B., *et al.* (1981). Exercise and sudden death. Part I. *Current Problems in Cardiology*, **6**, 1–89.

Meldgaard, K., Vesterby, A. & Østergaard, J. R. (1997). Sudden death due to rupture of a saccular intracranial aneurysm in a 13-year-old boy. *American Journal of Forensic Medicine and Pathology*, **18**, 342–4.

Melish, M. E. (1982). Kawasaki syndrome (the mucocutaneous lymph node syndrome). *Annual Review of Medicine*, **33**, 569–85.

Menahem, S. & Venables, A. W. (1987). Anomalous left coronary artery from the pulmonary artery: a 15 year sample. *British Heart Journal*, **58**, 378–84.

Menten, M. L. & Fetterman, G. H. (1948). Coronary sclerosis in infancy: report of three autopsied cases, two in siblings. *American Journal of Clinical Pathology*, **18**, 805–10.

Meradji, M., de Villeneuve, V. H., Huber, J., de Bruijn, W. C. & Pearse, R. G. (1978). Idiopathic infantile arterial calcification in siblings: radiologic diagnosis and successful treatment. *Journal of Pediatrics*, **92**, 401–5.

Meurman, L., Somersalo, O. & Tuuteri, L. (1965). Sudden death in infancy caused by idiopathic arterial calcification. *Annales Paediatriae Fenniae*, **11**, 19–24.

Meyer, W. W. & Lind, J. (1972a). Calcifications of iliac arteries in newborns and infants. *Archives of Disease in Childhood*, **47**, 364–72.

Meyer, W. W. & Lind, J. (1972b). Calcifications of the carotid siphon – a common finding in infancy and childhood. *Archives of Disease in Childhood*, **47**, 355–63.

Meyrick, B. & Reid, L. (1983). Pulmonary hypertension: anatomic and physiologic correlates. *Clinics in Chest Medicine*, **4**, 199–217.

Michael, J. R. & Summer, W. R. (1985). Pulmonary hypertension. *Lung*, **163**, 65–82.

Milner, L. S., Heitne, R., Thomson, P. D., Rothberg, A. D. & Ninin, D. T. (1984). Hypertension as the major problem of idiopathic arterial calcification of infancy. *Journal of Pediatrics*, **105**, 934–8.

Mintz, G. S., Iskandrian, A. S., Bemis, C. E., Mundith, E. D. & Owens, J. S. (1983). Myocardial ischemia in anomalous origin of the right coronary artery from the pulmonary trunk. Proof of a coronary steal. *American Journal of Cardiology*, **51**, 610–12.

Moerman, P., Goddeeris, P., Lauwerijns, J. & Van Der Hauwaert, L. G. (1980). Cardiovascular malformations in DiGeorge syndrome (congenital absence or hypoplasia of the thymus). *British Heart Journal*, **44**, 452–9.

Moore, L. & Byard, R. W. (1992a). Fatal paradoxical embolism to the left carotid artery during partial resection of Wilms' tumor. *Pediatric Pathology*, **12**, 551–6.

Moore, L. & Byard, R. W. (1992b). Sudden and unexpected death in infancy associated with a single coronary artery. *Pediatric Pathology*, **12**, 231–6.

Morales, A. R., Romanelli, R. & Boucek, R. J. (1980). The mural left anterior descending coronary artery, strenuous exercise and sudden death. *Circulation*, **62**, 230–37.

Moran, J. J. (1975). Idiopathic arterial calcification of infancy: a clinicopathologic study. *Pathology Annual*, **10**, 393–417.

Moran, J. J. & Becker, S. M. (1959). Idiopathic arterial calcification of infancy. Report of two cases occuring in siblings, and review of the literature. *American Journal of Clinical Pathology*, **31**, 517–29.

Moran, J. J. & Erickson, W. D. (1974). Idiopathic arterial calcification of infancy. *Pathology Annual*, **10**, 77–81.

Moran, J. J. & Steiner, G. C. (1962). Idiopathic arterial calcification in a 5-year-old child. *American Journal of Clinical Pathology*, **73**, 521–6.

Morgan, J. R., Forker, A. D., O'Sullivan, M. J., Jr & Fosburg, R. G. (1972). Coronary arterial fistulas. Seven cases with unusual features. *American Journal of Cardiology*, **30**, 432–6.

Morris, C. A. & Mervis, C. B. (2000). Williams syndrome and related disorders. *Annual Review of Genomics and Human Genetics*, **1**, 461–84.

Morris, C. A., Demsey, S. A., Leonard, C. O., Dilts, C. & Blackburn, B. L. (1988). Natural history of Williams syndrome: physical characteristics. *Journal of Pediatrics*, **113**, 318–26.

Morrow, A. G., Waldhausen, J. A., Peters, R. L., Bloodwell, R. D. & Braunwald, E. (1959). Supravalvular aortic stenosis: clinical, hemodynamic and pathologic observations. *Circulation*, **20**, 1003–10.

Morton, R. (1978). Idiopathic arterial calcification in infancy. *Histopathology*, **2**, 423–32.

Moscoso, G., Mieli-Vergani, G., Mowat, A. P. & Portmann, B. (1991). Sudden death caused by unsuspected pulmonary arterial hypertension, 10 years after surgery for extrahepatic biliary atresia. *Journal of Pediatric Gastroenterology and Nutrition*, **12**, 388–93.

Müller, K.-M. & Blaeser, B. (1976). Tödliche thrombembolische komplikationen nach zentralem venenkatheter. *Deutsche Medizinische Wochenschrift*, **101**, 411–13.

Murphy, J. D. (1991). Hypoplastic left-heart syndrome in children. *Current Opinion in Pediatrics*, **3**, 803–9.

Mustard, W. T., Bayliss, C. E., Fearon, B., Pelton, D. & Trusler, G. A. (1969). Tracheal compression by the innominate artery in children. *Annals of Thoracic Surgery*, **8**, 312–19.

Muster, A. J., Paul, M. H. & Nikaidoh, H. (1973). Tetralogy of Fallot associated with total anomalous pulmonary venous drainage. *Chest*, **64**, 323–7.

Muus, C. J. & McManus, B. M. (1984). Common origin of right and left coronary arteries from the region of left sinus of Valsalva: association with unexpected intrauterine fetal death. *American Heart Journal*, **107**, 1285–6.

Myerburg, R. J., Kessler, K. M. & Castellanos, A. (1992). Sudden cardiac death. Structure, function, and time-dependence of risk. *Circulation*, **85** (suppl 1), I-2-10.

Nadas, A. S., Alimurung, M. M. & Sieracki, L. A. (1951). Cardiac manifestations of Friedreich's ataxia. *New England Journal of Medicine*, **244**, 239–44.

Naeye, R. L. (1960). Advanced pulmonary vascular changes in schistosomal cor pulmonale. *American Journal of Tropical Medicine*, **10**, 191–9.

Nagao, G. I., Daoud, G. I., McAdams, A. J., Schwartz, D. C. & Kaplan, S. (1967). Cardiovascular anomalies associated with tetralogy of Fallot. *American Journal of Cardiology*, **20**, 206–15.

Nakamura, Y., Fujita, Y., Nagai, M., *et al.* (1991). Cardiac sequelae of Kawasaki disease in Japan: statistical analysis. *Pediatrics*, **88**, 1144–7.

Nakashima, Y., Kurozumi, T., Sueishi, K. & Tanaka, K. (1990). Dissecting aneurysm: a clinicopathologic and histopathologic study of 111 autopsied cases. *Human Pathology*, **21**, 291–6.

Navarro, C., Dickinson, P. C. T., Kondlapoodi, P. & Hagstrom, J. W. C. (1984). Mycotic aneurysms of the pulmonary arteries in intravenous drug addicts. Report of three cases and review of the literature. *American Journal of Medicine*, **76**, 1124–31.

Ness, M. J. & McManus, B. M. (1988). Anomalous right coronary artery origin in otherwise unexplained infant death. *Archives of Pathology and Laboratory Medicine*, **112**, 626–9.

Neufeld, H. N. & Blieden, L. C. (1975). Coronary artery disease in children. In *Progress in Cardiology*, ed. P. N. Yu & J. F. Goodwin. Philadelphia: Lea & Febiger, pp. 119–49.

Neufeld, H. N., Wagenvoort, C. A., Ongley, P. A. & Edwards, J. E. (1962). Hypoplasia of ascending aorta. An unusual form of supravalvular aortic stenosis with special reference to localized coronary arterial hypertension. *American Journal of Cardiology*, **10**, 746–51.

Newfeld, E. A., Paul, M. H., Muster, A. J. & Idriss, F. S. (1974). Pulmonary vascular disease in complete transposition of the great arteries: a study of 200 patients. *American Journal of Cardiology*, **34**, 75–82.

Newfeld, E. A., Paul, M. H., Muster, A. J. & Idriss, F. S. (1979). Pulmonary vascular disease in transposition of the great vessels and intact ventricular septum. *Circulation*, **59**, 525–30.

Newfeld, E. A., Wilson, A., Paul, M. H. & Reisch, J. S. (1980). Pulmonary vascular disease in total anomalous pulmonary venous drainage. *Circulation*, **61**, 103–9.

Nichols, M. M. & Tyson, K. R. T. (1978). Saddle embolus occluding pulmonary arteries. *American Journal of Diseases of Children*, **132**, 926.

Nicod, P., Bloor, C., Godfrey, M., *et al.* (1989). Familial aortic dissecting aneurysm. *Journal of the American College of Cardiology*, **13**, 811–19.

Nigro, G., Zerbini, M., Krzysztofiak, A., *et al.* (1994). Active or recent parvovirus B19 infection in children with Kawasaki disease. *Lancet*, **343**, 1260–61.

Nikaidoh, H., Idriss, F. S. & Riker, W. L. (1973). Aortic rupture in children as a complication of coarctation of the aorta. *Archives of Surgery*, **107**, 838–41.

Noonan, J. A., Cottrill, C. M. & O'Connor, W. N. (1982). Supravalvular aortic stenosis: a developmental complex with an increased risk of death at cardiac catheterization. *Pediatric Cardiology*, **3**, 342–3.

Nuss, R., Hays, T. & Manco-Johnson, M. (1995). Childhood thrombosis. *Pediatrics*, **96**, 291–4.

O'Connor, W. N., Davis, J. B., Jr, Geissler, R., *et al.* (1985). Supravalvular aortic stenosis. Clinical and pathologic observations in six patients. *Archives of Pathology and Laboratory Medicine*, **109**, 179–85.

Ogden, J. A. (1970). Congenital anomalies of the coronary arteries. *American Journal of Cardiology*, **25**, 474–9.

Ogden, J. A. & Goodyer, A. V. N. (1970). Patterns of distribution of the single coronary artery. *Yale Journal of Biology and Medicine*, **43**, 11–21.

Ogle, J. W., Waner, J. L., Joffe, L. S., *et al.* (1991). Absence of interferon in sera of patients with Kawasaki syndrome. *Pediatric Infectious Disease Journal*, **10**, 25–9.

Okuni, M. & Sumitomo, N. (1987). Sudden death of school children in Japan. *Japanese Circulation Journal*, **51**, 1397–9.

Page, H. L., Jr, Engel, H. J., Campbell, W. B. & Thomas, C. S., Jr (1974). Anomalous origin of the left circumflex coronary artery. Recognition, angiographic demonstration and clinical significance. *Circulation*, **50**, 768–73.

Paine, T. D. & Grafton, W. D. (1970). Calcification of the arteries in infancy: report of a case. *Journal of Louisiana State Medical Society*, **122**, 344–5.

Panja, M., Kumar, S., Panja, S. & Dutta, B. (1990). Aortic dissection in a non-Marfanoid child. *Journal of the Association of Physicians of India*, **38**, 369–71.

Pare, J. P., Cote, G. & Fraser, R. S. (1989). Long-term follow-up of drug abusers with intravenous talcosis. *American Review of Respiratory Disease*, **139**, 233–41.

Parker, R. J., Smith, E. H. & Stoneman, M. E. R. (1971). Generalised arterial calcification of infancy. *Clinical Radiology*, **22**, 69–73.

Patriarca, P. A., Rogers, M. F., Morens, D. M., Schonberger, L. B. & Kaminski, R. M. (1982). Kawasaki syndrome: association with the application of rug shampoo. *Lancet*, **ii**, 578–80.

Patterson, K., Kapur, S. P. & Chandra, R. S. (1988). Persistent pulmonary hypertension of the newborn: pulmonary pathologic aspects. *Cardiovascular Diseases*, **12**, 139–54.

Paz, J. E. & Castilla, E. E. (1971). Familial total anomalous pulmonary venous return. *Journal of Medical Genetics*, **8**, 312–14.

Perper, J. A., Rozin, L. & Williams, K. E. (1985). Sudden unexpected death following exercise and congenital anomalies of coronary arteries. A report of two cases. *American Journal of Forensic Medicine and Pathology*, **6**, 289–92.

Perrot, L. J. (1997). Malignant hemangioendothelioma: a case of sudden unexpected death in infancy. *American Journal of Forensic Medicine and Pathology*, **18**, 96–9.

Petersen, R. C. & Edwards, W. D. (1983). Pulmonary vascular disease in 57 necropsy cases of total anomalous pulmonary venous connection. *Histopathology*, **7**, 487–96.

Peterson, T. A., Todd, D. B. & Edwards, J. E. (1965). Supravalvular aortic stenosis. *Journal of Thoracic and Cardiovascular Surgery*, **50**, 734–41.

Pilz, P. & Hartjes, H. J. (1976). Fibromuscular dysplasia and multiple dissecting aneurysms of intracranial arteries. A further cause of Moyamoya syndrome. *Stroke*, **7**, 393–8.

Plunkett, J. (1999). Sudden death in an infant caused by rupture of a basilar artery aneurysm. *American Journal of Forensic Medicine and Pathology*, **20**, 45–7.

Pounder, D. J. (1985). Coronary artery aneurysms presenting as sudden death 14 years after Kawasaki disease in infancy. *Archives of Pathology and Laboratory Medicine*, **109**, 874–6.

Powell-Jackson, P. R., Melia, W., Canalese, J., *et al.* (1982). Budd–Chiari syndrome; clinical patterns and therapy. *Quarterly Journal of Medicine*, **201**, 79–88.

Prahlow, J. A., Rushing, E. J. & Barnard, J. J. (1998). Death due to a ruptured berry aneurysm in a 3. 5-year-old child. *American Journal of Forensic Medicine and Pathology*, **19**, 391–4.

Presbitero, P., Bull, C. & Macartney, F. J. (1983). Stenosis of pulmonary veins with ventricular septal defect: a cause of premature pulmonary hypertension in infancy. *British Heart Journal*, **49**, 600–603.

Price, R. A. & Vawter, G. F. (1972). Arterial fibromuscular dysplasia in infancy and childhood. *Archives of Pathology*, **93**, 419–26.

Punnett, H. H. & Zakai, E. H. (1990). Old syndromes and new cytogenetics. *Developmental Medicine and Child Neurology*, **32**, 824–31.

Quam, J. P., Edwards, W. D., Bambara, J. F. & Luzier, T. L. (1986). Sudden death in an adolescent four years after recovery from mucocutaneous lymph node syndrome (Kawasaki disease). *Journal of Forensic Sciences*, **31**, 1135–41.

Rabinovitch, M. & Reid, L. M. (1981). Quantitative structural analysis of the pulmonary vascular bed in congenital heart defects. In *Pediatric Cardiovascular Disease*, ed. M. A. Engle. Philadelphia: F. A. Davis, pp. 149–69.

Rabinovitch, M., Haworth, S. G., Castaneda, A. R., Nadas, A. S. & Reid, L. M. (1978). Lung biopsy in congenital heart disease: a morphometric approach to pulmonary vascular disease. *Circulation*, **58**, 1107–22.

Rabinovitch, M., Haworth, S. G., Vance, Z., *et al.* (1980). Early pulmonary vascular changes in congenital heart disease studied in biopsy tissue. *Human Pathology*, **11** (suppl), 499–509.

Rammos, S., Gittenberger-de Groot, A. C. & Oppenheimer-Dekker, A. (1990). The abnormal pulmonary venous connexion: a developmental approach. *International Journal of Cardiology*, **29**, 285–95.

Rauch, A. M., Glode, M. P., Wiggins, J. W., Jr, *et al.* (1991). Outbreak of Kawasaki syndrome in Denver, Colorado: association with rug and carpet cleaning. *Pediatrics*, **87**, 663–9.

Rauch, A. M., Kaplan, S., Nihill, M., *et al.* (1988). Kawasaki syndrome clusters in Harris County, Texas and Eastern North Carolina. A high endemic rate and a new environment risk factor. *American Journal of Diseases of Children*, **142**, 441–4.

Redington, A. N., Raine, J., Shinebourne, E. A. & Rigby, M. L. (1990). Tetralogy of Fallot with anomalous pulmonary venous connections: a rare but clinically important association. *British Heart Journal*, **64**, 325–8.

Reichel, W. & Garcia-Bunel, R. (1970). Pathologic findings in progeria: myocardial fibrosis and lipofuscin pigment. *American Journal of Clinical Pathology*, **53**, 243–53.

Reifenstein, G. H., Levine, S. A. & Gross, R. E. (1947). Coarctation of the aorta. A review of 104 autopsied cases of the "adult type", 2 years of age or older. *American Heart Journal*, **33**, 146–68.

Reyes-Mújica, M., López-Corella, E., Pérez-Fernández, L., Cuevas-Schacht, F. & Carillo-Farga, J. (1988). Osler-Weber-Rendu disease in an infant. *Human Pathology*, **19**, 1243–6.

Rich, S. & Brundage, B. H. (1984). Primary pulmonary hypertension. Current update. *Journal of the American Medical Association*, **281**, 2252–4.

Rich, S., Levitsky, S. & Brundage, B. H. (1988). Pulmonary hypertension from chronic pulmonary thromboembolism. *Annals of Internal Medicine*, **108**, 425–34.

Robbins, S. L., Cotran, R. S. & Kumar, V. (1984). *Pathologic Basis of Disease*, 3rd edn. Philadelphia: W. B. Saunders, p. 542.

Roberts, C. S. & Roberts, W. C. (1991). Dissection of the aorta associated with congenital malformation of the aortic valve. *Journal of the American College of Cardiology*, **17**, 712–16.

Roberts, W. C. (1978). Coronary embolism: a review of causes, consequences and diagnostic considerations. *Cardiovascular Medicine*, **3**, 699–710.

Roberts, W. C. & Robinowitz, M. (1984). Anomalous origin of the left anterior descending coronary artery from the pulmonary trunk with origin of the right and left circumflex coronary arteries from the aorta. *American Journal of Cardiology*, **54**, 1381–3.

Roberts, W. C., Dicicco, B. S., Waller, B. F., *et al.* (1982). Origin of the left main from the right coronary artery or from the right aortic sinus with intramyocardial tunneling to the left side of the heart via the ventricular septum: the case against clinical significance of myocardial bridge or coronary tunnel. *American Heart Journal*, **104**, 303–5.

Roberts, W. C., Siegel, R. J. & Zipes, D. P. (1982). Origin of the right coronary artery from the left sinus of Valsalva and its functional consequences: analysis of 10 necropsy patients. *American Journal of Cardiology*, **49**, 863–8.

Roberts, W. C., Silver, M. A. & Sapala, J. C. (1986). Intussusception of a coronary artery associated with sudden death in a college football player. *American Journal of Cardiology*, **57**, 179–80.

Robertson, B. (1971). Idiopathic pulmonary hypertension in infancy and childhood: microangiographic and histological observations in five cases. *Acta Pathologica et Microbiologica Scandinavica*, **79**, 217–27.

Robinowitz, M., Forman, M. B. & Virmani, R. (1989). Nonatherosclerotic coronary aneurysms. In *Nonatherosclerotic Ischemic Heart Disease*, ed. R. Virmani & M. B. Forman. New York: Raven Press, pp. 277–303.

Robinson, H. B., Jr (1975). DiGeorge's or the III-IV pharyngeal pouch syndrome: pathology and a theory of pathogenesis. In *Perspectives in Pediatric Pathology*, vol. 2, ed. H. S. Rosenberg & R. P. Bolande. Chicago: Year Book Medical Publishers, pp. 173–206.

Rogers, M. F., Kochel, R. L., Hurwitz, E. S., *et al.* (1985). Kawasaki syndrome: is exposure to rug shampoo important? *American Journal of Diseases of Children*, **139**, 777–9.

Rolfes, D. B., Towbin, R. & Bove, K. E. (1985). Vascular dysplasia in a child with tuberous sclerosis. *Pediatric Pathology*, **3**, 359–73.

Rosenberg, H. S. (1973). Coarctation of the aorta: morphology and pathogenetic considerations. In *Perspectives in Pediatric Pathology*, vol. 1, ed. H. S. Rosenberg & R. P. Bolande. Chicago: Year Book Medical Publishers, pp. 339–57.

Rosenberg, H. S. (1974). Systemic arterial disease and chronic arsenicism in infants. *Archives of Pathology*, **97**, 360–65.

Rossi, S. O., Gilbert-Barnes, E., Saari, T. & Corliss, R. (1992). Pulmonary hypertension with coexisting portal hypertension. *Pediatric Pathology*, **12**, 433–9.

Rotenstein, D., Gibbas, D. L., Majmudar, B. & Chastain, E. A. (1982). Familial granulomatous arteritis with polyarthritis of juvenile onset. *New England Journal of Medicine*, **306**, 86–90.

Rowley, A. H., Gonzalez-Crussi, F. & Shulman, S. T. (1988). Kawasaki disease. *Review of Infectious Diseases*, **10**, 1–15.

Rowley, A. H. & Shulman, S. T. (1999). Kawasaki syndrome. *Pediatric Clinics of North America*, **46**, 313–29.

Rubinstein, I., Murray, D. & Hoffstein, V. (1988). Fatal pulmonary emboli in hospitalized patients. An autopsy study. *Archives of Internal Medicine*, **148**, 1425–6.

Sahn, D. J., Goldberg, S. J., Allen, H. D. & Canale, J. M. (1981). Cross-sectional echocardiographic imaging of supracardiac total anomalous pulmonary venous drainage to a vertical vein in a patient with Holt-Oram syndrome. *Chest*, **79**, 113–15.

Samanek, M., Goetzova, J. & Benesova, D. (1985). Distribution of congenital heart malformations in an autopsied child population. *International Journal of Cardiology*, **8**, 235–48.

Sánchez-Torres, G., Pineda, C., Morales, E. & Martínez-Lavin, M. (1983). Takayasu's arteritis in children. *Arthritis and Rheumatism*, **26**, 535.

Sano, S., Brawn, W. J. & Mee, R. B. B. (1989). Total anomalous pulmonary venous drainage. *Journal of Thoracic and Cardiovascular Surgery*, **97**, 886–92.

Sasazuki, T., Harada, F. & Kawasaki, T. (1987). Genetic analysis of Kawasaki disease. *Progress in Clinical and Biological Research*, **250**, 251–5.

Saukko, P. & Lignitz, E. (1990). Plötzlicher tod durch malign hodentumoren. *Zeitschrift fur Rechtsmedizin*, **103**, 529–36.

Savage, C. O. S., Tizard, J., Jayne, D., Lockwood, C. M. & Dillon, M. J. (1989). Antineutrophil cytoplasm antibodies in Kawasaki disease. *Archives of Disease in Childhood*, **64**, 360–63.

Scambler, P. J., Kelly, D., Lindsay, E., *et al.* (1992). Velo-cardio-facial syndrome associated with chromosome 22 deletions encompassing the DiGeorge locus. *Lancet*, **339**, 1138–9.

Schimke, R. N., McKusick, V. A., Huang, T. & Pollack, A. D. (1965). Homocystinuria. Studies of 20 families with 38 affected members. *Journal of the American Medical Association*, **193**, 711–19.

Schmidt, R. E., Gilbert, E. F., Amend, T. C., Chamberlain, C. R. & Lucas, R. V., Jr (1969). Generalized arterial fibromuscular dysplasia and myocardial infarction in familial supravalvular aortic stenosis syndrome. *Journal of Pediatrics*, **74**, 576–84.

Schwartz, R. P. & Robicsek, F. (1971). An unusual anomaly of the coronary system: origin of the anterior (descending) interventricular artery from the pulmonary trunk. *Journal of Pediatrics*, **78**, 123–6.

Schwöbel, M. & Stauffer, U. G. (1983). Lungenembolien im kindesalter: pulmonary embolism in children. *Zeitschrift fur Kinderchirurgie*, **38**, 30–32.

Segel, G. B. & Francis, C. W. (2000). Anticoagulant proteins in childhood venous and arterial thrombosis: a review. *Blood Cells, Molecules, and Diseases*, **26**, 540–60.

Seguchi, M., Hino, Y., Aiba, S., *et al.* (1990). Ostial stenosis of the left coronary artery as a sole clinical manifestation of Takayasu's arteritis: a possible cause of unexpected sudden death. *Heart and Vessels*, **5**, 188–91.

Seo, J. W., Lee, H. J., Choi, J. Y., Choi, Y. H. & Lee, J. R. (1991). Pulmonary veins in total anomalous pulmonary venous connection with obstruction: demonstration using silicone rubber casts. *Pediatric Pathology*, **11**, 711–20.

Serry, C., Agomuoh, O. S. & Goldin, M. D. (1988). Review of Ehlers–Danlos syndrome. Successful repair of rupture and dissection of abdominal aorta. *Journal of Cardiovascular Surgery*, **29**, 530–34.

Sharbaugh, A. H. & White, R. S. (1974). Single coronary artery: analysis of the anatomic variation, clinical importance and report of five cases. *Journal of the American Medical Association*, **230**, 243–6.

Sharma, V. K. & Howden, C. W. (1998). Gastrointestinal and hepatic manifestations of hereditary hemorrhagic telangiectasia. *Digestive Diseases*, **16**, 169–74.

Shearer, W. T., Rutman, J. Y., Weinberg, W. A. & Goldring, D. (1970). Coarctation of the aorta and cerebrovascular accident: a proposal for early corrective surgery. *Journal of Pediatrics*, **77**, 1004–9.

Sholler, G. F., Yu, J. S., Bale, P. M., *et al.* (1984). Generalized arterial calcification of infancy: three case reports, including spontaneous regression with long-term survival. *Journal of Pediatrics*, **105**, 257–60.

Short, D. W. (1978). Multiple congenital aneurysms in childhood: report of a case. *British Journal of Surgery*, **65**, 509–12.

Shovlin, C. L. (1997). Molecular defects in rare bleeding disorders: hereditary haemorrhagic telangiectasia. *Thrombosis and Haemostasis*, **78**, 145–50.

Shovlin, C. L. & Letarte, M. (1999). Hereditary haemorrhagic telangiectasia and pulmonary arteriovenous malformations: issues in clinical management and review of pathogenic mechanisms. *Thorax*, **54**, 714–29.

Shprintzen, R. J., Goldberg, R. B., Young, D. & Wolford, L. (1981). The velo-cardio-facial syndrome: a clinical and genetic analysis. *Pediatrics*, **67**, 167–72.

Siegel, H. (1972). Human pulmonary pathology associated with narcotic and other addictive drugs. *Human Pathology*, **3**, 55–66.

Siegel, R. J. & Dunton, S. F. (1991). Systemic occlusive arteriopathy with sudden death in a 10-year-old boy. *Human Pathology*, **22**, 197–200.

Silver, M. M., Bohn, D., Shawn, D. H., *et al.* (1992). Association of pulmonary hypertension with congenital portal hypertension in a child. *Journal of Pediatrics*, **120**, 321–9.

Sissman, N. J., Neill, C. A., Spencer, F. C. & Taussig, H. B. (1959). Congenital aortic stenosis. *Circulation*, **19**, 458–68.

Slim, M. S. & Akel, S. R. (1982). Hydatidosis in children. *Progress in Pediatric Surgery*, **15**, 119–29.

Smith, J. C. (1950). Review of single coronary artery with report of 2 cases. *Circulation*, **1**, 1168–75.

Smith, R. J. H., Smith, M. C. F., Glossop, L. P., Bailey, C. M. & Evans, J. N. G. (1984). Congenital vascular anomalies causing tracheoesophageal compression. *Archives of Otolaryngology*, **110**, 82–7.

Solymar, L., Sabel, K.-G. & Zetterqvist, P. (1987). Total anomalous pulmonary venous connection in siblings. Report on three families. *Acta Paediatrica Scandinavica*, **76**, 124–7.

Sotrel, A., Lacson, A. G. & Huff, K. R. (1983). Childhood Köhlmeier–Degos disease with atypical skin lesions. *Neurology*, **33**, 1146–51.

Spach, M. S., Howell, D. A. & Harris, J. S. (1963). Myocardial infarction and multiple thromboses in a child with primary thrombocytosis. *Pediatrics*, **31**, 268–76.

Stahl, J., Santos, L. D. & Byard, R. W. (1995). Coronary artery thromboembolism and unexpected death in childhood and adolescence. *Journal of Forensic Sciences*, **40**, 599–601.

Stamm, C., Friehs, I., Ho, S. Y., *et al.* (2001). Congenital supravalvar aortic stenosis: a simple lesion? *European Journal of Cardiothoracic Surgery*, **19**, 195–202.

Steinberger, J., Lucas, R. V., Edwards, J. E. & Titus, J. L. (1996). Causes of sudden unexpected cardiac death in the first two decades of life. *American Journal of Cardiology*, **77**, 992–5.

Stoler, M. H., Anderson, V. M. & Stuard, L. D. (1982). A case of pulmonary veno-occlusive disease in infancy. *Archives of Pathology and Laboratory Medicine*, **106**, 645–7.

Strauss, A. W. & Johnson, M. C. (1996). The genetic basis of pediatric cardiovascular disease. *Seminars in Perinatology*, **20**, 564–76.

Strife, J. L., Baumel, A. S. & Dunbar, J. S. (1981). Tracheal compression by the innominate artery in infancy and childhood. *Pediatric Pathology*, **139**, 73–5.

Strole, W. E., Jr, Clark, W. H., Jr & Isselbacher, K. J. (1967). Progressive arterial occlusive disease (Kohlmeier–Degos). A frequently fatal cutaneosystemic disorder. *New England Journal of Medicine*, **276**, 195–201.

Strong, W. B., Perrin, E., Liebman, J. & Silbert, D. R. (1970). Systemic and pulmonary artery dysplasia associated with unexpected death in infancy. *Journal of Pediatrics*, **77**, 233–8.

Stryker, W. A. (1946). Arterial calcification in infancy with special reference to the coronary arteries. *American Journal of Pathology*, **22**, 1007–31.

Subramanyan, R., Joy, J. & Balakrishnan, K. G. (1989). Natural history of aortarteritis (Takayasu's disease). *Circulation*, **80**, 429–37.

Sullivan, K. E. (2001). DiGeorge syndrome/chromosome 22q11.2 deletion syndrome. *Current Allergy and Asthma Reports*, **1**, 438–44.

Sumboonnanonda, A., Robinson, B. L., Gedroyc, W. M. W., *et al.* (1992). Middle aortic syndrome: clinical and radiological findings. *Archives of Disease in Childhood*, **67**, 501–5.

Sun, C.-C. J., Jacot, J. & Brenner, J. I. (1992). Sudden death in supravalvular aortic stenosis: fusion of a coronary leaflet to the sinus ridge, dysplasia and stenosis of aortic and pulmonic valves. *Pediatric Pathology*, **12**, 751–9.

Takahashi, M., Mason, W. & Lewis, A. B. (1987). Regression of coronary aneurysms in patients with Kawasaki syndrome. *Circulation*, **75**, 387–94.

Tandon, H. D. & Kasturi, J. (1975). Pulmonary vascular changes associated with isolated mitral stenosis in India. *British Heart Journal*, **37**, 26–36.

Tasker, W. G., Mastri, A. R. & Gold, A. P. (1970). Chondrodystrophia calcificans congenita (dysplasia epiphysalis punctata). Recognition of the clinical picture. *American Journal of Diseases of Children*, **119**, 122–7.

Terasawa, K., Ichinose, E., Matsuishi, T. & Kato, H. (1983). Neurological complications in Kawasaki disease. *Brain and Development*, **5**, 371–4.

Terhune, P. E., Buchino, J. J. & Rees, A. H. (1985). Myocardial infarction associated with supravalvular aortic stenosis. *Pediatrics*, **106**, 251–4.

Thadani, U., Burrow, C., Whitaker, W. & Heath, D. (1975). Pulmonary veno-occlusive disease. *Quarterly Journal of Medicine*, **44**, 133–59.

Thomas, R. H. (2001). Hypercoagulability syndromes. *Archives of Internal Medicine*, **161**, 2433–9.

Thomas, W. A., Lee, K. T., McGavran, M. H. & Rabin, E. R. (1956). Endocardial fibroelastosis in infants associated with thrombosis and calcification of arteries and myocardial infarcts. *New England Journal of Medicine*, **255**, 464–8.

Thornback, P. & Fowler, R. S. (1975). Sudden unexpected death in children with congenital heart disease. *Canadian Medical Association Journal*, **113**, 745–8.

Tiefenbrunn, L. J. & Riemenschneider, T. A. (1986). Persistent pulmonary hypertension of the newborn. *American Heart Journal*, **111**, 564–72.

Tizard, E. J., Baguley, E., Hughes, G. R. V. & Dillon, M. J. (1991). Antiendothelial cell antibodies detected by a cellular based ELISA in Kawasaki disease. *Archives of Disease in Childhood*, **66**, 189–92.

Topaz, O., DeMarchena, E. J., Perin, E., *et al.* (1992). Anomalous coronary arteries: angiographic findings in 80 patients. *International Journal of Cardiology*, **34**, 129–38.

Towbin, J. A., Casey, B. & Belmont, J. (1999). Human genetics '99: the cardiovascular system. The molecular basis of vascular disorders. *American Journal of Human Genetics*, **64**, 678–84.

Toyama, M., Amano, A. & Kameda, T. (1989). Familial aortic dissection: a report of rare family cluster. *British Heart Journal*, **61**, 204–7.

Traisman, H. S., Limperis, N. M. & Traisman, A. S. (1956). Myocardial infarction due to calcification of the arteries in an infant. *American Journal of Diseases of Children*, **91**, 34–7.

Tri, T. B. & Combs, D. T. (1978). Congestive cardiomyopathy in Werner's syndrome. *Lancet*, **i**, 1052–3.

Trillo, A. A., Scharyj, M. & Prichard, R. W. (1980). Coronary artery aneurysm and myocardial infarction resulting in sudden death of a 6 year-old child. A case report. *American Journal of Forensic Medicine and Pathology*, **1**, 349–54.

Tron, V., Magee, F., Wright, J. L., Colby, T. & Churg, A. (1986). Pulmonary capillary hemangiomatosis. *Human Pathology*, **17**, 1144–50.

Turley, K., Tucker, W. Y., Ullyot, D. J. & Ebert, P. A. (1980). Total anomalous pulmonary venous connection in infancy: influence of age and type of lesion. *American Journal of Cardiology*, **45**, 92–7.

Van Dyck, M., Proesmans, W., Van Hollebeke, E., Marxhal, G. & Moerman, P. (1989). Idiopathic infantile arterial calcification with cardiac, renal and central nervous system involvement. *European Journal of Pediatrics*, **148**, 374–7.

Varghese, P. J., Izukawa, T. & Rowe, R. D. (1969). Supravalvular aortic stenosis as part of rubella syndrome, with discussion of pathogenesis. *British Heart Journal*, **31**, 59–62.

Vestermark, S. (1965). Single coronary artery. *Cardiologia*, **46**, 79–84.

Viles, P. H., Ongley, P. A. & Titus, J. L. (1969). The spectrum of pulmonary vascular disease in transposition of the great arteries. *Circulation*, **40**, 31–41.

Virmani, R. & Forman, M. B. (1989). Coronary artery dissections. In *Nonatherosclerotic Ischemic Heart Disease*, ed. R. Virmani & M. B. Foreman. New York: Raven Press, pp. 325–54.

Virmani, R., Chun, P. K. C., Goldstein, R. E., Robinowitz, M. & McAllister, H. A. (1984a). Acute takeoffs of the coronary arteries along the aortic wall and congenital coronary ostial valve-like ridges: association with sudden death. *Journal of the American College of Cardiology*, **3**, 766–71.

Virmani, R., Forman, M. B., Robinowitz, M. & McAllister, H. A., Jr (1984b). Coronary artery dissections. *Cardiology Clinics*, **2**, 633–46.

Virmani, R., Robinowitz, M. & Darcy, T. P. (1991). Coronary vasculitis. In *Cardiovascular Pathology, Major Problems in Pathology*, vol. 23, ed. R. Virmani, J. B. Atkinson & J. J. Fenoglio. Philadelphia: W. B. Saunders, pp. 166–202.

Virmani, R., Rogan, K. & Cheitlin, M. D. (1989). Congenital coronary artery anomolies: pathologic aspects. In *Nonatherosclerotic Ischemic Heart Disease*, ed. R. Virmani & M. B. Foreman. New York: Raven Press, pp. 153–83.

Virmani, R., Ursell, P. C. & Fenoglio, J. J. (1987). Examination of the heart. *Human Pathology*, **18**, 432–40.

Voordes, C. G., Kuipers, J. R. G. & Elema, J. D. (1977). Familial pulmonary veno-occlusive disease: a case report. *Thorax*, **32**, 763–6.

Wagenvoort, C. A. (1973). Hypertensive pulmonary vascular disease complicating congenital heart disease: a review. *Cardiovascular Clinics*, **5**, 43–60.

Wagenvoort, C. A. (1975). Pathology of congestive pulmonary hypertension. *Progressive Respiratory Research*, **9**, 195–202.

Wagenvoort, C. A. (1976). Pulmonary veno-occlusive disease: entity or syndrome? *Chest*, **69**, 82–6.

Wagenvoort, C. A. (1980). Lung biopsies in the differential diagnosis of thromboembolic versus primary pulmonary hypertension. *Progress in Respiratory Research*, **13**, 16–21.

Wagenvoort, C. A. & Wagenvoort, N. (1970). Primary pulmonary hypertension: a pathologic study of the lung vessels in 156 clinically diagnosed cases. *Circulation*, **42**, 1163–84.

Wagenvoort, C. A. & Wagenvoort, N. (1976). Pulmonary venous changes in chronic hypoxia. *Virchows Archive (Pathological Anatomy and Histology)*, **372**, 51–6.

Wagenvoort, C. A. & Wagenvoort, N. (1977). Pulmonary veno-occlusive disease. In *Pathology of Pulmonary Hypertension*. New York: John Wiley & Sons, pp. 217–31.

Wagenvoort, C. A., Harris, L. E., Brown, A. L., Jr & Veeneklaas, G. M. H. (1963). Giant-cell arteritis with aneurysm formation in children. *Pediatrics*, **32**, 861–7.

Wagenvoort, C. A., Losekoot, G. & Mulder, E. (1971). Pulmonary veno-occlusive disease of presumably intrauterine origin. *Thorax*, **26**, 429–34.

Wagenvoort, C. A., Neufeld, H. N., DuShane, J. W. & Edwards, J. E. (1961). The pulmonary arterial tree in atrial septal defect. A quantitative study of anatomic features in fetuses, infants, and children. *Circulation*, **23**, 733–9.

Walley, V. M., Virmani, R. & Silver, M. D. (1990). Pulmonary arterial dissections and ruptures: to be considered in patients with pulmonary arterial hypertension presenting with cardiogenic shock or sudden death. *Pathology*, **22**, 1–4.

Wallis, K., Deutsch, V. & Azizi, E. (1970). Hypertension in a case of von Recklinghausen's neurofibromatosis. *Helvetica Paediatrica Acta*, **2**, 147–53.

Weens, H. S. & Marin, C. A. (1956). Infantile arteriosclerosis. *Radiology*, **67**, 168–74.

Weik, C. & Greiner, L. (1999). The liver in hereditary hemorrhagic telangiectasia (Weber-Rendu-Osler disease). *Scandinavian Journal of Gastroenterology*, **34**, 1241–6.

Weisz, G. M., Schramkek, A., Abrahamson, J. & Barzilai, A. (1974). Fat embolism in children: tests for its early detection. *Journal of Pediatric Surgery*, **9**, 163–7.

Werner, B., Wróblewska-Kalużewska, M., Pleskot, M., Tarnowska, A. & Potocka, K. (2001). Anomalies of the coronary arteries in children. *Medical Science Monitor*, **7**, 1285–91.

Wesselhoeft, H., Fawcett, J. S. & Johnson, A. L. (1968). Anomalous origin of the left coronary artery from the pulmonary trunk. Its clinical spectrum, pathology, and pathophysiology, based on a review of 140 cases with seven further cases. *Circulation*, **38**, 403–25.

White, R. A., Preus, M., Watters, G. V. & Fraser, F. C. (1977). Familial occurrence of the Williams syndrome. *Journal of Pediatrics*, **91**, 614–16.

Wilkes, D., Donner, R., Black, I. & Carbello, B. A. (1985). Variant angina in an 11 year old boy. *Journal of the American College of Cardiology*, **5**, 761–4.

Wilson, C. L., Dlabal, P. W. & McGuire, S. A. (1979). Surgical treatment of anomalous left coronary artery from pulmonary artery: follow-up in teenagers and adults. *American Heart Journal*, **98**, 440–46.

Wilson, D. I., Goodship, J. A., Burn, J., Cross, I. E. & Scambler, P. J. (1992). Deletions within chromosome 22q11 in familial congenital heart disease. *Lancet*, **340**, 573–5.

Wilson, J. (1798). XIII. A description of a very unusual formation of the human heart. *Philosophical Transactions of the Royal Society of London*, **88**, 346–56.

Wreford, F. S., Conradi, S. E., Cohle, S. D., *et al.* (1991). Sudden death caused by coronary artery aneurysms: a late complication of Kawasaki disease. *Journal of Forensic Sciences*, **36**, 51–9.

Yamaki, S. & Wagenvoort, C. A. (1985). Comparison of primary plexogenic arteriopathy in adults and children: a morphometric study in 40 patients. *British Heart Journal*, **54**, 428–34.

Yamashita, M., Tanaka, K., Kishikawa, T. & Yokota, K. (1984). Moyamoya disease associated with renovascular hypertension. *Human Pathology*, **15**, 191–3.

Yanagawa, H., Nakamura, Y., Kawasaki, T. & Shigematsu, I. (1986). Nationwide epidemic of Kawasaki disease in Japan during winter of 1985–86. *Lancet*, **ii**, 1138–9.

York, M. J. & Dimon, J. H., III (1988). Idiopathic dissecting aortic aneurysm associated with pain in the back in an adolescent. *Journal of Bone and Joint Surgery*, **70-A**, 1418–21.

Zuccollo, J. M. & Byard, R. W. (2001). Sudden death in an infant (Kawasaki disease). *Pathology*, **33**, 235–8.

7

Respiratory conditions

Introduction

Respiratory causes of sudden and unexpected death are often due to acute obstruction of the airway by an impacted foreign body (as discussed in Chapter 2) or critical narrowing by an intrinsic lesion such as an inflamed epiglottis. Other major causes of sudden respiratory death are asthma and infective conditions, such as acute bronchopneumonia. These disorders are listed in Table 7.1.

In two studies of sudden death in children and young adults, respiratory disease was a cause of death in 10 of 31 (32%) cases (Molander, 1982) and in 12 of 78 cases (15%) (Siboni & Simonsen, 1986). Molander (1982) found four cases of bronchopneumonia, three cases of asthma, and three cases of acute epiglottitis, while Siboni & Simonsen found a greater number of cases of fulminant tracheobronchitis (five of the 12 cases of fatal respiratory disease), with four cases of acute epiglottitis, two of asthma, and a final case in which death was attributed to acute tonsillitis. Thus, acute respiratory disease accounts for a significant proportion of cases of sudden natural death in children and young adults. The proportion of cases of sudden childhood death due to respiratory obstruction has, however, changed in recent years. For example, there has been a reduction in the number of deaths due to acute epiglottitis in communities where immunization programs for *Hemophilus influenzae* have been instituted, and in the number of deaths due to foreign body inhalation when campaigns aimed at increasing parental awareness of the dangers of choking have been developed (Byard, 2000).

Asthma

Asthma is characterized by attacks of wheezy breathlessness due to paroxysmal narrowing of smaller airways triggered by a variety of specific allergenic materials. These include pollen, dust, chemical fumes, animal products, aspirin, and infectious agents such as viruses and *Aspergillus* sp. Physical stimuli such as cold temperatures may also induce an attack, as may exercise (McFadden & Gilbert, 1994). Asthma is the most common chronic lung disorder of childhood in a number of countries, including the USA, the UK, and Australia. Although asthma is associated only rarely with a fatal outcome (Friday & Fireman, 1988), the incidence of asthma-related deaths had been reported to be increasing (Larsen, 1992; Robin, 1988; Wasserfallen *et al.*, 1990). Death may occur during status asthmaticus, in which severe bronchospasm persists despite medical treatment, or it may be quite sudden and unexpected. In the pediatric age range, this tends to occur predominantly in older children and adolescents. For example, no children under three years of age were found in one series of 11 cases of sudden childhood death (age range 3 years, 10 months to 15 years, 2 months; mean 9 years, 9 months) (Champ & Byard, 1994).

Table 7.1. Respiratory causes of sudden pediatric death

Asthma
Upper airway obstruction
Bronchopulmonary dysplasia
Acute bronchopneumonia
Cystic fibrosis
Massive pulmonary hemorrhage
Idiopathic pulmonary hemosiderosis
Tension pneumothorax

Clinical features

Children with asthma have episodic wheezing, dyspnea, and hyperinflation of the chest. Individuals who are most likely to die are those with a long history of asthma and who have had episodes in the past that were life-threatening or that required hospitalization (Bateman & Clarke, 1979). Although sudden death has been reported in children who have presented with apparently only mild episodes, or without particularly severe histories (Hetzel, Clark & Branthwaite, 1977; Robertson, Rubinfeld & Bowes, 1992), analysis of one series revealed that significant growth retardation was present in the majority of children. This included a 14-year-old boy with reportedly "mild" asthma who also had extramedullary hematopoesis, indicating that there had been previous significant prolonged hypoxia (Champ & Byard, 1994). Delayed growth parameters may, therefore, be an additional useful morphological marker for the at-risk child.

It has been suggested that adolescence may be a time of increased risk of a lethal episode because of poor compliance with medication or abuse of certain prescribed drugs (Kravis & Kolski, 1985). Adolescents may also underestimate the severity of an attack (Zach & Karner, 1989). This was demonstrated clearly by a girl who booked in to a non-urgent clinic with central cyanosis, a quiet chest, and an FEV_1 of 0.15 l (Cushley & Tattersfield, 1983). A reduced perception of dyspnea may be associated with an impaired response to hypoxia (Barnes, 1994). Psychological factors such as deliberate denial of disease and depression may also be found in those at increased risk of sudden death (Rubinstein et al., 1984).

Occurrence of sudden death

The mechanisms of sudden death in an acute asthmatic attack are not understood completely. They include cardiac arrhythmias, hypokalemia, and asphyxia. Unfortunately, it has been difficult to obtain adequate data due to the rapidity of terminal episodes and their occurrence outside hospital. Asthma attacks in which the individual has progressed from minor symptoms to respiratory arrest within the space of one to two hours have been termed "sudden asphyxic asthma" (Wasserfallen et al., 1990). Death may also occur during sleep (Champ & Byard, 1994).

Bronchodilators have been implicated in the etiology of sudden death (Spitzer et al., 1992), possibly due to vasovagally mediated hypotension with bradycardia or cardiac arrhythmias (Grubb et al., 1992). Alternatively, bronchodilators may provide temporary symptomatic relief, resulting in a critical delay in presentation of the patient to hospital. Delay in seeking treatment for whatever reason has been found to be a significant factor in fatal episodes (Johnson et al., 1984). The possibility of pharyngeal irritation from inhalational agents inducing a vasovagal response and cardiac arrest has also been proposed (Morild & Giertsen, 1989).

Although cardiac arrhythmia exacerbated by anti-asthmatic drugs has been put forward as the most likely terminal event (Drislane et al., 1987; Wilson, Sutherland & Thomas, 1981), a clinical study of 10 adolescent and adult asthmatics who developed respiratory arrest before or soon after arrival at hospital failed to demonstrate significant disturbances of cardiac rhythm. It was concluded, therefore, that severe asphyxia rather than arrhythmia was the more important precipitating factor (Molfino et al., 1991). Sudden massive narrowing of the airways is certainly a well-recognized cause of collapse, based on observations of initially stable hospital asthmatic patients who suddenly deteriorate and require markedly increased ventilatory pressures (Wood & Lecks, 1976). The possibility of an alternative process such as pneumothorax should also be considered in this situation. This was found in two children in a series of 13 fatal cases (Kravis & Kolski, 1985). Pneumothorax may also be associated with fatal air embolism in status asthmaticus (Segal & Wasserman, 1971).

The possibility of electrolyte disturbance in fatal cases has been considered (Haalboom, Deenstra & Struyvenberg, 1985). In particular, hypokalemia due to the action of β-2 agonists may potentiate the irritative effects of hypoxia, acidosis, and of the β-2 agonists themselves on the myocardium. Hypokalemia may also induce muscle weakness (Knochel, 1982), which impedes chest wall and respiratory muscle actions.

Occasionally, the presence of other lung lesions may adversely affect the outcome of an acute attack. For example, bronchopneumonia and previous pulmonary thromboembolism were found in three of a series of 13 asthmatic children who died unexpectedly (Kravis & Kolski, 1985). Similarly, viral infection of the lungs may precipitate a lethal episode in predisposed children (Las Heras & Swanson, 1983). Along with bacterial infections, this may account for the seasonal variation in incidence of lethal episodes (Preston & Bowen, 1987). Drug hypersensitivity may also be a precipitating factor in a small number of cases (Benatar, 1986). Although children with acute asthmatic episodes often have nausea and vomiting, sometimes exacerbated by medications, aspiration of gastric contents has not been a significant contributor to death.

A final possibility that may increase the likelihood of sudden death is adrenal insufficiency (Las Heras & Swanson, 1983), which has been demonstrated in adolescent asthmatics secondary to prolonged steroid usage (Busuttil, 1991).

Pathological features

At autopsy, a history of rapidly progressive respiratory symptoms prior to collapse will enable clinicopathological correlation to be made in a child in whom fatal asthma is suspected. However, the time

from no apparent symptoms to death may be extremely short (Robin & Lewiston, 1989), and the presenting history may also be atypical in that hypoxia may induce seizures, with incontinence or impaired consciousness (Friday & Fireman, 1988).

The three main components in a fatal asthmatic attack are bronchospasm, plugging of airways by tenacious secretions, and edema of the mucosa, all of which may contribute to worsening hypoxia, resulting in cardiorespiratory arrest. Evidence of the latter two processes may be found at autopsy, with changes in the airways occurring in response to inflammatory mediators, such as histamine, prostaglandins, platelet activating factors, leukotrienes, and eosinophil cationic protein, which are released by mast cells and eosinophils (Champ & Byard, 1994). Tension pneumothorax, although rare, should always be considered in these children, and chest X-ray and/or opening of the chest under a water seal should be performed.

The lungs are usually markedly hyperinflated, often meeting in the midline and retaining their shape after evisceration (Color Plate 15). One of the most striking features on gross inspection of the opened airways and cut surface of the lungs may be the presence of thick tenacious mucus plugs filling bronchi and bronchioles (Figure 7.1). There may also be evidence of bronchiectasis and emphysema.

Classically, the microscopic features of asthma include edema of the bronchial walls, with an increase in inflammatory cells (particularly eosinophils), thickening of the subepithelial basement membrane, and hypertrophy of smooth muscle (Figure 7.2). There may also be hypertrophy of submucosal mucus glands (Figure 7.3), with generalized increased thickness of airway walls in fatal cases (Carroll *et al.*, 1993). The increase in submucosal chronic inflammatory cells may result from a viral infection that has triggered the lethal episode. Within the bronchial lumena there may be mucus plugs, which contain variable numbers of eosinophils and strands of desquamated ciliated respiratory epithelial cells forming Curshmann spirals. Charcot–Leyden crystals may be associated with eosinophils. Myocardial contraction band

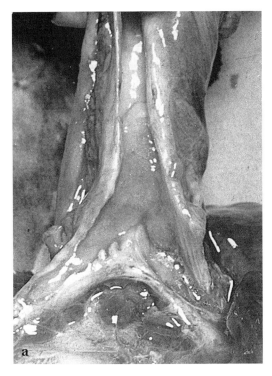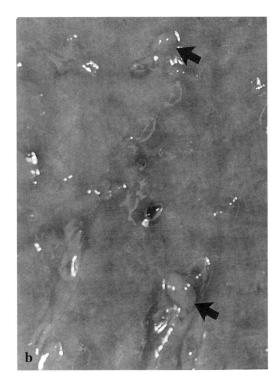

Figure 7.1 Tenacious mucus plugs filling the lower trachea and major bronchi may be found in asthma (a). The cut surface of the lung shows extruded mucus plugs (arrows) (b).

necrosis has also been reported in children who have died during status asthmaticus (Drislane *et al.*, 1987).

Although the histologic findings may be typical of asthma, there are no pathognomonic features unique to lethal cases, and lung sections may even appear reasonably normal (Robin & Lewiston, 1989). Also, features may be distributed variably, involving some but not necessarily all bronchi. Thus, there is a need to rely on an appropriate clinical history and on the exclusion of other possibilities.

Upper airway obstruction

While obstruction of the airways occurs most often in children as a result of foreign-body impaction, there are other intrinsic and extrinsic lesions that may also result in acute airway occlusion (Byard, 1993;

Byard, 1996). These can be classified according to their anatomical location and are listed in Table 7.2. Although not all of these lesions have been reported as causes of sudden death, it is reasonable to suppose that any lesion of the upper airway that causes significant dyspnea and stridor, and that requires urgent endotracheal intubation, is also capable of causing lethal airway occlusion. While a number of congenital abnormalities such as choanal atresia present within the neonatal period, occasional cases with incomplete airway occlusion may not be diagnosed until later in life.

Choanal atresia

Obstruction of the airway at the level of the choanae may be unilateral and partial, or bilateral and complete. When it is complete, either due

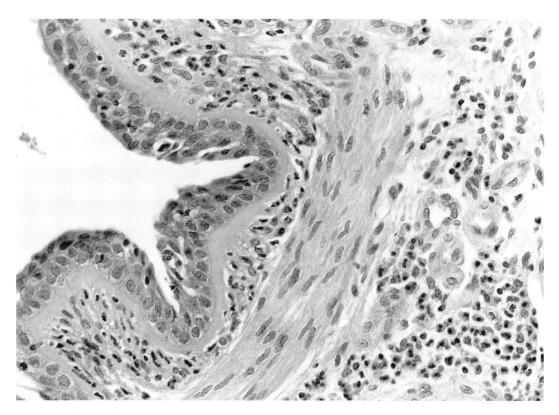

Figure 7.2 Thickening of the basement membrane and bronchiolar smooth muscle with an infiltrate of inflammatory cells containing a preponderance of eosinophils in a 10-year-old asthmatic girl who died suddenly (hematoxylin and eosin, ×440).

Table 7.2. Conditions associated with upper airway obstruction and sudden death in childhood

---

Choanal atresia

Nasopharyngeal tumors

Posterior lingual masses, e.g. thyroglossal duct cysts

Macroglossia

Micrognathic syndromes, e.g. Pierre–Robin, Goldenhar, Treacher–Collins, Apert, Crouzon

Heterotopic tissues

Upper airway infections

Structural airway defects, e.g. tracheomalacia, bronchomalacia

Tracheal stenosis

Vascular rings

Upper mediastinal tumors

Miscellaneous

---

to membranous or bony obstruction, symptoms of respiratory distress occur immediately after birth and may result in death (Canby, 1962). In incomplete cases, infants may survive longer, with signs of airway obstruction developing only during feeding (Strife, 1988). The cause of airway obstruction in these infants is similar to infants with Pierre–Robin anomalad and involves posterior displacement of the tongue, (Cozzi & Pierro, 1985).

In some cases, there may be functional nasal obstruction in the absence of definite choanal atresia, so-called congenital nasal stenosis (Knegt-Junk, Bos & Berkovits, 1988). The symptoms are similar to choanal atresia, suggesting that choanal atresia and congenital nasal stenosis represent different manifestations of the same disorder. Variable combinations of stenosis of the entire nasal cavity, the

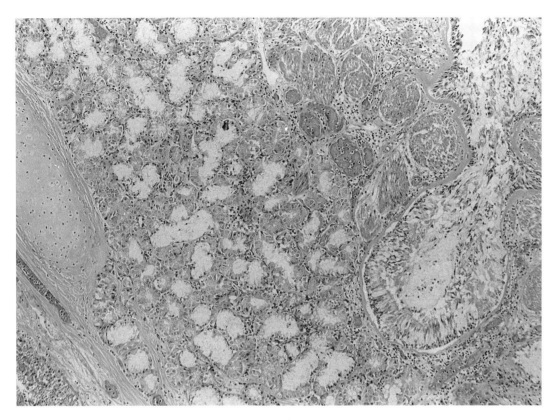

Figure 7.3 Mucus gland hyperplasia in an asthmatic child who died suddenly.

anterior portion of the nose, or the choanae characterize the latter entity (Leiberman *et al.*, 1992). A point to remember at autopsy in cases of possible congenital nasal stenosis is that functional airway obstruction may still have occurred even if it is possible to pass a probe from the nostrils into the nasopharynx.

Nasopharyngeal tumors

A variety of tumors and developmental anomalies such as teratomas and encephaloceles may impinge on the upper aerodigestive tract and cause obstruction (Richardson & Cotton, 1984). Congenital teratomas cause respiratory distress due to tracheal compression and deviation; they are usually symptomatic from the time of birth. They may be

associated with stillbirth and pulmonary hypoplasia and will require urgent surgical intervention if symptomatic (Byard *et al.*, 1990; Byard, Jimenez & Moore, 1992). Although these tumors are virtually always histologically benign (Figures 7.4 and 7.5), malignancy may develop subsequently (Byard, Smith & Chan, 1991).

Hypertrophy of the adenoids and tonsils may cause upper airway blockage, respiratory distress, and apnea, with some infants developing pulmonary hypertension and cor pulmonale from chronic hypoxia (Bland, Edwards & Brinsfield, 1969; Luke *et al.*, 1966; Suzuki, Yoshikawa & Ikeda, 1992). Other tumors unique to the neonatal period, such as salivary gland anlage tumor (congenital pleomorphic adenoma), may also cause airway obstruction (Dehner *et al.*, 1994).

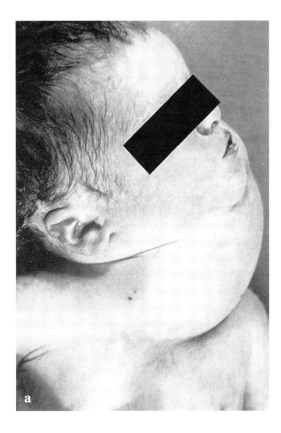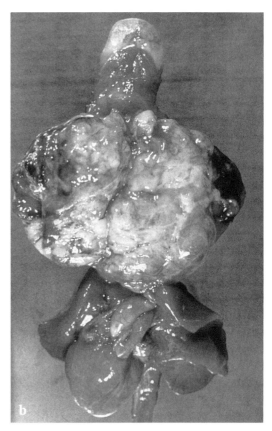

Figure 7.4 A congenital cervical teratoma that caused neonatal death from upper airway obstruction (a). The cut surface of the tumor, with the tongue above and the lungs below (b).

Lingual thyroglossal duct cysts

Thyroglossal duct remnants usually present in childhood as cystic midline swellings on the anterior aspect of the neck that are predisposed to recurrent infection and inflammation (Santiago, Rybak & Bass, 1985). Occasional remnants may be found close to the foramen cecum in the posterior portion of the tongue, where they may cause upper airway obstruction and sudden unexpected death in infancy due to their critical location (Byard, Bourne & Silver, 1990; Hanzlick, 1984; Müller-Holve *et al.*, 1975).

Infants with lingual thyroglossal duct cysts may have a history of positional dyspnea and stridor when placed in a supine position (Lewison & Lim, 1965; Paez, Warren & Srouji, 1974) or may have no apparent evidence of airway obstruction prior to the fatal episode. This rare lesion represents one condition in which the prone sleeping position is preferable to supine.

At autopsy in infants, it is important to dissect the upper aerodigestive tract carefully so that this lesion will not be overlooked. The characteristic features are of a centrally placed cystic mass at the level of the foramen cecum impinging on the epiglottis (Figure 7.6). Microscopic examination will reveal a unilocular cyst (Figure 7.7) with variable lining of respiratory or squamous epithelium.

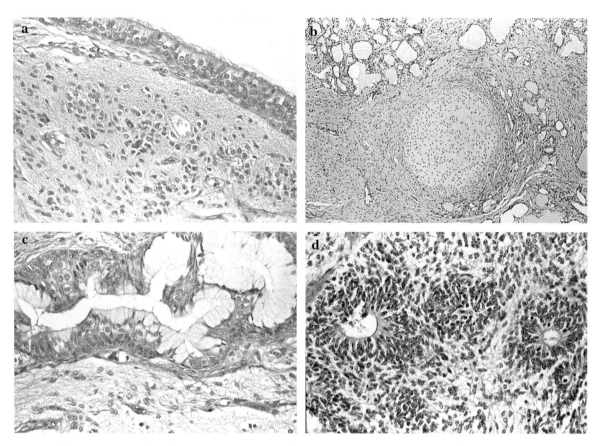

Figure 7.5 Characteristic tissues found in congenital teratomas: (a) ciliated respiratory epithelium overlying disorganized mature neural tissue (×220); (b) islands of hyaline cartilage within thyroid tissue (×56); (c) intestinal epithelium overlying disorganized neural tissue (×220); (d) immature neural tissue (hematoxylin and eosin, ×220).

Macroglossia

Macroglossia is defined as a resting tongue that protrudes beyond the teeth or alveolar ridge. It may be associated with life-threatening airway obstruction, particularly if there is generalized or posterior enlargement (Murthy & Laing, 1994). The author has reviewed a six-month-old girl with stigmata of congenital hypothyroidism who choked and died suddenly while being bottle-fed. No evidence of milk inhalation could be found; however, the infant's tongue was of considerable size, protruding from her mouth and causing the floor of the mouth to bulge inferiorly. It was considered likely that this had caused

upper airway obstruction and death. Enlargement of the tongue has also been reported as a possible contributing factor to airway narrowing in infants who die of SIDS (Siebert & Haas, 1991).

Micrognathism and associated syndromes

Infants suffering from a variety of syndromes characterized by micro/retrognathia are at risk of acute airway obstruction because of posterior displacement of the tongue (Figure 7.8). The anatomical effect of this arrangement on the upper airway is demonstrated well in Figure 7.9, which shows an en bloc

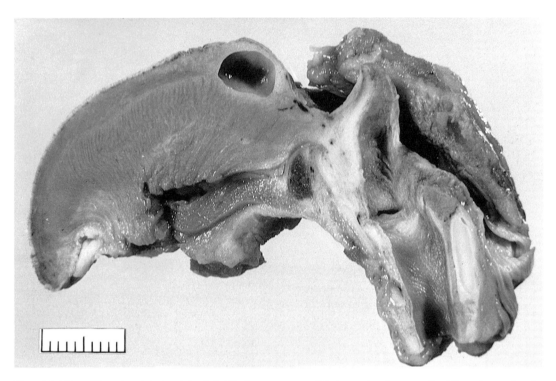

Figure 7.6 A lingual thyroglossal duct cyst situated at the foramen cecum of the tongue in a three-month-old boy who was found unexpectedly dead in his crib lying on his back.

dissection of the mandible and tongue in an infant with Pierre–Robin anomalad in which there is complete occlusion of the glottis by the tongue. Occasionally, there may also be an intrinsic abnormality of the epiglottis (Figure 7.10) or choanal narrowing, both of which exacerbate the tendency to airway obstruction (Byard & Kennedy, 1996).

Pierre–Robin anomalad is characterized by micrognathia and glossoptosis, with or without cleft palate (Figure 7.11). Anomalies of the limbs are also common, and congenital cardiac defects occur. Many infants with the Pierre–Robin complex also have an underlying syndrome, such as Stickler, Mobius, Joubert, Brachman de Lange, and Marden–Walker syndromes, the features of which should be checked for at autopsy (Sheffield *et al.*, 1987).

Sudden and unexpected death may occur even while the micrognathic infant is in hospital; although the cause may initially appear uncertain (Williams

et al., 1981), upper airway obstruction is most likely. Typical histories of choking, cyanosis, and difficulty in swallowing are supportive of this as the lethal mechanism. Infants with Pierre–Robin anomalad are also known to suffer central apneic episodes during sleep, which may contribute to the terminal episode (Guilleminault, 1989). Other conditions with fatal outcomes associated with micrognathia are Treacher–Collins and Goldenhar syndromes. Acute airway obstruction may also occur in infants with other types of facial skeletal abnormalities, such as maxillary hypoplasia in Crouzon and Apert syndromes.

Heterotopic tissues

Choristomas are aggregates of histologically unremarkable tissues found in heterotopic sites. These may be of minimal significance unless there is compromise of function due to critical location of the

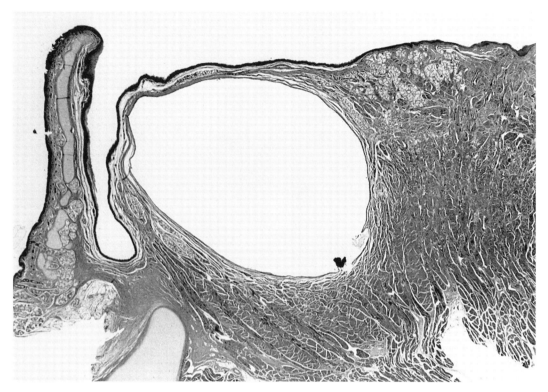

Figure 7.7 Cross-section of a lingual thyroglossal duct cyst in another three-month-old boy who presented with a history suggestive of SIDS (hematoxylin and eosin, ×7).

tissue, such as within the upper airway. Examples include thymus tissue within the trachea, thyroid tissue within the tongue, and gastric mucosa within the hypopharynx (Johnston *et al.*, 1989; Larochelle *et al.*, 1979; Martin & McAlister, 1987).

Upper airway infections

Examination of the epiglottis is a mandatory part of every pediatric autopsy. In cases of acute epiglottitis, the epiglottis is red and swollen and may completely occlude the laryngeal inlet (see Colour plate 6). Microscopic examination shows a florid neutrophil infiltrate, sometimes with bacterial colonies. Throat and blood cultures are an essential part of the autopsy and most often reveal *Hemophilus influenzae* type B. Acute hemorrhage into the soft tissues around the base of the epiglottis from other causes may also occlude the airway (see Figure 9.14).

Although much less common than fatal acute epiglottitis, other acute infections of the upper airway may cause sudden death due to airway occlusion. These include tonsillitis, peritonsillar abscess, retropharyngeal abscess, lingual tonsillitis, and posterior lingual abscess (Byard & Silver, 1994). Nonspecific symptoms and signs in infants with these conditions make careful examination of the upper airway essential at autopsy. Dissection should include en bloc removal of the tongue, tonsils, and Waldeyer's ring so that inflammatory pharyngeal lesions can be visualized adequately.

Tracheomalacia/bronchomalacia

These entities are grouped together as they represent conditions in which loss of structural integrity of the upper airway at various levels results in airway collapse and obstruction.

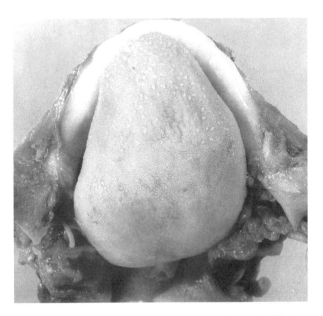

Figure 7.8 Superior view of the tongue in a five-week-old girl with Pierre–Robin anomalad, showing posterior displacement of the tongue.

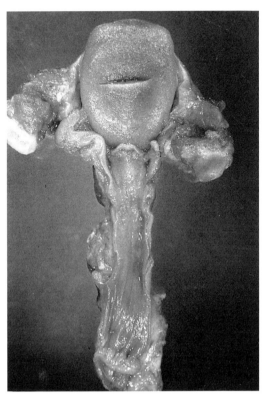

Figure 7.9 En bloc dissection of the tongue and upper airway in an infant with mandibular hypoplasia and recurrent cyanotic episodes, demonstrating clearly the effects on the laryngeal inlet of backward displacement of the tongue.

Tracheomalacia may be primary, or it may develop secondarily in infants with tracheo-esophageal fistulas and vascular rings, congenital chondromalacia, polychondritis, Ehlers–Danlos syndrome, and Larsen syndrome (Benjamin, 1984; Zalzal, 1989), or as a result of prolonged artificial ventilation (for example, in infants with bronchopulmonary dysplasia). It is characterized by a deficiency in tracheal cartilagenous rings, and although it is generally benign and undergoes spontaneous resolution, it may result in unexpected death in infancy due to airway compromise. (Emery, Nanayakkara & Wailoo, 1984; Jeffery, Rahilly & Read, 1983).

Bronchomalacia may also occur spontaneously or as part of a familial syndrome. It is characterized by incomplete development of cartilage, resulting in weakening and collapse of the walls of the lower airways. The presentation may be of respiratory distress soon after birth (Agosti *et al.*, 1974) or, rarely, as sudden infant death (Beal & Blundell, 1988).

Tracheal stenosis

Tracheal stenosis may predispose to sudden airway occlusion due to increased vulnerability to mucus plugging or to other conditions that may exacerbate luminal narrowing.

Vascular rings

Respiratory distress has been described in infants with aberrant vessels compressing the upper airway (Jeffery, Rahilly & Read, 1983; Strife, 1988) and also in acyanotic congenital cardiac disease due to bronchial compression by hypertensive pulmonary arteries. Occasionally, a massively enlarged heart may also compress the lungs (Stanger, Lucas &

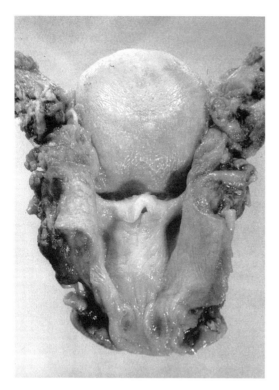

Figure 7.10 Thickening and deformation of the epiglottis contributing to airway obstruction in a 3.5-month-old boy with Pierre–Robin anomalad. The tongue was also displaced posteriorly.

Edwards, 1969). Vascular rings are discussed further in Chapter 6.

Mediastinal tumors

Compression of the trachea, major bronchi, and lungs may be caused by upper mediastinal tumors, resulting in acute upper airway obstruction and death. Symptoms of respiratory distress may be attributed incorrectly to asthma, as in a two-year-old girl with a mediastinal lymphoma described in Chapter 9 (see Figure 9.6). General anesthesia in these children may be fatal (Akhtar, Ridley & Best, 1991).

Miscellaneous

As well as external compression from aberrant vessels, the trachea may be compromised by food or

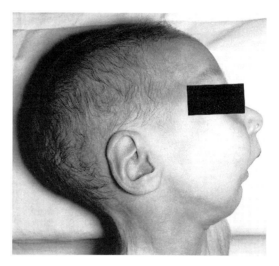

Figure 7.11 A three-month-old boy who was found dead in his bed, showing the typical facial profile of Pierre–Robin anomalad.

objects within the esophagus, or from neck and mediastinal masses (Byard, Moore & Bourne, 1990; Richardson & Cotton, 1984; Todres *et al.*, 1976). Tracheal compression resulting in stridor in a 7.5-year-old boy due to achalasia has been reported (Chapman *et al.*, 1989), and external pressure from esophageal duplication cysts may cause respiratory distress in neonates (Stewart, Bruce & Beasley, 1993).

Acute upper airway obstruction is a feature of a variety of other entities. Although some are exceedingly rare and are not usually associated with fatal airway compromise, they have been mentioned for completeness (Holinger & Brown, 1967; Kilham, Gillis & Benjamin, 1987). Any lesion that narrows the airways increases the risk of acute obstruction when more common coincident inflammatory conditions occur.

Vocal cord paralysis may be unilateral or bilateral, the latter more often associated with cerebral problems such as Arnold–Chiari malformation. While sudden death is not a feature of reports in the literature, airway obstruction may occur, necessitating tracheostomy (Richardson & Cotton, 1984).

Rheumatoid arthritis involving the cricoary-tenoid joint is found rarely in childhood, although

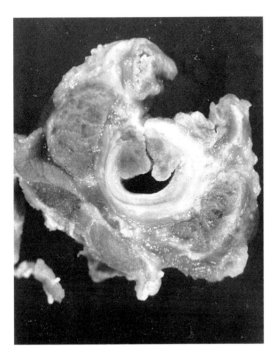

Figure 7.12 Marked obstruction of the airway due to an intraluminal hemangioma can be seen in this transverse section of the trachea.

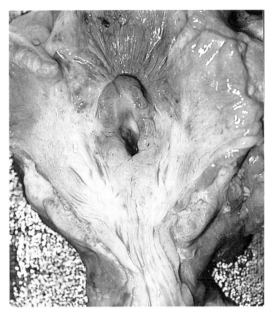

Figure 7.13 Narrowing of the laryngeal inlet due to an extensively infiltrating cystic hygroma.

occasional case reports have documented it as a cause of acute airway occlusion (Goldhagen, 1988).

Ligneous conjunctivitis is a rare, possibly familial condition of uncertain etiology in which recurrent pseudomembranes form on the conjunctivae and within the nasopharynx, larynx, trachea, and bronchi (Babcock, Bedford & Berry, 1987). Girls under the age of three years are most often affected, and significant airway obstruction may result. Histologically, there is pseudomembrane formation with chronic inflammation and neovascularization (Cohen, 1990).

Congenital subglottic stenosis is characterized by narrowing of the subglottic area, producing stridor and respiratory distress. There is an association with other congenital lesions and with Down syndrome. Acute airway obstruction may occur with minimal laryngeal inflammation, causing a significant percentage of affected infants to require tracheostomy (Holinger *et al.*, 1976), although the risk

of sudden death remains even if a tracheostomy has been performed. Histopathologically, the stenosis may be caused by either soft tissue or cartilagenous narrowing of the subglottic space (Tucker *et al.*, 1979).

Laryngomalacia is characterized by collapse of the epiglottis and adjacent airway. Although the possibility of laryngomalacia causing infantile apnea has been the subject of debate, Sivan, Ben-Ari & Schonfeld (1991) have documented a series of six infants with recurrent apnea of infancy who were found on fiber-optic endoscopy to have airway obstruction at the laryngeal orifice due to this condition.

Laryngeal webs and atresias are lesions that also cause airway obstruction. These usually present at or soon after birth (Richardson & Cotton, 1984).

Laryngeal papillomatosis is characterized by widely spreading exophytic papillomas within the larynx and pharynx that may rarely cause sudden death due to airway occlusion, sometimes in the absence of major symptoms (Sperry, 1994) (see Chapter 4).

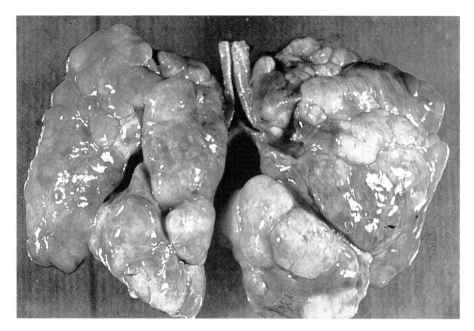

Figure 7.14 Irregular scarring and uneven expansion of the lungs in bronchopulmonary dysplasia.

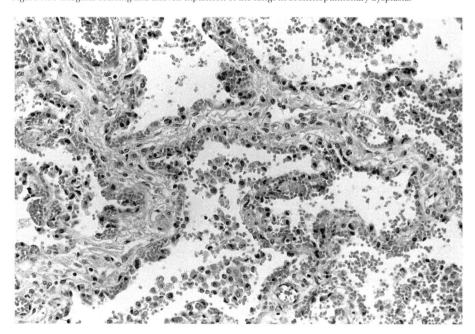

Figure 7.15 Prominant septal fibrosis due to bronchopulmonary dysplasia in a six-month-old boy who died unexpectedly. There was a history of prolonged ventilation following delivery at 26 weeks (hematoxylin and eosin, ×170).

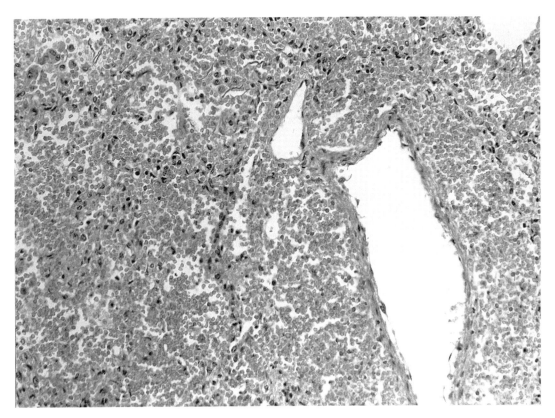

Figure 7.16 Microscopic section from the lungs of an 11-day-old girl who died from massive pulmonary hemorrhage, demonstrating filling of the alveoli with red blood cells (hematoxylin and eosin, ×170).

Subglottic hemangiomas are benign vascular lesions that may result in respiratory compromise due to their critical position (Figure 7.12). Respiratory symptoms again may be attributed incorrectly to asthma (Rodriguez *et al.*, 1992). As with hemangiomas in other parts of the body in early childhood, spontaneous resolution may occur, although surgery may be required if there are problems with airway obstruction (Leikensohn, Benton & Cotton, 1976; Rodriguez *et al.*, 1992). Other lesions such as extensive cystic hygromas may also compromise the upper airway if the epiglottis is involved (Figure 7.13).

Laryngeal cysts that fill with fluid and cause airway blockage may occur in neonates and young infants

(Vanhoucke & Minnigerode, 1989). Edema and hemorrhage associated with endoscopy in these cases may precipitate complete airway occlusion and sudden death (Richardson & Cotton, 1984).

Marshall–Smith syndrome is another exceedingly rare condition in which there is micrognathia, choanal atresia, laryngomalacia, and pulmonary hypertension, all of which may contribute to sudden death (Yoder *et al.*, 1988).

Harpey & Renault (1984) have postulated that an *excessively long uvula* may result in sudden infant death; however, confirmatory data are lacking.

As certain subtypes of *epidermolysis bullosa* produce blistering within the upper aerodigestive tract, it is conceivable that detachment of an inflammatory membrane could result in upper airway obstruction.

Bronchopulmonary dysplasia

Bronchopulmonary dysplasia refers to a chronic lung disease that was first reported in 1967 in infants with severe respiratory distress syndrome who had been treated with artificial ventilation and oxygen therapy (Northway, 1991). Subsequent studies have demonstrated a variety of contributing etiologic agents, including nutritional deficiencies and pulmonary edema (Northway, 1990).

Frequency

The frequency of bronchopulmonary dysplasia in ventilated infants has varied from a little over 4% to as high as 70% in infants ventilated for more than two weeks (Bancalari *et al.*, 1979; Greenough, 1990).

Occurrence of sudden death

Infants who have pulmonary changes of bronchopulmonary dysplasia are known to be at increased risk of sudden death, and this has led to diagnostic confusion with SIDS (Sauve & Singhal, 1985). The risk of sudden death has been estimated as seven times that of other infants in the population (Werthammer *et al.*, 1982). Sudden and unexpected death has also been reported in hospitalized infants with bronchopulmonary dysplasia, in spite of close cardiorespiratory monitoring (Abman *et al.*, 1989).

Pathological features

Pathologically, there are three distinct phases in the development of bronchopulmonary dysplasia: the acute, reparative, and chronic stages (Anderson, 1990). On gross examination, the lungs are initially smooth-surfaced, bulky, and increased in weight, but

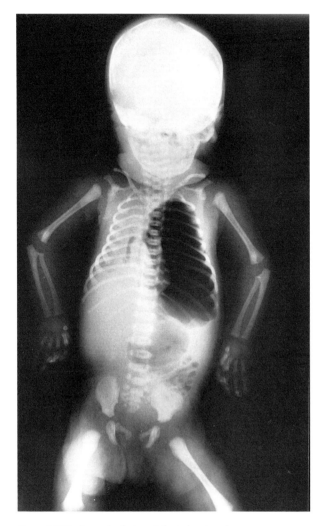

Figure 7.17 Radiograph of a term infant, showing a large left-sided tension pneumothorax secondary to failed resuscitation. There is mediastinal displacement to the right.

they progressively develop scarring so that the final stage is characterized by marked fissuring (Figure 7.14). There may also be evidence of cardiac hypertrophy in the later stages, involving both right and left ventricles (Stocker, 1986).

Microscopically, damage occurs from the trachea down to the alveoli, with the earliest changes being necrosis of the lining epithelial cells with ulceration.

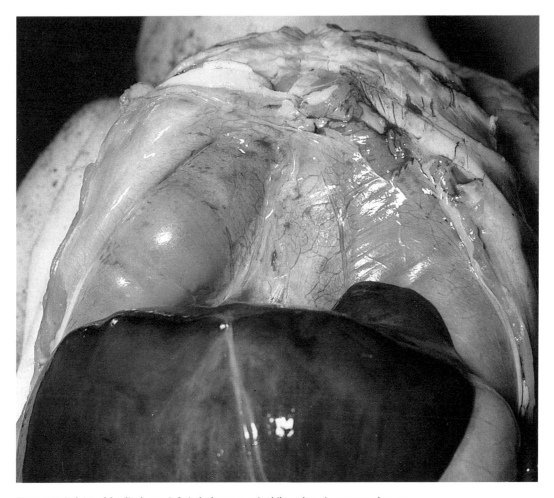

Figure 7.18 Bulging of the diaphragm inferiorly due to massive bilateral tension pneumothoraces.

In particularly severe cases, necrosis may involve the tracheal cartilage, causing tracheomalacia. As repair occurs, there may be squamous metaplasia, epithelial dysplasia, submucosal fibrosis, and muscular hypertrophy of smaller airways. In healed cases, evidence of damage may be patchy, with relatively normal-appearing hyperexpanded alveoli abutting alveoli that show prominent septal fibrosis with fibrous obliteration of distal airspaces. Alveolar septal fibrosis has been cited as the hallmark of healed bronchopulmonary dysplasia (Stocker, 1986) (Figure 7.15). Pulmonary arteries may show changes compatible with grade I–II hypertension, and within the heart there may be secondary hypertrophy of cardiac myocytes and interstitial fibrosis.

Pathophysiology

Infants who survive with moderate to severe bronchopulmonary dysplasia manifest a variety of abnormalities, including reduced head growth, general growth delay, pulmonary hypertension, increased airway resistance, reduced lung compliance, bronchial hyperreactivity, marked maldistribution of ventilation, carbon dioxide retention, hypochloremia with metabolic alkylosis, hypoxemia, sleep-related arterial oxygen desaturation, and neurodevelopmental deficits (Garg *et al.*, 1988; Northway *et al.*, 1990; Perlman *et al.*, 1986). Given the presence of these features and abnormal lungs on pathological examination, the diagnosis of SIDS in these infants cannot be sustained.

Acute pneumonia

Acute bacterial infection of the lungs and distal airways may cause sudden and unexpected death in children with relatively non-specific symptoms and signs. Diagnostic difficulties are discussed further in Chapter 4.

Cystic fibrosis

Cystic fibrosis is described in detail in Chapter 10. While the respiratory manifestations tend to be chronic, sudden death can occur in children due to electrolyte imbalances or to septic or gastrointestinal complications. Although the lungs in advanced cases may show extensive scarring with mucus plugging of bronchiectatic airways, this is not always the case in children who die early from the above complications. For example, a four-month-old boy who was brought to hospital after being discovered dead in his crib was found at autopsy to have undiagnosed cystic fibrosis, with marked atrophy and fibrosis of the pancreas, which contained residual ducts distended with typical inspissated eosinophilic secretions. The lungs were not particularly abnormal.

Massive pulmonary hemorrhage

Massive pulmonary hemorrhage of uncertain etiology may be responsible for sudden and unexpected death in severely growth-retarded infants (Figure 7.16). Risk factors include intrauterine growth retardation, infection, coagulation disorders, prematurity, birth asphyxia, breech or cesarian delivery,

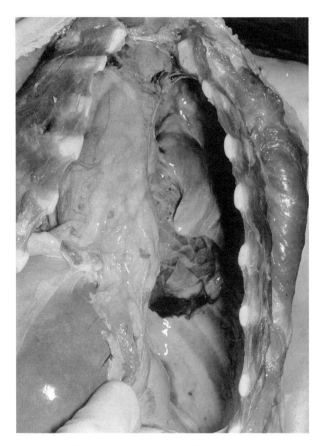

Figure 7.19 Collapse of the lung following a left-sided tension pneumothorax.

multiple births, the presence of a patent ductus arteriosus, and hyaline membrane disease (Coffin *et al.*, 1993; Sly & Drew, 1981). However, cases may occur in which none of these features are present. In older children, hereditary hemorrhagic telangiectasia (Osler–Weber–Rendu disease) may also result in death due to massive intrapulmonary hemorrhage (Byard, Schliebs & Koszyca, 2001; Reyes-Mújica *et al.*, 1988).

Idiopathic pulmonary hemosiderosis

Sudden death is a known complication of idiopathic pulmonary hemosiderosis (Jacobsen, 1971).

An example of this was a 7.5-year-old girl who had been investigated for idiopathic pulmonary hemosiderosis and who subsequently collapsed and died while walking in the street. The autopsy demonstrated typical features of chronic pulmonary hemorrhage with massive iron deposition.

Tension pneumothorax

This occurs in a number of conditions, such as asthma and staphylococcal pneumonia, when there is air-trapping with forcing of air under pressure into the pleural cavity. Sudden death results from compression of the lungs and shifting of the mediastinum (Figure 7.17). At autopsy, the most obvious initial finding may be ptosis of the abdominal organs and bulging of the diaphragmatic domes into the peritoneal cavity, with collapse of the lungs (Figures 7.18 and 7.19).

Pickwickian syndrome

Massive obesity that may cause sudden death from cardiorespiratory compromise due to chronic alveolar hypoventilation is discussed further in Chapter 10.

REFERENCES

Abman, S. H., Burchell, M. F., Schaffer, M. S. & Rosenberg, A. A. (1989). Late sudden unexpected deaths in hospitalized infants with bronchopulmonary dysplasia. *American Journal of Diseases of Children*, **143**, 815–19.

Agosti, E., De Filippi, G., Fior, R. & Chiussi, F. (1974). Generalized familial bronchomalacia. *Acta Paediatrica Scandinavica*, **63**, 616–18.

Akhtar, T. M., Ridley, S. & Best, C. J. (1991). Unusual presentation of acute upper airway obstruction caused by an anterior mediastinal mass. *British Journal of Anaesthesia*, **67**, 632–4.

Anderson, W. R. (1990). Bronchopulmonary dysplasia: a correlative study by light, scanning, and transmission electron microscopy. *Ultrastructural Pathology*, **14**, 221–32.

Babcock, M. F., Bedford, R. F. & Berry, F. A. (1987). Ligneous tracheobronchitis: an unusual cause of airway obstruction. *Anesthesiology*, **67**, 819–21.

Bancalari, E., Abdenour, G. E., Feller, R. & Gannon, J. (1979). Bronchopulmonary dysplasia: clinical presentation. *Journal of Pediatrics*, **95**, 819–23.

Barnes, P. J. (1994). Blunted perception and death from asthma. *New England Journal of Medicine*, **330**, 1383–4.

Bateman, J. R. M. & Clarke, S. W. (1979). Sudden death in asthma. *Thorax*, **34**, 40–44.

Beal, S. M. & Blundell, H. K. (1988). Recurrence incidence of sudden infant death syndrome. *Archives of Disease in Childhood*, **63**, 924–30.

Benatar, S. R. (1986). Fatal asthma. *New England Journal of Medicine*, **314**, 423–9.

Benjamin, B. (1984). Tracheomalacia in infants and children. *Annals of Otology, Rhinology and Laryngology*, **93**, 438–42.

Bland, J. W., Jr, Edwards, F. K. & Brinsfield, D. (1969). Pulmonary hypertension and congestive heart failure in children with chronic upper airway obstruction. New concepts of etiologic factors. *American Journal of Cardiology*, **23**, 830–37.

Busuttil, A. (1991). Adrenal atrophy at autopsy in two asthmatic children. *American Journal of Forensic Medicine and Pathology*, **12**, 36–9.

Byard, R. W. (1993). Mechanisms of laryngeal obstruction in cases of paediatric sudden death. *Pathology*, **28** (suppl 7).

Byard, R. W. (1996). Mechanisms of unexpected death in infants and young children following foreign body ingestion. *Journal of Forensic Sciences*, **41**, 438–41.

Byard, R. W. (2000). Accidental childhood death and the role of the pathologist. *Pediatric and Developmental Pathology*, **3**, 405–18.

Byard, R. W. & Kennedy, J. D. (1996). Diagnostic difficulties in cases of sudden death in infants with mandibular hypoplasia. *American Journal of Forensic Medicine and Pathology*, **17**, 255–9.

Byard, R. W. & Silver, M. M. (1994). Sudden infant death and acute posterior lingual inflammation. *International Journal of Pediatric Otorhinolaryngology*, **28**, 77–82.

Byard, R. W., Bourne, A. J. & Silver, M. M. (1990). The association of lingual thyroglossal duct remnants with sudden death in infancy. *International Journal of Pediatric Otorhinolaryngology*, **20**, 107–12.

Byard, R. W., Jimenez, C. L., Carpenter, B. F. & Smith, C. R. (1990). Congenital teratomas of the neck and nasopharynx: a clinical and pathological study of 18 cases. *Journal of Paediatrics and Child Health*, **26**, 12–16.

Byard, R. W., Jimenez, C. L. & Moore, L. (1992). Mechanisms of sudden death in patients with congenital teratoma. *Pediatric Surgery International*, **7**, 464–7.

Byard, R. W., Moore, L. & Bourne, A. J. (1990). Sudden and unexpected death. A late effect of occult intraesophageal foreign body. *Pediatric Pathology*, **10**, 837–41.

Byard, R. W., Schliebs, J. & Koszyca, B. A. (2001). Osler–Weber–Rendu syndrome – pathological manifestations and autopsy considerations. *Journal of Forensic Sciences*, **46**, 698–701.

Byard, R. W., Smith, C. R. & Chan, H. S. L. (1991). Endodermal sinus tumour of the nasopharynx and previous mature congenital teratoma. *Pediatric Pathology*, **11**, 297–302.

Canby, J. P. (1962). Choanal atresia and sudden death. *Medical Bulletin of the U. S. Army, Europe*, **19**, 57–8.

Carroll, N., Elliot, J., Morton, A. & James, A. (1993). The structure of large and small airways in nonfatal and fatal asthma. *American Reviews of Respiratory Disease*, **147**, 405–10.

Champ, C. S. & Byard, R. W. (1994). Sudden death in asthma in childhood. *Forensic Science International*, **66**, 117–27.

Chapman, S., Weller, P. H., Campbell, C. A. & Buick, R. G. (1989). Tracheal compression caused by achalasia. *Pediatric Pulmonology*, **7**, 49–51.

Coffin, C. M., Schechtman, K., Cole, F. S. & Dehner, L. P. (1993). Neonatal and infantile pulmonary hemorrhage: an autopsy study with clinical correlation. *Pediatric Pathology*, **13**, 583–9.

Cohen, S. R. (1990). Ligneous conjunctivitis: an ophthalmic disease with potentially fatal tracheobronchial obstruction. Laryngeal and tracheobronchial features. *Annals of Otology, Rhinology and Laryngology*, **99**, 509–12.

Cozzi, F. & Pierro, A. (1985). Glossoptosis-apnea syndrome in infancy. *Pediatrics*, **75**, 836–43.

Cushley, M. J. & Tattersfield, A. E. (1983). Sudden death in asthma: discussion paper. *Journal of the Royal Society of Medicine*, **76**, 662–6.

Dehner, L. P., Valbuena, L., Perez-Atayde, A., *et al.* (1994). Salivary gland anlage tumor ("congenital pleomorphic adenoma"). A clinicopathologic, immunohistochemical and ultrastructural study of nine cases. *American Journal of Surgical Pathology*, **18**, 25–36.

Drislane, F. W., Samuels, M. A., Kozakewich, H., Schoen, F. J. & Strunk, R. C. (1987). Myocardial contraction band lesions in patients with fatal asthma: possible neurocardiologic mechanisms. *American Review of Respiratory Disease*, **135**, 498–501.

Emery, J. L., Nanayakkara, C. F. & Wailoo, M. P. (1984). Tracheomalacia-lethal factor in a 17 month old child. *Pediatric Pathology*, **2**, 259–65.

Friday, G. A. & Fireman, P. (1988). Morbidity and mortality of asthma. *Pediatric Clinics of North America*, **35**, 1149–62.

Garg, M., Kurzner, S. I., Bautista, D. B. & Keens, T. G. (1988). Clinically unsuspected hypoxia during sleep and feeding in infants with bronchopulmonary dysplasia. *Pediatrics*, **81**, 635–42.

Goldhagen, J. L. (1988). Cricoarytenoiditis as a cause of acute airway obstruction in children. *Annals of Emergency Medicine*, **17**, 532–3.

Greenough, A. (1990). Bronchopulmonary dysplasia: early diagnosis, prophylaxis, and treatment. *Archives of Disease in Childhood*, **65**, 1082–8.

Grubb, B. P., Wolfe, D. A., Nelson, L. A. & Hennessy, J. R. (1992). Malignant vasovagally mediated hypotension and bradycardia: a possible cause of sudden death in young patients with asthma. *Pediatrics*, **90**, 983–6.

Guilleminault, C. (1989). Sleep-related respiratory function and dysfunction in postneonatal infantile apnea. In *Sudden Infant Death Syndrome. Medical Aspects and Psychological Management*, ed. J. L. Culbertson, H. K. Krous & R. D. Bendell. London: Edward Arnold, pp. 94–120.

Haalboom, J. R. E., Deenstra, M. & Struyvenberg, A. (1985). Hypokalaemia induced by inhalation of fenoterol. *Lancet*, **i**, 1125–7.

Hanzlick, R. L. (1984). Lingual thyroglossal duct cyst causing death in a four-week-old infant. *Journal of Forensic Sciences*, **29**, 345–8.

Harpey, J.-P. & Renault, F. (1984). The uvula and sudden infant death syndrome. *Pediatrics*, **74**, 319–20.

Hetzel, M. R., Clark, T. J. H. & Branthwaite, M. A. (1977). Asthma: analysis of sudden deaths and ventilatory arrests in hospital. *British Medical Journal*, **i**, 808–11.

Holinger, P. H. & Brown, W. T. (1967). Congenital webs, cysts, laryngoceles and other anomalies of the larynx. *Annals of Otology, Rhinology and Laryngology*, **76**, 744–52.

Holinger, P. H., Schild, J. A., Kutnick, S. L. & Holinger, L. D. (1976). Subglottic stenosis in infants and children. *Annals of Otolaryngology*, **85**, 591–9.

Jacobsen, K. B. (1971). Sudden death in idiopathic hemosiderosis. *Nordisk Medicin*, **86**, 978–80.

Jeffery, H. E., Rahilly, P. & Read, D. J. C. (1983). Multiple causes of asphyxia in infants at high risk for sudden infant death. *Archives of Disease in Childhood*, **58**, 92–100.

Johnson, A. J., Nunn, A. J., Somner, A. R., Stableforth, D. E. & Stewart, C. J. (1984). Circumstances of death from asthma. *British Medical Journal*, **288**, 1870–72.

Johnston, C., Benjamin, B., Harrison, H. & Kan, A. (1989). Gastric heterotopia causing airway obstruction. *International Journal of Pediatric Otorhinolaryngology*, **18**, 67–72.

Kilham, H., Gillis, J. & Benjamin, B. (1987). Severe upper airway obstruction. *Pediatric Clinics of North America*, **34**, 1–14.

Knegt-Junk, K. J., Bos, C. E. & Berkovits, R. N. P. (1988). Congenital nasal stenosis in neonates. *Journal of Laryngology and Otology*, **102**, 500–502.

Knochel, J. P. (1982). Neuromuscular manifestations of electrolyte disorders. *American Journal of Medicine*, **72**, 521–35.

Kravis, L. P. & Kolski, G. B. (1985). Unexpected death in childhood asthma. A review of 13 deaths in ambulatory patients. *American Journal of Diseases of Children*, **139**, 558–63.

Larochelle, D., Arcand, P., Belzile, M. & Gagnon, N.-B. (1979). Ectopic thyroid tissue – a review of the literature. *Journal of Otolaryngology*, **8**, 523–30.

Larsen, G. L. (1992). Asthma in children. *New England Journal of Medicine*, **326**, 1540–45.

Las Heras, J. & Swanson, V. L. (1983). Sudden death of an infant with rhinovirus infection complicating bronchial asthma: case report. *Pediatric Pathology*, **1**, 319–23.

Leiberman, A., Carmi, R., Bar-Ziv, Y. & Karplus, M. (1992). Congenital nasal stenosis in newborn infants. *Journal of Pediatrics*, **120**, 124–7.

Leikensohn, J. R., Benton, C. & Cotton, R. (1976). Subglottic hemangioma. *Journal of Otolaryngology*, **5**, 487–92.

Lewison, M. M. & Lim, D. T. (1965). Apnea in the supine position as an alerting symptom of a tumor at the base of the tongue in small infants. *Journal of Pediatrics*, **66**, 1092–3.

Luke, M. J., Mehrizi, A., Folger, G. M., Jr & Rowe, R. D. (1966). Chronic nasopharyngeal obstruction as a cause of cardiomegaly, cor pulmonale, and pulmonary edema. *Pediatrics*, **37**, 762–8.

Martin, K. W. & McAlister, W. H. (1987). Intratracheal thymus: a rare cause of airway obstruction. *American Journal of Roentgenology*, **149**, 1217–18.

McFadden, E. R. & Gilbert, I. A. (1994). Exercise-induced asthma. *New England Journal of Medicine*, **330**, 1362–7.

Molander, N. (1982). Sudden natural death in later childhood and adolescence. *Archives of Disease in Childhood*, **57**, 572–6.

Molfino, N. A., Nannini, L. J., Martelli, A. N. & Slutsky, A. S. (1991). Respiratory arrest in near-fatal asthma. *New England Journal of Medicine*, **324**, 285–8.

Morild, I. & Giertsen, J. C. (1989). Sudden death from asthma. *Forensic Science International*, **42**, 145–50.

Müller-Holve, W., Kirchschläger, H., Weber, J. & Saling, E. (1975). Neonatal asphyxia immediately following birth due to thyroglossal cyst blocking the larynx. *Zeitschrift fur Geburtshilfe und Perinatologie*, **179**, 147–50.

Murthy, P. & Laing, M. R. (1994). Macroglossia. *British Medical Journal*, **309**, 1386–7.

Northway, W. H., Jr (1990). Bronchopulmonary dysplasia: then and now. *Archives of Disease in Childhood*, **65**, 1076–81.

Northway, W. H., Jr (1991). Bronchopulmonary dysplasia and research in diagnostic radiology. *American Journal of Roentgenology*, **156**, 681–7.

Northway, W. H., Jr, Moss, R. B., Carlisle, K. B., *et al.* (1990). Late pulmonary sequelae of bronchopulmonary dysplasia. *New England Journal of Medicine*, **323**, 1793–9.

Paez, P., Warren, W. S. & Srouji, M. N. (1974). Stridor as the presenting symptom of lingual thyroglossal duct cyst in an infant. *Clinical Pediatrics*, **13**, 1077–8.

Perlman, J. M., Moore, V., Siegel, M. J. & Dawson, J. (1986). Is chloride depletion an important contributing cause of death in infants with bronchopulmonary dysplasia? *Pediatrics*, **77**, 212–16.

Preston, H. V. & Bowen, D. A. L. (1987). Asthma deaths: a review. *Medicine, Science and the Law*, **27**, 89–94.

Reyes-Mújica, M., López-Corella, E., Pérez-Fernández, L., Cuevas-Schacht, F. & Carillo-Farga, J. (1988). Osler–Weber–Rendu disease in an infant. *Human Pathology*, **19**, 1243–6.

Richardson, M. A. & Cotton, R. T. (1984). Anatomic abnormalities of the pediatric airway. *Pediatric Clinics of North America*, **31**, 821–34.

Robertson, C. F., Rubinfeld, A. R. & Bowes, G. (1992). Pediatric asthma deaths in Victoria: the mild are at risk. *Pediatric Pulmonology*, **13**, 95–100.

Robin, E. D. (1988). Death from bronchial asthma. *Chest*, **93**, 614–18.

Robin, E. D. & Lewiston, N. (1989). Unexpected, unexplained sudden death in young asthmatic subjects. *Chest*, **96**, 790–93.

Rodriguez, L. R., DiMaio, M., Kidron, D. & Kattan, M. (1992). Late presentation of a subglottic hemangioma masquerading as asthma. *Clinical Pediatrics*, **31**, 753–5.

Rubinstein, S., Hindi, R. D., Moss, R. B., Blessing-Moore, J. & Lewiston, N. J. (1984). Sudden death in adolescent asthma. *Annals of Allergy*, **53**, 311–18.

Santiago, W., Rybak, L. P. & Bass, R. M. (1985). Thyroglossal duct cyst of the tongue. *Journal of Otolaryngology*, **14**, 261–4.

Sauve, R. S. & Singhal, N. (1985). Long-term morbidity of infants with bronchopulmonary dysplasia. *Pediatrics*, **76**, 725–33.

Segal, A. J. & Wasserman, M. (1971). Arterial air embolism: a cause of sudden death in status asthmaticus. *Radiology*, **99**, 271–2.

Sheffield, L. J., Reiss, J. A., Strohm, K. & Gilding, M. (1987). A genetic follow-up study of 64 patients with the Pierre Robin complex. *American Journal of Medical Genetics*, **28**, 25–36.

Siboni, A. & Simonsen, J. (1986). Sudden unexpected natural death in young persons. *Forensic Science International*, **31**, 159–66.

Siebert, J. R. & Haas, J. E. (1991). Enlargement of the tongue in sudden infant death syndrome. *Pediatric Pathology*, **11**, 813–26.

Sivan, Y., Ben-Ari, J. & Schonfeld, T. M. (1991). Laryngomalacia: a cause for early near miss for SIDS. *International Journal of Pediatric Otorhinolaryngology*, **21**, 59–64.

Sly, P. D. & Drew, J. H. (1981). Massive pulmonary haemorrhage: a cause of sudden unexpected deaths in severely growth retarded infants. *Australian Paediatric Journal*, **17**, 32–4.

Sperry, K. (1994). Lethal asphyxiating juvenile laryngeal papillomatosis. A case report with human papillomavirus *in situ* hybridization analysis. *American Journal of Forensic Medicine and Pathology*, **15**, 146–50.

Spitzer, W. O., Suissa, S., Ernst, P., *et al.* (1992). The use of β-agonists and the risk of death and near death from asthma. *New England Journal of Medicine*, **326**, 501–6.

Stanger, P., Lucas, R. V., Jr & Edwards, J. E. (1969). Anatomic factors causing respiratory distress in acyanotic congenital cardiac disease. Special reference to bronchial obstruction. *Pediatrics*, **43**, 760–69.

Stewart, R. J., Bruce, J. & Beasley, S. W. (1993). Oesophageal duplication cyst: another cause of neonatal respiratory distress. *Journal of Paediatrics and Child Health*, **29**, 391–2.

Stocker, J. T. (1986). Pathologic features of long-standing "healed" bronchopulmonary dysplasia: a study of 28 3- to 40-month-old infants. *Human Pathology*, **17**, 943–61.

Strife, J. L. (1988). Upper airway and tracheal obstruction in infants and children. *Radiologic Clinics of North America*, **26**, 309–22.

Suzuki, T., Yoshikawa, K. & Ikeda, N. (1992) Sudden infant death syndrome and hypertrophy of the palatine tonsil: reports on two cases. *Forensic Science International*, **53**, 93–6.

Todres, I. D., Reppert, S. M., Walker, P. F. & Grillo, H. C. (1976). Management of critical airway obstruction in a child with a mediastinal tumor. *Anesthesiology*, **45**, 100–102.

Tucker, G. F., Ossoff, R. H., Newman, A. N. & Holinger, L. D. (1979). Histopathology of congenital subglottic stenosis. *Laryngoscope*, **89**, 866–77.

Vanhoucke, F. & Minnigerode, B. (1989). Plostselinge dood ten gevolge van een onopgemerkte congenitale larynxcyste. *Acta Otorhinolaryngology Belgica*, **43**, 125–9.

Wasserfallen, J.-B., Schaller, M.-D., Feihl, F. & Perret, C. H. (1990). Sudden asphyxic asthma: a distinct entity? *American Review of Respiratory Disease*, **142**, 108–11.

Werthammer, J., Brown, E. R., Neff, R. K. & Taeusch, H. W., Jr (1982). Sudden infant death syndrome in infants with bronchopulmonary dysplasia. *Pediatrics*, **69**, 301–4.

Williams, A. J., Williams, M. A., Walker, C. A. & Bush, P. G. (1981). The Robin anomalad (Pierre Robin syndrome) – a follow up study. *Archives of Disease in Childhood*, **56**, 663–8.

Wilson, J. D., Sutherland, D. C. & Thomas, A. C. (1981). Has the change to beta-agonists combined with oral theophylline increased cases of fatal asthma? *Lancet*, **i**, 1235–7.

Wood, D. W. & Lecks, H. J. (1976). Deaths due to childhood asthma. Are they preventable? *Clinical Pediatrics*, **15**, 677–87.

Yoder, C. C., Wiswell, T., Cornish, J. D., Cunningham, B. E. & Crumbaker, D. H. (1988). Marshall–Smith syndrome: further delineation. *Southern Medical Journal*, **81**, 1297–300.

Zach, M. S. & Karner, U. (1989). Sudden death in asthma. *Archives of Disease in Childhood*, **64**, 1446–51.

Zalzal, G. H. (1989). Stridor and airway compromise. *Pediatric Clinics of North America*, **36**, 1389–401.

8

Neurologic conditions

Introduction

This chapter deals with causes of sudden natural death in childhood involving the nervous system, a large number of which are due to vascular or infective disorders. It should be stressed, however, that trauma should be suspected if intracranial hemorrhage is found at autopsy. This is particularly so in infancy and early childhood. Detailed review of the presenting history should then be undertaken with a complete radiologic survey of the body. If a traumatic etiology can be excluded, then other conditions such as cerebrovascular disease may then be considered. Although fatal cerebrovascular disease in the pediatric age group is not common, it is possible that any of the causes of occlusive vascular disease that result in childhood stroke can also result in sudden death. Possible causes of sudden death and stroke in childhood can be found in Tables 8.1 and 8.2 (adapted from Ausman *et al.*, 1988; Harvey & Alvord, 1972; Pascual-Castroviejo, 1992; Raybaud *et al.*, 1985; Roach, Garcia & McLean, 1984; Ross, Curnes & Greenwood, 1987).

Hematologic conditions

Due to the rigidity of the skull after infancy and the relative plasticity of cerebral tissue, areas of significant hemorrhage tend to develop at the expense of the surrounding brain. Death may occur rapidly from resultant cerebral edema and brainstem herniation through the foramen magnum. Once occult trauma has been ruled out, there are a number of etiologically unrelated disorders with very different pathophysiologies responsible for intracranial hemorrhage in children.

Bleeding diatheses

Bleeding diatheses are dealt with in greater detail in Chapter 9; however, many conditions that predispose to spontaneous hemorrhage in other areas of the body may cause major problems with intracranial bleeding. One of the more common clinical scenarios resulting in sudden death in this situation involves a child who has acute leukemia with thrombocytopenia due to marrow infiltration by malignant cells or secondary to chemotherapy (see Figures 9.7–9.9). Spontaneous intracranial hemorrhage may also occur in other disorders where there is a reduction in the number of circulating platelets, such as aplastic anemia and Wiskott–Aldrich syndrome (see Figure 9.18).

Intracranial hemorrhage may follow relatively minor trauma in children with coagulation disorders such as hemophilia A, where there is a reduction in the amount of functional circulating factor VIII (Eyster *et al.*, 1978) (see Figure 9.13).

While intracranial hemorrhage may result from disseminated intravascular coagulation, bleeding tends to be more widespread and not necessarily unexpected, as patients are often already seriously ill from severe trauma or infection.

Table 8.1. Conditions associated with central nervous system causes of sudden pediatric death

---

Hematological conditions
    Bleeding diatheses
    Thrombotic disorders
    Hemoglobinopathies
Cardiovascular conditions
    Thromboembolism
    Vascular malformations
    Aneurysms
    Connective tissue disorders
    Moyamoya disease
    Fibromuscular dysplasia
    Vasculitides
Tumors
Epilepsy
Metabolic disorders
Infections
    Meningitis
    Encephalitis
    Poliomyelitis
Structural abnormalities
Friedreich ataxia
Tuberous sclerosis
Von Recklinghausen disease
Septo-optic dysplasia
Guillain–Barré syndrome
Déjérine–Sottas disease

Thrombotic disorders

Spontaneous thrombosis is also dealt with in Chapter 9, as certain inherited prothrombotic disorders may cause vascular thrombosis and ischemic stroke in children. Deficiencies in anti-thrombin III, plasminogen, and proteins C and S, or the presence of factor V Leiden, prothrombin gene 20210A, hyperhomocystinemia, antiphospholipid antibodies, dysfibrinogenemia, and elevated lipoprotein (a) may all result in arterial and venous thromboses (Abrantes *et al.*, 2002; Nestoridi *et al.*, 2002; Verdú *et al.*, 2001). Lupus anticoagulant syndrome has been associated with stroke in adolescence (Kelley & Berger, 1987). While family studies are indicated in such cases, many of these conditions are very rare, and the specific role of certain of these disorders in contributing

to childhood stroke remains to be defined (Chan & deVeber, 2000).

Hemoglobinopathies

Ischemic cerebral events are a known complication of sickle cell disease due to vascular obstruction by sickled red blood cells. This may lead to intracerebral and subarachnoid hemorrhage or to infarction with sudden death (Grotta *et al.*, 1986; Mills, 1985; Powars *et al.*, 1978). Cerebral vascular occlusion occurs in as many as 17% of children with sickle cell disease and may be exacerbated by hypercoagulable states in these patients if there is also factor V Leiden or plasminogen deficiency (Gerald, Sebes & Langston, 1980). Stroke in children with sickle cell disease has also been reported in association with fibrointimal proliferation of the carotid arteries (Seeler *et al.*, 1978; Stockman *et al.*, 1972). The extent of cerebral ischemia may be worsened significantly by the anemia that is present, as anemia on its own has been associated with symptomatic hypoxic episodes in children (Young *et al.*, 1983).

Cardiovascular conditions

Thromboembolism

Thrombosis of the cerebral veins or sinuses with stroke may occur in children with polycythemia and/or thrombocytosis secondary to cyanotic congenital heart disease (Figure 8.1) (Phornphutkul *et al.*, 1973). More rarely, venous thrombosis may be due to hypercoagulable states (as detailed above), which may be familial or result from sepsis (Figures 8.2 and 8.3 and Color Plate 16) (Berlin, 1975; Konishi *et al.*, 1987). Dehydration and anemia may be exacerbating factors, the former playing a major role in cases of cerebral venous thrombosis in children with profound gastroenteritis.

Local sepsis involving the middle ear or sinuses can erode the skull and extend into the adjacent cranial cavity, resulting in meningitis (see Figure 4.18) and venous sinus thrombosis (Janaki *et al.*,

Table 8.2. Conditions associated with cerebrovascular accidents in infancy and childhood

Hematologic
  Thrombocytopenia
  Thrombocytosis
  Polycythemia
  Leukemia
  Coagulation disorders
  Lupus anticoagulant
  Prothrombotic disorders
  Disseminated intravascular coagulation
  Hemoglobinopathies
  Marked anemia
  Hemolytic uremic syndrome
Cardiac
  Cyanotic congenital heart disease
  Infective endocarditis
  Myocarditis
  Rheumatic fever
  Myxomas
  Prosthetic valves
  Rhythm disorders
  Cardiomyopathies
  Myocardial infarction
  Mitral valve prolapse
Vascular
  Vascular malformations
  Arterial aneurysms
  Moyamoya disease
  Fibromuscular dysplasia
  Collagen vascular diseases
  Connective tissue disorders
  Takayasu disease
  Hypertension
  Acute hypotension
  Thromboembolism
  Hereditary hemorrhagic telangiectasia
  Neurocutaneous syndromes
  Arterial kinking
  Migraine
  External compression of vessels
  Superior vena cava syndrome
  Arterial agenesis or hypoplasia
Gastrointestinal
  Inflammatory bowel disease

Table 8.2. (*cont.*)

Metabolic
  Diabetes mellitus
  Homocystinuria
  Hyperlipidemia
  Fabry disease
  Congenital adrenal hyperplasia
  Scurvy
  Vitamin K deficiency
  Liver disease
  Congenital C2 deficiency
Microbiologic
  Local infection:
    ENT pyogenic infections
    Cavernous sinus thrombophlebitis
    Mucormycosis
    Meningitis
    Malaria
    Herpes ophthalmicum
  Generalized infection
    Viral disease
    Mycoplasma disease
    Bacterial disease
    Fungal disease
    Tuberculosis
    Syphilis
    Hydatid disease
Traumatic
  Closed head injury
  Neck or intraoral injury
  Foreign-body embolism
Drug-related
  Arterial spasm
  Necrotizing vasculitis
  Septic emboli
Skeletal
  Klippel–Feil anomaly
Iatrogenic
  Angiography
  Radiotherapy
Idiopathic

1975). In addition, infection may also cause arteritis, with subsequent occlusive thrombosis and stroke (Shillito, 1964). Although viral upper respiratory tract infection has been associated with cerebral arterial

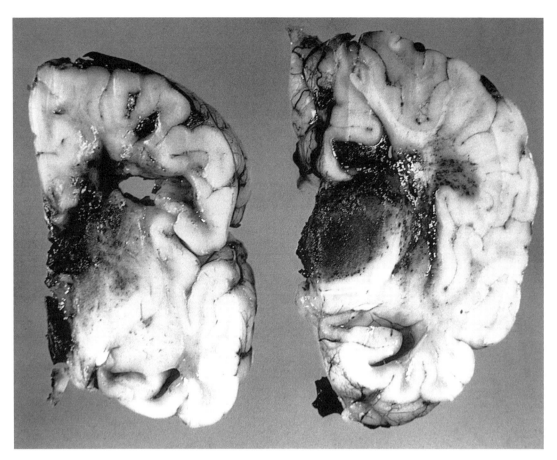

Figure 8.1 Cerebral infarction following cerebral venous thrombosis in a one-month-old boy with cyanotic congenital heart disease.

thrombosis (Blennow *et al.*, 1978; Eeg-Olofsson & Ringheim, 1983), its role in causing vascular occlusion is ill understood (Isler, 1984). On occasion, no apparent cause for spontaneous intracranial vessel thrombosis will be found despite careful pathologic examination (Fowler, 1961).

Intracranial embolism derives either from a left-sided intracardiac source or from paradoxical embolism. Bacterial endocarditis associated with congenital cardiac defects or prosthetic materials may result in cerebral embolism. Other lesions within the left atrium and ventricle that have led to cerebral ischemic events are those associated with rheumatic fever, myxomas, hydatid cysts, marantic

endocarditis, cardiomyopathy (Ausman *et al.*, 1988; Byard & Bourne, 1991; Kelley, 1986), and disorders associated with arrhythmias or infarction, including cardiac transplantation (Adair *et al.*, 1992). (Although the latter series included children, it is not certain whether any of them suffered cerebral events.)

Theoretically, any venous source of embolic material can lead to paradoxical embolism if there is a communication between the right and left sides of the heart, such as an atrial or ventricular septal defect. Embolized material may be thrombus, air, or even tumor, as was the case in an eight-year-old boy who suffered extensive cerebral infarction due to occlusion of his left internal carotid artery

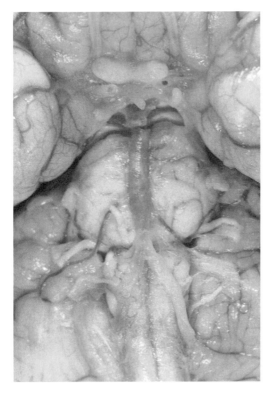

Figure 8.2 Basilar artery thrombosis with occipital lobe and cerebellar infarction in a one-year-old boy with viral pneumonia.

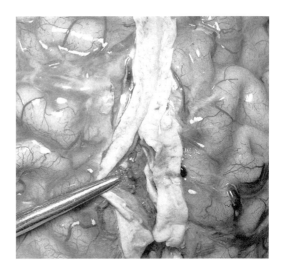

Figure 8.3 Opened superior sagittal sinus revealing an enclosed thrombus from a six-year-old boy with bacterial pneumonia.

by Wilms' tumor fragments that had passed through a ventricular septal defect during surgery (see Figure 10.25) (Moore & Byard, 1992). Pulmonary disorders such as hereditary hemorrhagic telangiectasia (Osler–Weber–Rendu syndrome) and arteriovenous fistulas may also lead to paradoxical cerebral embolism (Pellegrino, Zanesco & Battistella, 1992) (see Table 8.2).

Vascular malformations

In a review of 10 autopsy cases of sudden death involving non-traumatic intracranial hemorrhage from clinically unsuspected cerebral lesions in children, the most common findings were vascular malformations and tumors (Byard, Bourne & Hanieh, 1991–2). The clinicopathological features of these cases are summarized in Table 8.3.

Clinical features

Children bleeding from an intracranial vascular malformation tend not to die suddenly, the usual presentation being symptoms and signs of raised intracranial pressure, focal neurological deficits, or fitting (Mori *et al.*, 1980). Sudden and unexpected death may, however, be the presenting feature.

Pathological features

The first indication of a possible vascular malformation may be the presence of cerebral edema associated with localized subarachnoid hemorrhage around the base of the brain (Figure 8.4). Significant subdural hemorrhage may occur in these patients in association with intracranial hemorrhage without any apparent subarachnoid extension. Figure 8.5 demonstrates such a phenomenon in a three-year-old boy who died following hemorrhage from an intracerebral arteriovenous malformation.

One of the major problems in trying to provide confirmatory histologic evidence of a suspected vascular malformation at autopsy is that the lesions

Table 8.3. Clinicopathological features of 10 cases of sudden and unexpected pediatric death due to central nervous system hemorrhage

Case	Age (years)	Sex	Clinical course (h)	Prior symptoms	Location
1	3	M	22		AVM – parietal lobe
2	8	F	1.5	–	?VM – cerebellum
3	11.5	M	5	–	?VM – cerebellum
4	8	M	6	–	?VM – cerebellum
5	9	F	DIB	–	?VM – cerebellum
6	11.75	F	<1	–	Aneurysm – middle cerebral artery
7	7.25	F	8 (0 to arrest)	–	Medulloblastoma – cerebellum
8	5.25	F	17	–	Astrocytoma – optic chiasm
9	9	M	<10	1 year, mild headaches, sexual precocity	Teratoma – pineal gland
10	2.5	M	DIB	2 weeks' "breath holding episodes"	Ependymoma – 4th ventricle

AVM, arteriovenous malformation; DIB, dead in bed; VM, vascular malformation.

often self-destruct when hemorrhage occurs (Figure 8.6). It has been estimated that diagnostic material will be found in only 70–80% of cases (Dehner, 1987). It is important, therefore, to carefully sample as much of the loose and adherent blood clot as possible, as remnants of abnormal vessels may still be present within this material. Equally, it is also important to consider other possible etiologies when histologic confirmation of vascular malformation is lacking.

Vascular malformations may take a number of different histologic forms, with the most common being a tangle of disordered arterioles and venules. Histologically, a typical arteriovenous malformation can be recognized by the presence of abnormally dilated and irregularly shaped vascular channels composed of an intimate admixture of arterioles, venules, and capillaries, often with residual cerebral tissue interspersed between the vessels (Figure 8.7) (McCormick, 1966; Rosen, Armbrustmacher & Sampson, 2003). Hemosiderin deposition, calcification, demyelination, neuronal loss, and gliosis adjacent to vascular malformations occur when cases have had a more prolonged time course (Takashima & Becker, 1980). Osseous metaplasia has also been described (McCormick, Hardman & Boulter, 1968). Intracerebral vascular malformations may also be part of a more generalized condition such as Osler–Weber–Rendu syndrome (hereditary

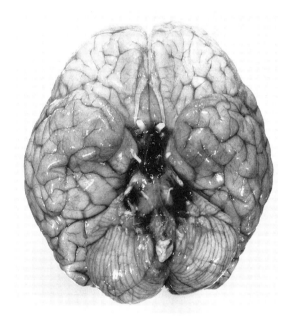

Figure 8.4 The first indication of the presence of extensive intracerebral hemorrhage due to a vascular malformation may be limited basal subarachnoid hemorrhage.

hemorrhagic telangiectasia), where vascular malformations may be found in a variety of organs including the brain, lungs, and gastrointestinal tract (Byard, Schliebs & Koszyca, 2001) (see Chapter 6).

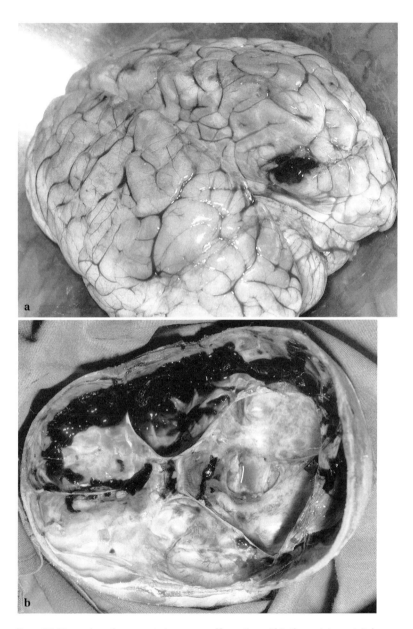

Figure 8.5 Hemorrhage from an arteriovenous malformation within the parieto-occipital lobes of the right cerebral hemisphere in a three-year-old boy with minimal subarachnoid extension (a) and a large amount of subdural clot (b).

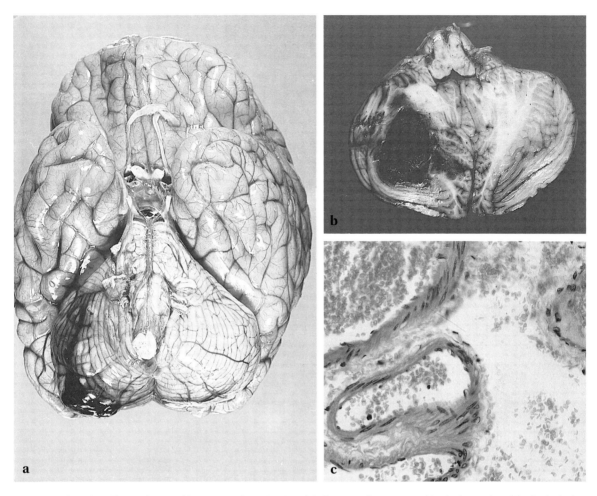

Figure 8.6 Subarachnoid hemorrhage visible on external examination of the brain (a) of a nine-year-old girl who was found dead in bed. The subarachnoid hemorrhage was in continuity with an area of extensive intracerebellar hemorrhage (b); however, the only residual vessels found were dilated but otherwise normal meningeal vessels (c).

Occurrence of sudden death

Byard, Bourne & Hanieh (1991–2) found that nearly one-half of their cases of probable bleeding cerebral vascular malformations presented acutely, with one patient surviving the onset of symptoms for less than one and a half hours, and another being found dead in bed having been apparently well the night before with no previous symptoms. Other authors have described similar cases of sudden death (Schejbal &

Oellig, 1979). Lesions that are within the posterior fossa or near the base of the brain, such as vascular malformations of the medulla, are more likely to be associated with sudden death (Demick, 1991) (Figure 8.8), although supratentorial lesions may also have a rapid course (Figure 8.9). Occasionally, sudden death occurs in children from bleeding vascular malformations of the choroid plexus (van Rybroek & Moore, 1990).

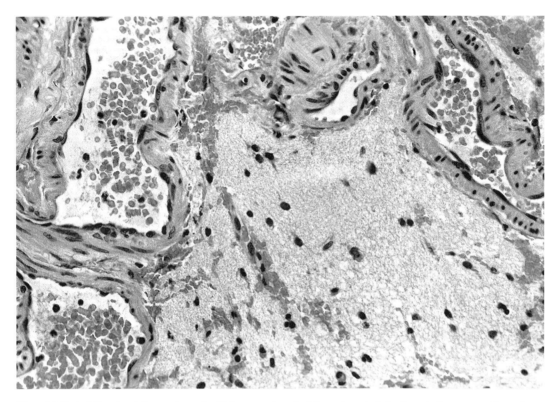

Figure 8.7 Typical dilated and abnormal vessels with interposed cerebral tissue characteristic of an arteriovenous malformation (hematoxylin and eosin, ×280).

Aneurysms

Death due to hemorrhage from a ruptured intracranial aneurysm is usually a condition of adults; however, sudden collapse and death may occur rarely in infants and children with this anomaly (Figure 8.10) (Byard, Bourne & Hanieh, 1991–2; Schulz, Hermann & Metter, 1981; Meldgaard, Vesterby & Østergaard, 1997; Plunkett, 1999). Individuals under the age of 20 years represented 1.5% of a series of 219 deaths from ruptured cerebral artery aneurysms (Gonsoulin, Barnard & Prahlow, 2002). Aneurysms are found more commonly in the vertebrobasilar system in children than around the circle of Willis, occur more often in males, and tend to be located more peripherally than in adults. Histologically, congenital aneurysms show absence or fragmentation of the elastic layers of the affected artery, with attenuation of smooth muscle and no inflammation (Prahlow, Rushing & Barnard, 1998).

An association exists mainly in adults between intracranial aneurysms and cystic renal and liver disease; thus, both the kidneys and liver should be carefully examined and sampled at autopsy. Intracranial aneurysms occur in individuals with adult polycystic disease in which the kidneys are enlarged and completely effaced by multiple cysts. Manifestations may appear in childhood and may be associated with polycystic liver disease in which there is hepatomegaly, with multiple cysts of varying sizes and Meyenberg complexes. The latter consist of aggregates of proliferating bile ductules surrounded by fibrous stroma. Inheritance of both adult polycystic kidney disease and polycystic liver disease is autosomal dominant (Geevarghese *et al.*, 1999; Schievink & Spetzler, 1998; Wakabayashi *et al.*, 1983).

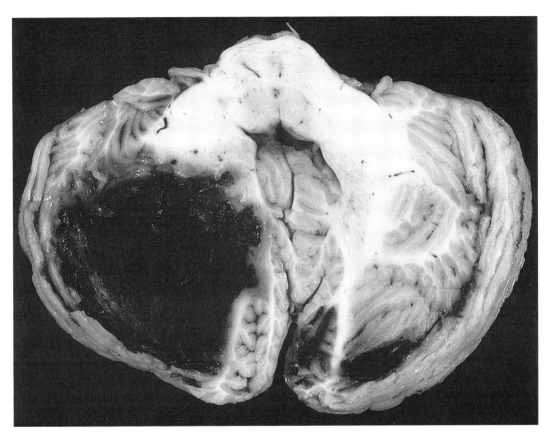

Figure 8.8 Massive intracerebellar hemorrhage due to a probable vascular malformation, resulting in sudden death of an eight-year-old girl.

There is also an increase in the incidence of intracranial aneurysms in children with coarctation of the aorta, collagen vascular disease, Marfan syndrome, Ehlers–Danlos syndrome, tuberous sclerosis, Moyamoya disease, fibromuscular dysplasia, tuberculosis, and syphilis (Choux, Lena & Genitori, 1992). Other heritable conditions that have been associated with intracranial aneurysms include achondroplasia, alkaptonuria, Cohen syndrome, Fabry disease, Kahn syndrome, Noonan syndrome, Osler–Weber–Rendu disease, osteogenesis imperfecta type 1, Pompe disease, pseudoxanthoma elasticum, Rambaud syndrome, Wermer syndrome, 3M syndrome, and alpha-1 anti-trypsin deficiency (Schievink, 1997). Aneurysms occurring in children

with these syndromes may be multiple (Kato *et al.*, 2001). Familial cases involving children are, however, rare (Graf, 1966; McKusick, 1964). Occasionally, dissecting aneurysms of the cerebral arteries will be found at autopsy, with no apparent predisposing disease (Manz, Vester & Lavenstein, 1979).

Intracranial aneurysms in children may also arise following trauma, such as closed head injury or projectile injury, and neurosurgery. Such aneurysms occur more often in males and are found at the skull base or on distal sections of the anterior and middle cerebral arteries. It has been claimed that traumatic aneurysms account for between 14% and 39% of all childhood intracranial aneurysms (Ventureyra & Higgins, 1994).

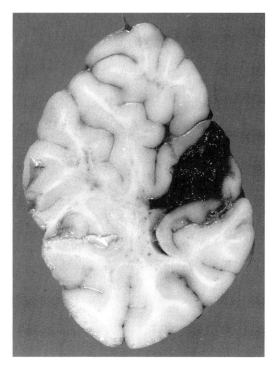

Figure 8.9 Sudden death due to intraparenchymal hemorrhage within the occipital lobe of a three-year-old boy caused by an arteriovenous malformation.

The so-called aneurysm of the vein of Galen is caused by direct shunting of branches of the internal carotid or posterior cerebral arteries into the vein of Galen. The presentation may be of high-output cardiac failure or hydrocephalus in early life, whereas older children and adolescents may present with subarachnoid hemorrhage.

Connective tissue disorders

Although rare, disorders of connective tissue should be considered in the differential diagnosis of cerebral hemorrhage at any age. These can be separated into primary and secondary groups, represented by disorders such as Ehlers–Danlos syndrome and scurvy, respectively. While patients with Ehlers–Danlos syndrome type IV often show general fragility of connective tissues, with easy bruisability (Hollister, 1978;

Owen & Durst, 1984), this is not always the case, and fatal intracranial hemorrhage may be the first manifestation of the disorder (Byard, Keeley & Smith, 1990) (see Figure 12.2). When the cause of intracranial bleeding is not immediately apparent at autopsy, the taking of fresh and frozen tissue (e.g. skin and aorta) will enable subsequent collagen analysis and cell culture studies, particularly if evidence of hemorrhage within other organs is found. DNA studies will also be required. Lack of type III collagen in analyses from a five-month-old girl enabled the diagnosis of type IV Ehlers–Danlos syndrome to be made, thus explaining the subarachnoid and multifocal visceral hemorrhages that had been found at autopsy (Byard, Keeley & Smith, 1990).

Moyamoya disease

In Moyamoya disease, a proliferative arterial lesion causes occlusion of intracranial arteries with, the development of a web-like net of vessels at the base of the brain. This creates the characteristic angiographic appearance of Moyamoya, "something hazy just like a puff of cigarette smoke drifting in the air" (Suzuki & Takaku, 1969) (Figure 8.11). Although originally described in Japan, it is now apparent that the condition has a worldwide distribution (Morgan, Besser & Procopis, 1987; Schoenberg, Mellinger & Schoenberg, 1978).

Clinical features

There are two clinical variants: one affects older children and causes subarachnoid hemorrhage, and the other affects younger children and causes exercise-related ischemia. The angiographic appearances are quite characteristic (Suzuki & Kodama, 1983) and usually allow the diagnosis to be established before death. The incidence of Moyamoya disease as a cause of childhood stroke varies with different series, from 4% to as high as 50%. Massive intracranial hemorrhage from collateral arteries (Oka *et al.*, 1981) or multiple dissecting aneurysms may also be found in affected children. The finding of a familial incidence of greater than 12% (Kitahara *et al.*, 1979) increases

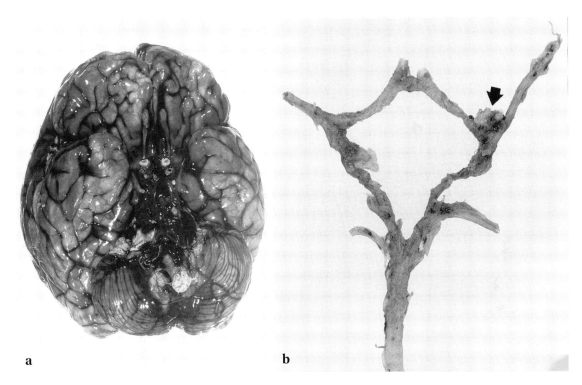

Figure 8.10 Predominantly basal subarachnoid hemorrhage (a) in a 12-year-old girl who collapsed and died within an hour of onset of symptoms. Dissection of the circle of Willis revealed a ruptured berry aneurysm (arrow) at the junction of the left middle and anterior cerebral arteries (b).

the importance of confirming the diagnosis at autopsy.

Pathological features

The major arteries that are affected are the internal carotid, anterior, and middle cerebral, the posterior communicating, and the anterior choroidal (Ausman *et al.*, 1988), all of which should be sampled at autopsy. Microscopically, affected vessels show splitting and reduplication of the internal elastic lamina, with eccentric intimal proliferation resulting in luminal narrowing (Yamashita, Oka & Tanaka, 1983). Vessels with microaneurysm formation show attenuation of the wall with focal fibrin deposition (Sato & Shimoji, 1992). Rarely, there may be an associated intracranial saccular aneurysm, although this is distinctly uncommon and tends to occur in older adolescents and adults (Adams *et al.*, 1979).

Differential diagnosis

To establish the diagnosis of Moyamoya disease, there has to be bilateral involvement of the cerebral vessels. If there is evidence of only unilateral disease, then the differential diagnosis would include the possibility of trauma, cerebral tumor, tuberculosis, von Recklinghausen disease, radiation effect, or fibromuscular dysplasia (although these may also have bilateral involvement) (Sato & Shimoji, 1992; Woody, Perrot & Beck, 1992). Moyamoya disease has also been associated with renovascular hypertension (Yamashita *et al.*, 1984).

Fibromuscular dysplasia

This is an uncommon condition that may involve the carotid arteries, resulting in vascular occlusion and ischemic cerebral events (Emparanza *et al.*, 1989; Pilz

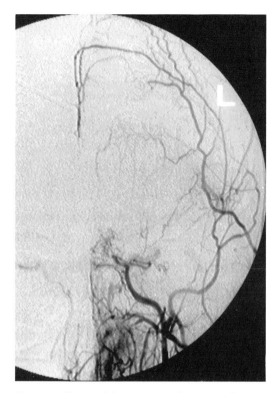

Figure 8.11 Characteristic appearance of Moyamoya disease on left internal carotid angiogram, showing a typical "puff of smoke" in the lower field.

& Hartjes, 1976). Angiographically, single or multiple stenoses as well as aneurysms are seen, giving the artery a beaded appearance (Lüscher *et al.*, 1987). Microscopically, there is marked hyperplasia of the arterial media, with disruption of the elastic laminae and adventitial fibrosis. Although generally a disorder of older age groups, cases in children have been reported (Lemahieu & Marchau, 1979; Shields *et al.*, 1977) involving both the carotid and vertebral artery systems. Affected children have had cerebral and cerebellar infarctions (Llorens-Terol, Sole-Llenas & Tura, 1983; Perez-Higueras *et al.*, 1988).

Vasculitides

Infectious vasculopathies

Involvement of cerebral vessels in bacterial meningitis may result in ischemic episodes, as detailed

in Chapter 4. Vasculitis and perivasculitis have also been found in children with AIDS in association with cerebral hemorrhage and stroke (Mizusawa *et al.*, 1988). Other viral infections such as herpes zoster may also be associated with vasculitis and stroke (Walker, El Gammal & Allen, 1973).

Inflammatory vasculopathies

While inflammatory vasculopathies of the cerebral circulation are exceedingly rare in the pediatric age range, several have been described that may have neurologic sequelae. These include systemic lupus erythematosis and granulomatous arteritis (Sabharwal *et al.*, 1982; Yancey, Doughty & Athreya, 1981). Kawasaki disease has been described occasionally as a cause of neurologic problems, but this is due to thromboembolism rather than direct involvement of the cerebral vessels (Lapointe *et al.*, 1984; Laxer, Dunn & Flodmark, 1984). Takayasu aortitis may rarely give rise to stroke in infancy (Kohrman & Huttenlocher, 1986). The neurologic complications of the vasculidites have been described in detail by Moore & Cupps (1983).

Miscellaneous

Arterial kinking

One controversial clinicoradiologic entity that has been described in association with cerebral infarction in children is arterial kinking. It has been proposed that coiling of the internal carotid artery in some children predisposes to temporary luminal occlusion, with resultant cerebral ischemia/infarction (Fisher, 1982; Parrish & Byrne, 1971; Sarkari, Holmes & Bickerstaff, 1970). However, not all investigators have commented on kinking in their series of children with strokes (Hilal *et al.*, 1971) or have found carotid artery elongation (Perdue *et al.*, 1975). Given the difficulties encountered at autopsy in examining portions of the internal carotid artery, it is unlikely that pathologic examination can contribute to this debate, except to exclude other etiologies.

Migraine

On very rare occasions, migraine has been reported as a cause of cerebral or cerebellar infarction in children (Barlow, 1984; Castaldo, Anderson & Reeves, 1982; Dorfman, Marshall & Enzmann, 1979; Dunn, 1985; Isler, 1992), sometimes resulting in death (Buckle, Du Boulay & Smith, 1964). There is also an association between migraine and epilepsy (Basser, 1969).

Sturge–Weber syndrome

Sturge–Weber syndrome is one of the neurocutaneous disorders characterized by cutaneous and leptomeningeal angiomatosis. Although the vast majority of cases present with epilepsy, subarachnoid hemorrhage may occur (Anderson & Duncan, 1974).

Mitral valve prolapse

A family has been reported in which there was an apparent association between mitral valve prolapse and embolic stroke at a young age. The two youngest members to manifest hemiplegias were aged six months and ten years, respectively (Rice *et al.*, 1980). Other reports have also documented an association of thromboembolic stroke in adolescence with mitral valve prolapse (Tharakan *et al.*, 1982).

Cardiac arrhythmias

Cardiac arrhythmias may rarely be responsible for the development of acute hemiplegia in children, most likely on an embolic basis (Atluru, Epstein & Gootman, 1985).

Drug overdose

The occurrence of hemorrhagic stroke in an adolescent due to phenylpropanolamine overdose (Forman *et al.*, 1989) and ischemic stroke in a 12-year-old after glue sniffing (Parker, Tarlow & Milne Anderson, 1984) suggests that toxicological screening at autopsy should be perfomed in cases of childhood stroke of uncertain etiology.

Other factors

Other, less common causes of hemorrhagic or ischemic cerebrovascular accidents in childhood include hypertension, acute hypotension, and collagen vascular diseases (Ausman *et al.*, 1988; Gold *et al.*, 1973). Finally, no cause will be found in a percentage

of ischemic strokes in children in spite of detailed investigation (Bates, Daniels & Benton, 1982).

Tumors

Generally, tumors of the brain and cranial contents produce symptoms and signs of raised intracranial pressure, with headache and alteration of conscious state. Occasionally, the presentation is more dramatic due to an acute disturbance in blood or cerebrospinal fluid flow (Abu al Ragheb, Koussous & Amr, 1986). Also, direct pressure on brainstem respiratory centers may cause sudden death in children with neoplasms located within the posterior fossa (Byard, Bourne & Hanieh, 1991–2; Gleckman & Smith, 1998; Nelson, Frost & Schochet, 1987; Rajs, Råsten-Almqvist & Nennesmo, 1997).

Metastatic tumors may also result in cerebrovascular accidents in children, particularly in the case of neuroblastoma. Other malignancy-related complications include intracranial hemorrhage or thrombosis due to disseminated intravascular coagulation or due to chemotherapy with L-asparginase (Packer *et al.*, 1985).

Hemorrhage

Hemorrhage has initiated the presentation in 3–10% of reported brain tumors in different series in the literature (Laurent, Bruce & Schut, 1981; Park *et al.*, 1983) and has a documented association with sudden death in both infancy and childhood (Aoki *et al.*, 1992; Poon & Solis, 1985).

Pathophysiology

Hemorrhage into a neoplasm may result in rapid expansion in size, with compression of the surrounding cerebral parenchyma. This is usually a complication of tumors, such as medulloblastoma, malignant astrocytoma, ependymoma, and oligodendroglioma (Park *et al.*, 1983; Poon & Solis, 1985), that have infiltrated and eroded a vessel wall or bled from rupture of delicate tumor neovasculature. Hemorrhage may also be precipitated by trauma (Torrey, 1983).

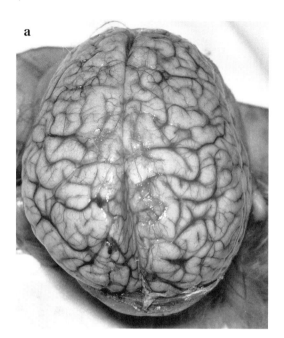
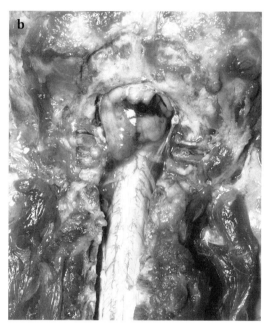

Figure 8.12 Marked cerebral edema in a 2.5-year-old boy with recent hemorrhage into a fourth ventricular ependymoma, showing flattening of gyri (a) and herniation of the cerebellar tonsils through the foramen magnum (b).

Pathological features

At autopsy, the presence of markedly increased intracranial pressure may be obvious as soon as the calvarium and dura are removed, as this will reveal prominent flattening of cerebral gyri. Other indicators of cerebral edema such as uncal grooving and herniation of the cerebellar tonsils may also be present (Figure 8.12).

The cases listed in Table 8.3 demonstrate the variety of tumor types that may result in massive intracranial hemorrhage, the variable location that includes both infra- and supratentorial compartments, and the minimal and often non-specific antemortem symptoms. The tumors are illustrated in the following figures: Figure 8.13 – cerebellar medulloblastoma in a seven-year-old girl (case 7); Figure 8.14 – optic chiasm astrocytoma in a five-year-old girl (case 8); Figure 8.15 – pineal teratoma in a nine-year-old boy with precocious sexuality (case 9); and Figure 8.16 – an ependymoma of the fourth ventricle in a 2.5-year-old boy (case 10) (Byard, Bourne & Hanieh, 1991–2).

It is apparent from these children that both low- and high-grade neoplasms may initiate intracranial hemorrhage.

Cerebrospinal fluid obstruction

Other rare cerebral lesions that may cause sudden death in childhood are tumors that cause obstruction to cerebrospinal fluid flow (Shemie *et al.*, 1997), such as colloid cyst of the third ventricle. These epithelial-lined cysts arise from the third ventricle in the midline and may obstruct the foramen of Monro. Their origin is uncertain, with derivation from neuroepithelial, ependymal, choroid plexus, and endodermal tissues being proposed (Aronica *at al.*, 1998).

Clinical features

The usual presentation of a colloid cyst is in later childhood or early adulthood with vomiting or headaches, which may be posture-related. These

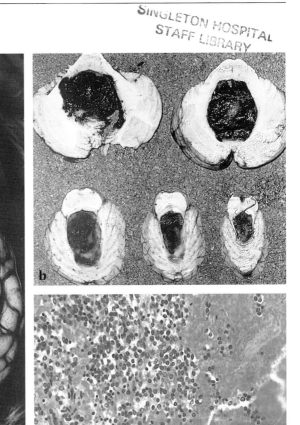

Figure 8.13 Cerebral edema (a) in a seven-year-old girl with intracerebellar hemorrhage (b) due to bleeding from a clinically unsuspected medulloblastoma (c) (hematoxylin and eosin, ×110).

features may also occur in younger children and in some cases have been attributed incorrectly to a minor viral infection or gastroenteritis (Byard & Moore, 1993; McDonald, 1982; Torrey, 1983).

Pathophysiology

Clinical symptoms are believed to be caused by blockage of the cerebral aqueduct due to the critical location of these lesions in the anterior portion of the third ventricle (Maeder *et al.*, 1990). This results in acute hydrocephalus as the cerebrospinal fluid pressure increases (Camacho *et al.*, 1989).

Occurrence of sudden death

Occasional cases of colloid cyst associated with sudden death in children have been reported, although there has usually been a history of the child being unwell in the days prior to death (Byard & Moore, 1993; Read, 1990; Saulsbury, Sullivan & Schmitt, 1981).

Pathological features

Symmetrical dilation of the lateral and third ventricles in association with a unilocular cystic mass at the entrance to the aqueduct is characteristic (Figure 8.17). The cysts are lined by flattened to cuboidal epithelium.

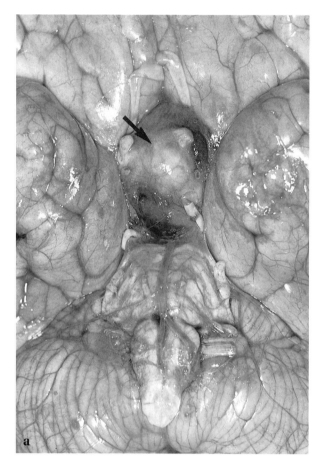

Figure 8.14 A low-grade astrocytoma of the optic chiasm (arrow) (a) with significant hemorrhage demonstrated on coronal sectioning (b). This was found in a previously asymptomatic five-year-old girl.

Other neoplasms that occur around the foramen of Monro may also cause obstructive hydrocephalus, although these often have a more prolonged time course (Ryder, Kleinschmidt-DeMasters & Keller, 1986). For example, sudden death occurred in a four-year-old boy who had a six-week history of increasing somnolence and weight gain. At autopsy, a pedunculated tumor arising from the wall of the third ventricle near the aqueduct was found that had caused acute obstruction. (Unfortunately, the results of histologic assessment were not available.) Obstruction to cerebrospinal fluid flow may also occur with other neoplasms at critically placed levels of the neuraxis, such as at the pontocerebellar angle (Buzzi *et al.*, 1998).

Miscellaneous

Peripheral neural tumors may also cause rapid deterioration due to interstitial hemorrhage, as was the case in a previously well 3.5-month-old girl who developed "colic" one evening. Her condition deteriorated rapidly, and she died within seven hours due to massive intraperitoneal hemorrhage caused by metastatic neuroblastoma infiltrating the liver. Another report has detailed the unexpected death of a 12-year-old boy who was found at autopsy to have lung and airway compression from a posterior mediastinal paraganglioma (Hutchins *et al.*, 1999).

Epilepsy

It is now well recognized that children with epilepsy have a higher mortality rate than unaffected individuals, although this proposal has not always been accepted (Cockerell *et al.*, 1994; Krohn, 1963). Death may occur due to an accident resulting from a seizure, a prime example of which would be drowning (Orlowski, Rothner & Lueders, 1982), or due to an associated disease process, such as tuberous sclerosis, or due to status epilepticus, or it may occur suddenly and unexpectedly for reasons that are not immediately obvious (Terrence, Wisotzkey & Perper, 1975). The final group is the most enigmatic, as the underlying mechanisms responsible for death are far from clear. For example, no mechanism of death could be determined at autopsy in 4–30% of reported cases reviewed by Terrence, Wisotzkey & Perper, (1975). The rarity of unexpected death during febrile convulsions in otherwise normal children also suggests that other mechanisms may be operating in children with epilepsy who die suddenly. A certain percentage of children who have febrile convulsions will, however, develop epilepsy later (Juul-Jensen & Foldspang, 1983).

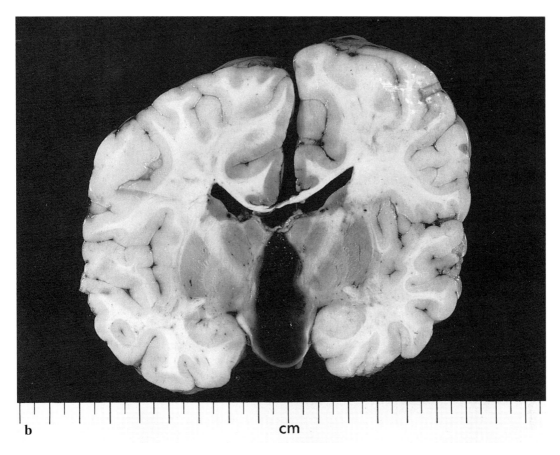

b   cm

Figure 8.14 (cont.)

Unfortunately, the problem of sudden death in epileptics has not been addressed extensively in the literature (Dasheiff, 1991). When it has been reviewed, the patient populations studied have tended to be adult and include a large number of alcohol abusers (Leestma *et al.*, 1989). Other authors have specifically excluded younger children from their analyses because of the occurrence of a wide variety of epileptogenic disorders that are associated with neural deficits (Hirsch & Martin, 1971). Conclusions based on this material are therefore not completely applicable to pediatric cases. More recent studies that have been undertaken in pediatric populations have confirmed an increased mortality risk, particularly in children with symptomatic epilepsy, although the risk factors may differ from those in adult populations (Breningstall, 2001; Callenbach *et al.*, 2001; Donner, Smith & Snead, 2001).

A classification system for sudden death in epilepsy (SUDEP) has been proposed, which defines SUDEP as "sudden, unexpected, witnessed or unwitnessed, non-traumatic, and non-drowning death in patients with epilepsy, with or without evidence for a seizure and excluding documented status epilepticus where necropsy examination does not reveal a toxicological or anatomical cause for death" (Nashef & Brown, 1996). Other deaths in epileptics in this classification are separated into those due to airway obstruction, aspiration, trauma, or drowning, and

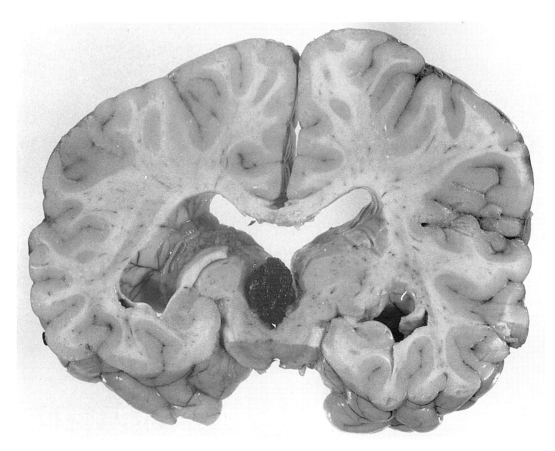

Figure 8.15 Coronal section of the brain from a nine-year-old boy with a history of mild headaches and precocious sexual development. Hemorrhage into a pineal teratoma with obstructive hydrocephalus can be seen.

those where there is significant underlying cardiorespiratory disease.

Frequency

The frequency of sudden and unexpected death in children with epilepsy is unknown; however, in general epileptic populations, it is estimated to range from one in 200 to one in 680 patients (Jay & Leestma, 1981). Sudden and unexpected death has accounted for between 10% and 30% of all epileptic deaths, representing 1–1.5% of all natural deaths and 8–12% of all sudden unexpected deaths (Leestma, 1988). (These latter data are again derived from predominantly adult cases.) The typical case of unexpected death encountered in pediatric autopsy practice is of an epileptic child, often with intellectual impairment, who is found dead in bed with minimal external or internal findings.

Pathophysiology of sudden death

The association of sudden death with sleep is noteworthy and most likely relates to reduction in seizure threshold that occurs with an increase in epileptic discharges (Hirsch & Martin, 1971; Schwender & Troncoso, 1986). For example, up to 79% of cases of sudden epileptic death have been found either in bed or in a bedroom (Schwender & Troncoso, 1986).

Table 8.4. Postulated causes of sudden death in epilepsy

Trauma
Suffocation
Asphyxia
Cardiac arrhythmia (sympathetically mediated)
Bradycardia/asystole (parasympathetically mediated)
Apnea/repiratory failure
Neurogenic pulmonary edema

A variety of theories have been proposed to explain the occurrence of sudden death in epilepsy (Table 8.4), including suffocation from bedding, asphyxia, pulmonary edema, and cardiac arrhythmia. Aspiration of food or foreign material is not usually found (Hirsch & Martin, 1971). Although supportive evidence for any of the categories is not great, Leestma (1988) has grouped the currently favored possibilities into (i) sympathetic induced cardiac arrhythmia, (ii) parasympathetic induced bradycardia/asystole, (iii) apnea/respiratory failure, (iv) a combination of arrhythmia and apnea, and (v) neurogenic pulmonary edema with cardiac failure.

The most popular theory to explain why apparently stable epileptic children are at increased risk of sudden death involves autonomic nervous system instability, with abnormal cardiac rhythms during seizure activity. This is supported by experimental data that show synchronization of vagal and sympathetic activity with cortical discharges in epileptic cats (Lathers & Schraeder, 1982; Schraeder & Lathers, 1983). It is proposed that an increase in predominantly sympathetic activity can result in tachycardias, ventricular arrhythmias, and asystole (Leestma et al., 1984). Overt muscle contractions are not necessary for this synchronization to occur. Vagally induced cardiac asystole or bradycardias are considered to be much less common than sympathetically induced arrhythmias (Leestma, 1988). The effects of this increased neural activity on the cardiac conduction system may also be exacerbated by coexistent hypoxia, and it is possible that laryngospasm, which has been documented in temporal lobe epilepsy (Ravindran, 1981), may also increase ictal

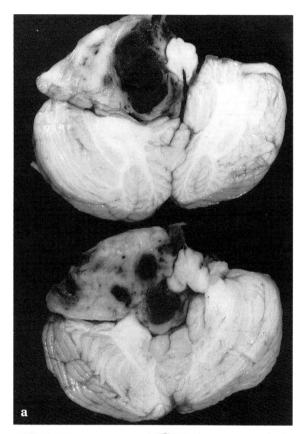

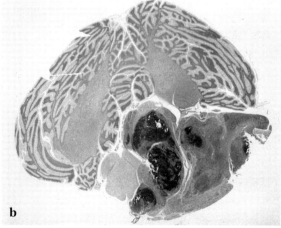

Figure 8.16 Cross-section of the cerebellum (a), with the corresponding whole mount (b), in a 2.5-year-old boy, showing extensive hemorrhage into a clinically undiagnosed ependymoma (c) (hematoxylin and eosin, ×100).

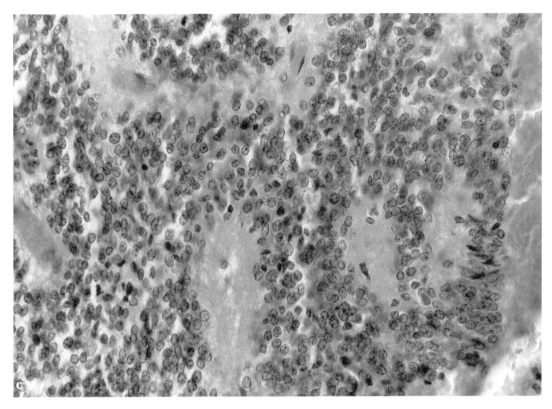

Figure 8.16 (cont.)

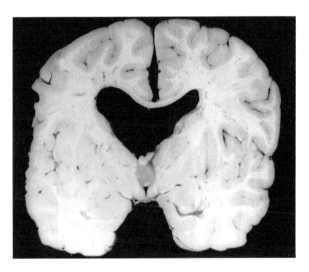

Figure 8.17 Colloid cyst of the third ventricle in a nine-year-old boy, with symmetrical ventricular dilation.

hypoxemia. However, there are very few cases of sudden death or cardiac arrest due to epilepsy in which an arrhythmia has actually been recorded (Dasheiff & Dickinson, 1986; Liedholm & Gudjonsson, 1992; Oppenheimer, 1990), and most reported clinical and experimental cases of arrhythmias associated with cerebral events have not been fatal (Dasheiff, 1991; Kiok *et al.*, 1986). Keilson and colleagues (1987, 1989) monitored 338 epileptic patients and found no increase in cardiac arrhythmias compared with the general population, with only 5% of patients showing high-risk patterns. There may also be a reverse association of cardiac arrhythmias with seizures, as there has been an increased incidence of epilepsy reported in patients with hereditary prolongation of the QT interval (Bricker, Garson & Gillette, 1984); i.e. seizures may be a secondary rather than a primary phenomenon resulting from cerebral hypoxia arising from ventricular tachycardia.

Determining the role of apnea in the terminal event is difficult, with some authors suggesting that seizures may be directly responsible for delayed respiratory arrest (Earnest *et al.*, 1992). This contrasts with the proposal that apnea plays only a secondary role during the tonic phase of the seizure (Leestma, 1988). As in other situations where complex pathophysiologic processes are acting, it may be that the end result is produced by integration of a number of predisposing factors rather than the effect of one element in isolation.

Autopsy findings

The absence of death scene and autopsy findings of disturbed bedding, urinary or fecal incontinence, bite marks on the tongue, and foam in the mouth or trachea does not mean that an epileptic episode did not occur, as these features have been absent in witnessed fatal episodes (Freytag & Lindenberg, 1964). As any type of fit (i.e. not only generalized tonic/clonic convulsions) may precede sudden death (Dasheiff, 1991), this could explain minimal external findings. In spite of this, bite marks on the tongue should always be looked for, although they are certainly not specific for epilepsy.

Autopsy investigations may show pre-existing chronic brain damage, developmental malformations, evidence of previous surgery, or neuronal depopulation and gliosis of the hippocampus secondary to past hypoxic episodes, usually with no evidence of an acute lesion. Relating these findings to autopsy data in the literature is complicated by the older age and previous alcohol intake of reported cases (Freytag & Lindenberg, 1964). For example, residual traumatic lesions, subdural hematomas, and Wernicke disease characterized the neuropathological findings in the series of Leestma and colleagues (1984). A study of 70 cases of unexpected death in epilepsy (age range 16–71 years) showed a higher incidence of gliosis, neuronal clusters, cystic gliotic lesions, increased perivascular oligodendroglia, decreased myelin, Bergmann's cerebellar astrogliosis, and folial atrophy compared with age- and sex-matched controls (Shields *et al.*, 2002).

The significance of cardiomegaly and interstitial and intra-arterial fibrosis within the heart (Falconer & Rajs, 1976; Leestma *et al.*, 1989) is difficult to determine given the medical histories and ages of the reported patients. It has, however, been suggested that prolonged sympathetic stimulation of the heart may result in similar lesions (Leestma *et al.*, 1989).

The presence of neurogenic pulmonary edema likely represents a secondary phenomenon rather than the cause of death and implies that death is not instantaneous, since edema takes some time to become established (Terrence, Rao & Perper, 1981). Occasionally, recent-onset epilepsy may be due to a neoplastic or infective space-occupying lesion.

It is important at autopsy to take serum for anticonvulsant drug levels, as poor compliance with medication has been reported (Leestma *et al.*, 1989; Terrence, Wisotzkey & Perper, 1975). However, therapeutic levels of anticonvulsants in 44% of Schwender & Troncoso's (1986) cases suggest that this does not exclude the occurrence of sudden death.

Associated features

A feature of pediatric cases of sudden death in epileptics is the number of infants and children who have associated severe neurologic handicaps. Whether this takes the form of profound intellectual impairment or merely motor difficulties, the most significant feature is that there is seizure activity present that may predispose to sudden death with minimal acute pathological findings. Examples of this occur in infants and children with cerebral palsy (Evans & Alberman, 1990). Rarely, epilepsy may also be associated with heritable connective tissue disorders such as Ehlers–Danlos syndrome (Jacome, 1999). Unfortunately, as there are usually no specific pathologic findings in cases of non-accidental asphyxia in young infants, this possibility should also be borne in mind in cases within that age group.

Conclusion

In summary, there is no doubt that children with epilepsy from any cause are at increased risk of sudden death. This often occurs during sleep, and often no major or acute lesions are found at autopsy. The absence of seizure-related phenomena such as disturbed bedding, incontinence, and tongue biting does not exclude an epileptic attack. While a likely terminal event is lethal cardiac arrhythmia, possibly exacerbated by hypoxia, it must be admitted that evidence for this in the literature is incomplete, and that many studies have involved adults rather than children. Given the absence of positive findings at autopsy, the diagnosis often becomes one of exclusion, which relies on clinicopathologic correlation, supported to a large degree by a past history of refractory epilepsy or a reliable description of the fatal episode.

Metabolic disorders

A variety of acquired and familial metabolic disorders have been associated with strokes in children, including diabetes mellitus, homocystinuria, congenital adrenal hyperplasia, Menkes kinky hair syndrome, familial hyperlipidemias, and Fabry disease.

Any condition that interferes with the adequate availability of vitamins necessary for hematopoiesis or in the maintenance of normal vascular integrity may also result in fatal hemorrhage. Examples include intrinsic liver disease causing deficient absorption of vitamin K, and dietary deficiency of vitamin C causing scurvy.

Scurvy

Children with scurvy tend to be irritable, with multiple mucosal and cutaneous petechial hemorrhages and pseudoparalysis due to bone pain. Although not seen so often today as in the past, scurvy still occurs in impoverished communities. Spontaneous intracranial hemorrhage may be a rare complication that results in sudden death from subdural or intracerebral collections. The underlying problem is a dietary deficiency of vitamin C that interferes with the normal process of hydroxylation of collagen with resultant vessel fragility. Color Plate 17 demonstrates such a case, showing a coronal section of brain from a 10-month-old scorbutic child who died due to hem-

orrhage into the right parietal lobe. Other findings at autopsy that may point to vitamin C deficiency are swollen, bleeding gums and swollen joints with widening of the costochondral joints producing the so-called scorbutic "rosary."

Homocystinuria

Homocystinuria is a heterogeneous metabolic disorder that may be caused by a deficiency in cystathionine synthetase. Patients with this disorder have variable degrees of intellectual impairment and cardiovascular disease, with a high rate of thromboembolism (Harker *et al.*, 1974). The basis for repeated thromboembolism is believed to be endothelial shedding, with exposure of subepithelial collagen, as well as reactive fibrointimal proliferation, which may also contribute to reduction in blood flow and peripheral organ ischemia. Abnormalities in blood clotting have also been documented (Palareti *et al.*, 1986), and cerebral thromboses and fatal cerebral infarcts are well-recognized complications (Harker *et al.*, 1974; Schwab, Peyster & Brill, 1987).

Fabry disease

Also known as angiokeratoma corporis diffusum universale, this is an X-linked recessive in-born error of metabolism caused by a deficiency of lysosomal alpha-galactosidase A (Dardir, Ferrans & Roberts, 1989). While cardiovascular involvement is a major feature of the disorder, death due to acute myocardial infarction appears to occur only in adults. Ischemic events involving the brain have been reported in childhood (Ausman *et al.*, 1988).

Leigh disease

Leigh disease, or subacute necrotizing encephalomyelopathy, is a heterogeneous, heritable, and progressive degenerative disorder of the brain characterized by capillary and glial proliferation within the medulla and thalamus, with neuronal degeneration (Figure 8.18) (Pincus, 1972). The

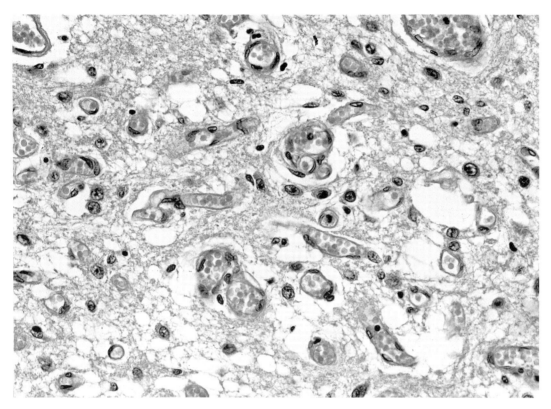

Figure 8.18 Capillary proliferation and gliosis in a case of Leigh disease (hematoxylin and eosin, ×200).

etiology involves disordered mitochondrial enzymes with pyruvate dehydrogenase deficiency (X-linked), cytochrome-c-oxidase deficiency (autosomal recessive) and OXPHOS defects (maternal inheritance). Mutations in the *Surf-1* gene on chromosome 9q34, in the *SDH* gene on chromosome 5p15, and in loci on chromosomes 5q11.1 and 11q13 have been identified (Gropman, 2001; Robinson, 2000; Schon *et al.*, 2001; Santorelli *et al.*, 1993). Affected children generally have a steadily downhill course, with developmental delay, psychomotor regression, ataxia, and seizures; hypertrophic cardiomyopathy (Figure 8.19) occasionally results in sudden death.

Miscellaneous

Children with diabetes mellitus or with congenital adrenal hyperplasia have been reported with acute cerebrovascular accidents (Atluru, 1986; Cleveland, Green & Wilkins, 1962). Ischemic cerebral events may also complicate familial hyperlipidemias due to premature atherosclerotic vascular occlusion (Daniels *et al.*, 1982; Glueck *et al.*, 1982).

Infections

Infectious agents that may cause sudden and unexpected death in children due to meningitis, encephalitis, or spinal cord involvement have been dealt with in Chapter 4. One of the most common agents in Western communities that causes fulminant meningitis, often resulting in death, is *Neisseria meningitidis*. Death in these cases may be caused by brainstem herniation due to massive cerebral edema.

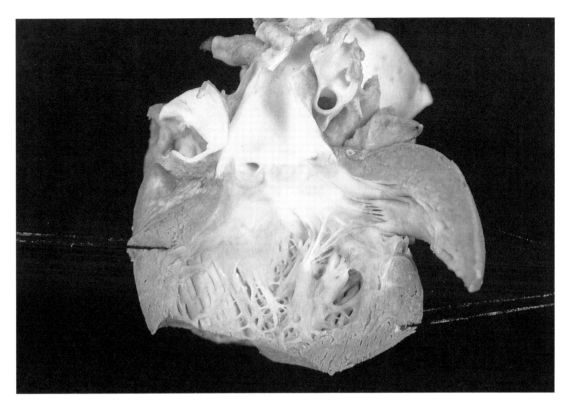

Figure 8.19 Left ventricular hypertrophy in a one-week-old girl dying unexpectedly from Leigh disease cardiomyopathy.

Structural abnormalities

It is often difficult to determine the mechanism of death in infants and children who die suddenly and who are found to have structural defects of the brain, such as microcephaly, hydrocephalus, pachygyria, or holoprosencephaly (Speights & Bauserman, 1991). Patients with abnormalities such as the Arnold–Chiari malformation, in which there is maldevelopment and downward displacement of portions of the medulla and cerebellum into the cervical spinal canal, have an increased incidence of sleep apnea (Ruff *et al.*, 1987) and are at risk of sudden death from brainstem compression (Byard, 1996; Friede & Roessmann, 1976; Tomaszek *et al.*, 1984) (Figure 8.20). Sudden death may be the first indication of an underlying Arnold–Chiari malformation (Martinot *et al.*, 1993). Other problems

that may be responsible for sudden death in children with Arnold–Chiari malformation are laryngeal obstruction due to recurrent laryngeal nerve paralysis.

In developmentally delayed children and children with cerebral palsy, aspiration of gastric contents and bacterial pneumonia may occur, with an associated reduction in life expectancy (Hutton, Cooke & Pharoah, 1994; Norman, Taylor & Clarke, 1990). Problems with swallowing, shallow respiration, disturbances of coughing or gagging reflexes, and immunological deficiencies may all predispose to lethal infection (Eyman *et al.*, 1990; Eyman *et al.*, 1993). It is also quite possible that defective autonomic control predisposes to cardiorespiratory arrest in such cases. Acute gastric dilation and rupture may occur in severely developmentally impaired individuals due to air swallowing and inadequate

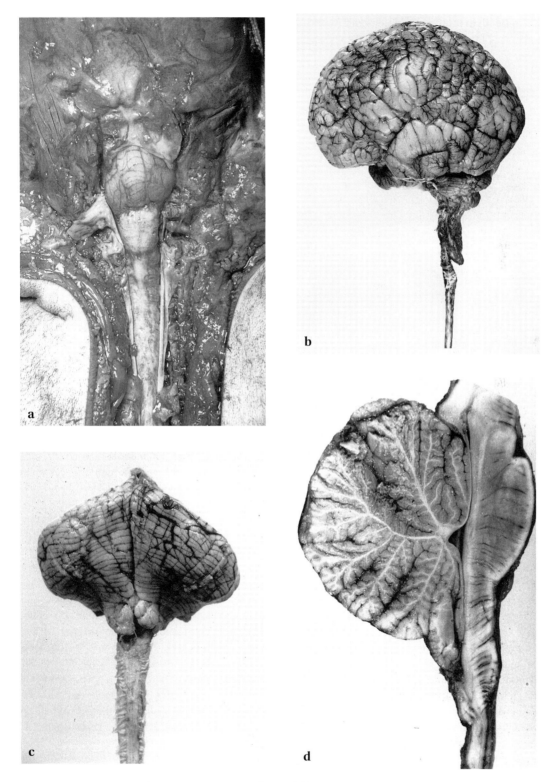

Figure 8.20 Posterior exposure demonstrating elongation of the medulla and cerebellar tonsils in a case of Arnold–Chiari malformation (a). Three separate views of cases of Arnold–Chiari malformation demonstrating variable elongation of the medulla and cerebellar tonsils (b–d).

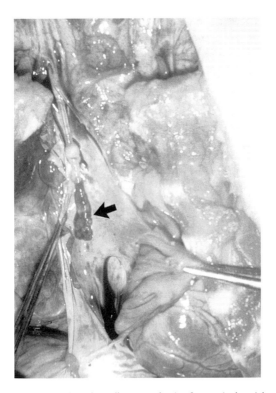

Figure 8.21 Thrombus adherent to the tip of a ventriculoatrial catheter (arrow) in a three-year-old girl with hydrocephalus and pulmonary hypertension secondary to recurrent pulmonary thromboembolism arising from the catheter tip.

gastric emptying (Byard & Couper, 2001; Byard, Couper & Cohle, 2001).

Sudden death due to ventriculovascular shunt-related pulmonary thromboembolism and shunt blockage was reported in 12 of 146 (8%) patients with hydrocephalic spina bifida (Figure 8.21) (Staal, Meihuizen-de Regt & Hess, 1987). Antemortem symptoms may be quite subtle, with chronic or only intermittent shunt malfunction (Tomlinson & Sugarman, 1995). Risk factors for pulmonary thromboembolism in children with shunts include both immobility and the presence of in-dwelling vascular catheters. Shunts not only are made out of thrombogenic material, but also damage the endothelial lining of vessels and disturb blood flow (David &

Andrew, 1993). The estimated five-year survival from pulmonary thromboembolism was 74% in one series of children receiving parenteral nutrition (Dollery *et al.*, 1994). Additional complicating factors in these children may be the presence of sepsis related to the in-dwelling shunt or catheter (Shiba *et al.*, 1992) or the development of pulmonary hypertension (Byard, 1996) (Figure 8.22). Cardiac catheterization may be dangerous in children with pulmonary hypertension and may precipitate sudden death (Byard 1996; Fuster *et al.*, 1984).

Other problems may arise from perforation of the intestine by ventriculoperitoneal shunt tips with ascending infection, as occurred in a 10-year-old boy with Arnold–Chiari malformation (Figure 8.23) (Byard, Koszyca & Qiao, 2001). Patency of a shunt on subsequent examination does not exclude previous malfunction (Sekhar, Moossy & Guthkelch, 1982).

Children with the Dandy–Walker malformation are also at risk of sudden death, either from tonsillar herniation or possibly from vascular compromise (Elterman, Bodensteiner & Barnard, 1995), in addition to the shunt-related problems detailed above. Dandy–Walker malformation is characterized by hydrocephalus with separation of the cerebellar hemispheres by a massively dilated fourth ventricle.

Friedreich ataxia

This rare hereditary spinocerebellar degenerative disorder usually manifests itself before adolescence with limb incoordination, dysarthria, scoliosis, pes cavus, and nystagmus. There is a strong association with cardiac problems and an increased risk of sudden death (Boyer, Chisholm & McKusick, 1962; Zimmermann *et al.*, 1986).

The inheritance is autosomal recessive, with 98% of mutations occurring in the *FRDA* gene located on chromosome 9q13, although there is evidence of genetic heterogeneity, with a further locus reported on chromosome 9p23-p11. The *FRDA* gene produces frataxin, a soluble protein found within mitochondria (Christodoulou *et al.*, 2001; Palau, 2001).

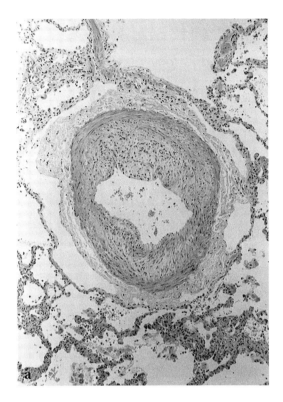
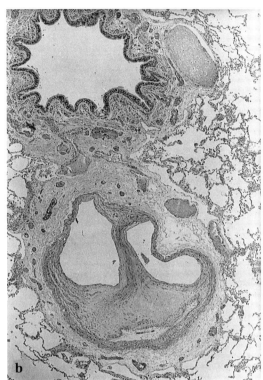

Figure 8.22 Sections of small pulmonary arteries from two cases of pulmonary hypertension secondary to recurrent thromboembolism from ventriculoatrial catheter tips showing prominent eccentric medial hypertrophy (×60) (a), and recanalization with multiple lumina (b) (hematoxylin and eosin, ×30).

Although death usually occurs in the fourth to fifth decades of life (Patel & Isaya, 2001), affected children may manifest rhythm disturbances, subaortic stenosis, and dilated or hypertrophic cardiomyopathy (Alboliras *et al.*, 1986; Boehm, Dickerson & Glasser, 1970; Child *et al.*, 1986). Microscopic changes in the heart are non-specific, with fibrointimal proliferation of the coronary arteries, diffuse myocardial fibrosis, and fatty change (Nadas, Alimurung & Sieracki, 1951).

There is a high incidence of diabetes mellitus in affected individuals, with an associated risk of ketoacidosis. Other documented causes of death are intracranial thromboembolism and hemorrhage (Hewer, 1968).

Tuberous sclerosis (Bourneville disease)

Tuberous sclerosis, or Bourneville disease, is an autosomal dominant condition characterized by mental retardation, epilepsy, and facial angiofibromas (so-called "adenoma sebaceum") (Byard *et al.*, 1991; Fryer & Osborne, 1987). It results from abnormalities in cellular migration, proliferation, and differentiation in a wide variety of tissue and organ systems (Byard, Blumbergs & James, 2003; Weiner *et al.*, 1998) and has quite variable penetrance with differing clinical manifestations (Al-Gazali *et al.*, 1989). The birth incidence is one in 6000, with the majority of cases being new mutations (O'Callaghan *et al.*, 1998).

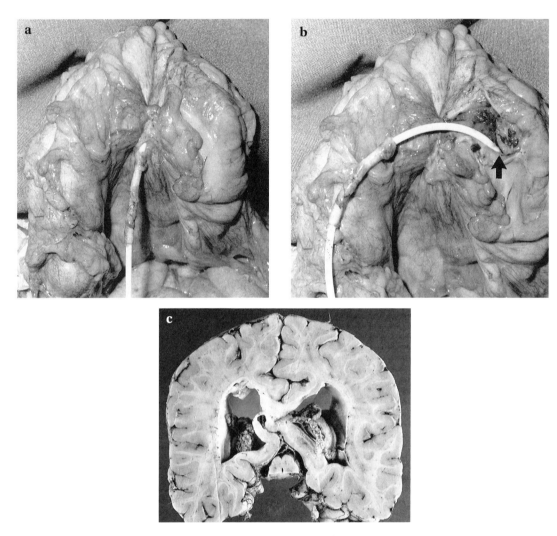

Figure 8.23 The midpoint of the transverse colon in a 10-year-old boy with hydrocephalus and ventriculoperitoneal shunting, showing the shunt firmly attached to the serosal surface (a). Further dissection revealed transmural penetration of the colonic wall (arrow) (b), with 34 cm of the catheter lying within the intestinal lumen. A coronal section of the brain revealed moderate ventricular dilation, with lining of the ventricles by a purulent exudate (c).

Clinical features

Major diagnostic features of tuberous sclerosis include facial angiofibromas or forehead plaques, hypomelanotic macules, non-traumatic ungual or periungual fibromas, cardiac rhabdomyomas, shagreen patches, retinal giant cell astrocytomas, nodular retinal hamartomas, subcortical glioneuronal hamartomas, cortical hamartomas (tubers), subependymal giant cell astrocytomas (SEGA), subependymal nodules, pulmonary lymphangiomyomatosis, and renal angiomyolipomas. Minor diagnostic criteria include cerebral white matter migration lines, bone cysts, dental enamel pits,

Table 8.5. Factors that may be associated with unexpected death in tuberous sclerosis

Cardiac	Cerebral	Renal	Vascular	Pulmonary
Arrhythmia	Epilepsy	Intratumoral hemorrhage	Aneurysm rupture	Pneumothorax
Outflow obstruction	Intratumoral hemorrhage			Chylous effusions
	Obstructive hydrocephalus			

Byard, Blumbergs & James (2003).

hamartomatous rectal polyps, gingival fibromas, non-renal hamartomas, "confetti" skin lesions, renal cysts, and retinal achromic patches (Roach, Gomez & Northrup, 1998; Weiner *et al.*, 1998). Rare cases have been reported with megacystis microcolon-intestinal hypoperistalsis syndrome, and aortic, peripheral, and intracranial aneurysms (Beltramello *et al.*, 1999; Couper *et al.*, 1991; Jost *et al.*, 2001). Convulsions are caused by central nervous system lesions such as cortical tubers (Bender & Yunis, 1982); however, cardiac rhabdomyomas are a more important finding in cases of sudden and unexpected death in childhood. Causes of sudden death in tuberous sclerosis are summarized in Table 8.5. Associated factors vary depending on age, with, for example, rhabdomyomas being more significant in the young and pulmonary lymphangiomatosis being mainly a disorder of adult females (Byard, Blumbergs & James, 2003).

Etiology

Two tuberous sclerosis genes have been identified: *TSC1* on chromosome 9q34 and *TSC2* on 16p13.3 (Cheadle *et al.*, 2000; Connor *et al.*, 1987), although there were initial suggestions of further heterogeneity with a possible locus on chromosome 11 (Smith & Simpson, 1989). *TSC1* and *TSC2* are tumor suppressor genes responsible for the production of the proteins hamartin and tuberin, which have both been demonstrated in neuroglial cells derived from cortical tubers (Johnson *et al.*, 1999).

Pathological features

At autopsy, a wide variety of lesions may be observed, as detailed above (Cassidy, 1984; Monaghan *et al.*,

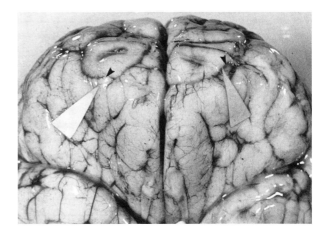

Figure 8.24 Two cortical tubers (arrowheads) in a child with unsuspected tuberous sclerosis, demonstrating how subtle an appearance they may have.

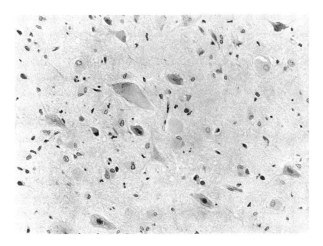

Figure 8.25 Large abnormal cells in a cortical tuber from a 13-month-old boy with tuberous sclerosis (hematoxylin and eosin, ×280).

1981), involving almost every tissue except skeletal muscle (Byard, Blumbergs & James, 2003; Sparagana & Roach, 2000). Cerebral findings consist of ventricular dilation, central demyelination, cortical tubers composed of aggregates of large bizarre cells interspersed with more normal appearing neurons and astrocytes, and subependymal nodules, sometimes with giant cell astrocytomas (Byard, Smith & Bourne, 1991; Fryer & Osborne, 1987) (Figures 8.24 & 8.25).

Rhabdomyomas are composed of markedly enlarged myocytes packed with glycogen (Byard, Smith & Bourne, 1991). Leaching out of glycogen during processing leaving strands of cytoplasmic material results in characteristic "spider" cells (see Figure 5.22). Rhabdomyomas are usually multiple and measure between 1 mm and 10 mm in diameter. They are found most often in the ventricles projecting into the cardiac cavity (Freedom *et al.*, 2000).

Occurrence of sudden death

Cardiac rhabdomyomas may be a "forme fruste" of tuberous sclerosis when multiple (Osborne, 1988), and either may be completely occult, representing an incidental finding at autopsy in early childhood (Byard, Smith & Bourne, 1991), or may be responsible for sudden death (Böhm & Krebs, 1980; Couper *et al.*, 1991; Rigle, Dexter & McGee, 1989; Williams *et al.*, 1972; Wilske, 1980; Winstanley, 1961). Rhabdomyomas may cause outflow obstruction, may obstruct coronary artery flow, or may involve conduction pathways resulting in arrhythmias (Fenoglio, McAllister & Ferrans, 1976; Gibbs, 1985; Smith *et al.*, 1989). An association with Wolff–Parkinson–White syndrome has been reported (O'Callaghan *et al.*, 1998). Rhabdomyomas may also lead to cerebral embolization, with resultant ischemia (Kandt, Gebarski & Goetting, 1985).

Sudden death has been described due to hemorrhage into a renal angiomyolipoma in a young woman with tuberous sclerosis (Byard, James & Blumbergs, 2003). Aortic rupture is another unusual cause of sudden death in young children with tuberous sclerosis (Freycon *et al.*, 1971; Larbre *et al.*, 1971),

although the exact reason for this association is unclear.

Autopsy investigation

The importance of accurately diagnosing cases at autopsy lies in the inherited nature of some cases. Although as many as 80% of cases have negative family histories and are assumed to represent new mutations, thorough clinical, echocardiographic, and radiological examination may reveal abnormalities compatible with tuberous sclerosis in apparently normal siblings or parents (Al-Gazali *et al.*, 1989). While not all studies have demonstrated this association (Fryer, Chalmers & Osborne, 1990), awareness of this possibility enables extra tissues to be taken for further investigation if needed. For example, cultured fibroblasts from affected patients have demonstrated consistent karyotypic variations (Scappaticci *et al.*, 1988). Given this finding and identification of gene loci, sterile skin for fibroblast culture and material for DNA studies should be taken at autopsy. As with all potentially heritable cases, liaison with a medical geneticist may be extremely useful.

Von Recklinghausen disease (neurofibromatosis)

Von Recklinghausen neurofibromatosis (NF1) is an autosomal dominant condition characterized by pigmented skin patches ("café-au-lait spots"), freckling, Lisch nodules of the iris, neurofibromas, optic gliomas, plexiform neurofibromas, and neurofibrosarcomas. It is found in approximately one in 3500 people. The *NF1* gene is a tumor suppressor gene located on chromosome 17q11.2 (Martin, 1993). Central neurofibromatosis (NF2) is characterized by meningiomas, acoustic neuromas, and spinal nerve root schwannomas, has a frequency of one in 50,000, and is linked to chromosome 22q12.2 (Martin, 1993).

While neurofibromatosis is not usually associated with sudden death in childhood or adolescence,

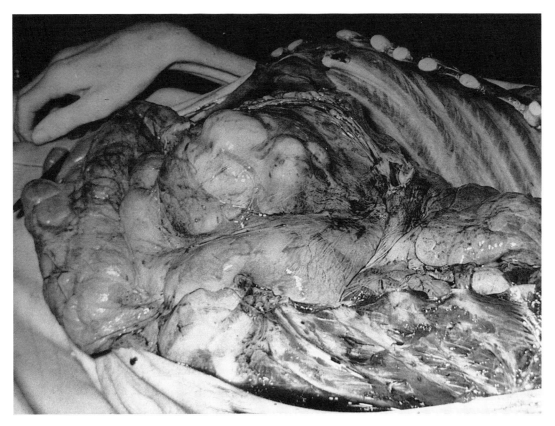

Figure 8.26 Large retroperitoneal neurofibroma in a 15-year-old boy with von Recklinghausen disease, with areas of malignant change that initiated substantial and lethal hemorrhage.

sudden death from an occult brain tumor has been reported (Unger *et al.*, 1984). Other extremely unusual cases of unexpected death in this condition have involved hemorrhage into the substance of a massive intrathoracic neurofibroma in a 15-year-old male (Koszyca *et al.*, 1993) (Figure 8.26) and a large neurofibroma of the vagus nerve in a 21-year-old male (Chow, Shum & Chow, 1993). Other potentially lethal abnormalities that have been reported in children with von Recklinghausen disease include fibromuscular dysplasia of the intracranial vessels, hypertensive stroke, hypertrophic cardiomyopathy, and right ventricular outflow obstruction (Erickson, Woolliscroft & Allen, 1980; Fitzpatrick & Emanuel, 1988; Pellock *et al.*, 1980; Rosenquist *et al.*, 1970). Cases of pe-

ripheral gangrene and vascular insufficiency have been reported in infants and children with neurofibromatosis and fibromuscular dysplasia (Kousseff & Gilbert-Barness, 1989). Hypertension may occur in affected children due to fibromuscular dysplasia of the renal arteries (Wallis, Deutsch & Azizi, 1970).

Septo-optic dysplasia

Septo-optic dysplasia (de Morsier syndrome) is a rare condition with variable manifestations caused by defects in cerebral midline structures, including hypothalamic abnormalities and optic nerve hypoplasia (Ouvrier & Billson, 1985; Morgan, Emsellem

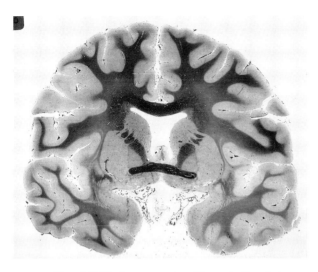

Figure 8.27 Wholemount section of the cerebral hemispheres in a case of septo-optic dysplasia (de Morsier syndrome), demonstrating absence of the interventricular septum and bilateral optic nerve atrophy (Weil stain).

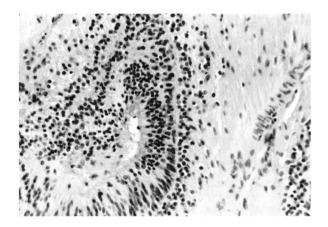

Figure 8.28 Disorganization and folding of the retina characteristic of retinal dysplasia in a four-year-old girl with septo-optic dysplasia (hematoxylin and eosin, ×200).

& Sandler, 1985). Severely affected individuals have short stature, blindness, psychomotor retardation, and hormone deficiencies (Gilbert, Scott & Byard, 2001). Although in many instances the etiology is unknown, rare cases are inherited, involving mutations

in the homeobox gene *HESX1* located on chromosome 3p21 (Dattani *et al.*, 1999; Parks *et al.*, 1999).

While unexpected death may be delayed until early adult life, it is more usual in children due to a complex interaction involving diabetes insipidus, corticotrophin deficiency, and unstable thermoregulation. Children may also suffer fatal hypoglycemia secondary to adrenal failure, often precipitated by viral infection (Brodsky *et al.*, 1997; Taback *et al.*, 1996). At autopsy, neuropathologic examination may reveal optic nerve atrophy, with absence of the interventricular septum, neuronal disruption, and gliosis of the hypothalamus, in addition to retinal dysplasia and cortical atrophy of the adrenal glands (Gilbert, Scott & Byard, 2001; Roessman *et al.*, 1987) (Figures 8.27–8.29).

As detailed medical histories are often not available at the time of non-hospital autopsies, it is worthwhile considering certain routine steps in children who appear dysmorphic, as these may be necessary if an accurate diagnosis is to be established. These include the taking of detailed external and internal photographs for later review by a medical geneticist if required, sterile skin and fresh tissues for cytogenetic and molecular studies, vitreous humor for biochemical and metabolic analyses, and the brain, spinal cord, eyes, and pituitary gland for histopathologic examination.

Guillain–Barré Syndrome

Guillain–Barré syndrome (infectious polyneuritis) is an acute demyelinating neuropathy characterized by rapidly progressive motor neuropathy with variable sensory changes. The etiology is not clear, although there is an association with preceding gastrointestinal or respiratory infection, immunization, and surgery (Thomas, Landon & King, 1992). In some cases, there is no apparent precipitating event. The clinical course varies from days to weeks; however, sudden death may occur in rare instances. This was the case in a 2.5-year-old boy who suffered an unexpected respiratory arrest following two days of leg weakness. On the day of his death, the weakness had progressed to involve his arms, and he had experienced difficulty in swallowing. On histologic examination of peripheral nerves, there is demyelination, with focal infiltrates of lymphocytes and macrophages (Thomas, Landon & King, 1992). Guillain–Barré syndrome should also be considered a possible cause of respiratory complications in infectious mononucleosis (Wolfe & Rowe, 1980).

Déjérine–Sottas disease

Déjérine–Sottas disease, or hereditary motor sensory neuropathy type III, is a rare disorder of peripheral nerves characterized by enlargement of peripheral nerves with sensorimotor neuropathy, ataxia, and skeletal deformity. It is an autosomal recessive condition that first manifests in childhood with early death occurring secondary to respiratory complications. Sudden death may occur rarely, as was the case of a 12-year-old girl with phrenic nerve involvement who died in her sleep (Felice *et al.*, 1994). Histologic examination reveals nerve fibers with abnormally thin myelin sheaths surrounded by "onion bulbs" composed of concentrically arranged double layers of basal lamina (Thomas, Landon & King, 1992). Although individuals with other types of hereditary motor sensory neuropathies, such as Charcot–Marie–Tooth disease, may also experience diaphragmatic impairment, this is not an acute phenomenon and occurs in adult life (Chan *et al.*, 1987; Hardie *et al.*, 1990).

Sudden infant death syndrome

There is evidence that subtle abnormalities of cerebral and neural biochemical and physiological function are involved in the etiology of this syndrome (Becker, 1990; Kinney & Filiano 2001; Kinney, Filiano & Harper, 1992). It is postulated that there is a defect in the brain and/or autonomic receptors and pathways that puts these infants at risk of sudden death during a particularly vulnerable period of their lives (between two and four months) (Byard, 1991).

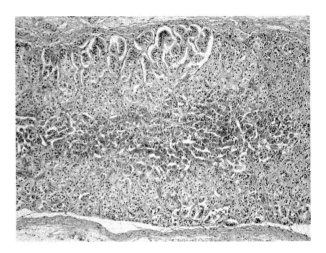

Figure 8.29 Section of the adrenal gland in a case of septo-optic dysplasia, demonstrating marked cortical atrophy (hematoxylin and eosin, ×30).

Whether the morphologic finding of increased brainstem gliosis has any relationship to this postulated malfunction awaits clarification. A review of possible neurologic mechanisms responsible for causing SIDS is provided in Chapter 13.

REFERENCES

Abrantes, M., Lacerda, A. F., Abreu, C. R., *et al.* (2002). Cerebral venous sinus thrombosis in a neonate due to factor V Leiden deficiency. *Acta Paediatrica*, **91**, 243–5.

Abu al Ragheb, S. Y. A., Koussous, K. J. & Amr, S. S. (1986). Intracranial neoplasms associated with sudden death: a report of seven cases and a review of the literature. *Medicine, Science and the Law*, **26**, 270–72.

Adair, J. C., Call, G. K., O'Connell, J. B. & Baringer, J. R. (1992). Cerebrovascular syndromes following cardiac transplantation. *Neurology*, **42**, 819–23.

Adams, H. P., Jr, Kassell, N. F., Wisoff, H. S. & Drake, C. G. (1979). Intracranial saccular aneurysm and Moyamoya disease. *Stroke*, **10**, 174–9.

Al-Gazali, L. I., Arthur, R. J., Lamb, J. T., *et al.* (1989). Diagnostic and counselling difficulties using a fully comprehensive screening protocol for families at risk for tuberous sclerosis. *Journal of Medical Genetics*, **26**, 694–703.

Alboliras, E. T., Shub, C., Gomez, M. R., *et al.* (1986). Spectrum of cardiac involvement in Friedreich's ataxia: clinical, electrocardiographic and echocardiographic observations. *American Journal of Cardiology*, **58**, 518–24.

Anderson, F. H. & Duncan, G. W. (1974). Sturge–Weber disease with subarachnoid hemorrhage. *Stroke*, **5**, 509–11.

Aoki, Y., Terunuma, H., Iwasaki, Y., Nata, M. & Sagisaka, K. (1992). A case of sudden infant death due to massive hemorrhage in primitive neuroectodermal tumor. *American Journal of Forensic Medicine and Pathology*, **13**, 199–203.

Aronica, P. A., Ahdab-Barmada, M., Rozin, L. & Wecht, C. H. (1998). Sudden death in an adolescent boy due to a colloid cyst of the third ventricle. *American Journal of Forensic Medicine and Pathology*, **19**, 119–22.

Atluru, V. L. (1986). Spontaneous intracerebral hematomas in juvenile diabetic ketoacidosis. *Pediatric Neurology*, **2**, 167–9.

Atluru, V. L., Epstein, L. G. & Gootman, N. (1985). Childhood stroke and supraventricular tachycardia. *Pediatric Neurology*, **1**, 54–6.

Ausman, J. I., Diaz, F. G., Ma, S. H., Dujovny, M. & Sadasivan, B. (1988). Cerebrovascular occlusive disease in children: a survey. *Acta Neurochirurgica*, **94**, 117–28.

Barlow, C. F. (1984). Migraine with seizures, stroke and syncope. In *Headaches and Migraine in Childhood*. Oxford: Blackwell Scientific Publications (Spastics International Medical Publications), pp. 146–51.

Basser, L. S. (1969). The relation of migraine and epilepsy. *Brain*, **92**, 285–300.

Bates, S. R., Daniels, S. R. & Benton, C. (1982). Childhood strokes. *Comprehensive Therapy*, **8**, 54–62.

Becker, L. E. (1990). Neural maturational delay as a link in the chain of events leading to SIDS. *Canadian Journal of Neurological Sciences*, **17**, 361–71.

Beltramello, A., Puppini, G., Bricolo, A., *et al.* (1999). Does the tuberous sclerosis complex include intracranial aneurysms? *Pediatric Radiology*, **29**, 206–11.

Bender, B. L. & Yunis, E. J. (1982). The pathology of tuberous sclerosis. *Pathology Annual*, **17** (part 1), 339–82.

Berlin, N. I. (1975). Diagnosis and classification of the polycythemias. *Seminars in Hematology*, **12**, 339–51.

Blennow, G., Cronqvist, S., Hindfelt, B. & Nilsson, O. (1978). On cerebral infarction in childhood and adolescence. *Acta Paediatrica Scandinavica*, **67**, 469–75.

Boehm, T. M., Dickerson, R. B. & Glasser, S. P. (1970). Hypertrophic subaortic stenosis occurring in a patient with Friedreich's ataxia. *American Journal of the Medical Sciences*, **260**, 279–84.

Böhm, N. & Krebs, G. (1980). Solitary rhabdomyoma of the heart. Clinically silent case with sudden, unexpected death in an 11-month-old boy. *European Journal of Pediatrics*, **134**, 167–72.

Boyer, S. H., IV, Chisholm, A. W. & McKusick, V. A. (1962). Cardiac aspects of Friedreich's ataxia. *Circulation*, **25**, 493–505.

Breningstall, G. N. (2001). Mortality in pediatric epilepsy. *Pediatric Neurology*, **25**, 9–16.

Bricker, J. T., Garson, A., Jr & Gillette, P. C. (1984). A family history of seizures associated with sudden cardiac deaths. *American Journal of Diseases of Children*, **138**, 866–8.

Brodsky, M. C., Conte, F. A., Taylor, D., Hoyt, C. S. & Mrak, R. E. (1997). Sudden death in septo-optic dysplasia. Report of 5 cases. *Archives of Ophthalmology*, **115**, 66–70.

Buckle, R. M., Du Boulay, G. & Smith, B. (1964). Death due to cerebral vasospasm. *Journal of Neurology, Neurosurgery and Psychiatry*, **27**, 440–44.

Buzzi, S., Verdura, C., Arlati, S. & Colecchia, M. (1998). Sudden death in a child due to rare endocranial neoformation. *Medicine, Science and the Law*, **38**, 176–8.

Byard, R. W. (1991). Possible mechanisms responsible for the sudden infant death syndrome. *Journal of Paediatrics and Child Health*, **27**, 147–57.

Byard, R. W. (1996). Mechanisms of sudden death and autopsy findings in patients with Arnold–Chiari malformation and ventriculoatrial catheters. *American Journal of Forensic Medicine and Pathology*, **17**, 260–3.

Byard, R. W. & Bourne, A. J. (1991). Cardiac echinococcosis with fatal intracerebral embolism. *Archives of Disease in Childhood*, **66**, 155–6.

Byard, R. W. & Couper, R. T. L. (2001). Acute gastric dilatation and spastic quadraparesis. *Journal of Pediatrics*, **139,** 166.

Byard, R. W. & Moore, L. (1993). Sudden and unexpected death in childhood due to a colloid cyst of the third ventricle. *Journal of Forensic Sciences*, **38**, 210–13.

Byard, R. W., Blumbergs, P. C. & James, R. A. (2003). Mechanisms of unexpected death in tuberous sclerosis. *Journal of Forensic Sciences*, **48**, 172–6.

Byard, R. W., Bourne, A. J. & Hanieh, A. (1991–2). Sudden and unexpected death due to hemorrhage from occult central nervous system lesions. A pediatric autopsy study. *Pediatric Neurosurgery*, **17**, 88–94.

Byard, R. W., Couper, R. T. L. & Cohle, S. D. (2001). Gastric distension, cerebral palsy and unexpected death. *Journal of Clinical Forensic Medicine*, **8,** 81–5.

Byard, R. W., Keeley, F. W. & Smith, C. R. (1990). Type IV Ehlers–Danlos syndrome presenting as sudden infant death. *American Journal of Clinical Pathology*, **93**, 579–82.

Byard, R. W., Koszyca, B. & Qiao, M. (2001). Unexpected childhood death due to a rare complication of ventriculoperitoneal shunting. *American Journal of Forensic Medicine and Pathology*, **22**, 207–10.

Byard, R. W., Phillips, G. E., Dardick, I., *et al.* (1991). Two unusual tumours of the gastrointestinal tract in a patient with tuberous sclerosis. *Journal of Paediatrics and Child Health*, **27**, 116–19.

Byard, R. W., Schliebs, J. & Koszyca, B. A. (2001). Osler–Weber–Rendu syndrome – pathological manifestations and autopsy considerations. *Journal of Forensic Sciences*, **46**, 274–7.

Byard, R. W., Smith, N. M. & Bourne, A. J. (1991). Incidental cardiac rhabdomyomas: a significant finding necessitating additional investigation at the time of autopsy. *Journal of Forensic Sciences*, **36**, 1229–33.

Callenbach, P. M. C., Westendorp, R. G. J., Geerts, A. T., *et al.* (2001). Mortality risk in children with epilepsy: the Dutch study of epilepsy in childhood. *Pediatrics*, **107**, 1259–63.

Camacho, A., Abernathey, C. D., Kelly, P. J. & Laws, E. R., Jr (1989). Colloid cysts: experience with the management of 84 cases since the introduction of computed tomography. *Neurosurgery*, **24**, 693–700.

Cassidy, S. B. (1984). Tuberous sclerosis in children: diagnosis and course. *Comprehensive Therapy*, **10**, 43–51.

Castaldo, J. E., Anderson, M. & Reeves, A. G. (1982). Middle cerebral artery occlusion with migraine. *Stroke*, **13**, 308–11.

Chan, A. K. C. & deVeber, G. (2000) Prothrombotic disorders and ischemic stroke in children. *Seminars in Pediatric Neurology*, **7**, 301–8.

Chan, C. K., Mohsenin, V., Loke, J., *et al.* (1987). Diaphragmatic dysfunction in siblings with hereditary motor sensory neuropathy (Charcot–Marie–Tooth disease). *Chest*, **91**, 567–70.

Cheadle, J. P., Reeve, M. P., Sampson, J. R. & Kwiatkowski, D. J. (2000). Molecular genetic advances in tuberous sclerosis. *Human Genetics*, **107**, 97–114.

Child, J. S., Perloff, J. K., Bach, P. M., *et al.* (1986). Cardiac involvement in Friedreich's ataxia: a clinical study of 75 patients. *Journal of the American College of Cardiology*, **7**, 1370–78.

Choux, M., Lena, G. & Genitori, L. (1992). Intracranial aneurysms in children. In *Cerebrovascular Diseases in Children*, ed. A. J. Raimondi, M. Choux & C. Di Rocco. New York: Springer-Verlag, pp. 123–31.

Chow, L. T.-C., Shum, B. S.-F. & Chow, W.-H. (1993). Intrathoracic vagus nerve neurofibroma and sudden death in a patient with neurofibromatosis. *Thorax*, **48**, 298–9.

Christodoulou, K., Deymeer, F., Serdaroglu, P., *et al.* (2001). Mapping of the second Friedreich's ataxia (FRDA2) locus to chromosome 9p23-p11: evidence for further locus heterogeneity. *Neurogenetics*, **3**, 127–32.

Cleveland, W. W., Green, O. C. & Wilkins, L. (1962). Deaths in congenital adrenal hyperplasia. *Pediatrics*, **29**, 3–17.

Cockerell, O. C., Johnson, A. L., Sander, J. W. A. S., *et al.* (1994). Mortality from epilepsy: results from a prospective population-based study. *Lancet*, **344**, 918–21.

Connor, J. M., Pirrit, L. A., Yates, J. R. W., Fryer, A. E. & Ferguson-Smith, M. A. (1987). Linkage of the tuberous sclerosis locus to a DNA polymorphism detected by v-abl. *Journal of Medical Genetics*, **24**, 544–6.

Couper, R. T. L., Byard, R. W., Cutz, E., Stringer, D. A. & Durie, P. R. (1991). Cardiac rhabdomyomata and megacystis-microcolon-intestinal hypoperistalsis syndrome. *Journal of Medical Genetics*, **28**, 274–6.

Daniels, S. R., Bates, S., Lukin, R. R., *et al.* (1982). Cerebrovascular arteriopathy (arteriosclerosis) and ischemic childhood stroke. *Stroke*, **13**, 360–65.

Dardir, M., Ferrans, V. J. & Roberts, W. C. (1989). Coronary artery disease in familial and metabolic disorders. In *Nonatherosclerotic Ischemic Heart Disease*, ed. R. Virmani & M. B. Forman. New York: Raven Press, pp. 185–235.

Dasheiff, R. M. (1991). Sudden unexpected death in epilepsy: a series from an epilepsy surgery program and speculation on the relationship to sudden cardiac death. *Journal of Clinical Neurophysiology*, **8**, 216–22.

Dasheiff, R. M. & Dickinson, L. J. (1986). Sudden unexpected death of epileptic patient due to cardiac arrhythmia after seizure. *Archives of Neurology*, **43**, 194–6.

Dattani, M. T., Martinez-Barbera, J. P., Thomas, P. Q., *et al.* (1999). HESX1: a novel gene implicated in a familial form of septo-optic dysplasia. *Acta Paediatrica Supplement*, **433**, 49–54.

David, M. & Andrew, M. (1993). Venous thromboembolic complications in children. *Journal of Pediatrics*, **123**, 337–46.

Dehner, L. P. (1987). *Pediatric Surgical Pathology*, 2nd edn. Baltimore: Williams & Wilkins, p. 1034.

Demick, D. A. (1991). Cerebrovascular malformation causing sudden death. Analysis of three cases and review of the literature. *American Journal of Forensic Medicine and Pathology*, **12**, 45–9.

Dollery, C. M., Sullivan, I. D., Bauraind, O., Bull, C. & Milla, P. J. (1994). Thrombosis and embolism in long-term central venous access for parenteral nutrition. *Lancet*, **344**, 1043–5.

Donner, E. J., Smith, C. R. & Snead, O. C. (2001). Sudden unexplained death in children with epilepsy. *Neurology*, **57**, 430–34.

Dorfman, L. J., Marshall, W. H. & Enzmann, D. R. (1979). Cerebral infarction and migraine: clinical and radiologic correlations. *Neurology*, **29**, 317–22.

Dunn, D. W. (1985). Vertebrobasilar occlusive disease and childhood migraine. *Pediatric Neurology*, **1**, 252–4.

Earnest, M. P., Thomas, G. E., Eden, R. A. & Hossack, K. F. (1992). The sudden unexplained death syndrome in epilepsy:

demographic, clinical, and postmortem features. *Epilepsia*, **33**, 310–16.

Eeg-Olofsson, O. & Ringheim, Y. (1983). Stroke in children. Clinical characteristics and prognosis. *Acta Paediatrica Scandinavica*, **72**, 391–5.

Elterman, R. D., Bodensteiner, J. B. & Barnard, J. J. (1995). Sudden unexpected death in patients with Dandy–Walker malformation. *Journal of Child Neurology*, **10**, 382–4.

Emparanza, J. I., Aldamiz-Echevarria, L., Perez-Yarza, E., *et al.* (1989). Ischemic stroke due to fibromuscular dysplasia. *Neuropediatrics*, **20**, 181–2.

Erickson, R. P., Woolliscroft, J. & Allen, R. J. (1980). Familial occurrence of intracranial arterial occlusive disease (Moyamoya) in neurofibromatosis. *Clinical Genetics*, **18**, 191–6.

Evans, P. M. & Alberman, E. (1990). Certified cause of death in children and young adults with cerebral palsy. *Archives of Disease in Childhood*, **65**, 325–9.

Eyman, R. K., Grossman, H. J., Chaney, R. H. & Call, T. L. (1990). The life expectancy of profoundly handicapped people with mental retardation. *New England Journal of Medicine*, **323**, 584–9.

Eyman, R. K., Grossman, H. J., Chaney, R. H. & Call, T. L. (1993). Survival of profoundly disabled people with severe mental retardation. *American Journal of Diseases of Children*, **147**, 329–36.

Eyster, M. E., Gill, F. M., Blatt, P. M., *et al.* (1978). Central nervous system bleeding in hemophiliacs. *Blood*, **51**, 1179–88.

Falconer, B. & Rajs, J. (1976). Post-mortem findings of cardiac lesions in epileptics: a preliminary report. *Forensic Science*, **8**, 63–71.

Felice, K. J., Fratkin, J. D., Feldman, E. L. & Sima, A. A. F. (1994). Phrenic nerve involvement in Déjérine–Sottas disease: a clinicopathological case study. *Pediatric Pathology*, **14**, 905–11.

Fenoglio, J. J., Jr, McAllister, H. A., Jr & Ferrans, V. J. (1976). Cardiac rhabdomyoma: a clinicopathologic and electron microscopic study. *American Journal of Cardiology*, **38**, 241–51.

Fisher, R. G. (1982). Strokes in children. Their relationship to intrinsic pathology of the carotid artery. *American Heart Journal*, **48**, 344–50.

Fitzpatrick, A. P. & Emanuel, R. W. (1988). Familial neurofibromatosis and hypertrophic cardiomyopathy. *British Heart Journal*, **60**, 247–51.

Forman, H. P., Levin, S., Stewart, B., Patel, M. & Feinstein, S. (1989). Cerebral vasculitis and hemorrhage in an adolescent taking diet pills containing phenylpropanolamine: case report and review of literature. *Pediatrics*, **83**, 737–41.

Fowler, M. (1961). Two cases of basilar artery occlusion in childhood. *Archives of Disease in Childhood*, **37**, 78–81.

Freedom, R. M., Lee, K.-J., MacDonald, C. & Taylor, G. (2000). Selected aspects of cardiac tumors in infancy and childhood. *Pediatric Cardiology*, **21**, 299–316.

Freycon, F., Mollard, P., Hermier, M., *et al.* (1971). Anévrysme de l'aorte abdominale au cours d'une sclérose tubéreuse de bourneville. *Pediatrie*, **26**, 421–7.

Freytag, E. & Lindenberg, R. (1964). 294 medicolegal autopsies on epileptics. *Archives of Pathology*, **78**, 274–86.

Friede, R. L. & Roessmann, U. (1976). Chronic tonsillar herniation. An attempt at classifying chronic herniations at the foramen magnum. *Acta Neuropathologica*. **34**, 219–35.

Fryer, A. E. & Osborne, J. P. (1987). Tuberous sclerosis – a clinical appraisal. *Pediatric Review Communication*, **1**, 239–55.

Fryer, A. E., Chalmers, A. H. & Osborne, J. P. (1990). The value of investigation for genetic counselling in tuberous sclerosis. *Journal of Medical Genetics*, **27**, 217–23.

Fuster, V., Steele, P. M., Edwards, W. D., *et al.* (1984). Primary pulmonary hypertension: natural history and importance of thrombosis. *Circulation*, **70**, 580–87.

Geevarghese, S. K., Powers, T., Marsh, J. W. & Pinson, C. W. (1999). Screening for cerebral aneurysm in patients with polycystic liver disease *Southern Medical Journal*, **92**, 1167–70.

Gerald, B., Sebes, J. I. & Langston, J. W. (1980). Cerebral infarction secondary to sickle cell disease: arteriographic findings. *American Journal of Roentgenology*, **134**, 1209–12.

Gibbs, J. L. (1985). The heart and tuberous sclerosis. An echocardiographic and electrocardiographic study. *British Heart Journal*, **54**, 596–9.

Gilbert, J. D., Scott, G. & Byard, R. W. (2001). Septo-optic dysplasia and unexpected adult death – an autopsy approach. *Journal of Forensic Sciences*, 46, 913–15.

Gleckman, A. M. & Smith, T. W. (1998) Sudden unexpected death from primary posterior fossa tumors. *American Journal of Forensic Medicine and Pathology*, **19**, 303–8.

Glueck, C. J., Daniels, S. R., Bates, S., *et al.* (1982). Pediatric victims of unexplained stroke and their families: familial lipid and lipoprotein abnormalities. *Pediatrics*, **69**, 308–16.

Gold, A. P., Challenor, Y. B., Gilles, F. H., *et al.* (1973). Report of joint committee for stroke facilities. IX. Strokes in children (part 1). *Stroke*, **4**, 834–93.

Gonsoulin, M., Barnard, J. J. & Prahlow, J. A. (2002). Death resulting from ruptured cerebral artery aneurysm in 219 cases. *American Journal of Forensic Medicine and Pathology*, **23**, 5–14.

Graf, C. J. (1966). Familial intracranial aneurysms. Report of four cases. *Journal of Neurosurgery*, **25**, 304–8.

Gropman, A. L. (2001). Diagnosis and treatment of childhood mitochondrial diseases. *Current Neurology and Neuroscience Reports*, **1**, 185–94.

Grotta, J. C., Manner, C., Pettigrew, L. C. & Yatsu, F. M. (1986). Red blood cell disorders and stroke. *Stroke*, **17**, 811–17.

Hardie, R., Harding, A. E., Hirsch, N., *et al.* (1990). Diaphragmatic weakness in hereditary motor and sensory neuropathy. *Journal of Neurology, Neurosurgery and Psychiatry*, **53**, 348–50.

Harker, L. A., Slichter, S. J., Scott, C. R. & Ross, R. (1974). Homocystinemia. Vascular injury and arterial thrombosis. *New England Journal of Medicine*, **291**, 537–43.

Harvey, F. H. & Alvord, E. C., Jr (1972). Juvenile cerebral arteriosclerosis and other cerebral arteriopathies of childhood – six autopsied cases. *Acta Neurologica Scandinavica*, **48**, 479–509.

Hewer, R. L. (1968). Study of fatal cases of Friedreich's ataxia. *British Medical Journal*, **3**, 649–52.

Hilal, S. K., Solomon, G. E., Gold, A. P. & Carter, S. (1971). Primary cerebral arterial occlusive disease in children. Part I. Acute acquired hemiplegia. *Radiology*, **99**, 71–86, 93–4.

Hirsch, C. S. & Martin, D. L. (1971). Unexpected death in young epileptics. *Neurology*, **21**, 682–90.

Hollister, D. W. (1978). Heritable disorders of connective tissue: Ehlers–Danlos syndrome. *Pediatric Clinics of North America*, **25**, 575–91.

Hutchins, K. D., Dickson, D., Hameed, M. & Natarajan, G. A. (1999). Sudden death in a child due to an intrathoracic paraganglioma. *American Journal of Forensic Medicine and Pathology*, **20**, 338–42.

Hutton, J. L., Cooke, T. & Pharoah, P. O. D. (1994). Life expectancy in children with cerebral palsy. *British Medical Journal*, **309**, 431–5.

Isler, W. (1984). Stroke in childhood and adolescence. *European Neurology*, **23**, 421–4.

Isler, W. (1992). Acute hemiplegia and migraine. In *Cerebrovascular Diseases in Children*, ed. A. J. Raimondi, M. Choux & C. Di Rocco. New York: Springer-Verlag, pp. 244–52.

Jacome, D. E. (1999). Epilepsy in Ehlers–Danlos syndrome. *Epilepsia*, **40**, 467–73.

Janaki, S., Baruah, J. K., Jayaram, S. R., *et al.* (1975). Stroke in the young: a four-year study, 1968 to 1972. *Stroke*, **6**, 318–20.

Jay, G. W. & Leestma, J. E. (1981). Sudden death in epilepsy. A comprehensive review of the literature and proposed mechanisms. *Acta Neurologica Scandinavica*, **63**, 1–66.

Johnson, M. W., Emelin, J. K., Park, S.-H. & Vinters, H. V. (1999). Co-localization of TSC1 and TSC2 gene products in tubers of patients with tuberous sclerosis. *Brain Pathology*, **9**, 45–54.

Jost, C. J., Gloviczki, P., Edwards, W. D., *et al.* (2001). Aortic aneurysms in children and young adults with tuberous sclerosis: report of two cases and review of the literature. *Journal of Vascular Surgery*, **33**, 639–42.

Juul-Jensen, P. & Foldspang, A. (1983). Natural history of epileptic seizures. *Epilepsia*, **24**, 297–312.

Kandt, R. S., Gebarski, S. S. & Goetting, M. G. (1985). Tuberous sclerosis with cardiogenic cerebral embolism: magnetic resonance imaging. *Neurology*, **35**, 1223–5.

Kato, T., Hattori, H., Yorifuji, T., Tashiro, Y. & Nakahata, T. (2001). Intracranial aneurysms in Ehlers-Danlos syndrome type IV in early childhood. *Pediatric Neurology*, **25**, 336–9.

Keilson, M. J., Hauser, W. A. & Magrill, J. P. (1989). Electrocardiographic change during electrographic seizures. *Archives of Neurology*, **46**, 1169–70.

Keilson, M. J., Hauser, W. A., Magrill, J. P. & Goldman, M. (1987). ECG abnormalities in patients with epilepsy. *Neurology*, **37**, 1624–6.

Kelley, R. E. (1986). Hemorrhagic cerebral infarction in pediatric patients. *Pediatric Neurology*, **2**, 111–14.

Kelley, R. E. & Berger, J. R. (1987). Ischemic stroke in a girl with lupus anticoagulant. *Pediatric Neurology*, **3**, 58–61.

Kinney, H. & Filiano, J. J. (2001). Brain research in SIDS. In *Sudden Infant Death Syndrome: Problems, Progress and Possibilities*, ed. R. W. Byard & H. F. Krous. London: Arnold, pp. 118–37.

Kinney, H. C., Filiano, J. J. & Harper, R. M. (1992). The neuropathology of the sudden infant death syndrome. A review. *Journal of Neuropathology and Experimental Neurology*, **51**, 115–26.

Kiok, M. C., Terrence, C. F., Fromm, G. H. & Lavine, S. (1986). Sinus arrest in epilepsy. *Neurology*, **36**, 115–16.

Kitahara, T., Ariga, N., Yamaura, A., Makino, H. & Maki, Y. (1979). Familial occurrence of Moya-moya disease: report of three Japanese families. *Journal of Neurology, Neurosurgery and Psychiatry*, **42**, 208–14.

Kohrman, M. H. & Huttenlocher, P. R. (1986). Takayasu arteritis: a treatable cause of stroke in infancy. *Pediatric Neurology*, **2**, 154–8.

Konishi, Y., Kuriyama, M., Sudo, M., *et al.* (1987). Superior sagittal sinus thrombosis in neonates. *Pediatric Neurology*, **3**, 222–5.

Koszyca, B., Moore, L. & Byard, R. W. (1993). Lethal manifestations of neurofibromatosis type-1 in childhood. *Pediatric Pathology*, **13**, 709–15.

Kousseff, B. G. & Gilbert-Barness, E. F. (1989). "Vascular neurofibromatosis" and infantile gangrene. *American Journal of Medical Genetics*, **34**, 221–6.

Krohn, W. (1963). Causes of death among epileptics. *Epilepsia*, **4**, 315–21.

Lapointe, J. S., Nugent, R. A., Graeb, D. A. & Robertson, W. D. (1984). Cerebral infarction and regression of widespread aneurysms in Kawasaki's disease: case report. *Pediatric Radiology*, **14**, 1–5.

Larbre, F., Loire, R., Guibaud, P., Lauras, B. & Weill, B. (1971). Observation clinique et anatomique d'un anevrysme de l'aorte au cours d'une sclerose tubereuse de Bourneville. *Archives Francaises De Pédiatrie.* **28**, 975–84.

Lathers, C. M. & Schraeder, P. L. (1982). Autonomic dysfunction in epilepsy: characterization of autonomic cardiac neural discharge associated with pentylenetetrazol-induced epileptogenic activity. *Epilepsia*, **23**, 633–47.

Laurent, J. P., Bruce, D. A. & Schut, L. (1981). Hemorrhagic brain tumors in pediatric patients. *Child's Brain*, **8**, 263–70.

Laxer, R. M., Dunn, H. G. & Flodmark, O. (1984). Acute hemiplegia in Kawasaki disease and infantile polyarteritis nodosa. *Developmental Medicine and Child Neurology*, **26**, 814–21.

Leestma, J. E. (1988). Forensic aspects of complex neural dysfunctions. In *Forensic Neuropathology*. New York: Raven Press, pp. 396–428.

Leestma, J. E., Kalelkar, M. B., Teas, S. S., Jay, G. W. & Hughes, J. R. (1984). Sudden unexpected death associated with seizures: analysis of 66 cases. *Epilepsia*, **25**, 84–8.

Leestma, J. E., Walczak, T., Hughes, J. R., Kalelkar, M. B. & Teas, S. S. (1989). A prospective study on sudden unexpected death in epilepsy. *Annals of Neurology*, **26**, 195–203.

Lemahieu, S. F. & Marchau, M. M. B. (1979). Intracranial fibromuscular dysplasia and stroke in children. *Neuroradiology*, **18**, 99–102.

Liedholm, L. J. & Gudjonsson, O. (1992). Cardiac arrest due to partial epileptic seizures. *Neurology*, **42**, 824–9.

Llorens-Terol, J., Sole-Llenas, J. & Tura, A. (1983). Stroke due to fibromuscular hyperplasia of the internal carotid artery. *Acta Paediatrica Scandinavica*, **72**, 299–301.

Lüscher, T. F., Lie, J. T., Stanson, A. W., *et al.* (1987). Arterial fibromuscular dysplasia. *Mayo Clinic Proceedings*, **62**, 931–52.

Maeder, P. P., Holtas, S. L., Basibuyuk L. N., *et al.* (1990). Colloid cysts of the third ventricle: correlation of MR and CT findings with histology and chemical analysis. *American Journal of Neuroradiology*, **11**, 575–81.

Manz, H. J., Vester, J. & Lavenstein, B. (1979). Dissecting aneurysm of cerebral arteries in childhood and adolescence. Case report and literature review of 20 cases. *Virchows Archive (Pathological Anatomy and Histology)*, **384**, 325–35.

Martin, J. B. (1993). Molecular genetics in neurology. *Annals of Neurology*, **34**, 757–73.

Martinot, A., Hue, V., Leclerc, F., *et al.* (1993). Sudden death revealing Chiari type 1 malformation in two children. *Intensive Care Medicine*, **19**, 73–4.

McCormick, W. F. (1966). The pathology of vascular ("arteriovenous") malformations. *Journal of Neurosurgery*, **24**, 807–16.

McCormick, W. F., Hardman, J. M. & Boulter, T. R. (1968). Vascular malformations ("angiomas") of the brain, with special reference to those occurring in the posterior fossa. *Journal of Neurosurgery*, **28**, 241–51.

McDonald, J. A. (1982). Colloid cyst of the third ventricle and sudden death. *Annals of Emergency Medicine*, **11**, 365–7.

McKusick, V. A. (1964). Intracranial aneurysm and heredity. *Journal of the American Medical Association*, **190**, 791.

Meldgaard, K., Vesterby, A. & Østergaard, J. R. (1997). Sudden death due to rupture of a saccular intracranial aneurysm in a 13-year-old boy. *American Journal of Forensic Medicine and Pathology*, **18**, 342–4.

Mills, M. L. (1985). Life threatening complications of sickle cell disease in children. *Journal of the American Medical Association*, **254**, 1487–91.

Mizusawa, H., Hirano, A., Llena, J. F., Shintaku, M. (1988). Cerebrovascular lesions in acquired immune deficiency syndrome (AIDS). *Acta Neuropathologica*, **76**, 451–7.

Monaghan, H. P., Krafchik, B. R., MacGregor, D. L. & Fitz, C. R. (1981). Tuberous sclerosis complex in children. *American Journal of Diseases of Children*, **135**, 912–17.

Moore, L. & Byard, R. W. (1992). Fatal paradoxical embolism to the left carotid artery during partial resection of Wilms' tumor. *Pediatric Pathology*, **12**, 371–6.

Moore, P. M. & Cupps, T. R. (1983). Neurological complications of vasculitis. *Annals of Neurology*, **14**, 155–67.

Morgan, M. K., Besser, M. & Procopis, P. G. (1987). Moyamoya disease: presentation and treatment of two cases by surgery. *Medical Journal of Australia*, **146**, 381–3.

Morgan, S. A., Emsellem, H. A. & Sandler, J. R. (1985). Absence of the septum pellucidum. Overlapping clinical syndromes. *Archives of Neurology*, **42**, 769–70.

Mori, K., Murata, T., Hashimoto, N. & Handa, H. (1980). Clinical analysis of arteriovenous malformations in children. *Child's Brain*, **6**, 13–25.

Nadas, A. S., Alimurung, M. M. & Sieracki, L. A. (1951). Cardiac manifestations of Friedreich's ataxia. *New England Journal of Medicine*, **244**, 239–44.

Nashef, L. & Brown, S. (1996). Epilepsy and sudden death. *Lancet*, **348**, 1324–5.

Nelson, J., Frost, J. L. & Schochet, S. S., Jr (1987). Sudden, unexpected death in a 5-year-old boy with an unusual primary intracranial neoplasm. *American Journal of Forensic Medicine and Pathology*, **8**, 148–52.

Nestoridi, E., Buonanno, F. S., Jones, R. M., *et al.* (2002). Arterial ischemic stroke in childhood: the role of plasma-phase risk factors. *Current Opinion in Neurology*, **15**, 139–44.

Norman, M. G., Taylor, G. P. & Clarke, L. A. (1990). Sudden, unexpected natural death in childhood. *Pediatric Pathology*, **10**, 769–84.

O'Callaghan, F. J. K., Clarke, A. C., Joffe, H., *et al.* (1998). Tuberous sclerosis complex and Wolf–Parkinson–White syndrome. *Archives of Disease in Childhood*, **78**, 159–62.

Oka, K., Yamashita, M., Sadoshima, S. & Tanaka, K. (1981). Cerebral haemorrhage in Moyamoya disease at autopsy. *Virchows Archive (Pathological Anatomy and Histology)*, **392**, 247–61.

Oppenheimer, S. (1990). Cardiac dysfunction during seizures and the sudden epileptic death syndrome. *Journal of the Royal Society of Medicine*, **83**, 134–6.

Orlowski, J. P., Rothner, A. D. & Lueders, H. (1982). Submersion accidents in children with epilepsy. *American Journal of Diseases of Children*, **136**, 777–80.

Osborne, J. P. (1988). Diagnosis of tuberous sclerosis. *Archives of Disease in Childhood*, **63**, 1423–5.

Ouvrier, R. & Billson, F. (1986). Optic nerve hypoplasia: a review. *Journal of Child Neurology*, **1**, 181–8.

Owen, S. M. & Durst, R. D. (1984). Ehlers–Danlos syndrome simulating child abuse. *Archives of Dermatology*, **120**, 97–101.

Packer, R. J., Rorke, L. B., Lange, B. J., Siegel, K. R. & Evans, A. E. (1985). Cerebrovascular accidents in children with cancer. *Pediatrics*, **76**, 194–201.

Palareti, G., Salardi, S., Piazzi, S., *et al.* (1986). Blood coagulation changes in homocystinuria: effects of pyridoxine and other specific therapy. *Journal of Pediatrics*, **109**, 1001–6.

Palau, F. (2001). Friedreich's ataxia and frataxin: molecular genetics, evolution and pathogenesis. *International Journal of Molecular Medicine*, **7**, 581–9.

Park, T. S., Hoffman, H. J., Hendrick, E. B., Humphreys, R. P. & Becker, L. E. (1983). Medulloblastoma: clinical presentation and management. Experience at the Hospital for Sick Children, Toronto 1950–1980. *Journal of Neurosurgery*, **58**, 543–52.

Parker, M. J., Tarlow, M. J. & Milne Anderson, J. (1984). Glue sniffing and cerebral infarction. *Archives of Disease in Childhood*, **59**, 675–7.

Parks, J. S., Brown, M. R., Hurley, D. L., Phelps, C. J. & Wajnrajch, M. P. (1999). Heritable disorders of pituitary development. *Journal of Clinical Endocrinology and Metabolism*, **84**, 4362–70.

Parrish, C. M. & Byrne, J. P., Jr (1971). Surgical correction of carotid artery obstruction in children. *Surgery*, **70**, 962–8.

Pascual-Castroviejo, I. (1992). Clinical pictures of vascular pathology in children. In *Cerebrovascular Diseases in Children*, ed. A. J. Raimondi, M. Choux & C. Di Rocco. New York: Springer-Verlag, pp. 38–49.

Patel, P. I. & Isaya, G. (2001). Friedreich ataxia: from GAA triplet-repeat expansion to frataxin deficiency. *American Journal of Human Genetics*, **69**, 15–24.

Pellegrino, P. A., Zanesco, L. & Battistella, P. A. (1992). Coagulopathies and vasculopathies. In *Cerebrovascular Diseases in Children*, ed. A. J. Raimondi, M. Choux & C. Di Rocco. New York: Springer-Verlag, pp. 189–204.

Pellock, J. M., Kleinman, P. K., McDonald, B. M. & Wixson, D. (1980). Childhood hypertensive stroke with neurofibromatosis. *Neurology*, **30**, 656–9.

Perdue, G. D., Barreca, J. P., Smith, R. B., III & King, O. W. (1975). The significance of elongation and angulation of the carotid artery: a negative view. *Surgery*, **77**, 45–52.

Perez-Higueras, A., Alvarez-Ruiz, F., Martinez-Bermejo, A., *et al.* (1988). Cerebellar infarction from fibromuscular dysplasia and dissecting aneursym of the vertebral artery. Report of a child. *Stroke*, **19**, 521–4.

Phornphutkul, C., Rosenthal, A., Nadas, A. S. & Berenberg, W. (1973). Cerebrovascular accidents in infants and children with cyanotic congenital heart disease. *American Journal of Cardiology*, **32**, 329–34.

Pilz, P. & Hartjes, H. J. (1976). Fibromuscular dysplasia and multiple dissecting aneurysms of intracranial arteries. A further case of Moyamoya syndrome. *Stroke*, **7**, 393–8.

Pincus, J. H. (1972). Subacute necrotizing encephalomyelopathy (Leigh's disease): a consideration of clinical features and etiology. *Developmental Medicine and Child Neurology*, **14**, 87–101.

Plunkett, J. (1999). Sudden death in an infant caused by rupture of a basilar artery aneurysm. *American Journal of Forensic Medicine and Pathology*, **20**, 211–14.

Poon, T. P. & Solis, O. G. (1985). Sudden death due to massive intraventricular hemorrhage into an unsuspected ependymoma. *Surgical Neurology*, **24**, 63–6.

Powars, D., Wilson, B., Imbus, C., Pegelow, C. & Allen, J. (1978). The natural history of stroke in sickle cell disease. *American Journal of Medicine*, **65**, 461–71.

Prahlow, J. A., Rushing, E. J. & Barnard, J. J. (1998). Death due to a ruptured berry aneurysm in a 3.5-year-old child. *American Journal of Forensic Medicine and Pathology*, **19**, 391–4.

Rajs, J., Råsten-Almqvist, P. & Nennesmo, I. (1997). Unexpected death in two young infants mimics SIDS. Autopsies demonstrate tumors of medulla and heart. *American Journal of Forensic Medicine and Pathology*, **18**, 384–90.

Ravindran, M. (1981). Temporal lobe seizure presenting as "laryngospasm". *Clinical Electroencephalography*, **12**, 139–40.

Raybaud, C. A., Livet, M.-O., Jiddane, M. & Pinsard, N. (1985). Radiology of ischemic strokes in children. *Neuroradiology*, **27**, 567–78.

Read, E. J., Jr (1990). Colloid cyst of the third ventricle. *Annals of Emergency Medicine*, **19**, 1060–62.

Rice, G. P. A., Boughner, D. R., Stiller, C. & Ebers, G. C. (1980). Familial stroke syndrome associated with mitral valve prolapse. *Annals of Neurology*, **7**, 130–34.

Rigle, D. A., Dexter, R. D. & McGee, M. B. (1989). Cardiac rhabdomyoma presenting as sudden infant death syndrome. *Journal of Forensic Sciences*, **34**, 694–8.

Roach, E. S., Garcia, J. C. & McLean, W. T., Jr (1984). Cerebrovascular disease in children. *American Family Physician*, **30**, 215–27.

Roach, E. S., Gomez, M. R., & Northrup, H. (1998). Tuberous Sclerosis Complex Consensus Conference: revised clinical diagnostic criteria. *Journal of Child Neurology*, **13**, 624–8.

Robinson, B. H. (2000). Human cytochrome oxidase deficiency. *Pediatric Research*, **48**, 581–5.

Roessman, U., Velasco, M. E., Small, E. J., & Hori, A. (1987). Neuropathology of "septo-optic dysplasia" (de Morsier syndrome) with immunohistochemical studies of the hypothalamus and pituitary gland. *Journal of Neuropathology and Experimental Neurology*, **46**, 597–608.

Rosen, R. S., Armbrustmacher, V. & Sampson, B. A. (2003). Spontaneous cerebellar hemorrhage in children. *Journal of Forensic Sciences*, **48**, 177–9.

Rosenquist, G. C., Krovetz, L. J., Haller, J. A., Jr, Simon, A. L. & Bannayan, G. A. (1970). Acquired right ventricular outflow obstruction in a child with neurofibromatosis. *American Heart Journal*, **79**, 103–8.

Ross, C. A., Curnes, J. T. & Greenwood, R. S. (1987). Recurrent vertebrobasilar embolism in an infant with Klippel–Feil anomaly. *Pediatric Neurology*, **3**, 181–3.

Ruff, M. E., Oakes, W. J., Fisher, S. R. & Spock, A. (1987). Sleep apnea and vocal cord paralysis secondary to type I Chiari malformation. *Pediatrics*, **80**, 231–4.

Ryder, J. W., Kleinschmidt-DeMasters, B. K. & Keller, T. S. (1986). Sudden deterioration and death in patients with benign tumors of the third ventricle area. *Journal of Neurosurgery*, **64**, 216–23.

Sabharwal, U. K., Keogh, L. H., Weisman, M. H. & Zvaifler, N. J. (1982). Granulomatous angitis of the nervous system: case report and review of the literature. *Arthritis and Rheumatism*, **25**, 342–5.

Santorelli, F. M., Shanske, S., Macaya, A., DeVivo, D. C. & DiMauro, S. (1993). The mutation at nt 8993 of mitochondrial DNA is a common cause of Leigh's syndrome. *Annals of Neurology*, **34**, 827–34.

Sarkari, N. B. S., Holmes, J. M. & Bickerstaff, E. R. (1970). Neurological manifestations associated with internal carotid loops and kinks in children. *Journal of Neurology, Neurosurgery and Psychiatry*, **33**, 194–200.

Sato, K. & Shimoji, T. (1992). Moyamoya disease. In *Cerebrovascular Diseases in Children*, ed. A. J. Raimondi, M. Choux & C. Di Rocco. New York: Springer-Verlag, pp. 227–43.

Saulsbury, F. T., Sullivan, J. S. & Schmitt, E. J. (1981). Sudden death due to colloid cyst of the third ventricle. *Clinical Pediatrics*, **20**, 218–19.

Scappaticci, S., Cerimele, D., Tondi, M., *et al.* (1988). Chromosome abnormalities in tuberous sclerosis. *Human Genetics*, **79**, 151–6.

Schejbal, V. & Oellig, W.-P. (1979). Sudden death of children by hemorrhage from a cerebral angioma. *Klinische Paediatrie*, **191**, 498–500.

Schievink, W. I. (1997). Genetics of intracranial aneurysms. *Neurosurgery*, **40**, 651–63.

Schievink, W. I. & Spetzler, R. F. (1998). Screening for intracranial aneurysms in patients with isolated polycystic liver disease. *J Neurosurgery*, **89**, 719–21.

Schoenberg, B. S., Mellinger, J. F. & Schoenberg, D. G. (1978). Moyamoya disease in children. *Southern Medical Journal*, **71**, 237–41.

Schon, E. A., Santra, S., Pallotti, F. & Girvin, M. E. (2001). Pathogenesis of primary defects in mitochondrial ATP synthesis. *Cell and Developmental Biology*, **12**, 441–8.

Schraeder, P. L. & Lathers, C. M. (1983). Cardiac neural discharge and epileptogenic activity in the cat: an animal model for unexplained death. *Life Sciences*, **32**, 1371–82.

Schulz, E., Hermann, G. & Metter, D. (1981). Sudden death from natural causes among children of preschool age and school age. *Munchener Medizinische Wochenschrift*, **123**, 1443–6.

Schwab, F. J., Peyster, R. G. & Brill, C. B. (1987). CT of cerebral venous sinus thrombosis in a child with homocystinuria. *Pediatric Radiology*, **17**, 244–5.

Schwender, L. A. & Troncoso, J. C. (1986). Evaluation of sudden death in epilepsy. *American Journal of Forensic Medicine and Pathology*, **7**, 283–7.

Seeler, R. A., Royal, J. E., Powe, L. & Goldbarg, H. R. (1978). Moyamoya in children with sickle cell anemia and cerebrovascular occlusion. *Journal of Pediatrics*, **93**, 808–10.

Sekhar, L. N., Moossy, J., Guthkelch, A. N. (1982). Malfunctioning ventriculoperitoneal shunts. Clinical and pathological features. *Journal of Neurosurgery*, **56**, 411–16.

Shemie S., Jay V., Rutka J. & Armstrong D. (1997). Acute obstructive hydrocephalus and sudden death in children. *Annals of Emergency Medicine*, **29**, 524–8.

Shiba, E., Kambayashi, J.-I., Sakon, M., *et al.* (1992). Septic pulmonary emboli after prolonged use of central venous catheter for parenteral nutrition. *European Journal of Surgery*, **158**, 59–61.

Shields, L. B. E., Hunsaker, D. M., Hunsaker, J. C. & Parker, J. C. (2002). Sudden unexpected death in epilepsy. Neuropathologic findings. *American Journal of Forensic Medicine and Pathology*, **23**, 307–14.

Shields, W. D., Ziter, F. A., Osborn, A. G. & Allen, J. (1977). Fibromuscular dysplasia as a cause of stroke in infancy and childhood. *Pediatrics*, **59**, 899–901.

Shillito, J., Jr (1964). Carotid arteritis: a cause of hemiplegia in childhood. *Journal of Neurosurgery*, **20**, 540–51.

Smith, H. C., Watson, G. H., Patel, R. G. & Super, M. (1989). Cardiac rhabdomyomata in tuberous sclerosis: their course and diagnostic value. *Archives of Disease in Childhood*, **64**, 196–200.

Smith, M. & Simpson, N. E. (1989). Report of the committee on the genetic constitution of chromosomes 9 and 10. *Cytogenetics and Cell Genetics*, **51**, 202–25.

Sparagana, S. P. & Roach, E. S. (2000). Tuberous sclerosis complex. *Current Opinion in Neurology*, **13**, 115–19.

Speights, V. O., Jr & Bauserman, S. C. (1991). Sudden death in an infant with central nervous system abnormalities. *Pediatric Pathology*, **11**, 751–8.

Staal, M. J., Meihuizen-de Regt, M. J. & Hess, J. (1987). Sudden death in hydrocephalic spina bifida aperta patients. *Pediatric Neuroscience*, **13**, 13–18.

Stockman, J. A., Nigro, M. A., Mishkin, M. M. & Oski, F. A. (1972). Occlusion of large cerebral vessels in sickle cell anemia. *New England Journal of Medicine*, **287**, 846–9.

Suzuki, J. & Kodama, N. (1983). Moyamoya disease – a review. *Stroke*, **14**, 104–9.

Suzuki, J. & Takaku, A. (1969). Cerebrovascular "Moyamoya" disease. *Archives of Neurology*, **20**, 288–99.

Taback, S. P., Dean, H. J. and members of the Canadian Growth Hormone Advisory Committee (1996). Mortality in Canadian children with growth hormone (GH) deficiency receiving GH therapy 1967–1992. *Journal of Clinical Endocrinology and Metabolism*, **81**, 1693–6.

Takashima, S. & Becker, L. E. (1980). Neuropathology of cerebral arteriovenous malformations in children. *Journal of Neurology, Neurosurgery and Psychiatry*, **43**, 380–85.

Terrence, C. F., Rao, G. R. & Perper, J. A. (1981). Neurogenic pulmonary edema in unexpected, unexplained death of epileptic patients. *Annals of Neurology*, **9**, 458–64.

Terrence, C. F., Jr, Wisotzkey, H. M. & Perper, J. A. (1975). Unexpected, unexplained death in epileptic patients. *Neurology*, **25**, 594–8.

Tharakan, J., Ahuja, G. K., Manchanda, S. C. & Khanna, A. (1982). Mitral valve prolapse and cerebrovascular accidents in the young. *Acta Neurologica Scandinavica*, **66**, 295–302.

Thomas, P. K., Landon, D. N. & King, R. H. M. (1992). Diseases of the peripheral nerves. In *Greenfield's Neuropathology*, 5th edn, ed. J. H. Adams & L. W. Duchen. London: Edward Arnold, pp. 1116–245.

Tomaszek, D. E., Tyson, G. W., Bouldin, T. & Hansen, A. R. (1984). Sudden death in a child with an occult hindbrain malformation. *Annals of Emergency Medicine*, **13**, 136–8.

Tomlinson, P. & Sugarman, I. D. (1995). Complications of shunts in adults with spina bifida. *British Medical Journal*, **311**, 286–7.

Torrey, J. (1983). Sudden death in an 11-year-old boy due to rupture of a colloid cyst of the third ventricle following disco-dancing. *Medicine, Science and the Law*, **23**, 114–16.

Unger, P. D., Song, S., Taff, M. L. & Schwartz, I. S. (1984). Sudden death in a patient with von Recklinghausen's neurofibromatosis. *American Journal of Forensic Medicine and Pathology*, **5**, 175–9.

Van Rybroek, J. J. & Moore, S. A. (1990). Sudden death from choroid plexus vascular malformation hemorrhage: case report and review of the literature. *Clinical Neuropathology*, **9**, 39–45.

Ventureyra, E. C. G. & Higgins, M. J. (1994). Traumatic intracranial aneurysms in childhood and adolescence. Case reports and review of the literature. *Child's Nervous System*, **10**, 361–79.

Verdú, A., Cazorla, M. R., Granados, M. A., (2001). Basilar artery thrombosis in a child heterozygous for factor V Leiden mutation. *Pediatric Neurology*, **24**, 69–71.

Wakabayashi, T., Fujita, S., Ohbora, Y., *et al.* (1983). Polycystic kidney disease and intracranial aneurysms. Early angiographic diagnosis and early operation for the unruptured aneurysm. *Journal of Neurosurgery*, **58**, 488–91.

Walker, R. J., III, El Gammal, T. & Allen, M. B., Jr (1973). Cranial arteritis associated with herpes zoster. Case report and angiographic findings. *Radiology*, **107**, 109–10.

Wallis, K., Deutsch, V. & Azizi, E. (1970). Hypertension in a case of von Recklinghausen's neurofibromatosis. *Helvetica Paediatrica Acta*, **2**, 147–53.

Weiner, D. M., Ewalt, D. H., Roach, E. S. & Hensle, T. W. (1998) The tuberous sclerosis complex: a comprehensive review. *Journal of the American College of Surgeons*, **187**, 548–61.

Williams, W. G., Trusler, G. A., Fowler, R. S., Scott, M. E. & Mustard, W. T. (1972). Left ventricular myocardial fibroma: a case report and review of cardiac tumors in children. *Journal of Pediatric Surgery*, **7**, 324–8.

Wilske, V. J. (1980). Tuberöse sklerose – ungewöhnlicher fall eines plötzlichen säuglingstodes. *Beitrage Zurgerichtlichen Medizin*, **38**, 451–6.

Winstanley, D. P. (1961). Sudden death from multiple rhabdomyomata of the heart. *Journal of Pathology and Bacteriology*, **81**, 249–51.

Wolfe, J. A. & Rowe, L. D. (1980). Upper airway obstruction in infectious mononucleosis. *Annals of Otology*, **89**, 430–33.

Woody, R. C., Perrot, L. J. & Beck, S. A. (1992). Neurofibromatosis cerebral vasculopathy in an infant: clinical, neuroradiographic, and neuropathologic studies. *Pediatric Pathology*, **12**, 613–19.

Yamashita, M., Oka, K. & Tanaka, K. (1983). Histopathology of the brain vascular network in Moyamoya disease. *Stroke*, **14**, 50–58.

Yamashita, M., Tanaka, K., Kishikawa, T. & Yokota, K. (1984). Moyamoya disease associated with renovascular hypertension. *Human Pathology*, **15**, 191–13.

Yancey, C. L., Doughty, R. A. & Athreya, B. H. (1981). Central nervous system involvement in childhood systemic lupus erythematosus. *Arthritis and Rheumatism*, **24**, 1389–95.

Young, R. S. K., Rannels, D. E., Hilmo, A., Gerson, J. M. & Goodrich, D. (1983). Severe anemia in childhood presenting as transient ischemic attacks. *Stroke*, **14**, 622–3.

Zimmermann, M., Gabathuler, J., Adamec, R. & Pinget, L. (1986). Unusual manifestations of heart involvement in Friedrich's ataxia. *American Heart Journal*, **111**, 184–7.

9

Hematologic conditions

Introduction

Hematologic disorders are not often considered in the differential diagnosis of unexpected death in infancy or childhood, although most physicians would be aware of sudden death as a potential complication of sickle cell anemia. While the mechanism of sudden death in sickle cell disease relates most often to splenic sequestration crisis, other complications may also result in quite rapid demise. Similarly, the range of lethal mechanisms in other forms of hematologic disorders may be more diverse than initial observations would suggest and includes massive hemorrhage, thromboses, stroke, overwhelming infection, airway obstruction and cardiac arrhythmia. A list of hematological conditions that may result in sudden pediatric death is provided in Table 9.1.

Hemoglobinopathies

Sickle cell anemia

Of all of the disorders caused by structural defects in the hemoglobin molecule, sickle cell disease is the most significant in terms of sudden death. Sickle cell anemia, which results from the replacement of glutamic acid by valine in the sixth position on the β-chain of the hemoglobin molecule (Nelson & Davey, 1984), is characterized by decreased plasticity of red blood cells, resulting in elongation and "sickling" (Figure 9.1). The sickled cells are no longer able to traverse normal vascular channels due to their altered configuration, and as such they are more susceptible to damage and more likely to obstruct blood vessels.

Clinical features

Homozygous patients develop a severe and chronic hemolytic anemia marked by episodic clinical deterioration in the form of "crises," several of which are potentially lethal (Powars, 1975). Sickle cell disease and trait are much more common in black than in white populations, possibly related to the partial protective effect that sickle cell trait has against malaria.

Although heterozygous patients generally have a more benign clinical course than homozygotes, under certain circumstances they have an increased risk of sudden death compared with the general population (Mease, Longo & Hakami, 1976; Ober et al., 1960). For example, sickle cell trait has been associated with an estimated 28–40 times increased risk of sudden death in black American military recruits during exercise (Kark et al., 1987). This phenomenon is more likely to occur in recruits over the age of 20 years. Exercise predisposes to acidosis and venous hypoxia, which, in combination with dehydration and hypotension, causes sickling (Jones, Binder & Donowho, 1970; Koppes et al., 1977). These factors may also precipitate sickling in infants with sickle cell trait (Ragab, Stein & Vietti, 1970) and have been associated with sudden death in heterozygous children following general anesthesia (McGarry & Duncan, 1973). Coagulopathy and exercise-induced rhabdomyolysis associated with unexpected death,

Table 9.1. Hematologic conditions associated with sudden pediatric death

Hemoglobinopathies
Hematologic malignancies
Disorders of coagulation
Platelet disorders
Anemia
Hemolytic-uremic syndrome
Polycythemia
Splenic disorders

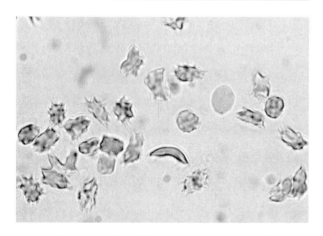

Figure 9.1 A sickle cell blood preparation demonstrating characteristic sickling (×1200).

as well as sequestration crisis, may occur in heterozygous adults (Dudley & Waddell, 1991; Hynd *et al.*, 1985; Rickles & O'Leary, 1974; Sateriale & Hart, 1985). Under the age of 20 years, the death rate peaks between one and three years of age, due predominantly to sepsis (Platt *et al.*, 1994). Sickle cell crisis is a term used for any new significant syndrome that develops in individuals with sickle cell disease, often precipitated by infection (Athanasou *et al.*, 1985).

Vaso-occlusive crisis

Vaso-occlusive, or painful, crises that occur relatively frequently in homozygous patients are often precipitated by infection and may be lethal in children. The underlying problem is small-vessel occlusion by deformed erythrocytes, resulting in peripheral ischemia and infarction. The extremities are most often involved (so-called hand–foot syndrome or sickle cell dactylitis), with infarction of the small bones of the hands and feet causing characteristic changes on X-ray (Nelson & Davey, 1984). Acute bone marrow infarcts have led to massive and fatal embolization of fat and necrotic marrow in adults (Garza, 1990).

Cerebral involvement is a more sinister potential complication occurring in approximately 7% of homozygous children and causing intracerebral hemorrhage, subarachnoid hemorrhage, and infarction with sudden death (Mills, 1985; Pellegrino, Zanesco & Battistella, 1992; Portnoy & Herion, 1972; Powars *et al.*, 1978). Cases of fatal intracranial sinus thromboses have also been reported in children (Schenk, 1964). Vaso-occlusion may be precipitated by the use of narcotic analgesia, resulting in respiratory depression with hypoxemia, and may occur in pregnancy (Gerber & Apseloff, 1993; Pastorek & Seiler, 1985).

Anaplastic crisis

In anaplastic crisis there is temporary cessation of red blood cell production, resulting in a marked fall in hemoglobin levels, which may be idiopathic or precipitated by infection, folic acid deficiency, or exposure to certain drugs (Nelson & Davey, 1984).

Hemolytic crisis

This may be induced by infection or may be precipitated by antioxidant drugs when there is an additional hematologic abnormality present, such as glucose-6-phosphate dehydrogenase deficiency. Hemolytic crisis may acutely exacerbate the effects of an already established hemolytic anemia.

Splenic sequestration crisis

One of the most feared complications of sickle cell disease is splenic sequestration crisis (Rogers *et al.*, 1978; Seeler & Shwiaki, 1972). When this occurs there is marked pooling of blood within the spleen and a danger that the patient may die very quickly of circulatory collapse (Emond *et al.*, 1985). Figure 9.2

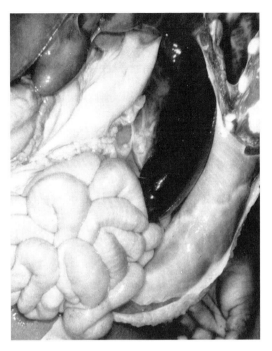

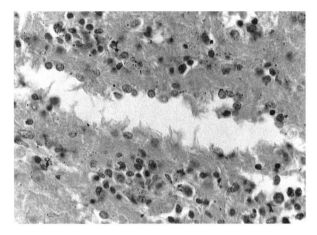

Figure 9.3 Engorgement of the splenic parenchyma by sickled red blood cells protruding into the lumen of a sinusoid in the boy illustrated in Figure 9.2 (hematoxylin and eosin, ×440).

Figure 9.2 Markedly enlarged spleen in a 21-month-old Jamaican boy who died from a sickle cell acute splenic sequestration crisis.

illustrates the massive splenic enlargement that may occur. Figure 9.3 shows a tangled array of erythrocytes clogging the splenic vascular channels taken from a 21-month-old Jamaican boy who was not known to have sickle cell disease (Byard *et al.*, 1991). He died suddenly in his mother's arms following a mild febrile illness. At autopsy, generalized pallor of all of the viscera was noted, except for the markedly enlarged, engorged spleen. Postmortem blood analysis revealed a hemoglobin of 18 g/l with 87% hemoglobin S (HbS). The presence of cardiomegaly with erythroid hyperplasia of the bone marrow suggested that significant anemia with a physiological response had been present for some time, in spite of his apparently normal health status and growth parameters.

The diagnosis of acute splenic sequestration should be suspected at autopsy when the spleen is markedly enlarged and has a purplish congested appearance due to engorgment with irreversibly sickled red blood cells. The remainder of the organs are unusually pale, giving the brain a "porcelain-like" appearance (Figure 9.4). Although the detection of sickled erythrocytes on microscopy does not necessarily imply that sickling was an antemortem phenomenon (Kark *et al.*, 1987; Sears, 1978), extensive sickling in acute sequestration should be readily demonstrable. Other autopsy findings in cases of fatal sickle cell disease include cerebral infarction, cardiomegaly, splenic infarction, and hyperplasia of bone marrow (Color Plate 18).

Splenic sequestration crisis is a particularly common presenting feature in children under the age of two years, accounting for a third of cases in one series (Bainbridge *et al.*, 1985). In this report, other presentations of sickle cell disease included pneumococcal sepsis and cerebrovascular accident. Twenty-four percent of their patients who died did so on first presentation, including 15% who were dead on arrival at hospital. The fact that sudden death may occur due to splenic sequestration in children with either no known history of sickle cell disease, or with only minimal symptoms (Topley *et al.*, 1981), may make the

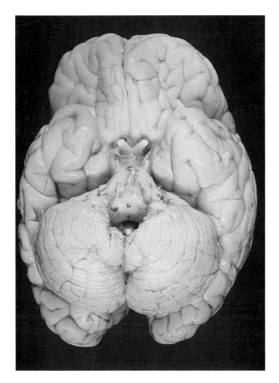

Figure 9.4 "porcelain brain," with marked pallor due to acute sickle cell sequestration.

autopsy examination crucial in the establishment of the diagnosis.

Cardiovascular complications

Proliferative lesions of the walls of the carotid arteries in patients with sickle cell disease that are associated with childhood stroke and death may be similar to arterial lesions of Moyamoya disease (Garza-Mercado, 1982; Seeler *et al.*, 1978; Stockman *et al.*, 1972). Thus, the carotid arteries should be sampled carefully in these cases as the brain pathology may not be due solely to local sickling and stasis.

Sudden death from coronary occlusion with acute myocardial infarction is a rare occurrence in childhood sickle cell disease, but it has been reported in young adults (Jenkins, Scott & Baird, 1960; Martin *et al.*, 1983). Cardiomegaly is a reasonably common finding in older children with sickle cell disease, as-

sociated with chronic anemia and high-output cardiac failure (Seeler, 1972). In cases of sudden death in which cardiomegaly is found at autopsy, it is possible that the underlying mechanism is ischemic arrhythmia rather than acute sequestration. However, the proposal that thrombotic occlusion of intramural coronary arteries in patients with sickle cell disease results in ischemic left ventricular dysfunction and cardiomyopathy has not been supported by later studies (Fleischer & Rubler, 1968; Gerry, Bulkley & Hutchins, 1978). The latter authors found no evidence of coronary occlusion or of ischemic myocardial damage in a series of 52 patients at autopsy. They concluded that there is no evidence for a specific "sickle cell cardiomyopathy," and that changes observed resulted from the effects of chronic anemia exacerbated by acute complications of the disease. Sudden death from pulmonary thromboembolism, possibly preceded by manifestations of "acute chest syndrome," appears to be a phenomenon that occurs predominantly in affected adults, along with pulmonary hypertension and cor pulmonale (Collins & Orringer, 1982; Rogers & Brunt, 1992; Rubler & Fleischer, 1967; Young *et al.*, 1981). Pulmonary vascular changes may, however, be found at earlier ages (Figure 9.5).

Infectious complications

Infections in children with sickle cell disease may be fulminant and may also result in sudden death (Roberts, Haas & King, 1973). There is a significantly increased risk of pneumococcal septicemia and meningitis, particularly in early childhood (Barrett-Connor, 1971; Powars *et al.*, 1981). This is thought to be due to a combination of reduced splenic function associated with repeated episodes of infarction, which ultimately results in functional asplenia, a defect in the alternate pathway of complement activation, altered neutrophil activity, reduced serum opsonizing activity for pneumococcus, and reticuloendothelial dysfunction due to chronic hemolysis (Johnston, Newman & Struth, 1973; Overturf, Powars & Baraff, 1977; Pearson, Spencer & Cornelius, 1969; Pegelow *et al.*, 1980; Winkelstein & Drachman, 1968). Parvovirus B19 infection may also be rapidly fatal in

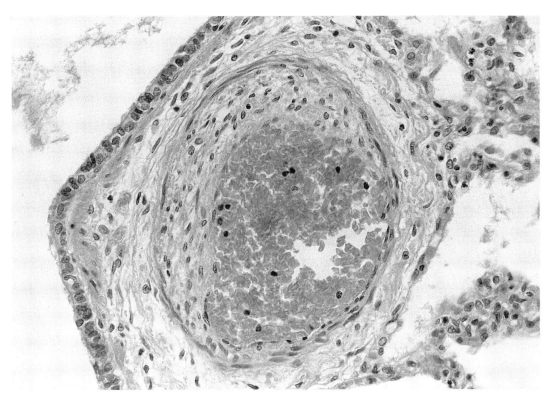

Figure 9.5 Eccentric fibrointimal proliferation of a small pulmonary artery in a nine-year-old girl who died suddenly with sickle cell disease/thalassemia (hematoxylin and eosin, ×280).

children with hemoglobinopathies due to massive sickling or to fat embolism from massive bone marrow necrosis (Kolquist *et al.*, 1996).

Respiratory complications

Acute sickle chest syndrome refers to acute pulmonary symptoms characterized by chest pain and shortness of breath, which may lead to unexpected cardiac arrest. Although pathologic examination may reveal extensive pulmonary infarcts, there is debate as to whether the underlying mechanism is intravascular sickling, infection, or vasospasm, as thrombi are not always found (Athanasou *et al.*, 1985).

Chronic sickle cell lung disease occurs in adults from episodes of acute chest syndrome. It is charac-

terized by pulmonary hypertension and fibrosis with cor pulmonale, and is a major cause of death (Powars *et al.*, 1988). However, studies in children do not usually show these underlying pulmonary abnormalities (Pianosi *et al.*, 1993).

Autopsy investigations

Sickle cell disease should be suspected in any infant or young child who suddenly collapses and dies, particularly if there is African or Mediterranean heritage. Investigations at the time of autopsy include a full septic work-up with cerebrospinal fluid and blood cultures, hematocrit, hemoglobin, and hemoglobin electrophoresis (if possible). Although it has been claimed that the incidence of SIDS is higher in affected infants (Vix *et al.*, 1987), the diagnosis of SIDS should not be entertained in these cases given the possibility of sudden and unexpected death from a variety of mechanisms and the presence of underlying pathology. In the absence of a clear cause of death at autopsy, the author would designate such cases as "sudden death in an infant with sickle cell disease." Other authors who have accepted a diagnosis of SIDS in these infants have not found the incidence of "SIDS" to be higher (Gozal *et al.*, 1994).

Other hemoglobinopathies

The association of sudden death with other hemoglobinopathies is not as well recognized, although sudden death in childhood may occur with hemoglobin CS (HbCS) (Tuttle & Koch, 1960) and in sickle-*β* thalassemia. The presence of the latter combination in populations around the Mediterranean means that a caucasian background does not exclude the possibility of acute splenic sequestration at autopsy (Color Plate 19). Intractable cardiac failure with arrhythmias due to iron overload may occur in children with thalassemia; however, the terminal episode usually extends over one to two days (Modell & Berdoukas, 1984).

Hematologic malignancies

Lymphomas

The clinical course of children with hematologic malignancies that fail to respond to therapy is usually protracted, with death being neither sudden nor unexpected. When unexpected death does occur, it may be due to fungal thromboembolism following immunosuppressive therapy. A clinical history of prolonged fever, antibiotic and corticosteroid administration, and profound neutropenia may be clues to the presence of fungal sepsis prior to performance of an autopsy. Overwhelming bacterial sepsis and hemorrhage are also potentially lethal complications that may result in rapid demise.

A less common cause of death or life-threatening respiratory compromise may, however, be acute up-

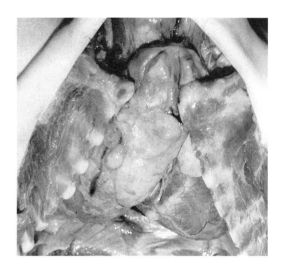

Figure 9.6 An unsuspected mediastinal lymphoma that caused fatal compression of the lungs and airways in a two-year-old girl.

per airway obstruction due to a local mass effect from mediastinal lymphoma (Jeffery, Mead & Whitehouse, 1991). A case such as this occurred in a two-year-old intellectually impaired girl thought to have asthma, who was found at autopsy to have a large, clinically unsuspected anterior mediastinal large-cell lymphoma compressing her larger airways (Figure 9.6). In this case, other medical problems had made accurate clinical assessment difficult. Airway obstruction in children with mediastinal tumors may also occur following the induction of anesthesia (Bray & Fernandes, 1982; Keon, 1981), and children with this problem are also at risk of sudden death from cardiac compression, or from compression of the pulmonary artery in the supine position (Halpern *et al.*, 1983; Levin, Bursztein & Heifetz, 1985; Yamashita *et al.*, 1990).

Another potential cause of sudden death in children with lymphoma is marked metabolic disturbance (Robertson, Stiller & Kingston, 1992). This may occur following chemotherapy in sensitive tumors if there has been rapid tumor lysis with marked hyperkalemia and hypocalcemia (Cohen *et al.*, 1980).

Rarely, rupture of the spleen resulting in rapid death may be the first presentation of lymphoma, as was reported in a 15-year-old girl who died soon after the onset of abdominal pain. Hodgkin's disease was discovered at autopsy (Schulz, 1969).

Leukemias

The usual cause of unexpected death in children with leukemia is intracranial hemorrhage due to primary or secondary thrombocytopenia. Children with acute promyelocytic leukemia are particularly prone to developing hemorrhagic complications. Other mechanisms may involve local cerebral leukemic infiltration, or hyperviscosity and leukostasis in acute disease. Fungal disease may also result in occlusive thromboemboli (Byard *et al.*, 1987), and certain types of chemotherapy, such as aspariginase and methotrexate, can cause thromboses and hemorrhage (Pellegrino, Zanesco & Battistella, 1992).

The author has reviewed several patients in whom the diagnosis of acute leukemia was made only at postmortem following clinical presentations of sudden collapse. A nine-year-old boy who had been drowsy and irritable on the day of admission died soon after the onset of coma. Autopsy revealed multifocal white-matter hemorrhages in association with an acute myeloid leukemia. Extensive hemorrhage within the pons had compressed surrounding structures. Another patient, a three-year-old girl who had been treated with antibiotics for cervical lymphadenopathy and an upper respiratory tract infection, collapsed and died suddenly. At autopsy, massive intrapontine hemorrhage was found in association with an acute myeloid leukemia (Figure 9.7 and Color Plate 20). Fatal cerebral hemorrhage was also the mode of presentation of acute lymphoblastic leukemia in a 13-year-old boy (Figures 9.8 and 9.9). Thus, death may occur rapidly in young patients with leukemia, even if they appear medically stable and sometimes even before the clinical diagnosis has been established.

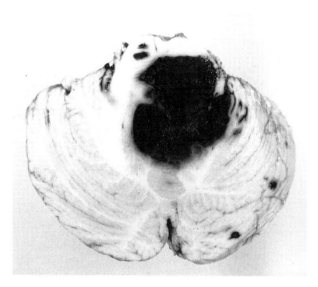

Figure 9.7 Hemorrhage into the brainstem with compression of adjacent vital centers, which caused sudden death in a three-year-old girl due to clinically unsuspected acute myeloid leukemia.

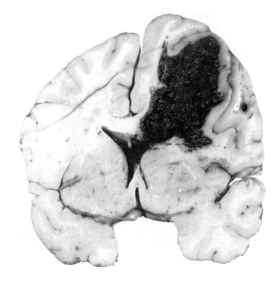

Figure 9.8 Massive hemorrhage into the frontoparietal region in a 13-year-old boy with acute lymphoblastic leukemia associated with sudden onset of coma and death.

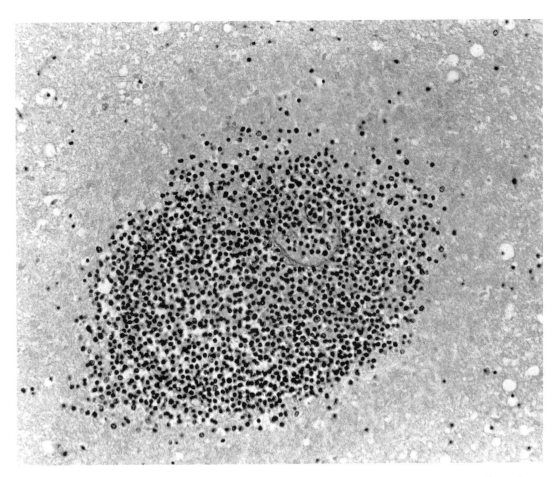

Figure 9.9 Perivascular infiltrate of leukemic cells with surrounding intracerebral hemorrhage precipitating massive hemorrhage in the case shown in Figure 9.8 (hematoxylin and eosin, ×280).

Death may also occur rapidly if there has been myocardial infiltration by leukemic cells. This was responsible for the demise of a 16-week-old boy who was found at autopsy to have a pre-B-cell-type lymphoblastic leukemia infiltrating a variety of organs (Whybourne *et al.*, 2001) (Figures 9.10–9.12).

Disorders of coagulation

Disorders of the coagulation pathways may be inherited, such as deficiencies of factors VIII and IX, or acquired, due to liver disease or to inadequate dietary intake of vitamin K, resulting in low levels of factors II, VII, IX, and X. Independent of the underlying etiology, patients with any of these conditions are at risk of significant hemorrhage, either spontaneously or following minimal trauma.

Primary deficiencies

Inherited disorders of coagulation usually involve factor VIII (hemophilia A), factor IX (hemophilia B or Christmas disease), or von Willebrand factor, although a number of other less common deficiencies have been described, hematological details of which have been reviewed by Miller (1984a). Hemophilia A is the most common hereditary disorder of coagulation. It is X-linked and has an incidence of approximately 20 per 100 000 male births (Hoyer, 1994).

While patients with hemophilia A or B tend to bleed spontaneously into the soft tissues and joints, intracranial hemorrhage remains the major cause of premature mortality (Miller, 1984a) and has been reported in 2.2–7.8% of affected individuals, accounting for 25–30% of deaths overall (Eyster *et al.*, 1978). There are also significantly increased risks associated with surgical and dental procedures and with minor trauma. Damage to the posterior pharynx, as may occur in a child who falls with an object such as a pencil in the mouth, may result in massive retropharyngeal hemorrhage, with life-threatening upper airway obstruction. Intracranial hemorrhage is much less common in von Willebrand disease but remains a potentially fatal complication (Zimmerman & Ruggeri, 1987).

The following case of a 14-year-old boy with known hemophilia A illustrates how insidious hemorrhage in these children may be. The boy had suffered mild concussion with no loss of consciousness following a fall from his bicycle. Skull radiographs revealed no evidence of fractures; however, in view of his underlying coagulopathy, he was admitted to hospital and observed for three days. At the end of that time, he appeared quite well and so was sent home, only to appear at the end of the first week with an acute onset of reduced consciousness, hemiparesis, and death within 24 hours. There was no history of additional head trauma, although this cannot be excluded. At autopsy, extensive hemorrhage into his left frontal lobe with intraventricular extension was found (Figure 9.13).

As well as being associated with a bleeding tendency, von Willebrand syndrome has been linked with mitral valve prolapse (Pickering, Brody & Barrett, 1981). However, as this study dealt only with one living adolescent and 14 adults, the relationship of this phenomenon to sudden death, and specifically to pediatric sudden death, is uncertain. Other coagulation disorders such as congenital afibrinogenemia and factor VII and XIII deficiencies may re-

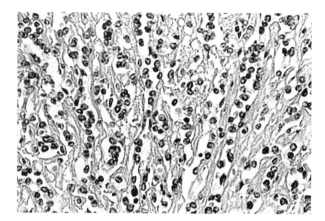

Figure 9.10 Infiltration of myocardium by leukemic cells in a four-month-old boy who was found moribund in his crib (hematoxylin and eosin, ×300).

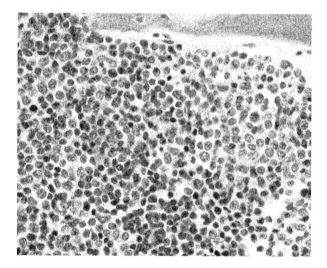

Figure 9.11 Effacement of bone marrow in a four-month old boy (illustrated in Figure 9.10) by malignant hematopoetic cells, which were subsequently shown on immunohistochemical staining to have a pre-B-cell phenotype (hematoxylin and eosin, ×400).

sult in intracranial bleeding in childhood (Pellegrino, Zanesco & Battistella, 1992).

Secondary deficiencies

There is a variety of acquired disorders of coagulation, the most common being disseminated

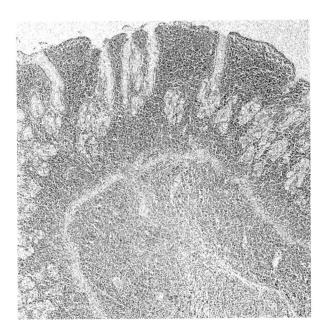

Figure 9.12 Widespread tissue and organ infiltration in the case illustrated in Figures 9.10 and 9.11 included the mucosa and submucosa of the stomach (hematoxylin and eosin, ×80).

intravascular coagulation associated with sepsis, malignancy, trauma, or obstetric complications. In most of these conditions, the patient is in a critical state, and hemorrhage is often terminal, multifocal, and associated with a range of hemodynamic and metabolic disruptions.

Thrombotic conditions

Thromboses in infants may be associated with septicemia, peripartum asphyxia, maternal diabetes, cardiac disease, in-dwelling central lines, and familial hypercoagulable syndromes (Gaston, 1966; Heller *et al.*, 2000; Atalay *et al.*, 2002). It is now recognized that children with mutations in the factor V Leiden and prothrombin genes, or deficiencies in anti-thrombin III, plasminogen, and proteins C and S, or lupus anticoagulant are at increased risk of vascular thrombosis (Nuss, Hays & Manco-Johnson, 1995; Thomas, 2001). Thrombotic events may be arterial or venous, and may occur within the lung, heart, brain, and abdomen. Intracranial thrombosis

Table 9.2. Causes of thrombocytopenia

Decreased production
  Decreased megakaryopoiesis, e.g. aplastic anemia, drugs, chemicals, marrow replacement from leukemia/lymphoma, solid tumors such as neuroblastoma, osteopetrosis, and storage disorders
  Ineffective thrombopoiesis, e.g. megaloblastic anemia, hereditary thrombocytopenias
Abnormal distribution or dilution
  Pooling in cases of splenomegaly
  Following transfusion of stored blood
Increased destruction
  Immunological, e.g. idiopathic thrombocytopenia purpura
  Non-immunological, e.g. thrombotic thrombocytopenia, disseminated intravascular coagulation, hemolytic-uremic syndrome, cardiac prostheses

has been associated with ischemic stroke (Abrantes *et al.*, 2002; Atalay *et al.*, 2002; Chan & deVeber, 2000; Nestoridi *et al.*, 2002; Verdú *et al.*, 2001). The risk of thrombosis for children with heterozygous deficiencies remains poorly defined (Segel & Francis, 2000).

Platelet disorders

Thrombocytopenia from any cause may result in spontaneous hemorrhage. A list of possible causes of thrombocytopenia is given in Table 9.2

Occurrence of sudden death

Sudden death may occur in children with any of these entities if bleeding occurs in a vital location, such as within the cranial cavity. Rarely, hemorrhage into soft tissues around the laryngeal inlet may also result in death from airway obstruction. Figure 9.14 illustrates such a case in a one-year-old girl with treated neuroblastoma, marrow aplasia, and *Pseudomonas* sepsis and who suffered airway compromise from spontaneous pharyngeal hemorrhage.

The usual conditions associated with sudden lethal intracranial hemorrhage in childhood in this collection of disorders are the acute leukemias.

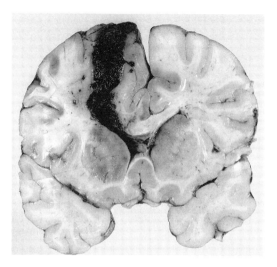

Figure 9.13 Intracerebral hemorrhage resulting in the sudden onset of a reduced conscious state followed by death within 24 hours in a 14-year-old boy with hemophilia A. This occurred one week after apparently minor head trauma.

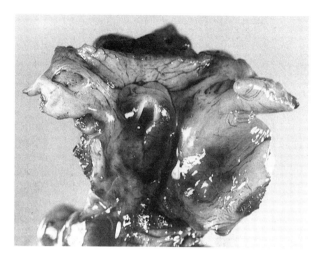

Figure 9.14 Obstruction of the laryngeal inlet due to interstitial hemorrhage resulted in sudden onset of inspiratory stridor, cyanosis, and death in a one-year-old girl with treated neuroblastoma and chemotherapy-induced thrombocytopenia.

This is due to either replacement of marrow hematopoietic cells by malignant cells, or treatment-induced marrow aplasia, with reduction in circulating platelet numbers.

In a number of childhood malignancies, there may be several contributing factors to spontaneous hemorrhage as well as thrombocytopenia. These include reduced clotting factors from an inadequate diet associated with the underlying malignancy and chemotherapy, or disseminated intravascular coagulation due to concurrent sepsis.

Inherited platelet abnormalities

Inherited disorders of platelets involving abnormal function or reduced numbers are less common than acquired disorders but may also result in lethal hemorrhage at an early age. Miller (1984b) has separated these conditions into five main groups: (i) defects of the platelet surface membrane, (ii) platelet-type von Willebrand disease, (iii) granule defects, e.g. Wiskott–Aldrich syndrome (X-linked thrombocytopenia with eczema), (iv) defective arachidonic metabolism, and (v) a miscellaneous group that is quite heterogeneous, including platelet abnormalities associated with congenital heart disease, Down syndrome, and metabolic disorders.

An example of sudden death in one of these conditions occurred in a five-month-old boy with Wiskott–Aldrich syndrome and who was in hospital for a platelet transfusion when he suffered sudden deterioration and death. Intracerebellar and diffuse basal subarachnoid hemorrhage were found at autopsy.

Idiopathic thrombocytopenic purpura

This is the most common childhood thrombocytopenic purpura. It is characterized by decreased circulating platelets, increased marrow megakaryocytes, and mucocutaneous bleeding. The underlying etiology is believed to be an autoimmune response to platelets, often triggered by a preceding viral infection. Although mucosal bleeding may be quite profound, intracranial hemorrhage occurs in only 1–2% of cases (Pellegrino, Zanesco & Battistella, 1992).

Thrombotic thrombocytopenic purpura

This is a rare disorder in childhood of uncertain etiology. It bears certain similarities to the hemolytic-uremic syndrome and is characterized by fever, renal dysfunction, thrombocytopenic purpura, microangiopathic hemolytic anemia, and neurologic manifestations that may include convulsions, stroke, and death (Amorosi & Ultmann, 1966). Rapid death has been reported in adolescents and young adults with this condition, which may complicate pregnancy (Bell, Barnhart & Martin, 1990; Kemp, Barnard & Prahlow, 1999; Khoo, Dickens & Cheung, 1992; Ross, Newton & Stivers, 1987). The peripheral blood smear (if available) shows features of microangiopathic hemolytic anemia, with schistocytes (helmet cells) and thrombocytopenia; the autopsy will reveal widespread hyalinized thrombi within arterioles of the bone marrow, pancreas, lymph nodes, spleen, liver, ovaries, adrenal gland, heart, kidneys, and brain (Ross, Newton & Stivers, 1987).

Kasabach–Merritt syndrome

This syndrome is characterized by consumption coagulopathy with reduction in platelet numbers due to trapping and destruction of platelets within large vascular neoplasms (Sencer et al., 1987). Although the underlying lesions are classified as hemangiomas, they are thought to be different from the more typical involuting hemangiomas of childhood by some authors, who consider them to be more like tufted angiomas or kaposiform hemangioendotheliomas (Enjolras et al., 1997; Powell, 1999). The hemangiomas occur in all parts of the body. While most infants and children with this condition survive, this is not always the case, as

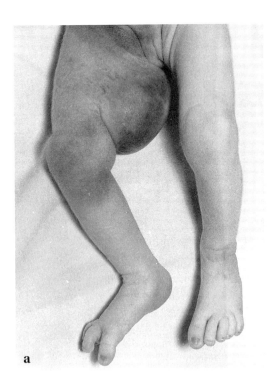
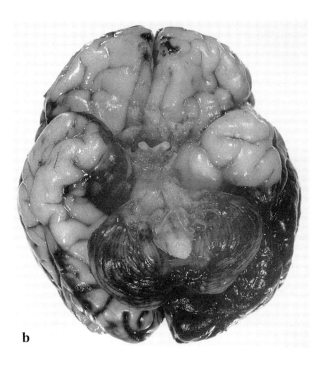

Figure 9.15 Large hemangioma (a) of the upper thigh of a four-day-old girl, causing Kasabach–Merritt syndrome, with thrombocytopenia and resultant fatal subarachnoid hemorrhage (b).

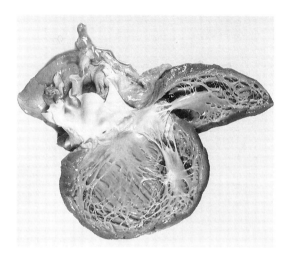

Figure 9.16 Massive cardiomegaly with chamber dilation in a seven-year-old boy with thalassemia.

demonstrated in Figure 9.15. This shows a large cavernous hemangioma of the leg in a four-day-old infant that was associated with thrombocytopenia and unexpected death from subarachnoid hemorrhage. Hyperkalemia secondary to excessive red blood cell destruction in Kasabach–Merritt syndrome has also been reported as a rare cause of potentially fatal cardiac arrhythmias in this age group (Vellodi & Bini, 1988).

Primary thrombocytosis

Although primary thrombocytosis, which is usually related to myeloproliferative disorders, is extremely rare and tolerated better in children than in adults, cases have been described in which non-fatal acute myocardial infarction has occurred. One such report involved an eight-year-old girl, and another a 17-year-old adolescent (Høst, Hasselbalch & Feldt-Rasmussen, 1988; Spach, Howell & Harris, 1963). Secondary thrombocytosis is generally a benign condition (Vora & Lilleyman, 1993).

Anemia

Unless there is postmortem evidence of previous high-output cardiac failure with marked cardiomegaly (Figure 9.16) and erythroid hyperplasia of the bone marrow, it may be difficult to determine the significance of an antemortem diagnosis of anemia. However, if these findings are present, it is reasonable to suggest that anemia of whatever etiology may have contributed to sudden death, given the known association of cardiac arrhythmias with hypoxia and cardiomegaly. Other cardiac findings in cases of severe anemia include chamber dilation, myocardial infarction/ischemia, and fatty infiltration, with a "thrush breast" pattern of the myocardium (Color Plate 21) (Bor, 1969; Ferrans & Boyce, 1983). It would not be possible to support a diagnosis of SIDS in infants who are found to have these changes. The case of a four-month-old boy with hereditary spherocytosis (Figure 9.17) who was thought initially to have succumbed to SIDS illustrates this point. He had required blood transfusions because of ongoing hemolysis, and at autopsy he was found to have marked cardiomegaly and marrow erythroid hyperplasia, thus precluding the diagnosis of SIDS. An additional reason for clearly separating infants who die with anemia from infants who die of SIDS is the known association of acute life-threatening events (ALTEs) with anemia in infancy (Kelly & Shannon, 1988).

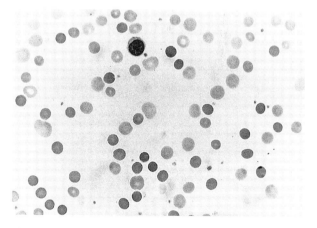

Figure 9.17 Multiple dense hyperchromic microspherocytes typical of hereditary spherocytosis in a four-month–old boy who died suddenly with spherocytosis and cardiomegaly (Giemsa, ×1100).

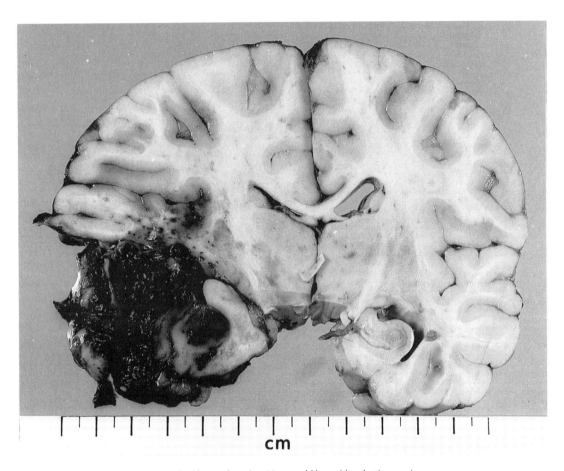

Figure 9.18 Spontaneous fatal intracerebral hemorrhage in a 10-year-old boy with aplastic anemia.

Other possible mechanisms relating anemia and sudden death are those of cerebral ischemia (Young *et al.*, 1983) and increased numbers of cyanotic breath-holding episodes (Poets *et al.*, 1992). Also, while anemia may not be solely responsible for the lethal event, it may serve to exacerbate pre-existing conditions. An example of this was a 13-month-old boy who had a cardiac arrest and was found to have both severe anemia and a solitary coronary artery (Gonzalez-Angulo, Reyes & Wallace, 1966).

Anemia may also be associated with reduction in platelet numbers, as in aplastic and megaloblastic anemias, which may result in death from spontaneous hemorrhage (Arey & Sotos, 1956). This was the case in a 10-year-old boy with a past history of intracranial hemorrhage and who was known to have aplastic anemia. He presented to hospital dead on arrival following the acute onset of headache that had progressed rapidly to coma. At autopsy, extensive intracerebral hemorrhage involving the left parietotemporal lobes with extension into the subarachnoid space was found (Figure 9.18).

Hemolytic-uremic syndrome

This disorder is characterized by the sudden onset of hemolytic anemia, thrombocytopenia, and uremia, with underlying endothelial damage. Clinically, approximately one-third of patients have neurological complications, with coma, seizures, and hemiparesis resulting from thrombosis of the microvasculature, metabolic abnormalities, or systemic hypertension (Sheth, Swick & Haworth, 1986; Steinberg *et al.*, 1986). Intracranial hemorrhage (Crisp *et al.*, 1981) and status epilepticus (Pellegrino, Zanesco & Battistella, 1992) are two manifestations that have a known association with sudden death (see Figure 10.26). Further details are given in Chapter 10.

Polycythemia

The most common forms of polycythemia in children are secondary to cyanotic congenital heart disease or chronic pulmonary disease. Primary polycythemia occurs much less often. Other disorders such as cystic renal disease, cerebellar hemangioblastomas, and the Pickwickian syndrome may also result in marked polycythemia (Berlin, 1975; Grotta *et al.*, 1986), all of which may predispose to lethal thrombotic cerebral events.

Splenic disorders

Asplenia/hyposplenia

Asplenia may be congenital, acquired, or functional, with congenital asplenia being syndromal or non-syndromal. Non-syndromal congenital asplenia may be either sporadic or familial (Kanthan, Moyana & Nyssen, 1999). Absence or marked hypoplasia of the spleen (Figure 9.19) may be associated with cardiovascular abnormalities and an increased risk of fulminant sepsis. The most common associated cardiac anomalies are transposition of the great vessels, pulmonary stenosis, or atresia and total anomalous pulmonary venous drainage (Rose, Izukawa & Moës, 1975). Details of associated infectious and vascular complications are dealt with in Chapters 4 and 6, respectively.

Splenic rupture

Although often related to hematologic disorders, splenomegaly from any cause may be associated

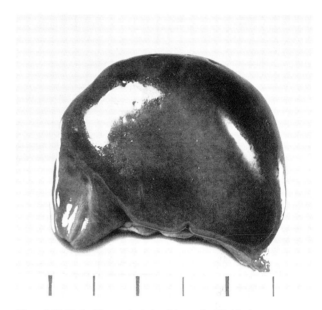

Figure 9.19 Marked hyposplenia in a 14-month-old girl who died of complex congenital heart disease. The spleen weighed only 3 g (normal for age ≈ 26 g). (scale = 5 mm)

with rupture and sudden death due to exsanguination. While malaria is a more frequent cause of splenomegaly on a global scale, infectious mononucleosis and leukemias are more common causes of splenic enlargement in Western countries. Even relatively mild trauma may cause rupture when the spleen is significantly enlarged. This was the case in an adolescent girl with infectious mononucleosis (Figure 9.20), who died quite suddenly due to massive intraperitoneal hemorrhage with no history of trauma. Minor trauma resulting in splenic rupture in individuals with infectious mononucleosis has included straining at stool, vomiting, coughing, exercise, and medical examination (Bell & Mason, 1980; Molander, 1982; Springate & Adelson, 1966). Rupture of the spleen as the initial presentation of Hodgkin's disease has also been reported in adolescence (Schulz, 1969). Hemangiomas, cysts, and Ehlers–Danlos syndrome are other extremely rare causes of spontaneous splenic rupture (Harris, Slater & Austin, 1985).

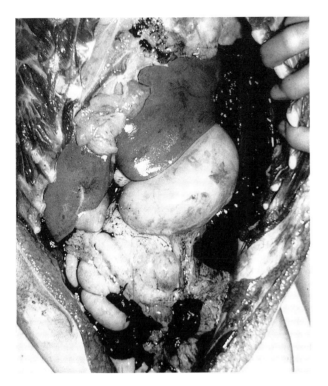

Figure 9.20 Traumatic rupture of the spleen resulting in sudden death in an adolescent girl with splenomegaly due to infectious mononucleosis.

REFERENCES

Abrantes, M., Lacerda, A. F., Abreu, C. R., Levy, A., Azevedo, A. & Da Silva, L. J. (2002). Cerebral venous sinus thrombosis in a neonate due to factor V Leiden deficiency. *Acta Paediatrica*, **91**, 243–5.

Amorosi, E. L. & Ultmann, J. E. (1966). Thrombotic thrombocytopenic purpura: report of 16 cases and review of the literature. *Medicine*, **45**, 139–59.

Arey, J. B. & Sotos, J. (1956). Unexpected death in early life. *Journal of Pediatrics*, **49**, 523–39.

Atalay, S., Akar, N., Tutar, H. E. & Yilmaz, E. (2002). Factor V 1691 G-A mutation in children with intracardiac thrombosis: a prospective study. *Acta Paediatrica*, **91**, 168–71.

Athanasou, N. A., Hatton, C., McGee, J. O. & Weatherall, D. J. (1985). Vascular occlusion and infarction in sickle cell crisis and sickle chest syndrome. *Journal of Clinical Pathology*, **38**, 659–64.

Bainbridge, R., Higgs, D. R., Maude, G. H. & Serjeant, G. R. (1985). Clinical presentation of homozygous sickle cell disease. *Journal of Pediatrics*, **106**, 881–5.

Barrett-Connor, E. (1971). Bacterial infection and sickle cell anemia. An analysis of 250 infections in 166 patients and a review of the literature. *Medicine*, **50**, 97–112.

Bell, J. S. & Mason, J. M. (1980). Sudden death due to spontaneous rupture of the spleen from infectious mononucleosis. *Journal of Forensic Sciences*, **25**, 20–24.

Bell, M. D., Barnhart, J. S., Jr & Martin, J. M. (1990). Thrombotic thrombocytopenic purpura causing sudden, unexpected death – a series of eight patients. *Journal of Forensic Sciences*, **35**, 601–13.

Berlin, N. I. (1975). Diagnosis and classification of the polycythemias. *Seminars in Hematology*, **12**, 339–51.

Bor, I. (1969). Myocardial infarction and ischaemic heart disease in infants and children. Analysis of 29 cases and review of the literature. *Archives of Disease in Childhood*, **44**, 268–81.

Bray, R. J. & Fernandes, F. J. (1982). Mediastinal tumour causing airway obstruction in anaesthetised children. *Anaesthesia*, **37**, 571–5.

Byard, R. W., Jimenez, C. L., Carpenter, B. F., Cutz, E. & Smith, C. R. (1991). Four unusual cases of sudden and unexpected cardiovascular death in infancy and childhood. *Medicine, Science and the Law*, **31**, 157–61.

Byard, R. W., Jimenez, C. L., Carpenter, B. F. & Hsu, E. (1987). Aspergillus-related aortic thrombosis. *Canadian Medical Association Journal*, **136**, 155–6.

Chan, A. K. C. & deVeber, G. (2000). Prothrombotic disorders and ischemic stroke in children. *Seminars in Pediatric Neurology*, **7**, 301–8.

Cohen, L. F., Balow, J. E., Magrath, I. T., Poplack, D. G. & Ziegler, J. L. (1980). Acute tumor lysis syndrome. A review of 37 patients with Burkitt's lymphoma. *American Journal of Medicine*, **68**, 486–91.

Collins, F. S. & Orringer, E. P. (1982). Pulmonary hypertension and cor pulmonale in the sickle hemoglobinopathies. *American Journal of Medicine*, **73**, 814–21.

Crisp, D. E., Siegler, R. L., Bale, J. F. & Thompson, J. A. (1981). Hemorrhagic cerebral infarction in the hemolytic-uremic syndrome. *Journal of Pediatrics*, **99**, 273–6.

Dudley, A. W., Jr & Waddell, C. C. (1991). Crisis in sickle cell trait. *Human Pathology*, **22**, 616–18.

Emond, A. M., Collis, R., Darvill, D., Higgs, D. R., Maude, G. H. & Sergeant, G. R. (1985). Acute splenic sequestration in homozygous sickle cell disease: natural history and management. *Journal of Pediatrics*, **107**, 201–6.

Enjolras, O., Wassef, M., Mazoyer, E., *et al.* (1997). Infants with Kasabach-Merritt syndrome do not have "true" hemangiomas. *Journal of Pediatrics*, **130**, 631–40.

Eyster, M. E., Gill, F. M., Blatt, P. M., *et al.* (1978). Central nervous system bleeding in hemophiliacs. *Blood*, **51**, 1179–88.

Ferrans, V. J. & Boyce, S. W. (1983). Metabolic and familial diseases. In *Cardiovascular Pathology*, vol. 2, ed. M. D. Silver. New York: Churchill Livingstone, pp. 945–1004.

Fleischer, R. A. & Rubler, S. (1968). Primary cardiomyopathy in nonanemic patients. Association with sickle cell trait. *American Journal of Cardiology*, **22**, 532–7.

Garza, J. A. (1990). Massive fat and necrotic bone marrow embolization in a previously undiagnosed patient with sickle cell disease. *American Journal of Forensic Medicine and Pathology*, **11**, 83–8.

Garza-Mercado, R. (1982). Pseudomoyamoya in sickle cell anemia. *Surgical Neurology*, **18**, 425–31.

Gaston, L. W. (1966). Studies on a family with an elevated plasma level of factor V (proaccelerin) and a tendency to thrombosis. *Journal of Pediatrics*, **68**, 367–73.

Gerber, N. & Apseloff, G. (1993). Death from a morphine infusion during a sickle cell crisis. *Journal of Pediatrics*, **123**, 322–5.

Gerry, J. L., Jr, Bulkley, B. H. & Hutchins, G. M. (1978). Clinicopathologic analysis of cardiac dysfunction in 52 patients with sickle cell anemia. *American Journal of Cardiology*, **42**, 211–16.

Gonzalez-Angulo, A., Reyes, H. A. & Wallace, S. A. (1966). Anomalies of the origin of coronary arteries (special reference to single coronary artery). *Angiology*, **17**, 96–103.

Gozal, D., Lorey, F. W., Chandler, D., *et al.* (1994). Incidence of sudden infant death syndrome in infants with sickle cell trait. *Journal of Pediatrics*, **124**, 211–14.

Grotta, J. C., Manner, C., Pettigrew, L. C. & Yatsu, F. M. (1986). Red blood cell disorders and stroke. *Stroke*, **17**, 811–17.

Halpern, S., Chatten, J., Meadows, A. T., Byrd, R. & Lange, B. (1983). Anterior mediastinal masses: anesthesia hazards and other problems. *Journal of Pediatrics*, **102**, 407–10.

Harris, S. C., Slater, D. N. & Austin, C. A. (1985). Fatal splenic rupture in Ehlers-Danlos syndrome. *Postgraduate Medical Journal*, **61**, 259–60.

Heller, C., Schobess, R., Kurnik, K., *et al.* (2000). Abdominal venous thrombosis in neonates and infants: role of prothrombotic risk factors – a multicentre case-control study. *British Journal of Haematology*, **111**, 543–9.

Høst, N. B., Hasselbalch, H. & Feldt-Rasmussen, B. (1988). Letter to editor. *European Journal of Haematology*, **141**, 511.

Hoyer, L. W. (1994). Hemophilia A. *New England Journal of Medicine*, **330**, 38–47.

Hynd, R. F., Bharadwaja, K., Mitas, J. A. & Lord, J. T. (1985). Rhabdomyolysis, acute renal failure, and disseminated intravascular coagulation in a man with sickle cell trait. *Southern Medical Journal*, **78**, 890–91.

Jeffery, G. M, Mead, G. M. & Whitehouse, J. M. A. (1991). Life-threatening airway obstruction at the presentation of Hodgkin's disease. *Cancer*, **67**, 506–10.

Jenkins, M. E., Scott, R. B. & Baird, R. L. (1960). Studies in sickle cell anemia. XVI. Sudden death during sickle cell anemia crises in young children. *Journal of Pediatrics*, **56**, 30–38.

Johnston, R. B., Jr, Newman, S. L. & Struth, A. G. (1973). An abnormality of the alternative pathway of complement activation in sickle-cell disease. *New England Journal of Medicine*, **288**, 803–8.

Jones, S. R., Binder, R. A. & Donowho, E. M., Jr (1970). Sudden death in sickle-cell trait. *New England Journal of Medicine*, **282**, 323–5.

Kanthan, R., Moyana, T. & Nyssen, J. (1999). Asplenia as a cause of sudden unexpected death in childhood. *American Journal of Forensic Medicine and Pathology*, **20**, 57–9.

Kark, J. A., Posey, D. M., Schumacher, H. R. & Ruehle, C. J. (1987). Sickle-cell trait as a risk factor for sudden death in physical training. *New England Journal of Medicine*, **317**, 781–7.

Kelly, D. H. & Shannon, D. C. (1988). The medical management of cardiorespiratory monitoring in infantile apnea. In *Sudden Infant Death Syndrome. Medical Aspects and Psychological Management*, ed. J. L. Culbertson, H. F. Krous & R. D. Bendell. London: Edward Arnold, pp. 139–54.

Kemp, W. L., Barnard, J. J. & Prahlow, J. A. (1999). Death due to thrombotic thrombocytopenic purpura during pregnancy. Case report with review of thrombotic microangiopathies of pregnancy. *American Journal of Forensic Medicine and Pathology*, **20**, 189–98.

Keon, T. P. (1981). Death on induction of anesthesia for cervical node biopsy. *Anesthesiology*, **55**, 471–2.

Khoo, U. S., Dickens, P. & Cheung, A. N. Y. (1992). Rapid death from thrombotic thrombocytopenic purpura following Caesarian section. *Forensic Science International*, **54**, 75–80.

Kolquist, K. A., Vnencak-Jones, C. L., Swift, L., Page, D. L., Johnson, J. E. & Denison, M. R. (1996). Fatal fat embolism syndrome in a child with undiagnosed hemoglobin S/beta+ thalassemia: a complication of acute parvovirus B19 infection. *Pediatric Pathology and Laboratory Medicine*, **16**, 71–82.

Koppes, G. M., Daly, J. J., Coltman, C. A., Jr & Butkus, D. E. (1977). Exertion-induced rhabdomyolysis with acute renal failure and disseminated intravascular coagulation in sickle cell trait. *American Journal of Medicine*, **63**, 313–17.

Levin, H., Bursztein, S. & Heifetz, M. (1985). Cardiac arrest in a child with an anterior mediastinal mass. *Anesthesia and Analgesia*, **64**, 1129–30.

Martin, C. R., Cobb, C., Tatter, D., Johnson, C. & Haywood, L. J. (1983). Acute myocardial infarction in sickle cell anemia. *Archives of Internal Medicine*, **143**, 830–31.

McGarry, P. & Duncan, C. (1973). Anesthetic risks in sickle cell trait. *Pediatrics*, **51**, 507–12.

Mease, A. D., Longo, D. L. & Hakami, N. (1976). Sicklemia and unexpected death in sickle cell trait: observations of five cases. *Military Medicine*, **141**, 470–74.

Miller, J. L. (1984a). Blood coagulation and fibrinolysis. In *Clinical Diagnosis and Management by Laboratory Methods*, 17th edn, ed. J. B. Henry. Philadelphia: W. B. Saunders, pp. 765–87.

Miller, J. L. (1984b). Blood platelets. In *Clinical Diagnosis and Management by Laboratory Methods*, 17th edn, ed. J. B. Henry. Philadelphia: W. B. Saunders, pp. 749–64.

Mills, M. L. (1985). Life-threatening complications of sickle cell disease in children. *Journal of the American Medical Association*, **254**, 1487–91.

Modell, B. & Berdoukas, V. (1984). Death and survival. In *The Clinical Approach to Thalassaemia*. London: Grune & Stratton, p. 161.

Molander, N. (1982). Sudden natural death in later childhood and adolescence. *Archives of Disease in Childhood*, **57**, 572–6.

Nelson, D. A. & Davey, F. R. (1984). Erythrocytic disorders. In *Clinical Diagnosis and Management by Laboratory Methods*, 17th edn, ed. J. B. Henry. Philadelphia: W. B. Saunders, pp. 652–703.

Nestoridi, E., Buonanno, F. S., Jones, R. M., *et al.* (2002). Arterial ischemic stroke in childhood: the role of plasma-phase risk factors. *Current Opinion in Neurology*, **15**, 139–44.

Nuss, R., Hays, T. & Manco-Johnson, M. (1995). Childhood thrombosis. *Pediatrics*, **96**, 291–4.

Ober, W. B., Bruno, M. S., Weinberg, S. B., Jones, F. M., Jr & Weiner, L. (1960). Fatal intravascular sickling in a patient with sickle-cell trait. *New England Journal of Medicine*, **263**, 947–9.

Overturf, G. D., Powars, D. & Baraff, L. J. (1977). Bacterial meningitis and septicemia in sickle cell disease. *American Journal of Diseases of Children*, **131**, 784–7.

Pastorek, J. G. & Seiler, B. (1985). Maternal death associated with sickle cell trait. *American Journal of Obstetrics and Gynecology*, **151**, 295–7.

Pearson, H. A., Spencer, R. P. & Cornelius, E. A. (1969). Functional asplenia in sickle-cell anemia. *New England Journal of Medicine*, **281**, 923–6.

Pegelow, C. H., Wilson, B., Overturf, G. D., Tigner-Weekes, L. & Powars, D. (1980). Infection in splenectomized sickle cell disease patients. *Clinical Pediatrics*, **19**, 102–5.

Pellegrino, P. A., Zanesco, L. & Battistella, P. A. (1992). Coagulopathies and vasculopathies. In *Cerebrovascular Diseases in Children*, ed. A. J. Raimondi, M. Choux & C. Di Rocco. New York: Springer-Verlag, pp. 188–203.

Pianosi, P., D'Souza, S. J. A., Charge, T. D., Esseltine, D. E. & Coates, A. L. (1993). Pulmonary function abnormalities in childhood sickle cell disease. *Journal of Pediatrics*, **122**, 366–71.

Pickering, N. J., Brody, J. I. & Barrett, M. J. (1981). Von Willebrand syndromes and mitral-valve prolapse. Linked mesenchymal dysplasias. *New England Journal of Medicine*, **305**, 131–4.

Platt, O. S., Brambilla, D. J., Rosse, W. F., *et al.* (1994). Mortality in sickle cell disease. Life expectancy and risk factors for early death. *New England Journal of Medicine*, **330**, 1639–44.

Poets, C. F., Samuels, M. P., Wardrop, C. A. J., Picton-Jones, E. & Southall, D. P. (1992). Reduced haemoglobin levels in infants presenting with apparent life-threatening events – a retrospective investigation. *Acta Paediatrica*, **81**, 319–21.

Portnoy, B. A. & Herion, J. C. (1972). Neurological manifestations in sickle-cell disease. With a review of the literature and emphasis on the prevalence of hemiplegia. *Annals of Internal Medicine*, **76**, 643–52.

Powars, D. R. (1975). Natural history of sickle cell disease – the first ten years. *Seminars in Hematology*, **12**, 267–85.

Powars, D., Overturf, G., Weiss, J., Lee, S. & Chan, L. (1981). Pneumococcal septicemia in children with sickle cell anemia. Changing trend of survival. *Journal of the American Medical Association*, **245**, 1839–42.

Powars, D., Weidman, J. A., Odom-Maryon, T., Niland, J. C. & Johnson, C. (1988). Sickle cell chronic lung disease: prior morbidity and the risk of pulmonary failure. *Medicine*, **67**, 66–76.

Powars, D., Wilson, B., Imbus, C., Pegelow, C. & Allen, J. (1978). The natural history of stroke in sickle cell disease. *American Journal of Medicine*, **65**, 461–71.

Powell, J. (1999). Update on hemangiomas and vascular malformations. *Current Opinion in Pediatrics*, **11**, 457–63.

Ragab, A.-S. H., Stein, M. R. & Vietti, T. J. (1970). Severe complications in an infant due to sickle-cell trait. *Clinical Pediatrics*, **9**, 416–18.

Rickles, F. R. & O'Leary, D. S. (1974). Role of coagulation system in pathophysiology of sickle cell disease. *Archives of Internal Medicine*, **133**, 635–41.

Roberts, G. J., Haas, R. A. & King, F. M. (1973). Emergency-room crises in sickle-cell disease. *Lancet*, **i**, 1511.

Robertson, C. M., Stiller, C. A. & Kingston, J. E. (1992). Causes of death in children diagnosed with non-Hodgkin's lymphoma between 1974 and 1985. *Archives of Disease in Childhood*, **67**, 1378–83.

Rogers, D. W., Clarke, J. M., Cupidore, L., Ramlal, A. M., Sparke, B. R. & Serjeant, G. R. (1978). Early deaths in Jamaican children with sickle cell disease. *British Medical Journal*, **i**, 1515–16.

Rogers, J. & Brunt, E. N. (1992). Sudden death in a young woman with sickle cell anemia. *American Journal of Medicine*, **92**, 556–60.

Rose, V., Izukawa, T. & Moës, C. A. F. (1975). Syndromes of asplenia and polysplenia. A review of cardiac and non-cardiac malformations in 60 cases with special reference to diagnosis and prognosis. *British Heart Journal*, **37**, 840–52.

Ross, W. K., Newton, N. E. & Stivers, R. R. (1987). Sudden death due to thrombotic thrombocytopenic pupura. *American Journal of Forensic Medicine and Pathology*, **8**, 158–63.

Rubler, S. & Fleischer, R. A. (1967). Sickle cell states and cardiomyopathy. Sudden death due to pulmonary thrombosis and infarction. *American Journal of Cardiology*, **19**, 867–73.

Sateriale, M. & Hart, P. (1985). Unexpected death in a black military recruit with sickle cell trait: case report. *Military Medicine*, **150**, 602–5.

Schenk, E. A. (1964). Sickle cell trait and superior longitudinal sinus thrombosis. *Annals of Internal Medicine*, **60**, 465–70.

Schulz, E. V. (1969). Uber besondere falle von plotzlichem naturlichem tod im jugend – und erwachsenenalter. *Beitrage zur gerichtlichen Medizin*, **30**, 400–402.

Sears, D. A. (1978). The morbidity of sickle cell trait. A review of the literature. *American Journal of Medicine*, **64**, 1021–36.

Seeler, R. A. (1972). Deaths in children with sickle cell anemia. A clinical analysis of 19 fatal instances in Chicago. *Clinical Pediatrics*, **11**, 634–7.

Seeler, R. A. & Shwiaki, M. Z. (1972). Acute splenic sequestration crises (ASSC) in young children with sickle cell anemia. Clinical observations in 20 episodes in 14 children. *Clinical Pediatrics*, **11**, 701–4.

Seeler, R. A., Royal, J. E., Powe, L. & Goldbarg, H. R. (1978). Moyamoya in children with sickle cell anemia and cerebrovascular occlusion. *Journal of Pediatrics*, **93**, 808–10.

Segel, G. B. & Francis, C. A. (2000). Anticoagulant proteins in childhood venous and arterial thrombosis: a review. *Blood, Cells, Molecules and Diseases*, **26**, 540–60.

Sencer, S., Coulter-Knoff, A., Day, D., Foker, J., Thompson, T. & Burke, B. (1987). Splenic hemangioma with thrombocytopenia in a newborn. *Pediatrics*, **79**, 960–66.

Sheth, K. J., Swick, H. M. & Haworth, N. (1986). Neurological involvement in hemolytic-uremic syndrome. *Annals of Neurology*, **19**, 90–93.

Spach, M. S., Howell, D. A. & Harris, J. S. (1963). Myocardial infarction and multiple thromboses in a child with primary thrombocytosis. *Pediatrics*, **31**, 268–76.

Springate, C. S., II & Adelson, L. (1966). Sudden and unexpected death due to splenic rupture in infectious mononucleosis. *Medicine, Science and the Law*, **6**, 215–16.

Steinberg, A., Ish-Horowitcz, M., El-Peleg, O., Mor, J. & Branski, D. (1986). Stroke in a patient with hemolytic-uremic syndrome with a good outcome. *Brain & Development*, **8**, 70–72.

Stockman, J. A., Nigro, M. A., Mishkin, M. M. & Oski, F. A. (1972). Occlusion of large cerebral vessels in sickle-cell anemia. *New England Journal of Medicine*, **287**, 846–9.

Thomas, R. H. (2001). Hypercoagulability syndromes. *Archives of Internal Medicine*, **161**, 2433–9.

Topley, J. M., Rogers, D. W., Stevens, M. C. G. & Serjeant, G. R. (1981). Acute splenic sequestration and hypersplenism in the first five years in homozygous sickle cell disease. *Archives of Disease in Childhood*, **56**, 765–9.

Tuttle, A. H. & Koch, B. (1960). Clinical and hematological manifestations of hemoglobin CS disease in children. *Journal of Pediatrics*, **56**, 331–42.

Vellodi, A. & Bini, R. M. (1988). Malignant ventricular arrhythmias caused by hyperkalaemia complicating the Kasabach-Merritt syndrome. *Journal of the Royal Society of Medicine*, **81**, 167–8.

Verdú, A., Cazorla, M. R., Granados, M. A., Alonso, J. A. & Casado, L. F. (2001). Basilar artery thrombosis in a child heterozygous for factor V Leiden mutation. *Pediatric Neurology*, **24**, 69–71.

Vix, J., Buguet, A., Staboni, S. & Beidari, H. (1987). Sudden infant death syndrome and sickle cell anemia in Sahelian Africa. *Medecine Tropicale*, **47**, 153–9.

Vora, A. J. & Lilleyman, J. S. (1993). Secondary thrombocytosis. *Archives of Disease in Childhood*, **68**, 88–90.

Whybourne, A., Zillman, M. A., Miliauskas, J., & Byard, R. W. (2001). Sudden and unexpected infant death due to occult lymphoblastic leukaemia. *Journal of Clinical Forensic Medicine*, **8**, 160–62.

Winkelstein, J. A. & Drachman, R. H. (1968). Deficiency of pneumococcal serum opsonizing activity in sickle-cell disease. *New England Journal of Medicine*, **279**, 459–66.

Yamashita, M., Chin, I., Horigome, H., Umesato, Y. & Tsuchida, M. (1990). Sudden fatal cardiac arrest in a child with an unrecognised anterior mediastinal mass. *Resuscitation*, **19**, 175–7.

Young, R. S. K., Rannels, E., Hilmo, A., Gerson, J. M. & Goodrich, D. (1983). Severe anemia in childhood presenting as transient ischemic attacks. *Stroke*, **14**, 622–3.

Young, R. C., Jr, Castro, O., Baxter, R. P., *et al.* (1981). The lung in sickle cell disease: a clinical overview of common vascular, infectious, and other problems. *Journal of the National Medical Association*, **73**, 19–26.

Zimmerman, T. S. & Ruggeri, Z. M. (1987). Von Willebrand disease. *Human Pathology*, **18**, 140–52.

10

Gastrointestinal and genitourinary conditions

Gastrointestinal conditions

Introduction

Gastrointestinal causes of sudden and unexpected death in childhood, such as intussusception, volvulus, and small-intestinal obstruction, are uncommon (Jorgensen & Gregersen, 1990) (Table 10.1). As the clinical presentation of these disorders may be nonspecific, the diagnosis may not have been established prior to autopsy. However, the cause of death usually becomes obvious once the peritoneal cavity has been opened. Delay in diagnosis may be a particular problem in intellectually impaired children.

Gastroenteritis

Gastroenteritis resulting in dehydration and electrolyte imbalance may cause sudden death, particularly in early life. The causative agents are often viral infections, and the effects of fluid depletion may be exacerbated by hot weather and parental inattention (Whitehead *et al.*, 1996). Further discussion on the role of gastroenteritis in sudden death may be found in Chapter 4.

Intestinal obstruction

Acute intestinal obstruction in children may be caused by intussusception or volvulus, with rare lethal episodes resulting from electrolyte imbalance and intestinal perforation with sepsis. Obstruction may also be caused by incarcerated external or internal hernias, which may infarct (Figure 10.1). As obstruction causes a characteristic clinical picture of colicky abdominal pain and vomiting over some time, it is usually not considered a cause of unexpected death. However, occasional cases of bowel obstruction presenting in a fulminant manner have been reported (Pershad *et al.*, 1998; Powley, 1965; Pfalzgraf, Zumwalt & Kenny, 1988). In addition, cases are encountered occasionally in which either delay by parents in seeking treatment or the provision of inadequate medical treatment has resulted in early death. For example, in the following two cases, death occurred during or shortly after transfer from the country to a tertiary center: in the first case, a 17-month-old boy suddenly collapsed and died from peritonitis associated with ischemic necrosis of the small intestine due to obstruction from a congenital band (an example of which is shown in Figure 10.2); in the second case, a five-year-old girl died suddenly from dehydration due to small-bowel obstruction caused by postsurgical adhesions. Unfortunately, a simple change in management strategies may have altered the outcome in both cases.

Intussusception

Intussusception refers to telescoping of a proximal segment of intestine into the adjacent distal intestine (Figure 10.3). It is a major cause of bowel obstruction in childhood (DiFiore, 1999). Males are affected more often than females, with most cases occurring in infancy. While intussusception is rarely fatal, cases of unexpected death have been reported (Atkinson & Busuttil, 1994; Byard & Simpson, 2001). The

Table 10.1. Gastrointestinal causes of sudden pediatric death

Gastroenteritis
Intestinal obstruction
   Intussusception
   Volvulus
Acute gastric dilation and perforation
Intestinal perforation
Duplication cysts
Gastroesophageal reflux/aspiration
Late-presenting congenital diaphragmatic hernia
Gastrointestinal hemorrhage
Cystic fibrosis
Pancreatitis
Anorexia nervosa/malnutrition
Microvillus inclusion disease
Pickwickian syndrome

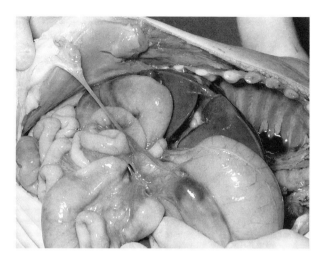

Figure 10.2 An intestinal band that had caused bowel obstruction on several occasions in a three-month-old boy.

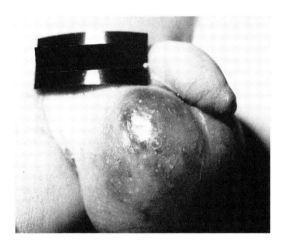

Figure 10.1 Swelling of the scrotum due to an incarcerated and infarcted small-intestinal hernia that resulted in the death of a young infant.

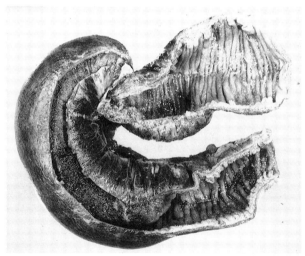

Figure 10.3 A typical case of intussusception in which the specimen has been opened to reveal distension and mottling of the distal intestine (the intussuscepiens), which has enveloped the invaginated portion of proximal intestine (the intussusceptum).

presenting features are usually abdominal pain, vomiting, rectal bleeding, or an abdominal mass (Pollack & Pender, 1991). However, symptoms may be absent or quite subtle, making diagnosis difficult, with 13–20% of affected children presenting as "painless intussusception," having no significant abdominal pain or discomfort (Pollack & Pender, 1991; Stringer, Pledger & Drake, 1992).

Intussusception may be caused by local structures, conditions, or diseases, including hyperplastic Peyer patches, Meckel diverticulum, duplication cysts, surgical suture lines, the appendix, mesenteric cysts, omphalomesenteric duct abnormalities, mesenteric defects, polyps, neoplasms, and mural hematomas (Ein, 1976; Little & Danzl, 1991; Ong & Beasley, 1990; St-Vil *et al.*, 1991). Most cases are ileocolic, with ileo-ileal, jejunojejunal, and colocolic occurring less often (Alford & McIlhenny, 1992). In addition, intussusception may be a manifestation of more generalized conditions, including cystic fibrosis, Henoch–Schönlein purpura, hemophilia, and hematopoetic malignancy (Ein & Stephens, 1971; Ein *et al.*, 1986; Holmes *et al.*, 1991; Lipsett & Byard, 1995). Accuracy of diagnosis is important to enable genetic counselling of the family, as some of these conditions may be inherited.

If the presenting symptoms are relatively non-specific, then there is a possibility that intussusception will remain undetected, allowing progression to intestinal infarction from vascular compromise. In these rare cases, there may be precipitate clinical deterioration, with unexpected death secondary to the development of septicemia. Two fatal cases of ileo-ileal and ileocolic intussusception are illustrated in Figures 10.4 and 10.5, respectively, in two infants aged five and six months, respectively, both of whom presented with sudden collapse and death following non-specific symptoms and signs attributed incorrectly to minor upper respiratory tract infection.

Autopsy examination of cases of fatal intussusception includes determination of the level of the obstruction and identification of any local or more generalized precipitating factors. Blood cultures are useful in demonstrating sepsis, and vitreous humor electrolyte measurements may reveal dehydration. Careful assessment of the presenting history is also required to determine the quality of both domestic and medical care received by the child during the terminal illness (Byard & Simpson, 2001).

A comment should be made regarding agonal intussusception. This is an unrelated and incidental finding at autopsy in infants that should be distinguished clearly from the above situation. It is believed to be caused by terminal intestinal dysmotility and peristaltic incoordination and is not a rare finding. There is no evidence of vascular obstruction, disseminated sepsis, intestinal infarction, or obstruc-

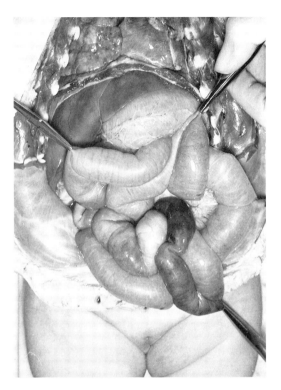

Figure 10.4 A necrotic segment of distal ileum associated with an ileo-ileal intussusception in a five-month-old girl who suddenly developed respiratory distress and died.

tion, and the bowel appears quite viable (Figure 10.6). Although agonal intussusception has been held responsible for death (Cox, 1997), the author finds it difficult to justify this conclusion in the absence of plausible lethal mechanisms.

Volvulus

This is a rare event in childhood that may involve any portion of the gastrointestinal tract, from the stomach to the sigmoid colon. Children with gastric or small-intestinal volvulus may present with bilious vomiting; however, clinical symptoms may be non-specific with volvulus of the large intestine (Andersen, Eklöf & Thomasson, 1981), leading to a delay in treatment. In most cases, the predisposing factors are unknown, although unusually long loops of colon, intestinal duplication cysts, mesenteric cysts and defects, and chronic constipation have been reported (Byard, 2000; Campbell & Blank, 1974; Wong & Gardner, 1992). Volvulus may also complicate meconium ileus in patients with cystic fibrosis. Death may occur very rapidly in a child with volvulus (Wong & Gardner, 1992) due to vascular compromise of the twisted bowel with ischemic necrosis and resultant septicemia.

Figure 10.7 demonstrates a dilated and dusky-appearing colon caused by a right-sided colonic volvulus in a seven-week-old boy who had appeared quite well several hours before he was found moribund in his crib. His only significant past history was of minimal episodic vomiting after feeding in the preceding two weeks of life. Blood, cerebrospinal fluid, and lung cultures all grew *Clostridium perfringens*.

Acute gastric dilation and perforation

Acute gastric dilation with infarction or rupture is a rare condition occurring mainly in adults and associated with a wide variety of predisposing factors, including excessive eating, air swallowing, ingestion of sodium bicarbonate, and pregnancy (Abdu, Garritano & Culver, 1987; Byard, Couper & Cohle, 2001; Lazebnik, Iellin & Michowitz, 1986; Wharton *et al.*, 1997). Gastric rupture may also be due to trauma and has occurred following cardiopulmonary resuscitation, the Heimlich maneuver, and inflicted injury (Reiger *et al.*, 1997; Schechner & Ehrlich, 1974; van der Ham & Lange, 1990). Even with surgical treatment a mortality rate of 65% in adults has been reported.

Gastric dilation with rupture may also occur in individuals with cerebral palsy (Figures 10.8–10.10), possibly related to air swallowing due to neuromuscular incoordination, and autonomic neuropathy. In these cases malposition of the stomach may prevent spontaneous decompression, and as assessment of the clinical status may be difficult, symptoms and signs may not be obvious until terminal stages have been reached (Byard & Couper, 2001). Death in children with severe spastic quadraparesis following gastric distention and/or rupture may be due to a combination of respiratory compromise and

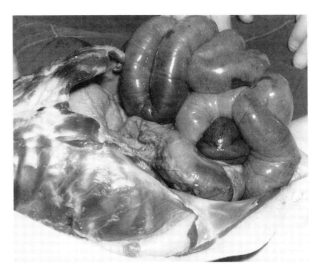

Figure 10.5 Marked intestinal dilation with necrosis of the distal ileum was the first indication of an ileocolic intussusception in this six-month-old girl who died suddenly en route to hospital after blood was noted in her diaper.

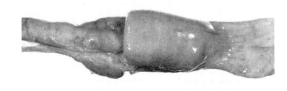

Figure 10.6 Agonal intussusception unrelated to the cause of death in a young child.

sepsis (Byard, Couper & Cohle, 2001; Del Beccaro, McLaughlin & Polage, 1991). Ingested foreign bodies are another possible cause of gastric perforation in intellectually impaired children (Byard, 1996). Individuals with Prader–Willi syndrome may develop acute gastric dilation due to a combination of excessive appetite, reduced vomiting, and high pain thresholds (Wharton *et al.*, 1997).

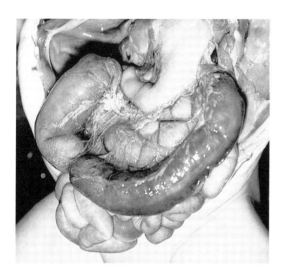

Figure 10.7 Colonic dilation due to a right-sided volvulus in a seven-week-old boy who had appeared quite well prior to being put to bed. Blood, cerebraspinal fluid, and lung cultures all grew *Clostridium perfringens*.

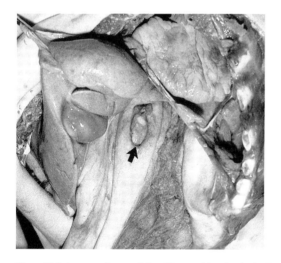

Figure 10.8 A ruptured stomach in a 20-year-old male who had severe spastic quadraparesis and mental retardation. The liver and gallbladder have been lifted to one side to better expose the defect (arrow). The deceased had presented with marked gastric dilation and at autopsy there was 1500 ml of dark brown fluid and food material within the peritoneal cavity (see also Figures 10.9 and 10.10).

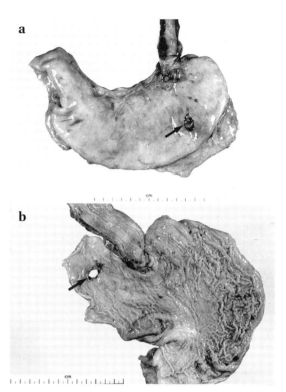

Figure 10.9 Eviscerated stomach from the patient illustrated in Figure 10.8, demonstrating the defect in the unopened (a) and opened (b) stomach (arrows).

Intestinal perforation

Non-traumatic perforation of the intestine may result from ischemic necrosis due to mechanical obstruction, or from localized inflammation, such as that associated with acute appendicitis (Arey & Sotos, 1956). Alternatively, traumatic perforation may occur from objects that have been ingested (Byard, 1996).

Perforation with fulminant sepsis may also occur in children with distension of the bowel from impacted material, such as in untreated Hirschprung disease (Figure 10.11) or with trichobezoars (hair balls) in the Rapunzel syndrome. Trichobezoars (Figure 10.12) may extend from the stomach or proximal small intestine into the colon. This

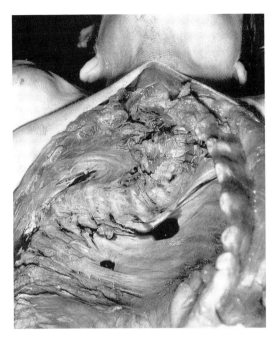

Figure 10.10 Marked kyphoscoliosis in the case illustrated in Figures 10.8 and 10.9 caused severe deformation of both the pleural and peritoneal cavities.

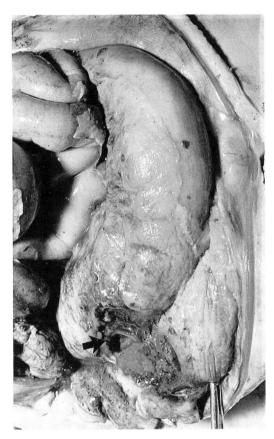

Figure 10.11 Markedly dilated descending colon with distal perforation (arrow) in a fatal case of untreated Hirschprung disease.

condition is named after Rapunzel, a young woman with particularly long tresses who was a character in a Grimm Brothers' fairytale. In contrast to Rapunzel's golden tresses, the hair forming bezoars becomes blackened (Vaughan, Sawyers & Scott, 1968). Perforation is believed to result from pressure necrosis of the distended bowel wall from the impacted material and is associated with a mortality rate of 83%. The clinical symptoms may be non-specific, particularly in intellectually impaired children (Avissar, Goldberg & Lernau, 1994). Unexpected cardiac arrest and death due to duodenal perforation during medical treatment have been reported in a 14-year-old girl with a trichobezoar that extended from the stomach into the transverse colon (Deslypere, Praet & Verdonk, 1982).

Other causes of intestinal perforation in infancy and childhood include necrotizing enterocolitis, der-matomyositis, Ehlers–Danlos syndrome, and congenital absence of small-intestinal musculature.

Duplication cysts

Intestinal duplication cysts are developmental defects that arise when the foregut and notochord separate incompletely. They may be single or multiple and have been associated with intestinal obstruction. Although it is possible that sudden death may occur following the development of intussusception or volvulus, this is extremely rare (Byard 2000; Byard

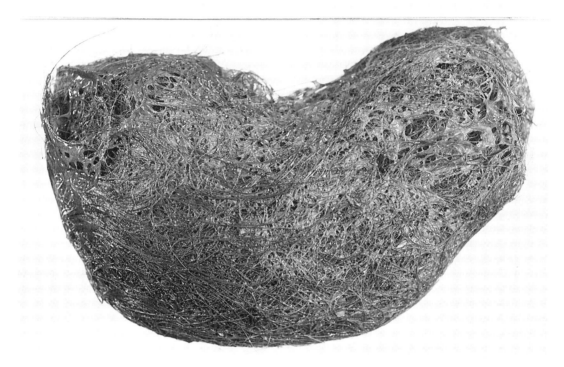

Figure 10.12 A large gastric bezoar composed of malodorous matted hair from a young girl retained the shape of the stomach after removal.

& Simpson, 2001). Neonatal respiratory distress has been caused by duplication cysts of the esophagus (Stewart, Bruce & Beasley, 1993).

Gastroeosophageal reflux/aspiration

Mechanisms by which gastroesophageal reflux might cause sudden death in infancy such as reflex apnea, bradycardia, and anaphylaxis are discussed in Chapter 13.

The contribution of gastric aspiration to sudden death in other cases is often difficult to determine, since reflux of stomach contents has been produced experimentally within cadavers (Gardner, 1958) and may also occur as an agonal event in a variety of disorders (Knight, 1975). While large amounts of food within the major airways extending into the smaller air passages are compatible with a lethal episode of airway obstruction due to gastric aspiration, clinico-pathological correlation is required before this can be accepted as a cause of death (Arey & Sotos, 1956). Histories of sudden collapse while vomiting, of swallowing incoordination in cerebral palsy, or of mental retardation may lend weight to the possibility of genuine aspiration (Einfeld *et al.*, 1987). A history of acute alcohol intoxication may also be present in adolescents. Gastric aspiration becomes more plausible if other causes of death have been excluded, although it may be hard to accept as a cause of death in a previously apparently healthy child with no known neurologic impairments or illnesses unless it is florid.

Concerns were raised initially that the recommendation of supine sleeping position for infants would result in an increase in deaths due to gastric aspiration, but this has not occurred. In fact, a study of 196 cases of infant and early childhood deaths under the age of three years found only three cases where death had been attributed to aspiration, and these were all in infants and young children who were sleeping face down (Byard & Beal, 2000).

Occasionally, a bolus of solid food may be found lodged within the airway or esophagus in cases of sudden childhood death. A large portion of sausage (Figure 10.13) retrieved from the esophagus of a 19-month-old child who collapsed suddenly while eating his lunch at a childcare center demonstrates this phenomenon (Byard, 1994). Similarities in predisposing factors to café coronary such as inadequate dentition, underappreciation of appropriate food bolus size, and failure to chew food adequately has caused this event in childcare centers to be termed "crèche coronary."

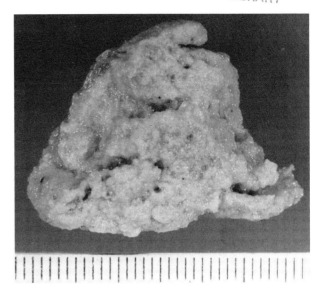

Figure 10.13 A large portion of partially chewed sausage retrieved from the esophagus of a 19-month-old boy who collapsed and died while eating (scale = mm).

Late-presenting congenital diaphragmatic hernia

Embryology

The diaphragm forms during intrauterine life from fusion of tissue aggregates that line the pleuroperitoneal canal. Failure of complete fusion leaves a hiatus through which the intestinal organs may herniate, resulting in interference with lung growth (Kluth *et al.*, 1989). Most herniae occur on the left posterolateral aspect of the diaphragm through the foramen of Bochdalek and usually lead to clinical presentation within hours of birth.

Clinical features

Affected infants usually show symptoms and signs of marked respiratory distress due to lung compression and pulmonary hypoplasia, exacerbated by persistant fetal circulation (Cullen, Klein & Philippart, 1985). These infants often have a scaphoid abdomen. However, occasional children do not present classically, either because a membrane covers the defect preventing intestinal herniation or because the defect has been plugged by one of the abdominal organs such as the spleen (Lynch, Adkins & Wiener, 1982). These children are at risk of developing herniation at a later age, sometimes even delayed until adulthood.

Children with diaphragmatic herniae presenting after the neonatal period are usually considered to have an excellent prognosis, responding well to surgical repair (Hight *et al.*, 1982; Storm, Gisbertz & Steiger, 1987). While this is generally true, occasional children may suffer a precipitate clinical deterioration with sudden death (Byard, Bourne & Cockington, 1991; Byard *et al.*, 1990; Chhanabhai, Avis & Hutton, 1995). Clinical symptoms and signs in the late-presenting group tend to be non-specific, often resulting in misdiagnosis. Presenting problems include failure to thrive, recurrent chest infections, episodic dyspnea, diarrhea, constipation, vomiting, dysphagia, and colicky upper-abdominal pain. On occasion, thoracentesis has been performed due to a mistaken clinical diagnosis of pneumothorax (Berman *et al.*, 1988).

Table 10.2. Clinicopathological features of six cases of late-presenting congenital diaphragmatic hernias with sudden death

Case	Age	Sex	Initial presentation	Clinical diagnosis	Autopsy findings
1	2 months	M	"Colic"	SIDS	2-cm defect in left diaphragm
2	3 months	M	Vomiting	Croup	3-cm defect in left diaphragm
3	4 months	M	Irritability	Cardiac arrest	3-cm defect in left diaphragm
4	2 years	F	"Flu" with vomiting – 1 day	–	No autopsy, CXR hernia, left diaphragm
5	4 years	M	Lethargy, vomiting, abdominal pain – 2 days	Otitis media	4-cm defect in left diaphragm
6	13 years	F	Abdominal pain – 1 week, vomiting – 1 day	Gastroenteritis	Postsurgical hernia repair, left diaphragm

Table 10.2 lists the clinicopathological features of six children who suffered unexpected cardiac arrest caused by gut herniation through unsuspected diaphragmatic hernias. These cases further demonstrate the diversity of presenting symptoms, signs, and clinical diagnoses, the latter including croup, otitis media, and SIDS. In four children, the diagnosis was not suspected until autopsy, a feature that

has been noted in other series (Booker, Meerstadt & Bush, 1981). In some cases, the clinical symptoms of coughing or vomiting have been due to an unrelated respiratory or gastrointestinal disorder that preceded, and most likely initiated, herniation by increasing intra-abdominal pressure on the diaphragmatic defect (Byard *et al.*, 1990). A case has also been reported of a 19-year-old female who was 25 weeks

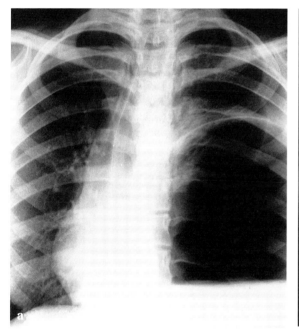 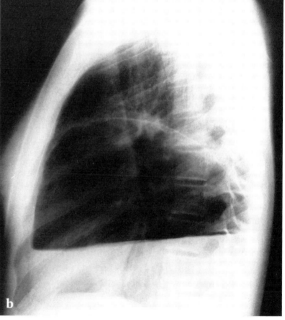

Figure 10.14 Marked mediastinal deviation to the right in a 13-year-old girl who presented with relatively non-specific symptoms prior to terminal collapse from a late-presenting diaphragmatic hernia (a). The lateral radiograph demonstrates clearly the fluid level in the grossly distended stomach within the left pleural cavity (b) (Case 6 in Table 10.2).

pregnant and who died after her intestinal contents herniated through a congenital diaphragmatic defect (Browning, 1973).

Pathological features

At autopsy, the usual finding is of small- and large-intestinal herniation into the chest cavity (Color Plate 22) through relatively small diaphragmatic defects (Color Plates 23 and 24). This causes considerable mediastinal shift, usually to the right, as can be seen in the chest radiograph from the 13-year-old girl described in Table 10.2 (Figure 10.14). Atelectasis of the ipsilateral lung occurs, and a complicating factor may be massive gastric dilation (Figure 10.15).

Pathophysiology

While the usual mechanism of death is similar to that of untreated tension pneumothorax, cases with a more prolonged course may develop ischemic necrosis of the herniated segments of intestine with perforation and sepsis (Figure 10.16).

Gastrointestinal hemorrhage

Massive hemorrhage from the gastrointestinal tract during childhood may result from systemic disease or from localized lesions. Terminal hemorrhage into the bowel is seen occasionally in malignant disease, particularly in leukemias and lymphomas, but it is usually the final manifestation of a generalized decline with multiorgan failure.

Brisk hemorrhage may result from upper-gastrointestinal peptic ulcer disease in children who require emergency surgery. In contrast, the bleeding associated with ulcers due to heterotopic gastric mucosa in a Meckel diverticulum tends to be less florid. Both hemorrhage from and perforation of peptic ulcers may result in death in childhood (Seagram, Stephens & Cumming, 1973).

Esophageal varices may cause fatal hemorrhage in children with portal hypertension (Color Plate 25), and an unusual variant of the Mallory–Weiss phenomenon has been described in a young adult with esophageal varices due to congenital portal vein

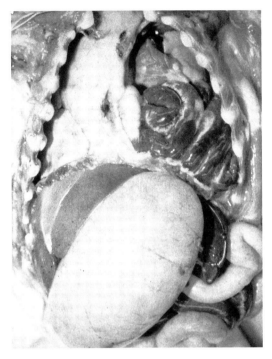

Figure 10.15 Marked dilation of the stomach may be found in cases of late-presenting diaphragmatic hernias, which exacerbates respiratory difficulties.

atresia (Bramwell & Byard, 1989). The young woman, who had recently received sclerotherapy, collapsed and died due to hemorrhage into the chest cavity from a linear tear in the external wall of the esophagus following vomiting (Figure 10.17).

Profuse gastrointestinal hemorrhage may also complicate arteriovenous malformations such as those found in Osler–Weber–Rendu syndrome and angiodysplasia, although significant hemorrhage is not usually a problem until later in life (Byard, Schliebs & Koszyca, 2001).

Cystic fibrosis

Cystic fibrosis is an autosomal recessive disorder caused by a defect in the cystic fibrosis transmembrane conductance regulator (CFTR) gene located on the long arm of chromosome 7. Over 1000 unique mutations have been reported (Brennan & Geddes,

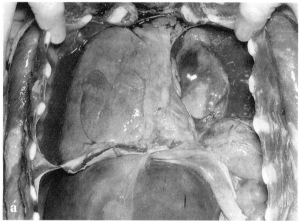

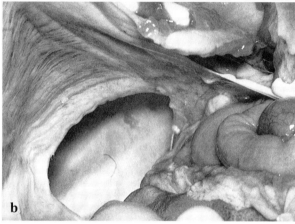

Figure 10.16 Perforation of the stomach (a), which had herniated through a small left-sided diaphragmatic hernia (b), resulted in fulminant sepsis in a four-year-old boy.

2002; Riordan *et al.*, 1989; Rommens *et al.*, 1989). The defect results in increased viscosity of exocrine secretions, with particularly severe effects noted in the pancreas, liver, gastrointestinal tract, and lungs. Major pulmonary problems are caused by recurrent and persistent bacterial and fungal infections, which result in progressive bronchiectasis and destruction of lung parenchyma. Common infections involve bacteria such as *Staphylococcus aureus*, *Hemophilus influenzae*, and *Pseudomonas aeruginosa* (Brennan & Geddes, 2002).

Occurrence of sudden death

Sudden and unexpected death may occur in the neonatal period due to intestinal volvulus, infarction, and perforation from meconium ileus, or later in life due to electrolyte imbalance and dehydration. Affected children are particularly vulnerable to dehydration during hot weather as they lose excessive amounts of sodium in their sweat (Morales, Kulesh & Valdes-Dapena, 1984). Occasional children may present with collapse in hot weather before the diagnosis has been established clinically. Thus, the presence of inspissated secretions within the intestinal mucosal, pancreatic, and salivary glands at autopsy may be the first indication of the diagnosis (Figures 10.18 and 10.19).

Figure 10.20 shows a volvulus in a 11-day-old infant who died unexpectedly following a short history of vomiting and drawing up of the knees. The autopsy findings were of small intestinal volvulus with infarction associated with meconium ileus and inspissation of secretions characteristic of cystic fibrosis within the remainder of the bowel, pancreas, and submandibular gland.

Pancreatitis

Acute pancreatitis is rare in childhood, although sudden death associated with pancreatitis has been reported in a 10-year-old steroid-dependent asthmatic, most likely related to prednisone intake (Richards & Patrick, 1965). Unexpected death with acute pancreatitis, not always related to steroid therapy (Tada *et al.*, 1982), has also been reported in other infants and children (Marczynska-Robowska, 1957).

Anorexia nervosa/malnutrition

It is probable that only a pathologist would classify anorexia nervosa as a gastrointestinal disorder. However, while this eating disorder is obviously of psychiatric origin, the physical changes and causes of sudden death result from chronic undernutrition. A lethal outcome has been reported in 10–20% of cases, with the exact mechanism of death remaining obscure in some cases even after the performance of an autopsy (Bruch 1971; Cooke *et al.*, 1994).

Clinical features

As noted by Sir William Gull in 1874, the usual clinical course is one of relapsing episodes of food refusal, most often in adolescent girls, associated with a marked reduction in body weight.

Occurrence of sudden death

Rarely, sudden death has been described in emaciated anorexic patients due to cardiac arrhythmia, most likely associated with diet-induced prolongation of the QT interval (Cooke *et al.*, 1994; Isner *et al.*, 1985; Thurston & Marks, 1974). Similar electrocardiographic (ECG) changes have been observed in other forms of malnutrition (Isner *et al.*, 1979). While the ECG changes may occur in the absence of electrolyte disturbance, abnormal potassium levels from vomiting or laxative abuse may exacerbate myocardial irritability. Cardiac size is also reduced in patients with anorexia nervosa (Gottdiener *et al.*, 1978). Rarely, death may result from sudden severe hypoglycemia or sepsis (Ratcliffe & Bevan, 1985; Rich *et al.*, 1990; Warren & Vande Wiele, 1973). Fatal gastric necrosis and rupture have also been reported in girls with eating disorders following an excessive intake of food ("binge" eating) (Abdu, Garritano & Culver, 1987).

Microvillus inclusion disease

Microvillus inclusion disease is characterized by severe secretory diarrhea presenting soon after birth and worsened by oral feeding (Davidson *et al.*, 1978). The etiology is uncertain, but there appears to be disturbance of cytoskeletal function within intestinal mucosal cells, with failure of transport of plasma membrane proteins (Cutz *et al.*, 1989). Familial cases occur with an autosomal recessive mode of inheritance, although the gene locus has not yet been identified (Candy *et al.*, 1981). While the clinical course is usually chronic, with rare cases showing improvement over time (Croft *et al.*, 2000), respiratory distress and severe metabolic acidosis may

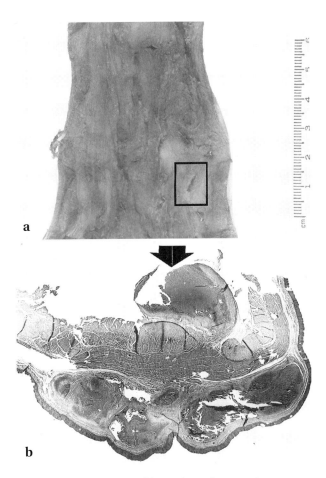

Figure 10.17 External surface of the esophagus demonstrating a linear tear in a 20-year-old woman with esophageal varices following congenital portal vein atresia (a). The tear corresponds to a defect visible in a dilated adventitial vein (arrow) (b), which was responsible for her sudden death by exsanguination (hematoxylin and eosin, ×9).

develop precipitately in previously stable neonates (Byard *et al.*, 1992), and sudden death has occurred rarely.

Histologically, there may be difficulties in demonstrating the characteristic features of diffuse thinning of the small-intestinal mucosa, with villus atrophy, crypt hypoplasia, and disorganization of surface enterocytes in postmortem material. Ultrastructural examination is essential for confirmation of the

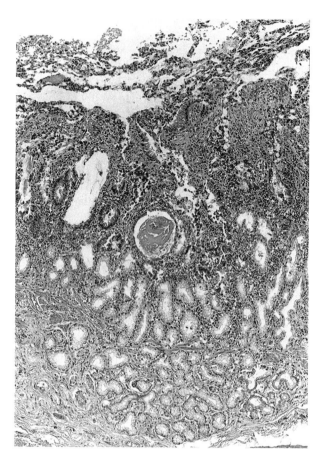

Figure 10.18 Inspissated mucus within duodenal crypts suggestive of cystic fibrosis (hematoxylin and eosin, ×110).

diagnosis, with electron microscopy showing increased numbers of apical electron-dense secretory granules in enterocytes with typical microvillus inclusions (Figure 10.21) (Byard *et al.*, 1992; Cutz *et al.*, 1989). Again, this may not be possible if there has been postmortem tissue breakdown.

Pickwickian syndrome

Extreme obesity may be associated rarely with alveolar hypoventilation, somnolence, secondary polycythemia, cyanosis, cor pulmonale, and right ventricular hypertrophy (MacGregor, Block & Ball, 1970). Termed the "Pickwickian syndrome" after the

Table 10.3. Genitourinary causes of sudden pediatric death

Primary renal disease
Urinary tract obstruction
Wilms tumor
  Hemorrhage
  Embolism
Hemolytic-uremic syndrome
Ovarian torsion
Complications of pregnancy
  Pulmonary thromboembolism
  Eclampsia with intracerebral hemorrhage
  Ruptured ectopic/intraperitoneal pregnancy
  Amniotic fluid embolism
  Placenta previa/accreta
  Peripartum cardiomyopathy
  Air embolism
  Sepsis
  Metastatic choriocarcinoma

obese boy in Dicken's *Pickwick Papers*, it has caused sudden death from cardiorespiratory failure in children as young as six years of age (Jenab *et al.*, 1959).

Genitourinary conditions

Primary renal disease

Although diseases of the urinary tract in children have been cited as causes of sudden death (Table 10.3), detailed clinicopathologic information on affected children is generally not available (Canby & Jaffurs, 1963; Rabson, 1949). The author has one case, that of a six-year-old girl who presented with a one-day history of vomiting and who died of acute renal failure within hours. At autopsy, the kidneys were pale, and microscopy revealed hypercellular glomeruli typical of acute proliferative glomerulonephritis.

Sudden death may result rarely from a hypertensive crisis in children with chronic renal insufficiency, and may also occur in apparently stable children with nephrotic syndrome due to marked hyponatremia resulting from a combination of salt restriction,

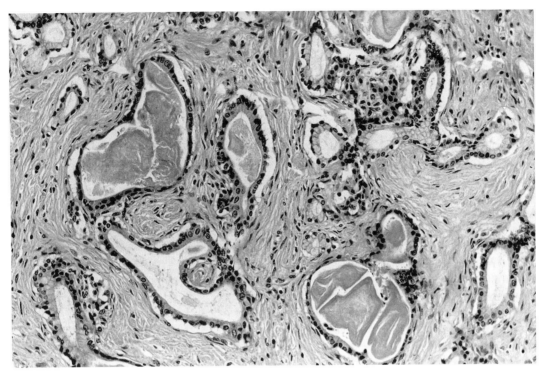

Figure 10.19 Characteristic inspissated eosinophilic concretions with fibrous scarring of the pancreas in a five-year-old boy with occult cystic fibrosis who collapsed after being left in a motor vehicle cabin for a number of hours (hematoxylin and eosin, ×140).

vomiting, and hot weather (Hagge, Burke & Stickler, 1967). Vitreous electrolyte levels are mandatory in such cases.

Urinary tract obstruction

Untreated urinary tract obstruction usually results in progressive loss of renal function with associated symptoms and signs of chronic renal failure. However, occasional cases may have the diagnosis made at autopsy following precipitate clinical deterioration. Male infants with posterior urethral valves may also present in this manner (Figure 10.22).

Wilms tumor

Wilms tumor or nephroblastoma, a primary tumor of the kidney, is the most common childhood malignancy, arising in one in 10,000 children under the age of 15 years. Most cases occur before the age of four years, and there is an association with aniridia, trisomy syndromes, urogenital anomalies, and hemihypertrophy in the Beckwith–Wiedeman, Frasier, WAGR (Wilms tumor, aniridia, genitourinary malformations, and mental retardation) and Denys–Drash syndromes. Familial, multifocal, and bilateral cases occur. The genetic background is complex, with WT1 and WT2 representing the first two Wilms tumor genes identified on chromosomes 11p13 and 11p15, respectively. FWT1 and FWT2 are additional familial Wilms tumor loci on chromosomes 17q and 19q, and further abnormalites have been identified in chromosomes 1p, 7p, and 16q, suggesting that these sites may also be involved. Mutations have also been found in beta-catenin, a cellular adhesion protein involved in the genesis of

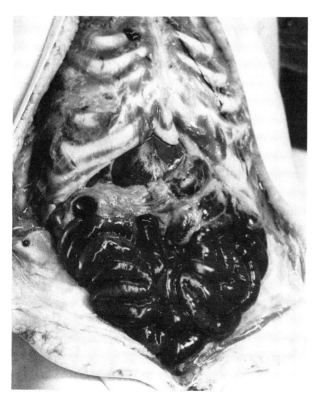

Figure 10.20 Intestinal infarction following a small-intestinal volvulus in an infant with cystic fibrosis and meconium ileus.

other malignancies (Dome & Coppes, 2002; McLorie, 2001).

While the prognosis of treated Wilms tumor is usually very good, sudden and unexpected death may occur due to secondary hemorrhage or to tumor embolism. Massive hemorrhage from a Wilms tumor may occur into the parenchyma of the tumor itself or into the adjacent retroperitoneal tissues and abdominal cavity. Hypovolemic shock may ensue, followed by death, if fluid replacement and urgent surgery are not undertaken. Figure 10.23 illustrates a Wilms tumor with extensive intraparenchymal hemorrhage in an infant who died of shock. Hemorrhage may result from erosion of the tumor into vessels, and may be exacerbated by an accompanying consumption coagulopathy secondary to disseminated intravascular coagulation.

Embolization of tumor fragments is a particular problem in Wilms tumor due to its angioinvasive qualities (Zakowski, Edwards & McDonough, 1990). Figure 10.24 shows a sectioned Wilms tumor that had invaded the adjacent inferior vena cava and embolized to the main pulmonary trunk in a three-year-old girl. Portions of necrotic tumor may lodge more distally in branches of the pulmonary arteries, and paradoxical embolization may occur if there is communication between the right and left sides of the heart. Figure 10.25 illustrates cerebral infarction in an eight-year-old boy due to a paradoxical tumor embolus that had passed through a ventricular septal defect (Moore & Byard, 1992).

Hemolytic-uremic syndrome

Hemolytic-uremic syndrome is characterized by an acute onset of microangiopathic hemolytic anemia, thrombocytopenia, and renal insufficiency caused by a systemic thrombotic microangiopathy (Gallo & Gianantonio, 1995). It often follows an infectious illness such as gastrointestinal infection with verotoxin-producing *Escherichia coli* (most commonly 0157:H7), but it has also been linked to drugs, tumors, other infectious agents, and immunization (although the latter association is speculative) (Gianantonio *et al.*, 1973; Manton, Smith & Byard, 2000). Children under the age of five years are at particular risk. The mechanism of tissue injury remains obscure, with endotoxemia being proposed as the initiating event (Richardson *et al.*, 1988).

Most patients recover, although a small percentage develop chronic renal disease or relapse (Habib *et al.*, 1982). Central nervous system manifestations such as respiratory deregulation, seizures, and coma may result from vascular thrombosis, systemic hypertension, or metabolic derangements such as hypocalcemia and hyponatremia (Sheth, Swick & Haworth, 1986). Death occurs in as many as 10% of cases. Robson, Leung & Montgomery (1991) have attributed death to central nervous system complications (47%), uncertain causes (16%), shock and sepsis (12%), cardiovascular complications (6%), gastrointestinal complications (6%), and iatrogenic causes

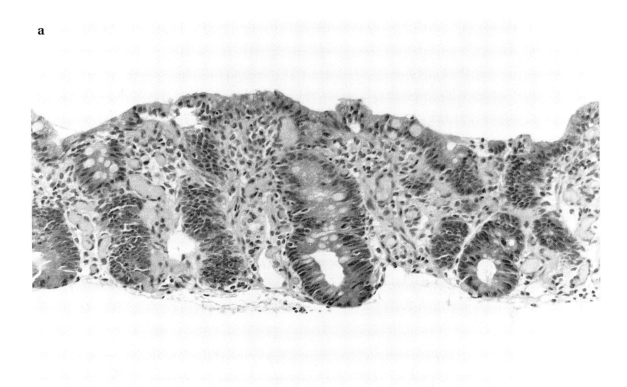

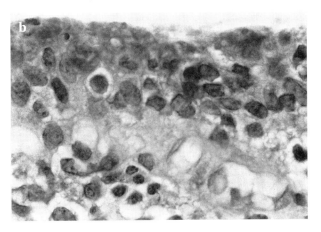

Figure 10.21 Biopsy material from a case of microvillus inclusion disease showing thinning of the small-intestinal mucosa with villus atrophy and crypt hypoplasia. There was no increase in inflammatory cells within the lamina propria (a) (hematoxylin and eosin, ×180). Higher power of the mucosa in an affected individual (b) showed surface enterocyte disorganization contrasting with normal duodenal mucosa (c) (hematoxylin and eosin, ×800). Ultrastructural examination demonstrated reduction in surface microvilli, with a characteristic intracytoplasmic inclusion (d) (×14 000).

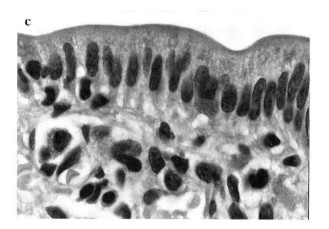

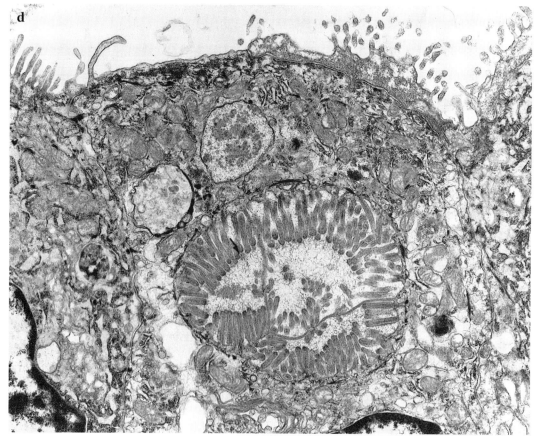

Figure 10.21 (cont.)

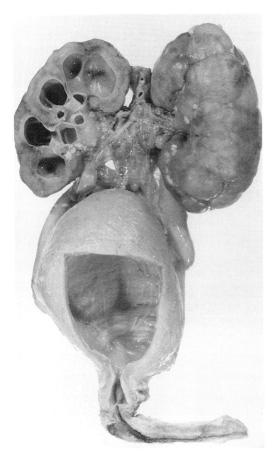

Figure 10.22 Hypertrophied bladder with bilateral hydroureteronephroses due to posterior urethral valves in a four-month-old boy. His final presentation was of fulminant metabolic acidosis with death within 12 hours, which was attributed to probable meningitis before autopsy.

(6%). While sudden death is uncommon, it may result from myocarditis, cardiomyopathy, epilepsy, or intracranial hemorrhagic infarction (Abu-Arafeh *et al.*, 1995; Crisp *et al.*, 1981; Manton, Smith & Byard, 2000) (Figure 10.26).

Ovarian torsion

Torsion and infarction of ovaries is a well-recognized although rare cause of sudden death in neonates and infants. Massive hemorrhage into cystic ovarian

tissue may occur, as may intraoperative rupture (Alrabeeah *et al.*, 1988). Predisposing factors include ovarian cysts and neoplasms, hydro- or pyosalpinx, long or redundant fallopian tubes, and abdominal trauma. Torsion involves both the ovary and adjacent fallopian tube rotating on their attachments and is usually unilateral (Havlik & Nolte, 2002). It has also been suggested that pain in the absense of rupture or infarction might precipitate reflex apnea or bradycardia, with lethal consequences (Kasian *et al.*, 1986).

Complications of pregnancy

As a number of the complications of pregnancy may result in unexpected death, evidence of pregnancy should be sought in all sexually mature females who die suddenly. The possibility of an illegal abortion should also be considered. Sudden death during pregnancy may be due to conditions that are unique to pregnancy, although some of these disorders tend to be more of a problem in older mothers. Amniotic fluid or air embolism, rupture of an ectopic or intraperitoneal pregnancy, hemorrhage from uterine rupture, placenta previa or placenta accreta,

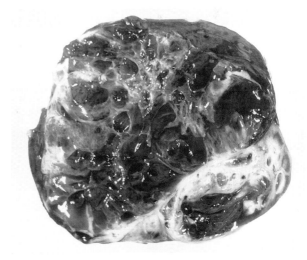

Figure 10.23 Extensive intraparenchymal hemorrhage into a cystic congenital Wilms tumor resulted in sudden death.

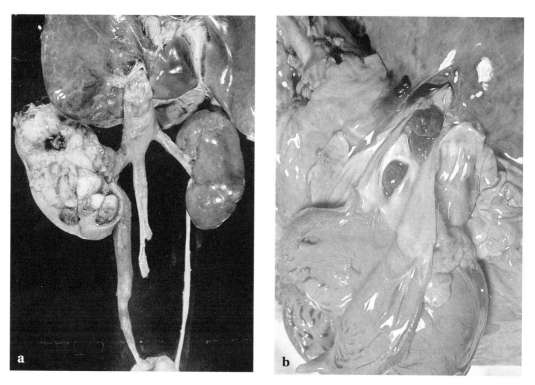

Figure 10.24 Wilms tumor extending along the renal vein into the inferior vena cava (a), with sudden death in a three-year-old girl due to a saddle tumor embolism blocking the pulmonary outflow tract (b).

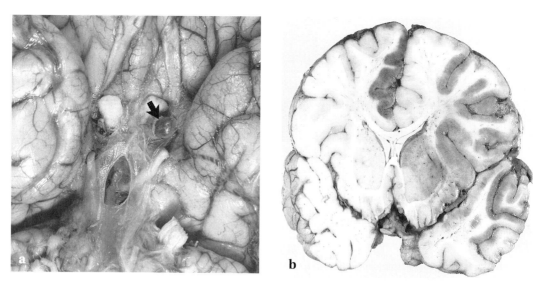

Figure 10.25 Base of the brain in an eight-year-old boy who died postoperatively following attempted resection of a large Wilms tumor. A portion of tumor that had paradoxically embolized through a ventricular septal defect can be seen protruding from the left middle cerebral artery (arrow) (a). Coronal section of the brain revealing recent infarcts in the areas of the left middle cerebral and right anterior cerebral arteries due to Wilms tumor emboli (b).

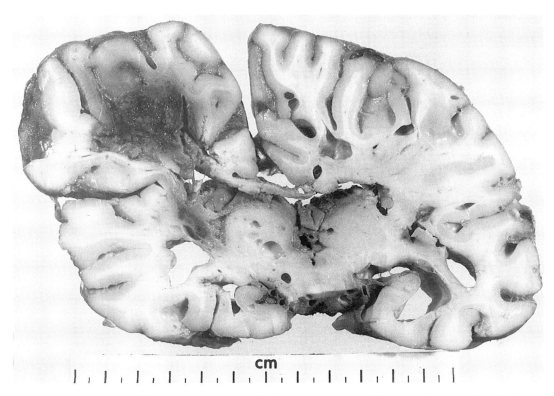

Figure 10.26 Coronal section of the brain from a four-year-old girl showed hemorrhagic infarction of the posterior frontal lobe due to hemolytic-uremic syndrome associated with verocytotoxin-producing *Escherichia coli.*

peripartum cardiomyopathy, metastatic choriocarcinoma, and intracerebral hemorrhage associated with eclampsia may all be associated with sudden and unexpected death (Biller & Adams, 1986; Clark & McMillan, 1974; Filkins, Kalelkar & Chambliss, 1998; Gibb, 1990; Gravanis & Ansari, 1987; Jehle, Krause & Braen, 1994; Lau, 1994; Matthews, McCowan & Patten 1996; Maymon & Fejgin, 1990).

Pregnancy may also exacerbate underlying conditions, such as cardiac valvular disease, aortic coarctation, epilepsy, connective tissue disorders, and cerebral aneurysms or arteriovenous malformations, and should be avoided in cases of Marfan syndrome with significant aortic root or aortic valve involvement, severe aortic stenosis, significant pulmonary hypertension, and severe left ventricular dysfunction.

Pulmonary thromboembolism may occur, and rarely problems may arise with congenital diaphragmatic hernias, pheochromocytomas, and sickle cell disease (Biller & Adams, 1986; Browning, 1973; Clark, 1991; Colman *et al.*, 2000; Lau *et al,*. 1996; Grimes, 1994; Pastorek & Seiler, 1985; Pyeritz, 1981; Snyder, Gilstrap & Hauth, 1983).

Mortality risks associated with particular cardiovascular conditions during pregnancy are summarized in Table 10.4. Clark (1991) attributes a mortality risk of <1% for the low-risk group, which includes septal defects, a mortality risk of 5–15% for the intermediate group, which includes mitral and aortic valve stenoses, and a mortality risk of 25–50% for the high-risk, group which includes marked pulmonary hypertension and severe outflow obstruction.

Table 10.4. Cardiovascular conditions associated with increased mortality during pregnancy

Low risk	Intermediate risk	High risk
Uncomplicated septal defects	Mitral stenosis	Marked pulmonary hypertension
Uncomplicated ductus arteriosus	Aortic stenosis	Marked aortic stenosis
Uncomplicated bicuspid aortic valve	Uncorrected cyanotic conditions	Complicated aortic coarctation
Repaired lesions with normal cardiac function	Aortic coarctation	Marfan syndrome with aortic root
Mitral valve prolapse	Prosthetic valves	or valve involvement.
Pulmonary or tricuspid valve disease	Marked pulmonary stenosis	
Aortic or mitral regurgitation with intact	Uncorrected tetralogy of Fallot	
ventricular function	Previous myocardial infarction	
Small left-to-right shunts	Marfan syndrome with normal aorta	
	Large left-to-right shunts	

Derived from Clark (1991) and Colman *et al.* (2000).

Although death may occur in patients with pre-eclampsia and HELLP (hemolysis, elevated liver enzymes, low platelets) syndrome, this is usually due to complications of renal failure, adult respiratory distress syndrome, cerebral edema, and hypoglycemia (Catanzarite *et al.*, 1995). Sepsis may also cause death but is usually clinically symptomatic.

An intraperitoneal collection of blood may be the first indication of a ruptured ectopic pregnancy. Examination of the fallopian tubes in such a case will localize the site of rupture, and careful sectioning of the tube and adherent blood clot may reveal products of conception. Specific techniques for maternal autopsies have been described elsewhere (Rushton & Dawson, 1982).

Sudden collapse and death during or soon after delivery must raise the possibility of amniotic fluid embolism (Ziadlourad & Conklin, 1987). This can be confirmed on histologic examination of the lungs, when fetal squames, lanugo, and intestinal mucin are detected within the pulmonary vessels (Lau, 1994; Price, Baker & Cefalo, 1985). Anti-keratin or fetal isoantigen immunohistochemical staining may be of assistance in delineating intravascular fetal material (Garland & Thompson, 1983; Ishiyama *et al.*, 1986). Embolization of trophoblastic tissue from a hydatidiform mole has also been documented in a 16-year-old patient during hysterotomy and curettage,

resulting in sudden death (Cohle & Petty, 1985), and may follow cesarian section for placenta accreta (Rashid, Moir & Butt, 1994).

Fatal disseminated intravascular coagulation may occur during pregnancy due to retention of a dead fetus, sepsis, eclampsia, multiple transfusions, placental abruption, and amniotic fluid or trophoblastic tissue embolism. Other causes of thrombotic microangiopathy in pregnancy are thrombotic thrombocytopenic purpura, hemolytic-uremic syndrome, systemic lupus erythematosis, eclampsia, and acute fatty liver of pregnancy (Kemp, Barnard & Prahlow, 1999).

Air embolism is another possible cause of sudden death during pregnancy. It may result from surgical procedures such as cesarian section, from criminal abortion, and from certain kinds of sexual or drug-taking activities (Collins, Davis & Lantz, 1994; Fatteh, Leach & Wilkinson, 1973). Deaths during pregnancy may also be due to disease or trauma that is completely unrelated to the underlying gestation (Fildes *et al.*, 1992). While users of oral contraceptives have an increased risk of sudden death from pulmonary embolism, myocardial infarction, and subarachnoid and intracerebral hemorrhage, this does not usually occur in adolescence (Layde, Beral & Kay, 1981; Stadel, 1981a; Stadel, 1981b).

REFERENCES

Abdu, R. A., Garritano, D. & Culver, O. (1987). Acute gastric necrosis in anorexia nervosa and bulimia. *Archives of Surgery*, **122**, 830–32.

Abu-Arafeh, I., Gray, E., Youngson, G., Auchterlonie, I. & Russell, G. (1995). Myocarditis and haemolytic uraemic syndrome. *Archives of Disease in Childhood*, **72**, 46–7.

Alford, B. A. & McIlhenny, J. (1992). The child with acute abdominal pain and vomiting. *Radiologic Clinics of North America*, **30**, 441–53.

Alrabeeah, A., Galliani, C. A., Giacomantonio, M., Heifetz, S. A. & Lau, H. (1988). Neonatal ovarian torsion: report of three cases and review of the literature. *Pediatric Pathology*, **8**, 143–9.

Andersen, J. F., Eklöf, O. & Thomasson, B. (1981). Large bowel volvulus in children. Review of case material and the literature. *Pediatric Radiology*, **11**, 129–38.

Arey, J. B. & Sotos, J. (1956). Unexpected death in early life. *Journal of Pediatrics*, **49**, 523–39.

Atkinson, M. C. & Busuttil, A. (1994). Two undiagnosed cases of intussusception. *Medicine, Science and the Law*, **34**, 337–9.

Avissar, E., Goldberg, M. & Lernau, O. (1994). Bezoar-induced ulceration and perforation of the upper gastrointestinal tract in mentally retarded patients. *Pediatric Surgery International*, **9**, 279–80.

Berman, L., Stringer, D. A., Ein, S. & Shandling, B. (1988). Childhood diaphragmatic hernias presenting after the neonatal period. *Clinical Radiology*, **39**, 237–44.

Biller, J. & Adams, H. P. (1986). Cerebrovascular disorders associated with pregnancy. *American Family Physician*, **33**, 125–32.

Booker, P. D., Meerstadt, P. W. D. & Bush, G. H. (1981). Congenital diaphragmatic hernia in the older child. *Archives of Disease in Childhood*, **56**, 253–7.

Bramwell, N. H. & Byard, R. W. (1989). Hemothorax from external rupture of esophageal varices: an unusual fatal complication. *Canadian Journal of Gastroenterology*, **3**, 58–60.

Brennan, A. L. & Geddes, D. M. (2002). Cystic fibrosis. *Current Opinion in Infectious Diseases*, **15**, 175–82.

Browning, D. J. (1973). Maternal death and diaphragmatic hernia. *Medical Journal of Australia*, **2**, 297.

Bruch, H. (1971). Death in anorexia nervosa. *Psychosomatic Medicine*, **33**, 135–44.

Byard, R. W. (1994). Unexpected death due to acute airway obstruction in daycare centers. *Pediatrics*, **94**, 113–14.

Byard, R. W. (1996). Mechanisms of unexpected death in infants and young children following foreign body ingestion. *Journal of Forensic Sciences*, **41**, 438–41.

Byard, R. W. (2000). Sudden infant death, large intestinal volvulus, and a duplication cyst of the terminal ileum. *American Journal of Forensic Medicine and Pathology*, **21**, 62–4.

Byard, R. W. & Beal, S. M. (2000). Gastric aspiration and sleeping position in infancy and early childhood. *Journal of Paediatrics and Child Health*, **36**, 403–5.

Byard, R. W. & Couper, R. T. L. (2001). Acute gastric dilatation and spastic quadraparesis. *Journal of Pediatrics*, **139**, 166.

Byard, R. W. & Simpson, A. (2001). Sudden death and intussusception in infancy and childhood – autopsy considerations. *Medicine, Science and the Law*, **41**, 41–5.

Byard, R. W., Bohn, D. J., Wilson, G., Smith, C. R. & Ein, S. H. (1990). Unsuspected diaphragmatic hernia: a potential cause of sudden and unexpected death in infancy and early childhood. *Journal of Pediatric Surgery*, **25**, 1166–8.

Byard, R. W., Bourne, A. J. & Cockington, R. A. (1991). Fatal gastric perforation in a 4-year-old child with a late-presenting congenital diaphragmatic hernia. *Pediatric Surgery International*, **6**, 44–6.

Byard, R. W., Couper, R. T. L. & Cohle, S. D. (2001). Gastric distension, cerebral palsy and unexpected death. *Journal of Clinical Forensic Medicine*, **8**, 81–5.

Byard, R. W., Moore, L., Jaunzems, A. & Davidson, G. P. (1992). Test and teach number 68 (microvillus inclusion disease). *Pathology*, **24**, 170–1, 224–5.

Byard, R. W., Schliebs, J. & Koszyca, B. A. (2001). Osler–Weber–Rendu syndrome – pathological manifestations and autopsy considerations. *Journal of Forensic Sciences*, **46**, 698–701.

Campbell, J. R. & Blank, E. (1974). Sigmoid volvulus in children. *Pediatrics*, **53**, 702–5.

Canby, J. P. & Jaffurs, W. J. (1963). Sudden and unexpected death in childhood. A four year study in a United States Army station hospital in Germany. *Military Medicine*, **128**, 613–16.

Candy, D. C. A., Larcher, V. F., Cameron, D. J. S., *et al.* (1981). Lethal familial protracted diarrhoea. *Archives of Disease in Childhood*, **56**, 15–23.

Catanzarite, V. A., Steinberg, S. M., Mosley, C. A., Landers, C. F., Cousins, L. M. & Schneider, J. M. (1995). Severe preeclampsia with fulminant and extreme elevation of aspartate aminotransferase and lactate dehydrogenase levels: high risk for maternal death. *American Journal of Perinatology*, **12**, 310–13.

Chhanabhai, M., Avis, S. P. & Hutton, C. J. (1995). Congenital diaphragmatic hernia. A case of sudden unexpected death in childhood. *American Journal of Forensic Medicine and Pathology*, **16**, 27–9.

Clark, S. L. (1991). Cardiac disease in pregnancy. *Obstetrics and Gynecology Clinics of North America*, **18**, 237–56.

Clark, A. D. & McMillan, J. A. (1974). Maternal death due to primary peritoneal pregnancy. *Journal of Obstetrics and Gynaecology of the British Commonwealth*, **81**, 652–4.

Cohle, S. D. & Petty, C. S. (1985). Sudden death caused by embolization of trophoblast from hydatidiform mole. *Journal of Forensic Sciences*, **30**, 1279–83.

Collins, K. A., Davis, G. J. & Lantz, P. E. (1994). An unusual case of maternal-fetal death due to vaginal insufflation of cocaine. *American Journal of Forensic Medicine and Pathology*, **15**, 335–9.

Colman, J. M., Sermer, M. S., Seaward, P. G. R. & Siu, S. C. (2000). Congenital heart disease in pregnancy. *Cardiology in Review*, **8**, 166–73.

Cooke, R. A., Chambers, J. B., Singh, R., *et al.* (1994). QT interval in anorexia nervosa. *British Heart Journal*, **72**, 69–73.

Cox, D. E. (1997). Intussusception: agonal phenomenon or cause of death? *Medicine, Science and the Law*, **37**, 355–8.

Crisp, D. E., Siegler, R. L., Bale, J. F. & Thompson, J. A. (1981). Hemorrhagic cerebral infarction in the hemolytic-uremic syndrome. *Journal of Pediatrics*, **99**, 273–6.

Croft, N. M., Howatson, A. G., Ling, S. C., Nairn, L., Evans, T. J. & Weaver, L. T. (2000). Microvillous inclusion disease: an evolving condition. *Journal of Pediatric Gastroenterology and Nutrition*, **31**, 185–9.

Cullen, M. L., Klein, M. D. & Philippart, A. I. (1985). Congenital diaphragmatic hernia. *Surgical Clinics of North America*, **65**, 1115–39.

Cutz, E., Rhoads, J. M., Drumm, B., Sherman, P. M., Durie, P. R. & Forstner, G. G. (1989). Microvillus inclusion disease: an inherited defect of brush-border assembly and differentiation. *New England Journal of Medicine*, **320**, 646–51.

Davidson, G. P., Cutz, E., Hamilton, J. R. & Gall, D. G. (1978). Familial enteropathy: a syndrome of protracted diarrhea from birth, failure to thrive, and hypoplastic villus atrophy. *Gastroenterology*, **75**, 783–90.

Del Beccaro, M. A., McLaughlin, J. F. & Polage, D. L. (1991). Severe gastric distension in seven patients with cerebral palsy. *Developmental Medicine and Child Neurology*, **33**, 912–29.

Deslypere, J. P., Praet, M. & Verdonk, G. (1982). An unusual case of trichobezoar: the Rapunzel syndrome. *American Journal of Gastroenterology*, **77**, 467–70.

DiFiore, J. W. (1999). Intussusception. *Seminars in Pediatric Surgery*, **8**, 214–20.

Dome, J. S. & Coppes, M. J. (2002). Recent advances in Wilms tumor genetics. *Current Opinion in Pediatrics*, **14**, 5–11.

Ein, S. H. (1976). Leading points in childhood intussusception. *Journal of Pediatric Surgery*, **11**, 209–11.

Ein, S. H. & Stephens, C. A. (1971). Intussusception: 354 cases in 10 years. *Journal of Pediatric Surgery*, **6**, 16–27.

Ein, S. H., Stephens, C. A., Shandling, B. & Filler, R. M. (1986). Intussusception due to lymphoma. *Journal of Pediatric Surgery*, **21**, 786–8.

Einfeld, S. L., Fairley, M. J., Green, B. F. & Opitz, J. M. (1987). Sudden death in childhood in a case of the G syndrome. *American Journal of Medical Genetics*, **28**, 293–6.

Fatteh, A., Leach, W. B. & Wilkinson, C. A. (1973). Fatal air embolism in pregnancy resulting from orogenital sex play. *Forensic Science*, **2**, 247–50.

Fildes, J., Reed, L., Jones, N., Martin, M. & Barrett, J. (1992). Trauma: the leading cause of maternal death. *Journal of Trauma*, **32**, 643–5.

Filkins, J. A., Kalelkar, M. B. & Chambliss, M. J. (1998). Unexpected death due to gestational choriocarcinoma. A report of two cases. *American Journal of Forensic Medicine and Pathology*, **19**, 387–90.

Gallo, G. E. & Gianantonio, C. A. (1995). Extrarenal involvement in diarrhoea-associated haemolytic-uraemic syndrome. *Pediatric Nephrology*, **9**, 117–19.

Gardner, A. M. N. (1958). Aspiration of food and vomit. *Quarterly Journal of Medicine*, **27**, 227–42.

Garland, I. W. C. & Thompson, W. D. (1983). Diagnosis of amniotic fluid embolism using an antiserum to human keratin. *Journal of Clinical Pathology*, **36**, 625–7.

Gianantonio, C. A., Vitacco, M., Mendilaharzu, F., Gallo, G. E. & Sojo, E. T. (1973). The hemolytic-uremic syndrome. *Nephron*, **11**, 174–92.

Gibb, D. (1990). Confidential inquiry into maternal death. *British Journal of Obstetrics and Gynaecology*, **97**, 97–101.

Gottdiener, J. S., Gross, H. A., Henry, W. L., Borer, J. S. & Ebert, M. H. (1978). Effects of self-induced starvation on cardiac size and function in anorexia nervosa. *Circulation*, **58**, 425–33.

Gravanis, M. B. & Ansari, A. A. (1987). Idiopathic cardiomyopathies. A review of pathologic studies and mechanisms of pathogenesis. *Archives of Pathology and Laboratory Medicine*, **111**, 915–29.

Grimes, D. A. (1994). The morbidity and mortality of pregnancy: still risky business. *American Journal of Obstetrics and Gynecology*, **170**, 1489–94.

Gull, W. W. (1874). Anorexia nervosa. *Transactions of the Clinical Society*, **7**, 22–8.

Habib, R., Lévy, M., Gagnadoux, M.-F. & Broyer, M. (1982). Progress of the hemolytic uremic syndrome in children. *Advances in Nephrology*, **11**, 99–128.

Hagge, W. W., Burke, E. C. & Stickler, G. B. (1967). Sudden death in the nephrotic syndrome: salt depletion as a probable mechanism. *Clinical Pediatrics*, **6**, 524–7.

Havlik, D. M. & Nolte, K. B. (2002). Sudden death in an infant resulting from torsion of the uterine adnexa. *American Journal of Forensic Medicine and Pathology*, **23**, 289–91.

Hight, D. W., Hixon, S. D., Reed, J. O. Watts, F. B., Jr & Hertzler, J. H. (1982). Intermittent diaphragmatic hernia of Bochdalek: report of a case and literature review. *Pediatrics*, **69**, 601–4.

Holmes, M., Murphy, V., Taylor, M. & Denham, B. (1991). Intussusception in cystic fibrosis. *Archives of Disease in Childhood*, **66**, 726–7.

Ishiyama, I., Mukaida, M., Komuro, E. & Keil, W. (1986). Analysis of a case of generalized amniotic fluid embolism by demonstrating the fetal isoantigen (A blood type) in maternal tissues of B blood type, using immunoperoxidase staining. *American Journal of Clinical Pathology*, **85**, 239–41.

Isner, J. M., Roberts, W. C., Heymsfield, S. B. & Yager, J. (1985). Anorexia nervosa and sudden death. *Annals of Internal Medicine*, **102**, 49–52.

Isner, J. M., Sours, H. E., Paris, A. L., Ferrans, V. J. & Roberts, W. C. (1979). Sudden, unexpected death in avid dieters using the liquid-protein-modified-fast diet. Observations in 17 patients and the role of the prolonged QT interval. *Circulation*, **60**, 1401–12.

Jehle, D., Krause, R. & Braen, G. R. (1994). Ectopic pregnancy. *Emergency Medicine Clinics of North America*, **12**, 55–71.

Jenab, M., Lade, R. I., Chiga, M. & Diehl, A. M. (1959). Cardiorespiratory syndrome of obesity in a child. Case report and necropsy findings. *Pediatrics*, **24**, 23–30.

Jorgensen, I. M. & Gregersen, M. (1990). Sudden death in children with gastrointestinal disease. Reports of 24 medico-legal cases. *Ugeskrift Laeger*, **152**, 2233–7.

Kasian, G. F., Taylor, B. W., Sugarman, R. G. & Nyssen, J. N. (1986). Ovarian torsion related to sudden infant death. *Canadian Medical Association Journal*, **135**, 1373.

Kemp, W. L., Barnard, J. J. & Prahlow, J. A. (1999). Death due to thrombotic thrombocytopenic purpura during pregnancy. Case report with review of thrombotic microangiopathies of pregnancy. *American Journal of Forensic Medicine and Pathology*, **20**, 189–98.

Kluth, D., Peterson, C., Zimmerman, H. J. & Muhlhaus, K. (1989). The embryology of congenital diaphragmatic hernia. *Modern Problems in Paediatrics*, **24**, 7–21.

Knight, B. H. (1975). The significance of the post mortem discovery of gastric contents in the air passages. *Forensic Science*, **6**, 229–34.

Lau, G. (1994). Amniotic fluid embolism as a cause of sudden maternal death. *Medicine, Science and the Law*, **34**, 213–20.

Lau, P., Permezel, M., Dawson, P., Chester, S., Collier, N. & Forbes, I. (1996). Phaeochromocytoma in pregnancy. *Australian and New Zealand Journal of Obstetrics and Gynaecology*, **36**, 472–6.

Layde, P. M., Beral, V. & Kay, C. R. (1981). Further analyses of mortality in oral contraceptive users. Royal College of General Practitioners' oral contraceptive study. *Lancet*, **i**, 541–6.

Lazebnik, N., Iellin, A. & Michowitz, M. (1986). Spontaneous rupture of the normal stomach after sodium bicarbonate ingestion. *Journal of Clinical Gastroenterology*, **8**, 454–6.

Lipsett, J. & Byard, R. W. (1995). Small bowel stricture due to vascular compromise: a late complication of Henoch–Schönlein purpura. *Pediatric Pathology and Laboratory Medicine*, **15**, 333–40.

Little, K. J. & Danzl, D. F. (1991). Intussusception associated with Henoch–Schonlein purpura. *Journal of Emergency Medicine*, **9**, 29–32.

Lynch, J. M., Adkins, J. C. & Wiener, E. S. (1982). Incarcerated congenital diaphragmatic hernias with bowel obstruction (Bochdalek). *Journal of Pediatric Surgery*, **17**, 537–40.

MacGregor, M. I., Block, A. J. & Ball, W. C., Jr (1970). Serious complications and sudden death in the Pickwickian syndrome. *Hopkins Medical Journal*, **126**, 279–95.

Manton, N., Smith, N. M. & Byard, R. W. (2000). Unexpected death due to hemolytic uremic syndrome. *American Journal of Forensic Medicine and Pathology*, **21**, 90–92.

Marczynska-Robowska, M. (1957). Pancreatic necrosis in a case of Still's disease. *Lancet*, **i**, 815–16.

Matthews, N. M., McCowan, L. M. E. & Patten, P. (1996). Placenta praevia accreta with delayed hysterectomy. *Australian and New Zealand Journal of Obstetrics and Gynaecology*, **36**, 476–9.

Maymon, R. & Fejgin, M. (1990). Intracranial hemorrhage during pregnancy and puerperium. *Obstetrical and Gynecological Survey*, **45**, 157–9.

McLorie, G. A. (2001). Wilms tumor (nephroblastoma). *Current Opinion in Urology*, **11**, 567–70.

Moore, L. & Byard, R. W. (1992). Fatal paradoxical embolism to the left carotid artery during partial resection of Wilms tumor. *Pediatric Pathology*, **12**, 371–6.

Morales, A. R., Kulesh, M. & Valdes-Dapena, M. (1984). Maximising the effectiveness of the autopsy in cases of sudden death. *Archives of Pathology and Laboratory Medicine*, **108**, 460–61.

Ong, N.-T. & Beasley, S. W. (1990). The leadpoint in intussusception. *Journal of Pediatric Surgery*, **25**, 640–43.

Pastorek, J. G. & Seiler, B. (1985). Maternal death associated with sickle cell trait. *American Journal of Obstetrics and Gynecology*, **151**, 295–7.

Pershad, J., Simmons, G. T., Chung, D., Frye, T. & Marques, M. B. (1998). Two acute pediatric abdominal catastrophes from strangulated left paraduodenal hernias. *Pediatric Emergency Care*, **14**, 347–9.

Pfalzgraf, R. R., Zumwalt, R. E. & Kenny, M. R. (1988). Mesodiverticular band and sudden death in children. A report of two cases. *Archives of Pathology and Laboratory Medicine*, **112**, 182–4.

Pollack, C. V. Jr. & Pender, E. S. (1991). Unusual cases of intussusception. *Journal of Emergency Medicine*, **9**, 347–55.

Powley, J. M. (1965). Unexpected deaths from small bowel obstruction. *Proceedings of the Royal Society of Medicine*, **58**, 870–73.

Price, T. M., Baker, V. V. & Cefalo, R. C. (1985). Amniotic fluid embolism. Three case reports with a review of the literature. *Obstetrical and Gynaecological Survey*, **40**, 462–75.

Pyeritz, R. E. (1981). Maternal and fetal complications of pregnancy in the Marfan syndrome. *American Journal of Medicine*, **71**, 784–90.

Rabson, S. M. (1949). Sudden and unexpected natural death. IV. Sudden and unexpected natural death in infants and young children. *Journal of Pediatrics*, **34**, 166–73.

Rashid, A.-M. H., Moir, C. L. & Butt, J. C. (1994). Sudden death following cesarian section for placenta previa and accreta. *American Journal of Forensic Medicine and Pathology*, **15**, 32–5.

Ratcliffe, P. J. & Bevan, J. S. (1985). Severe hypoglycaemia and sudden death in anorexia nervosa. *Psychological Medicine*, **15**, 679–81.

Reiger, J., Eritscher, C., Laubreiter, K., Trattnig, J., Sterz, F. & Grimm, G. (1997). Gastric rupture – an uncommon complication after successful cardiopulmonary resuscitation: report of two cases. *Resuscitation*, **35**, 175–8.

Rich, L. M., Caine, M. R., Findling, J. W. & Shaker, J. L. (1990). Hypoglycemic coma in anorexia nervosa. Case report and review of the literature. *Archives of Internal Medicine*, **150**, 894–5.

Richards, W. & Patrick, J. R. (1965). Death from asthma in children. *American Journal of Diseases of Children*, **110**, 4–20.

Richardson, S. E., Karmali, M. A., Becker, L. E. & Smith, C. R. (1988). The histopathology of the hemolytic uremic syndrome associated with verocytotoxin-producing *Escherichia coli* infections. *Human Pathology*, **19**, 1102–8.

Riordan, J. R., Rommens, J. M., Kerem, B.-S., *et al.* (1989). Identification of the cystic fibrosis gene: cloning and characterization of complementary DNA. *Science*, **245**, 1066–73.

Robson, W. L. M., Leung, A. K. C. & Montgomery, M. D. (1991). Causes of death in hemolytic uremic syndrome. *Child Nephrology and Urology*, **11**, 228–33.

Rommens, J. M., Iannuzzi, M. C., Kerem, B.-S., *et al.* (1989). Identification of the cystic fibrosis gene: chromosome walking and jumping. *Science*, **245**, 1059–65.

Rushton, D. I. & Dawson, I. M. P. (1982). The maternal autopsy. *Journal of Clinical Pathology*, **35**, 909–21.

Schechner, S. A. & Ehrlich, F. E. (1974). Gastric perforation and child abuse. *Journal of Trauma*, **14**, 723–5.

Seagram, C. G. F., Stephens, C. A. & Cumming, W. A. (1973). Peptic ulceration at the Hospital for Sick Children, Toronto, during the 20-year period 1949–1969. *Journal of Pediatric Surgery*, **8**, 407–13.

Sheth, K. J., Swick, H. M. & Haworth, N. (1986). Neurological involvement in hemolytic-uremic syndrome. *Annals of Neurology*, **19**, 90–93.

Snyder, R. R., Gilstrap, L. C. & Hauth, J. C. (1983). Ehlers–Danlos syndrome and pregnancy. *Obstetrics and Gynecology*, **61**, 649–51.

Stadel, B. V. (1981a). Oral contraceptives and cardiovascular disease (first of two parts). *New England Journal of Medicine*, **305**, 612–18.

Stadel, B. V. (1981b). Oral contraceptives and cardiovascular disease (second of two parts). *New England Journal of Medicine*, **305**, 672–7.

Stewart, R. J., Bruce, J. & Beasley, S. W. (1993). Oesophageal duplication cyst: another cause of neonatal respiratory distress. *Journal of Paediatrics and Child Health*, **29**, 391–2.

Storm, W., Gisbertz, K. H. & Steiger, H. (1987). Delayed onset of left-sided diaphragmatic hernia in a newborn. *Acta Paediatrica Hungarica*, **28**, 261–6.

Stringer, M. D., Pledger, G. & Drake, D. P. (1992). Childhood deaths from intussusception in England and Wales, 1984–9. *British Medical Journal*, **304**, 737–9.

St-Vil, D., Brandt, M. L., Panic, S., Bensoussan, A. L. & Blanchard, H. (1991). Meckel's diverticulum in children: a 20-year review. *Journal of Pediatric Surgery*, **26**, 1289–92.

Tada, T., Wakabayashi, T., Kishimoto, H., Nishino, R. & Hayashi, K. (1982). Sudden death due to infantile pancreatitis. *Acta Pathologica Japonica*, **32**, 917–23.

Thurston, J. & Marks, P. (1974). Electrocardiographic abnormalities in patients with anorexia nervosa. *British Heart Journal*, **36**, 719–23.

Van der Ham, A. C. & Lange, J. F. (1990). Traumatic rupture of the stomach after Heimlich maneuver. *Journal of Emergency Medicine*, **8**, 713–15.

Vaughan, E. D., Jr, Sawyers, J. L. & Scott, H. W., Jr (1968). The Rapunzel syndrome: an unusual complication of intestinal bezoar. *Surgery*, **63**, 339–43.

Warren, M. P. & Vande Wiele, R. L. (1973). Clinical and metabolic features of anorexia nervosa. *American Journal of Obstetrics and Gynecology*, **117**, 435–49.

Wharton, R. H., Wang, T., Graeme-Cook, F., Briggs, S. & Cole, R. E. (1997). Acute idiopathic gastric dilation with gastric necrosis in individuals with Prader–Willi syndrome. *American Journal of Medical Genetics*, **73**, 437–41.

Whitehead, F. J., Couper, R. T. L., Moore, L., Bourne, A. J. & Byard, R. W. (1996). Dehydration deaths in infants and children. *American Journal of Forensic Medicine and Pathology*, **17**, 73–8.

Wong, S. W. & Gardner, V. (1992). Sudden death in children due to mesenteric defect and mesenteric cyst. *American Journal of Forensic Medicine and Pathology*, **13**, 214–16.

Zakowski, M. F., Edwards, R. H. & McDonough, E. T. (1990). Wilms tumor presenting as sudden death due to tumor embolism. *Archives of Pathology and Laboratory Medicine*, **114**, 605–8.

Ziadlourad, F. & Conklin, K. A. (1987). Amniotic fluid embolism. *Seminars in Anesthesia*, **6**, 171–5.

11

Metabolic and endocrine conditions

Introduction

A variety of inborn errors of metabolism listed in Table 11.1 may cause unexpected death in infancy and childhood. Clinical presentations include failure to thrive, hypotonia, psychomotor delay, seizures, unusual odors, vomiting, and diarrhea, sometimes with a family history of an inherited metabolic disorder or previous infant or childhood deaths. As inborn errors of metabolism represent a very heterogeneous group of rare disorders (Dionisi-Vici *et al.*, 2002), only the more "common" conditions are dealt with in detail in this text, which also includes acquired metabolic disorders. The diagnosis of a metabolic disorder is more likely to be known in older children than in infants, and so the autopsy may assume particular importance in establishing the diagnosis in very early life. Occasional cases may remain undiagnosed until adult life (Pien *et al.*, 2002).

Pathological features

Findings at autopsy are quite variable because of the disparate nature of these disorders. However, in infancy certain features should suggest an underlying metabolic defect. These are summarized in Table 11.2 and include cardiomegaly and fatty change in the liver, heart, smooth and skeletal muscle, and renal tubules (Emery *et al.*, 1988) (Figure 11.1 and Color Plate 26). Unfortunately, autopsy findings are often not specific. Cerebral swelling is found in many conditions, ranging from trauma to sudden infant death syndrome (SIDS). Additionally, fatty change

within the myocardium occurs in a wide range of disorders, including infections and congenital malformations (Carter & Variend, 1992). Hypertrophic or dilated cardiomyopathies are also not specific to any particular metabolic disorder (Kohlschütter & Hausdorf, 1986) (Table 11.3).

Autopsy sampling

Specimens that need to be taken at autopsy in cases of suspected metabolic conditions, along with appropriate sampling methods, are listed in Appendix VI. Further details of the laboratory diagnosis of these disorders have been reviewed by Applegarth, Dimmick & Toone (1989).

Frequency

The estimated frequency of metabolic disease in infants dying suddenly and unexpectedly has been controversial, with some authors claiming that between 5 and 20% of cases result from metabolic defects (Emery, Chandra & Gilbert-Barness, 1988; Harpey, Charpentier & Paturneau-Jouas, 1990; Vawter *et al.*, 1986). However, these high figures do not appear to reflect general experience (Arens *et al.*, 1993; Holton *et al.*, 1991; Rebuffat *et al.*, 1991). For example, no cases of medium-chain acyl-CoA dehydrogenase (MCAD) deficiency were identified on fibroblast culture in one study of 70 cases of SIDS, and no abnormal organic acid metabolites were found on examination of urine, cerebrospinal fluid, and vitreous humor from 88 SIDS cases in

Table 11.1. Inborn errors of metabolism that have been associated with sudden or unexpected deaths in infancy and childhood

Fatty acid oxidation disorders	Carbohydrate disorders	Amino acid disorders	Urea cycle disorders	Organic acid disorders	Miscellaneous disorders
Acyl-CoA dehydrogenase deficiencies (medium-chain acyl-CoA dehydrogenase (MCAD), very-long-chain acyl-CoA dehydrogenase (VLCAD), long-chain acyl-CoA dehydrogenase (LCAD))	Fructose-1,6-diphosphatase deficiency	Homocystinuria	Argininosuccinate lyase deficiency	Glutaric aciduria type 2	Biotinidase deficiency
	Galactosemia	Isovaleric acidemia	Argininosuccinate synthetase deficiency	Glutaconic aciduria	Cytochrome oxidase deficiency
	Glycogen storage diseases	Lysinuric protein intolerance	Carbamylphosphate synthetase deficiency	Hydroxycarboxylic aciduria	Electron transfer flavoprotein deficiency
	Hereditary fructose intolerance	Maple syrup urine disease	Ornithine carbamoyltransferase deficiency	3-Hydroxy-2-methylbutyric aciduria	Electron transfer flavoprotein dehydrogenase deficiency
	Mitochondrial phosphoenolpyruvate carboxykinase deficiency	Tyrosinemia		3-Hydroxy-3-methyl-glutaryl-CoA lyase deficiency	Glycerol kinase deficiency
Primary carnitine deficiency (carnitine transporter deficiency)				Propionic acidemia	GM$_1$ gangliosidosis
Carnitine-acylcarnitine translocase deficiency				Lactate dehydrogenase complex defects	Holocarboxylase synthetase deficiency
Carnitine palmitoyltransferase II deficiency				3-Methylcrotonyl-CoA carboxylase deficiency	Mucopolysaccharidoses
Ethylmalonic adipic aciduria				Methylmalonic acidemia	Niemann–Pick disease type C
					Phosphoenolpyruvate carboxykinase deficiency

Clayton *et al.* (1986), Emery *et al.* (1988), and Norman, Taylor & Clarke (1990).

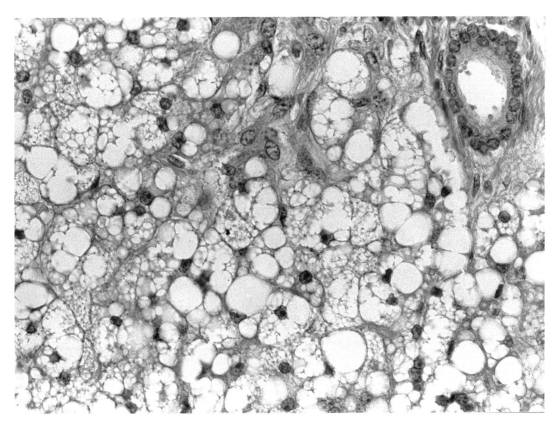

Figure 11.1 Mixed macro- and microvesicular steatosis of the liver, suggesting a possible underlying metabolic disorder in an infant who died suddenly and unexpectedly (hematoxylin and eosin, ×440).

Table 11.2. Autopsy findings that may indicate an inborn error of metabolism

Family history of similar sudden death, particularly in siblings
Dysmorphic features
Enlargement of liver, spleen, heart
Pallor of liver, heart, muscles
Cerebral edema
Fatty change in liver, heart, muscle, kidney

the same report (Holton *et al.*, 1991). Similarly, another study of 47 SIDS cases failed to identify any evidence of organic acidemias (Divry *et al.*, 1990). Miller *et al.* (1992) did not find any infants homozygous for the common G-985 mutation of MCAD deficiency in a retrospective examination of DNA taken from 67 SIDS infants. It seems likely that the number of cases of sudden infant death caused by metabolic disease is closer to 1–2% or less, although the possibility of underdiagnosis must be considered in smaller, non-specialized centers (Bennett & Powell, 1994).

Fatty acid oxidation disorders

At least 12 disorders of fatty acid oxidation have been reported as causes of sudden and unexpected death in infancy and early childhood (Boles *et al.*, 1994).

Table 11.3. Inborn errors of metabolism associated with cardiomyopathy in children

Mucopolysaccharidoses
    Type I (Hurler syndrome) – hypertrophic and dilated
    Type II (Hunter syndrome) – hypertrophic
    Type III (Sanfilippo syndrome) – hypertrophic
    Type IV (Morquio syndrome) – hypertrophic
    Type VI (Marateaux–Lamy syndrome) – dilated
    Type VII (Sly syndrome) – hypertrophic
Glycogen storage diseases (GSDs)
    Type II (Pompe disease) – hypertrophic
    Type III (Cori disease) – hypertrophic
    Type IV (Andersen disease) – dilated
    Type IX (cardiac phosphorylase kinase deficiency) – hypertrophic
    GSD without acid maltase deficiency – hypertrophic
Combined ganglioside/mucopolysaccharide/oligosaccharide degradation disorders
    GM_1 gangliosidosis – hypertrophic and dilated
    GM_2 gangliosidosis (Sandhoff disease) – hypertrophic and dilated
Phytanic acid oxidation disorder (Refsum disease) – hypertrophic and dilated
Fatty acid disorders
    Primary carnitine deficiency – hypertrophic and dilated
    Muscle carnitine deficiency – hypertrophic and dilated
    Very-long-chain acyl-CoA dehydrogenase (VLCAD) deficiency – hypertrophic and dilated
    Long-chain acyl-CoA dehydrogenase (LCAD) deficiency – hypertrophic
    Long-chain 3-hydroxyacyl-CoA dehydrogenase deficiency – hypertrophic and dilated
    Carnitine acylcarnitine translocase deficiency – hypertrophic
    Carnitine palmitoyl transferase type II deficiency
Pyruvate metabolic disorders
    Pyruvate dehydrogenase complex deficiency (Leigh disease) – hypertrophic
Oxidative phosphorylation disorders
    Complex I deficiency – dilated
    Complex II deficiency
    Complex III deficiency (histiocytoid cardiomyopathy) – hypertrophic
    Complex IV deficiency (muscle and Leigh disease forms) – hypertrophic
    Complex V deficiency – hypertrophic
    Combined respiratory chain deficiencies
        Mitochondrial DNA deletions and duplications
            Kearns–Sayre syndrome – hypertrophic
        Mitochondrial transfer RNA mutations
            MERRF (myoclonic epilepsy with ragged red fibers) syndrome – hypertrophic and dilated
            MELAS (mitochondrial myopathy, encephalopathy, lactic acidosis, and stroke) syndrome – hypertrophic
        Senger syndrome – hypertrophic
        Barth syndrome (3-methylglutaconic aciduria type II) – hypertrophic and dilated
Aminoacid metabolic disorders
    Propionic acidemia
Miscellaneous

Antozzi & Zeviani (1997), Guertl, Noehammer & Hoefler (2000), Kohlschütter & Hausdorf (1986), Pande (1999), and Schwartz *et al.* (1996).

Acyl-CoA dehydrogenase deficiencies

Metabolic defects involving fat oxidation have received particular attention due to the possibility of sudden and unexpected death in infancy producing a clinical picture identical to SIDS. The enzymes concerned are dehydrogenases involved in the progressive mitochondrial β-oxidation of long-chain fatty acids mobilized from adipose tissue (Anonymous, 1986). Hypoglycemia results when glycogen stores are depleted, as the deficiency of acyl-CoA dehydrogenases hinders gluconeogenesis from fat deposits (Howat *et al.*, 1985).

Medium-chain acyl-CoA dehydrogenase deficiency

MCAD deficiency interferes with β-oxidation of fatty acids, causing episodic hypoglycemia, lethargy, vomiting, seizures, coma, respiratory depression/apnea, and sudden death (Iafolla, Thompson & Roe, 1994). Hepatomegaly due to marked hepatic steatosis and encephalopathy may have been detected clinically, but in some infants sudden and unexpected death may be the first indication of an underlying problem (Roe *et al.*, 1986).

Frequency
MCAD deficiency is one of the most common inborn metabolic errors and has an estimated frequency of one per 20,000 newborns. There is a higher frequency among people of northern European descent (Touma & Charpentier, 1992; Wang *et al.*, 1999).

Etiology
Inheritance of the acyl-CoA dehydrogenase deficiencies is autosomal recessive, and the gene for MCAD has been fully characterized on chromosome 1p31 (Matsubara, Narisawa & Tada, 1992). The most common mutation, found in nearly 89% of patients, involves an A-to-G nucleotide replacement at position 985, resulting in a substitution of glutamate for lysine at position 329 of the MCAD precursor protein (Anonymous, 1991; Gregersen, Andresen & Bross, 2000).

Pathophysiology

Metabolic crises are often precipitated by viral infection or fasting, and result in hypoglycemia and hypoketonemia, sometimes with metabolic acidosis (Touma & Charpentier, 1992). This may occur after immunization (Harpey, Charpentier & Paturneau-Jouas, 1987; Harpey *et al.*, 1987), and may be heralded by episodic diarrhea and vomiting (Allison *et al.*, 1988). The first episode of metabolic decompensation usually occurs in the second year (Duran *et al.*, 1986), although it may occur much earlier in neonatal life (Wilcken, Carpenter & Hammond, 1993).

Pathological features
The autopsy findings in the acyl-CoA dehydrogenase deficiencies are variable. Although lipid accumulation within hepatocytes and cardiac myocytes is characteristic (Figure 11.2), it cannot be relied upon. Carter & Variend (1992) found fatty change within the heart in only one of three cases with proven MCAD deficiency. Similarly, while diffuse hepatic steatosis has been accepted as a marker for β-oxidative defects, it may also not be present in fatal cases (Losty *et al.*, 1991). Fatty change in the liver may be found in so many children dying of non-metabolic conditions that Bonnel & Beckwith (1986) describe it as "ubiquitous," and consider that it is a non-specific finding of little use in isolation. Thus, diagnosis of the acyl-CoA dehydrogenase deficiencies depends on other investigations.

Diagnosis
Traditionally, the diagnosis of acyl-CoA dehydrogenase deficiencies has been made by identifying urinary dicarboxylic acids on gas chromatography–mass spectrometry or by measuring enzyme activity in cultured skin fibroblasts (Treem *et al.*, 1986). While measuring blood dodecanoic acid levels has been proposed as a screening test for family members (Kemp *et al.*, 1996), molecular analysis of DNA can also be performed. In postmortem cases, DNA can be extracted from frozen blood, from liver extract, from paraffin-embedded formalin-fixed material, and from stored neonatal blood cards

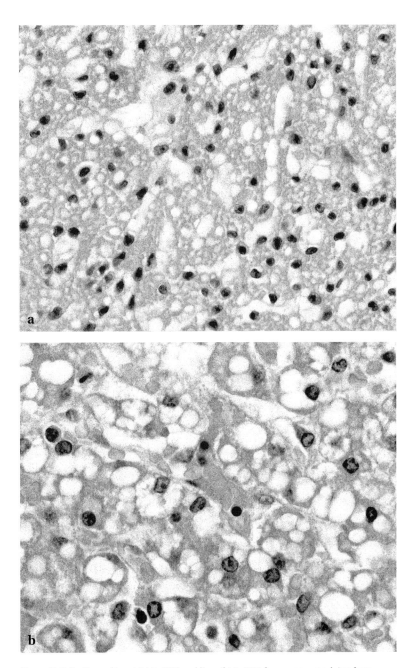

Figure 11.2 Sections of heart (a) (×280) and liver (b) (×320) from a neonate dying from MCAD deficiency, demonstrating marked lipid droplet accumulation (hematoxylin and eosin)

(Bennett *et al.*, 1991; Ding *et al.*, 1991; Kelly *et al.*, 1992; Matsubara, Narisawa & Tada, 1992).

Miscellaneous acyl-CoA dehydrogenase deficiencies

Very-long-chain acyl-CoA dehydrogenase (VLCAD) deficiency may be associated with both hypertrophic and dilated cardiomyopathy (see Table 11.3) and may lead to arrhythmias and cardiac arrest in infancy. The mutation responsible for the defect has been mapped to chromosome 17p11.13-p11.2 (Antozzi & Zeviani, 1997; Guertl, Noehammer & Hoefler, 2000; Treem, 2000). Long-chain acyl-CoA dehydrogenase (LCAD) deficiency occurs less frequently than MCAD deficiency, but may also result in a SIDS-like picture. Other manifestations include neonatal hypoglycemia, hypotonia, cardiomyopathy, and encephalopathy (Duran *et al.*, 1991; Treem *et al.*, 1991), although these may not always be present (Elpeleg, 1992). While long-chain 3-hydroxyacyl-CoA dehydrogenase has also been implicated in sudden infant death (Pollitt, 1993), the much rarer short-chain acyl-CoA dehydrogenase (SCAD) deficiency has not.

Primary carnitine deficiency

This is a disorder of fatty acid metabolism in which there is defective fatty acid transport across mitochondrial membranes due to a lack of functional carnitine receptors. It may be myopathic or systemic (Breningstall, 1990). Inheritance is autosomal recessive, although autosomal dominant forms have also been reported (Antozzi & Zeviani, 1997). Multiple mutations have been found in the OCTN2 gene on chromosome 5q31.2-32 in affected individuals (Treem, 2000).

Clinical features

The clinical presentation of systemic carnitine deficiency may mimic features of Reye syndrome (*vide infra*), with an acute encephalopathy (Chapoy *et al.*, 1980), or there may be evidence of cardiac involvement with cardiomegaly (Ino *et al.*, 1988), heart failure, and endocardial fibroelastosis. Sudden death

may occur following prolonged illness (Legge, 1985; Tripp *et al.*, 1981).

Pathological features

At autopsy there may be a dilated or hypertrophic cardiomyopathy with lipid accumulation within myocytes on microscopy (Antozzi & Zeviani, 1997; Gilbert, 1985), although occasionally the myocardium may be spared (Karpati *et al.*, 1975).

Carnitine-acylcarnitine translocase deficiency

This is another autosomal recessively inherited defect of mitochondrial fatty acid oxidation. Affected infants present with hypoglycemia, lethargy, arrhythmias, coma, and convulsions. Sudden death may occur, and at autopsy hypertrophic cardiomyopathy may be found, with fatty infiltration of the kidney, liver, and muscle (Pande, 1999; Stanley *et al.*, 1992).

Carnitine palmitoyltransferase II deficiency

Carnitine palmitoyltransferase is an enzyme involved in transporting long-chain fatty acids across the mitochondrial membrane. Although carnitine palmitoyltransferase II deficiency is usually characterized by recurrent episodes of exercise-induced rhabdomyolysis occurring in adolescence or early adulthood, rare cases have been reported with hypoglycemia, arrhythmias, cardiomyopathy, and sudden death in infancy (Demaugre *et al.*, 1991). Fatty infiltration of the heart, liver, kidneys, and skeletal muscle may be seen on autopsy histology (Hug, Bove & Soukup, 1991) (Figure 11.3).

Carbohydrate disorders

Glycogen storage diseases

Sudden and unexpected death has been reported in both types Ic and II glycogen storage disease, with SIDS being a differential diagnosis in infancy (Berry, 1989; Holton *et al.*, 1991). Although in one series of

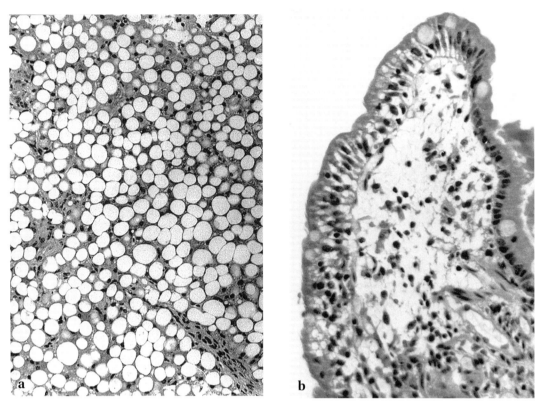

Figure 11.3 Marked macrovesicular steatosis in the liver of a 4.5-month-old girl with carnitine palmityltransferase II deficiency who died suddenly following a seizure (a) (hematoxylin and eosin, ×200). Previous duodenal biopsy had shown lipid accumulation within the tips of villi (b) (hematoxylin and eosin, ×220).

38 infants diagnosed as having died of SIDS, eight were reported to have glucose-6-phosphatase deficiency (type Ia glycogen storage disease), with two having transport protein T2 deficiency (type Ic glycogen storage disease) (Burchell *et al.*, 1989), doubts have been raised as to the reliability of these results (Rebuffat *et al.*, 1991). Cardiomyopathies may occur in types II, III, IV, and IX, in addition to glycogen storage disease with normal acid maltase levels (Schwartz *et al.*, 1996) (see Table 11.3).

Type II glycogen storage disease
Type II glycogen storage (Pompe) disease is an autosomal recessive disorder caused by acid alpha-glucosidase (acid maltase) deficiency. The clinical expression is varied, with both infantile and adolescent/adult types being recognized. In the classic infantile form (type IIa), affected infants are profoundly hypotonic with cardiomegaly and usually die within the first year of life (McKusick, 1990) (Figure 11.4). This contrasts with the more benign muscular form, which is associated with longer survival. The underlying gene mapped to chromosome 17q25.2-25.3 has over 30 mutations (Elpeleg, 1999).

Sudden death is a known complication of type IIa (Berry, 1989), most likely due to metabolic or cardiac sequelae (Bulkley & Hutchins, 1978; Tripathy *et al.*, 1988). A family has been reported in which unexpected death occurred in two siblings with acid maltase deficiency due to rupture of basilar artery aneurysms (Makos *et al.*, 1987), although the

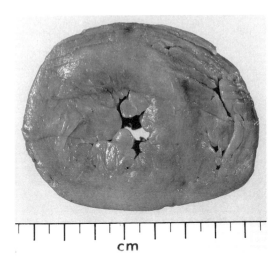

Figure 11.4 Cross-section of the heart in a five-month-old girl with Pompe (type II glycogen storage) disease, demonstrating massive cardiomegaly.

relationship between the vascular abnormalities and the metabolic disorder is unclear.

Clinical features
The characteristic finding in this disorder is failure to thrive, with skeletal muscle involvement, hepatomegaly, and cardiomegaly, the latter being profound enough to cause outflow obstruction. Within skeletal and cardiac muscle, there is an increase in membrane-bound intracytoplasmic glycogen as well as an increase in free cytoplasmic glycogen within cardiac myocytes (Figure 11.5).

Diagnosis
As increased cellular glycogen stores are not always present, diagnosis requires biochemical testing for specific enzyme deficiencies or molecular analysis (Ferrans & Boyce, 1983; Raben, Plotz & Byrne, 2002).

Amino acid disorders

Homocystinuria

Homocystinuria may be caused by any one of several enzyme defects, including cystathionine synthetase

deficiency. This autosomal recessive defect results in increased levels of serum and urine homocystine (Carson *et al.*, 1965) and is characterized by a phenotype similar to Marfan syndrome. Features that separate homocystinuria from Marfan syndrome are the finding of homocystine in plasma and urine, variable intellectual impairment, generalized osteoporosis, malar flushing, and alternative vascular complications (Schimke *et al.*, 1965).

Occurrence of sudden death
Myocardial infarction, cerebrovascular accident, and pulmonary thromboembolism are complications of homozygous homocystinuria that may result in premature death in childhood and adolescence. Up to 50% of these patients in some series have died before the age of 20 years (Dettmeyer, Varchmin-Schultheiss & Medea, 1998; Grieco, 1977; James, Carson & Froggatt, 1974; Schimke *et al.*, 1965). Cerebral arteries, veins, and sinuses are all at increased risk of thrombosis.

Pathophysiology
The cause of thromboembolic phenomenon in homocystinuria is an increase in fragility of endothelial cells (Almgren *et al.*, 1978), with desquamation and exposure of subendothelial connective tissue. Similar changes have been produced in experimental animals exposed to increased levels of homocystine (Harker *et al.*, 1974; McCully & Wilson, 1975). Blood coagulation abnormalities have also been reported, which may contribute to the thrombotic tendency (Palareti *et al.*, 1986). Also, there is fibromuscular thickening of the intima of vessels (Figure 11.6), with premature atherosclerosis and endocardial fibroelastosis of the heart (Gibson, Carson & Neill, 1964). Premature atherosclerosis has been found in heterozygous adults but does not appear to be a major problem in children (Mudd *et al.*, 1985).

Maple syrup urine disease

While the usual presentation of maple syrup urine disease is of anorexia, vomiting, and convulsions during the neonatal period, a late-onset form is recognized. It is possible for apparently healthy infants

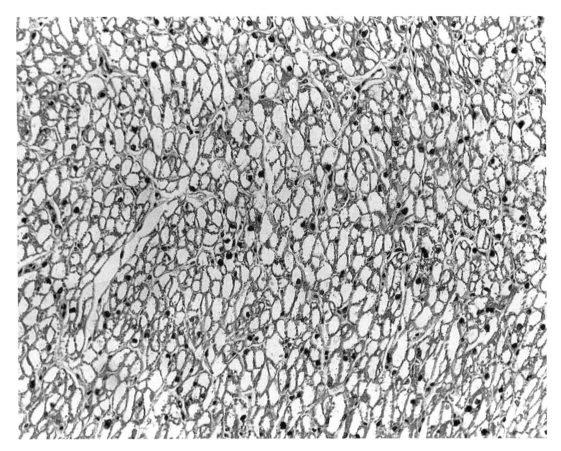

Figure 11.5 Microscopy of the heart in Pompe disease, showing extensive vacuolation of myocytes due to leaching out of glycogen during processing (hematoxylin and eosin, ×280).

with this condition to present with unexpected cardiorespiratory arrest (Hallock *et al.*, 1969).

Miscellaneous

Biotinidase deficiency

Biotinidase deficiency is the major defect in children with late-onset multiple carboxylase deficiency. Features include convulsions, developmental delay, hypotonia, hearing loss, alopecia, ataxia, and rashes (Wolf *et al.*, 1985). However, the clinical presentation may be variable. Metabolic acidosis may occur in undiagnosed cases, resulting in sudden and unexpected death (Burton & Wolf, 1987).

Gangliosidoses

These disorders are characterized by abnormalities in the metabolic handling of complex sugar-containing cerebrosides. While a chronic clinical course is more typical, with progressive dementia from cerebral storage, sudden death due to cardic arrhythmia may occur in GM_1 gangliosidosis (Patterson, Donnelly & Dehner, 1992). Cardiomyopathies may occur in both GM_1 and GM_2 gangliosidoses (see Table 11.3).

Mucopolysaccharidoses

This heterogeneous collection of lysosomal enzyme disorders is characterized by abnormal

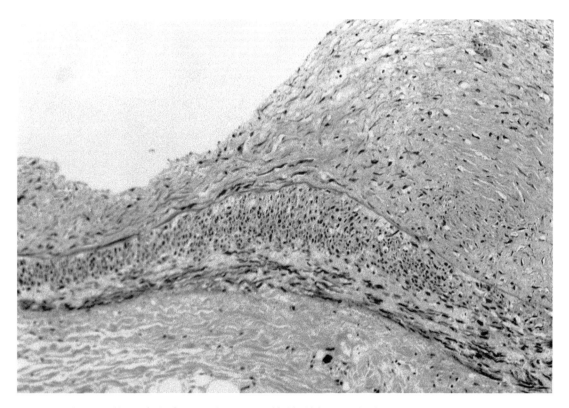

Figure 11.6 Fibrointimal hyperplasia of an artery in a 14-year-old girl with homocystinuria.

accumulation of acid mucopolysaccharides within a variety of tissues. Six main types with a number of subtypes have been identified, the features of which have been well described elsewhere (Dardir, Ferrans & Roberts, 1989). Hurler, Sanfilippo, Morquio, and Marateaux–Lamy syndromes are inherited on an autosomal recessive basis, Sly syndrome is autosomal recessive, and Hunter syndrome is a sex-linked recessive trait. Cardiomyopathies may occur in each subtype (see Table 11.3).

As the most severe cardiovascular abnormalities are found in Hurler syndrome, which is due to a deficiency of alpha-L-iduronidase, the following discussion will concentrate predominantly on children with this variant, although similar changes may be found in the other types of mucopolysaccharidoses (Factor, Biempica & Goldfischer, 1978).

Pathological features

At autopsy, lesions may be found within a variety of tissues, including the coronary arteries, elastic arteries, endocardium, myocardium, and the heart valves, all of which show infiltration by storage cells (Figure 11.7). The coronary arteries may be prominent on gross examination and show marked diffuse luminal narrowing due to concentric thickening of the intima, which contains numerous clear cells, collagen fibers, and increased amounts of acid mucopolysaccharide (Brosius & Roberts, 1981). The media may also be involved, and some of the intramural arteries may be affected similarly. The absence of cholesterol deposits and the concentric nature of the luminal narrowing help to differentiate the arterial lesions from those seen in premature atherosclerosis (Dardir, Ferrans & Roberts, 1989). The degree

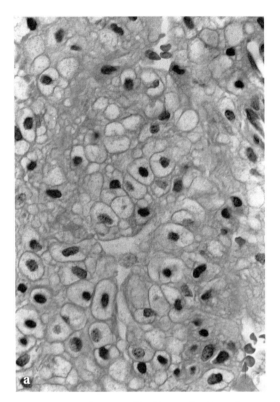
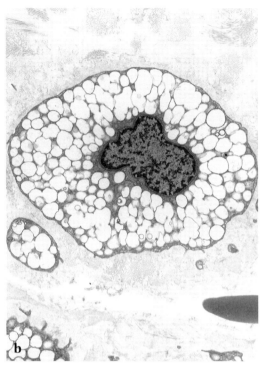

Figure 11.7 Typical storage cells with vacuolated cytoplasm (a) (hematoxylin and eosin, ×480), filled with dilated lysosomes (b) in a case of mucopolysaccharidosis (electronmicroscopy ×6000).

of narrowing is marked, with 71% of arteries in one study showing 76–100% stenosis on cross-sectional study (Brosius & Roberts, 1981). Very occasionally, calcification occurs within coronary arteries, and focal intimal changes have also been reported in both the aorta and the pulmonary artery (Krovetz & Schiebler, 1972).

Although the heart weight may not necessarily be increased in these disorders, there is diffuse thickening of the endocardium, resulting in a lack of compliance in the ventricular walls, particularly within the left ventricle. Microscopic examination reveals typical large vacuolated cells and collagen deposition within the ventricular myocardium (Renteria, Ferrans & Roberts, 1976). Both hypertrophic and dilated cardiomyopathies have been described.

Valvular lesions result from the same underlying process and involve particularly the mitral valve (Goldfischer *et al.*, 1975). All of the cardiac valves may be involved with the development of mitral stenosis, aortic stenosis, and aortic incompetence (Krovetz, Lorincz & Schiebler, 1965; Krovetz & Schiebler, 1972). Visual inspection of the cardiac valves may reveal thickened leaflets and shortening of the chordae tendinae (Figure 11.8).

Occurrence of sudden death

Although recognized more for severe mental retardation, hepatosplenomegaly, and skeletal abnormalities, the presence of cardiovascular disease and upper airway narrowing may predispose affected children to sudden death (Lindsay, 1950; Shapiro, Strome & Crocker, 1985). Ten of 87 (12%) deaths in children with Hunter–Hurler syndrome were sudden, although the pathophysiology was often not clear (Krovetz & Schiebler, 1972).

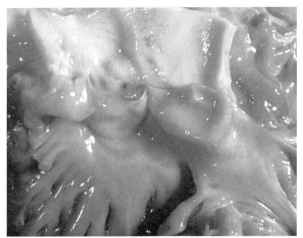

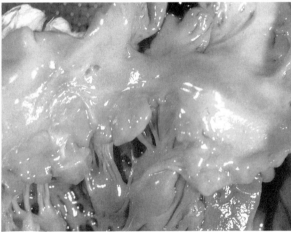

Figure 11.8 Thickening of aortic and mitral valves in a case of Hurler syndrome.

Pathophysiology

The cause of sudden death might seem straightforward given the degree of coronary arterial narrowing, but affected children usually do not show evidence of myocardial ischemia (Brosius & Roberts, 1981; Dardir, Ferrans & Roberts, 1989). This may be due to death occurring before the development of histologic changes within the myocardium, or to lethal arrhythmias occurring in the absence of permanent ischemic damage. It is also thought that other factors such as valve disease, aortic narrowing, myocardial infiltration by storage cells, systemic hypertension, respiratory insufficiency, and nutritional anemia are all contributors to myocardial instability (Hayflick *et al.*, 1992; Renteria, Ferrans & Roberts, 1976; Taylor *et al.*, 1991). Pulmonary hypertension has also been described in these children (Emanuel, 1954), in one case associated with acute postoperative death (Schenk & Haggerty, 1964).

Upper airway narrowing is another risk factor that may cause particular difficulties during intubation for general anesthesia. It also results in sleep apnea. Abnormalities such as deformation of tracheal and bronchial cartilages, and enlargment of the tonsils, adenoids, and tongue may narrow the airways (Shapiro, Strome & Crocker, 1985). Krovetz & Schiebler (1972) describe two of 87 children who died during anesthetic induction due to this problem.

Hyperlipidemias

The hyperlipidemias may be inherited or acquired and are divided into five categories according to the Frederickson classification, each of which is biochemically and etiologically heterogeneous. Sudden childhood death may occur in types I and II. Ischemic cerebrovascular strokes in infants and children have been associated with low levels of high-density lipoprotein cholesterol, sometimes occurring with high levels of triglycerides (Daniels *et al.*, 1982; Glueck *et al.*, 1982).

Type I hyperlipidemia

This is the rarest of the inherited hyperlipidemias and is believed to be due to a defect in extrahepatic lipoprotein lipase or its activator, apoprotein C-II, resulting in delayed clearance of chylomicrons from the blood. While patients with this condition do not have accelerated atherosclerosis, cerebral infarction has been reported in a six-year-old child (Berger & Bonnici, 1977) and in a two-month-old infant (Potter & Hilton, 1983). Sudden death occurred in the latter case due to cerebral infarction from excessive blood viscosity associated with marked chylomicronemia. Subsequent investigation of other family members demonstrated occult lipid abnormalities compatible with lipoprotein lipase deficiency.

Type II hyperlipidemia

Familial hypercholesterolemia is characterized by elevated low-density lipoproteins and cholesterol due to a deficiency of low-density lipoprotein receptors. It has an autosomal dominant inheritance pattern. The homozygous form is clinically the most severe, with manifestations of accelerated atherosclerosis developing in childhood, which may result in death from myocardial infarction at an early age (Mabuchi *et al.*, 1986; Sprecher *et al.*, 1984). In some cases, death is sudden and unexpected (Williams, 1989).

At autopsy, the ascending aorta shows more severe atherosclerosis than the abdominal aorta. This may be sufficiently florid to produce an angiographic appearance of supravalvular stenosis. Involvement of the coronary ostia (Allen *et al.*, 1980) may precipitate myocardial infarction, even in the absence of coronary artery disease, although the coronary arteries usually show diffuse involvement with atherosclerotic narrowing. Involvement of the aortic and mitral valves with significant stenosis is also characteristic, along with atherosclerotic deposits in the pulmonary artery. Microscopically, atherosclerotic plaques are similar to the more usual atheromas that occur with aging.

Clues to the presence of familial hypercholesterolemia prior to the commencement of autopsy include orange-yellow cutaneous xanthomas, which may develop in early childhood, and tendon xanthomas and arcus senilis, which are more common in older adolescents.

Types III–V hyperlipidemia

Type III and type IV hyperlipoproteinemias are characterized by abnormal beta very-low-density lipoproteins and elevated very-low-density lipoproteins, respectively. Although both are associated with a high incidence of atherosclerosis, sudden death in childhood is not a feature of these disorders (Morganroth, Levy & Fredrickson, 1975; Roberts *et al.*, 1973). Similarly, sudden childhood death has not been found in type V hyperlipoproteinemia, in which there is elevation of plasma very-low-density lipoproteins and chylomicrons (Ferrans & Boyce, 1983; Roberts *et al.*, 1973).

Miscellaneous

Sudden cardiac death during late adolescence may occur rarely in populations predisposed to premature atherosclerosis, such as in Finland, without any evidence of the above hyperlipoproteinemias (Koskenvuo, Karvonen & Rissanen, 1978). Premature atherosclerosis is also a feature of Cockayne, Hutchinson–Gilford (progeria), and Werner syndromes (Dardir, Ferrans & Roberts, 1989).

Menkes kinky hair syndrome

This X-linked recessive disorder is characterized by mental and growth retardation, abnormal hair growth producing the characteristic "pili torti" (Figure 11.9), and progressive neurologic deterioration, with death within one or two years. Other features include hypothermia, convulsions, subdural hematomas, aneurysms, arterial stenoses, and

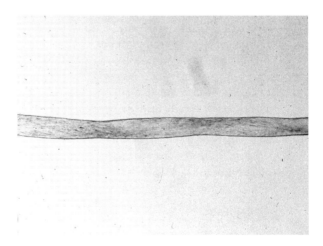

Figure 11.9 Typical axial twisting of a hair shaft with pili torti in Menkes syndrome.

thromboses (Pellegrino, Zanesco & Battistella, 1992). The incidence is estimated to be between one in 100,000 to one in 250,000 live births (Kodama, Murata & Kobayashi, 1999). Sudden death may occur, however, and was present in two of six cases reported by Danks and colleagues (1972).

A variety of molecular mutations have been identified at the ATP7A locus on the X chromosome that are responsible for the manifestations of Menkes disease. The result of this is a defect in copper-transporting P-type ATPase, which affects copper absorption, causing low serum copper and ceruloplasmin levels (Kaler, 1998). Vascular changes are common, and superficial vessels may be aneurysmally dilated and tortuous. Microscopically, there is fibromuscular intimal proliferation with fragmentation of the internal elastic lamina (Martin *et al.*, 1978) and decreased numbers of medial smooth muscle cells in a variety of vessels, including the coronary arteries (Uno *et al.*, 1983). Veins as well as arteries are affected (Wheeler & Roberts, 1976), with arterial changes resulting in obliteration of vessel lumena (Danks *et al.*, 1972; Pellegrino, Zanesco & Battistella, 1992).

Reye syndrome

Reye syndrome is characterized by an acute onset of encephalopathy often associated with hypoglycemia and/or hyperammonemia, liver dysfunction, and fatty change in the viscera associated with mitochondrial malfunction (Larsen, 1997; Starko *et al.*, 1980). Although once considered a defined entity, nowadays it is regarded as a non-specific term covering a variety of heterogeneous infectious, toxic, and metabolic etiologies (Casteels-Van Daele *et al.*, 2000). However, there remains a concurrence of characteristic clinical and pathologic features.

Clinical features

The clinical course may be fulminant, usually occurring in children under 10 years of age. It often follows a viral illness, particularly influenza and chickenpox,

although occasionally sudden death may occur with relatively non-specific symptoms and signs that were not thought to be significant at the time (Young, 1992). Features of vomiting, lethargy, irritability, delirium, and coma have raised the possibility of a toxic etiology. Aspirin was once the chief suspect, as it was recognized that children who were on salicylate medication for other diseases had an increased risk of Reye syndrome; however, there is also an association with phenothiazine and antiemetic use (Casteels-Van Daele *et al.*, 2000; Halpin *et al.*, 1982; Meier, Baron & Greenberg, 1983; Rennebohm *et al.*, 1985; Starko & Mullick, 1983). The decline in incidence of the syndrome is believed to be due to more accurate clinical detection of possible precipitating factors (Casteels-Van Daele *et al.*, 2000) and identification of cases where there is a specific underlying metabolic abnormality.

In reviewing the clinical presentation, the diagnosis of Reye syndrome is less likely in younger children who have had previous episodes of hypoglycemia or acidosis precipitated by minor illness or fasting. An inherited metabolic disorder is more probable if there has been a similar sibling death.

Pathological features

At autopsy, the liver may be enlarged and on cut section will show yellowish coloration (Figure 11.10). Quite marked cerebral edema may be noted when the calvarium is removed (Figure 11.11). Microscopically, the pattern of hepatic steatosis may not be helpful, because a number of conditions may result in microvesicular lipid deposition. Certain features may be found on electron microscopy if tissue preservation is adequate. Unfortunately, swelling of mitochondria with accumulation of flocculent matrix material and loss of intramitochondrial dense bodies (Partin, Schubert & Partin, 1971) may be more discernable in biopsy than in autopsy material. These features are not present in the livers of children with MCAD or LCAD deficiencies (Treem *et al.*, 1986). Lipid deposits may be found in other organs, such as in the heart or within the renal tubules (Figures 11.12).

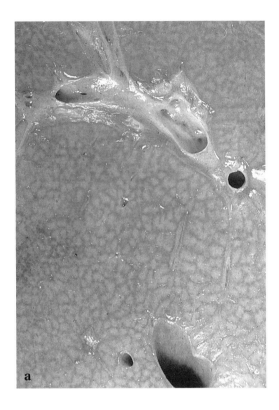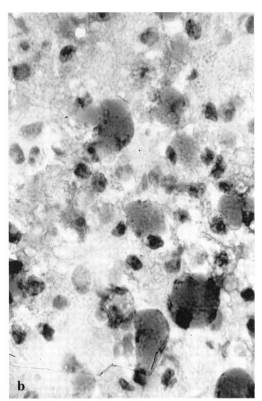

Figure 11.10 Cut surface of the liver in a six-year-old girl who died from Reye syndrome, showing diffuse mottling from lipid accumulation (a). Microscopy revealed lipid deposition within hepatocytes (b) (oil-red O, ×440).

Occurrence of sudden death

Sudden death in fulminant cases may lead to confusion with acyl-CoA dehydrogenase deficiencies or with SIDS (Glasgow & Moore, 1993; Mason & Bain, 1982). Usually, however, a history of progressive neurologic deterioration can be elicited.

Autopsy investigation

Meier, Baron & Greenberg (1983) recommended that postmortem levels of serum transaminases, creatinine kinase, and blood ammonia be measured in suspected cases as they are elevated, whereas serum alkaline phosphatase, gamma glutamyl transpeptidase, and bilirubin are within the normal range.

Further investigative protocols for Reye syndrome and metabolic disorders with similar presentations have been outlined by Green & Hall (1992).

Hemorrhagic shock and encephalopathy syndrome

Hemorrhagic shock and encephalopathy syndrome is a devastating disorder affecting infants and young children; it was first described in 1983 by Levin and colleagues. Although many of the manifestations involve the central nervous system, the etiology remains unclear. The syndrome has been included in this chapter as the manifestations are similar to certain inborn errors of metabolism and it has been proposed that defective protease inhibitor production

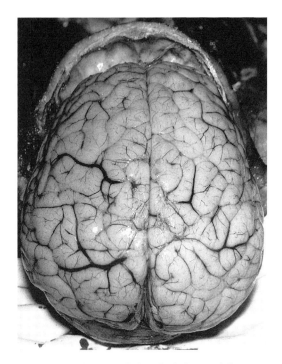

Figure 11.11 Although marked cerebral edema with flattening of gyri is a non-specific finding, it may indicate metabolic encephalopathy.

or release may be involved in the pathogenesis (Levin *et al.*, 1989).

Clinical features

Affected infants and children are usually healthy before the illness when they present with the sudden onset of fever, diarrhea, convulsions, coma, and shock. There may be severe metabolic acidosis with hepatorenal failure and hemorrhagic manifestations (Ince, Kuloglu & Akinci, 2000). While there is generalized multiorgan failure, lethal manifestations generally arise from cerebral involvement, with seizures and cerebral edema resulting in rapid death (Levin *et al.*, 1989; Trounce *et al.*, 1991).

The differential diagnosis includes fulminant sepsis, toxic shock syndrome, hemolytic-uremic syndrome, Reye syndrome, and certain inborn errors of metabolism. Microbiologic and metabolic investigations have failed to find a cause, and no drugs, poisons, or toxins have been detected. While similar findings may occur in infants with heatstroke, overwrapping and overheating have not been features of reported cases (Bacon & Hall, 1992; Levin *et al.*, 1989). It is possible that hemorrhagic shock and encephalopathy syndrome may be initiated by a variety of environmental factors or may represent a final common pathway for a number of disorders (Chesney & Chesney, 1989; Little & Wilkins, 1997).

Pathological features

The autopsy findings are non-specific and relate to shock, hypoxia, and disseminated intravascular coagulation. Cerebral edema with widespread intravascular microthrombi and hemorrhage is present, and there may be extensive infarction. The liver shows centrilobular necrosis, with mixed micro- and macrovesicular steatosis. There may be inflammation, hemorrhage, and villus atophy within the intestine, with adrenal hemorrhage, pituitary necrosis, and acute renal tubular necrosis (Bratton & Jardine, 1992; Chaves-Carballo *et al.*, 1990; Levin *et al.*, 1989; Little & Wilkins, 1997).

Occurrence of sudden death

The clinical course of this disorder is rapid, with significant morbidity and mortality. Sudden collapse and death have been described in both infants and young children (Little & Wilkins, 1997; Pollack & Pender, 1991; Weibley, Pimental & Ackerman, 1989).

Autopsy investigation

The diagnosis of hemorrhagic shock and encephalopathy syndrome remains one of exclusion. Scene examination and review of bedding, household heating, and medications that may predispose to hyperthermia are required to exclude heat shock. Full microbiologic assessment is required to exclude viral or bacterial sepsis. Toxic shock syndrome can be eliminated if there are no skin or mucosal lesions and *Staphylococcus aureus* is not cultured.

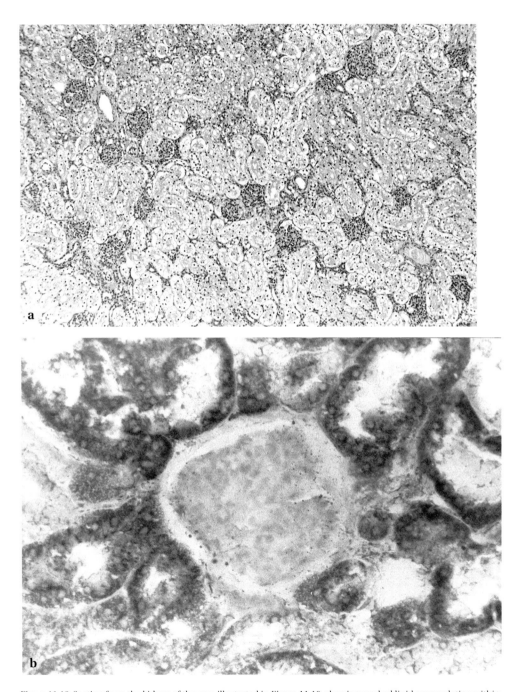

Figure 11.12 Section from the kidney of the case illustrated in Figure 11.10, showing marked lipid accumulation within renal tubular epithelial cells (a) (hematoxylin and eosin, ×110). Oil-red O staining demonstrated lipid droplets within tubules surrounding an uninvolved glomerulus (b) (×440).

Hyperpyrexia is not usually a feature of inborn errors of metabolism, such as urea cycle defects, organic acidurias, and fatty acid oxidation disorders. The age range, presentation, and histology differ from those of Reye syndrome and hemolytic-uremic syndrome. Toxicologic screening of blood or serum is required to determine whether there are any drugs, toxins, or poisons present (Little & Wilkins, 1997).

Miscellaneous disorders

Mitochondrial encephalomyelopathies are a diverse group of conditions in which there are structurally abnormal mitochondria with defects in mitochondrial aerobic oxidative metabolism. While the clinical course is usually chronic with hypotonia, the association with cardiomyopathies (see Table 11.3), convulsions, and stroke-like episodes raises the possibility of rapid terminal decline (Cornelio & DiDonato, 1985; Pavlakis *et al.*, 1984).

Although cardiomyopathy or cardiac involvement may be present in a range of other inherited metabolic disorders, such as Fabry disease (angiokeratoma corporis diffusum universale), Leigh disease (subacute necrotising encephalomyelopathy), Refsum disease (phytanic acid alpha-hydroxylase deficiency), Cori–Forbes disease (type III glycogen storage disease, amylo-1,6-glycosidase deficiency), and primary oxalosis (Allen *et al.*, 1978; Colucci *et al.*, 1982; Coltart & Hudson, 1971; Dardir, Ferrans & Roberts, 1989), the clinical courses tend to be chronic, the cardiac lesions are of secondary importance, and death does not usually occur until adulthood.

Endocrine disorders

Endocrine disorders are not usually considered in the differential diagnosis of sudden and unexpected deaths in children, since the clinical courses are often prolonged, occurring in children with established diagnoses. Very occasionally, however, death can occur unexpectedly at the time of first presentation, or

Table 11.4. Endocrine conditions potentially associated with sudden death in childhood

Insulin-dependent diabetes mellitus
Hyper/hypoadrenalism
Pheochromocytoma
Nesiodioblastosis
Hyper/hypothyroidism
Multiple endocrine neoplasia

when coincidental stresses result in a fulminant and fatal episode in a child who was thought to be clinically stable. Potential endocrine causes of sudden childhood death are listed in Table 11.4.

Insulin-dependent diabetes mellitus

Although children may die on their initial presentation with insulin-dependent diabetes mellitus (Neuspiel & Kuller, 1985; Rozin *et al.*, 1994), reports of sudden death in previously undiagnosed individuals due to ketoacidosis have occurred mainly in adults (DiMaio, Sturner & Coe, 1977; Irwin & Cohle, 1988). Unexpected death has, however, been described in diabetic children who were thought to be responding appropriately to treatment for ketoacidosis (Hayes & Woods, 1968). The mechanisms for this are not well understood, but may involve cerebral edema not related to excessive rehydration, or hypokalemia with cardiac arrhythmia (Buchino, Corey & Montgomery, 2002; Edge, Ford-Adams & Dunger, 1999; Glaser *et al.*, 2001).

The diagnosis of diabetes mellitus with hyperglycemia/ketoacidosis at autopsy is difficult. Postmortem blood and cerebrospinal fluid glucose levels are unreliable, as there may be a substantial reduction in glucose levels due to bacterial action and continued tissue glycolysis, or an increase due to postmortem hepatic glycogenolysis (Rozin *et al.*, 1994). Analysis of vitreous humor provides more reliable estimates of elevated glucose and beta-hydroxy butyrate levels in cases of possible hyperglycemic ketoacidosis (DiMaio, Sturner & Coe, 1977). Ketones may also be present in the urine.

Certain morphologic findings of hyperglycemia, such as vacuolization of renal tubular epithelium – so-called Armanni–Ebstein nephropathy (Figure 11.13) – may assist in making the diagnosis, although this is not specific for diabetes. The liver may also show non-specific microvesicular steatosis with glycogenation of nuclei. Pancreatic autolysis usually precludes proper histologic assessment; however, a reduction in the number and size of the islets of Langerhans and interstitial fibrosis have been described (Rozin *et al.*, 1994). Vascular complications may occur infrequently in childhood, resulting in myocardial or cerebral infarction (Atluru, 1986; Molander, 1982; Shivelhood, 1947).

Sudden death may also occur from excessive insulin administration with hypoglycemia. This may have been intentional or inadvertent. Assessment of such a case will require measurement of serum insulin levels, possibly with comparisons of insulin levels from injection sites and control tissues. Measurement of C-peptide levels will help to differentiate endogenous from therapeutic animal insulin (Knight, 1996).

An unusual group of young diabetics has been described where deaths have occurred unexpectedly in bed, the so-called "dead in bed syndrome" (Sartor & Dahlquist, 1995; Thordarson & Søvik, 1995). These individuals characteristically are in good health with uncomplicated diabetes and no recent changes in insulin therapy. As the deaths all occur during sleep, suggestions have been made that nocturnal hypoglycemia may be a problem (Tattersall & Gill, 1991). Unfortunately, vitreous humor glucose levels also fall after death and so cannot be used to confirm hypoglycemia (Edge, Ford-Adams & Dunger, 1999).

Adrenal hypoplasia

Hypoplasia or atrophy of the adrenal glands may result in sudden and unexpected death in infants and children due to Addisonian crises, which may mimic SIDS (Batch *et al.*, 1991; Favara, Franciosi & Miles, 1972; Jindrich, 1984; O'Donohoe & Holland, 1968; Russell *et al.*, 1977; Sperling, Wolfsen & Fisher, 1973).

Two types of congenital adrenal hypoplasia have been identified. In the first, the adrenal gland is morphologically similar to the adult adrenal gland but is considerably reduced in size. This type may be associated with pituitary hypoplasia and anencephaly and may be inherited in an autosomal recessive manner. The second type shows remnants of the fetal cortex in the form of cytomegaly, is associated with a much longer survival (Kerenyi, 1961), and may be inherited in an X-linked recessive manner. There is, however, considerable variation in clinical expression, and there may be a degree of histologic overlap between the two types.

Addison disease in later life may be asymptomatic until exertion precipitates sudden collapse and death. Such was the case in a 19-year-old youth who collapsed during a cross-country race (Molander, 1982). The only significant finding at autopsy was fibrosis and calcification of the adrenal glands. There may be a history of weakness, lethargy, and diarrhea prior to death (al Sabri, Smith & Busuttil, 1997; Russell *et al.*, 1977). An association with Duchenne muscular dystrophy has been reported in the X-linked variant (Stuhrmann *et al.*, 1991).

Adrenal hyperplasia

There are a group of enzymatic defects in the cortisol synthetic pathway that result in congenital adrenal hyperplasia due to increased stimulation of the adrenal gland by elevated levels of adrenocorticotrophic hormone (ACTH) (New & Levine, 1981).

Etiology

These inborn errors of metabolism are autosomal recessively inherited, with the most common defect involving a deficiency in 21-hydroxylase. This results in excessive loss of sodium due to aldosterone deficiency, which may lead to rapidly developing shock and death (Cleveland, Green & Wilkins, 1962).

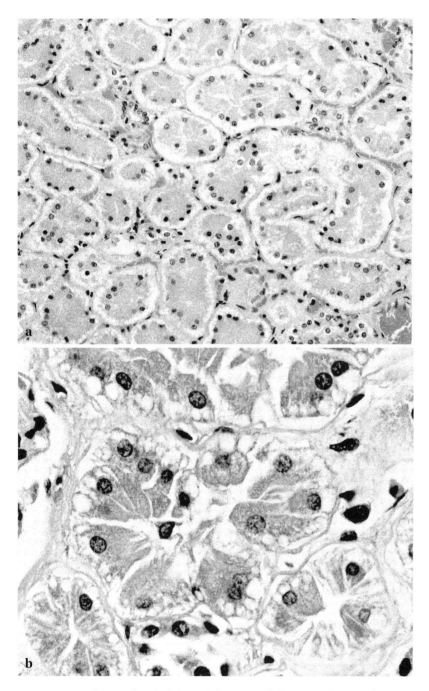

Figure 11.13 Vacuolization of renal tubular epithelium – so-called Armanni–Ebstein nephropathy – in a 16-year-old male dying of diabetic ketoacidosis (a, hematoxylin and eosin, ×150; b, hematoxylin and eosin, ×350).

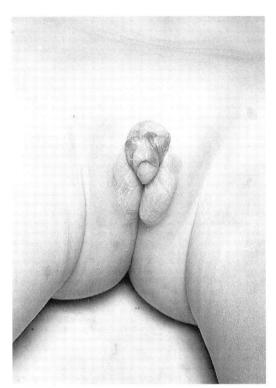 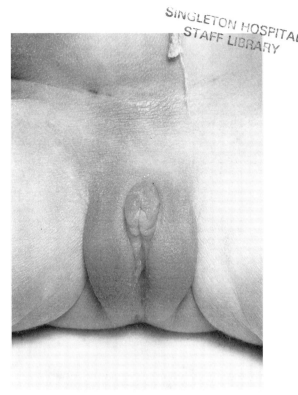

Figure 11.14 Examples of virulization with clitoral enlargement in two infants with congenital adrenal hyperplasia.

Clinical features

Female infants are usually diagnosed at a younger age than males because of virilization with variable clitoral enlargement and fusion of the labioscrotal folds (Marshall & Lightner, 1980; New & Levine, 1984) (Figure 11.14). Males may remain undiagnosed until a fatal episode occurs, although in retrospect there may have been a history of anorexia, failure to thrive, or vomiting. Cardiac tachyarrhthymias may have been noted prior to collapse. Hypertension, a feature of 11-β-hydroxylase deficiency, may be associated with stroke at an early age (Cleveland, Green & Wilkins, 1962).

Pathological features

At autopsy, infants and children may be dehydrated, with female infants showing evidence of masculinization, sometimes with polycystic ovaries. The internal genitalia are otherwise normal in appearance.

Male infants may have undescended testes and hypospadius, and boys may show signs of sexual precocity (White, New & Dupont, 1987). The adrenal glands are enlarged, with nodular or diffuse cortical hyperplasia. Histologically, the cortex appears homogeneous, with loss of distinction between the zona fasciculata and reticularis.

Pheochromocytoma

This catecholamine-producing tumor of the adrenal medulla may occur in childhood and may be a potential cause of unexpected death due to uncontrolled hypertension. Intracerebral hemorrhage and embolism, cardiomyopathy, cardiac failure, and myocardial infarction may also occur (Dagartzikas *et al.*, 2002). There is an association with multiple endocrine neoplasia syndromes, neurofibromatosis (von Recklinghausen disease), and von

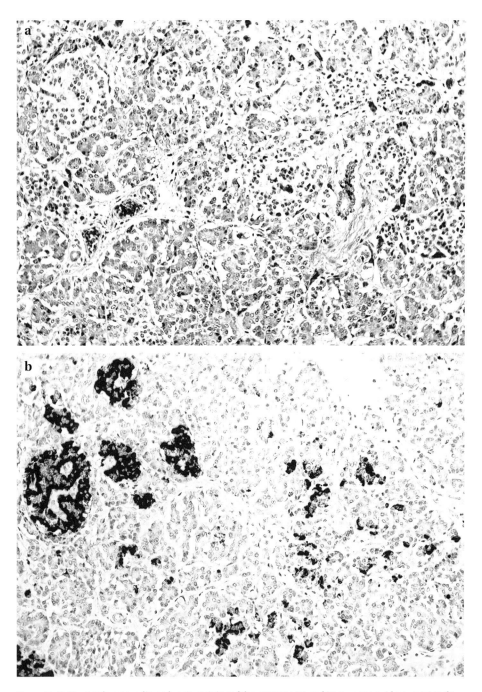

Figure 11.15 Routine hematoxylin and eosin staining of the pancreas (a) and immunoperoxidase staining (b) for insulin, demonstrating diffuse dispersion of endocrine cells throughout the pancreatic parenchyma in a three-month-old boy with recurrent hypoglycemia (×110).

Hipple–Lindau disease, with the possibility of a family history even in the absence of a defined syndrome (Inabnet, Caragliano & Pertsemlidis, 2000; Reddy *et al.*, 2000). Pheochromocytoma in pregnancy is associated with an increased risk of both maternal and fetal mortality, possibly exacerbated by concurrent prothrombotic conditions (Botchan *et al.*, 1995; Jessurun *et al.*, 1993; Zangrillo *et al.*, 1999).

Nesidioblastosis

Nesidioblastosis complex, also known as islet cell dysmaturational syndrome, refers to the range of histologic changes that may be found in the pancreas in association with hyperinsulinemic hypoglycemia (Jaffe, Hashida & Yunis, 1982). Histologic findings in infants with infantile hyperinsulinemic hypoglycemia are variable, consisting of apparently normal pancreatic morphology, hyperplasia, adenoma, or nesidioblastosis (Thomas *et al.*, 1977). The latter entity is a proliferation of islet cells from small ducts and acini, with scattering of endocrine cells throughout the pancreatic parenchyma (Gould *et al.*, 1983) (Figure 11.15).

While nesidioblastosis was once claimed to be a factor in certain deaths ascribed to SIDS (Hirvonen *et al.*, 1980), it is now apparent that "disorganization" of islet cells is probably a normal phenomenon related to maturation (Jaffe, Hashida & Yunis, 1982). Certainly a number of infants examined by the author and with otherwise typical features of SIDS have had this finding (see Figure 13.28). It has been suggested, therefore, that this finding is of significance only if hyperinsulinemia and hypoglycemia can be demonstrated. Nesidioblastosis has also been associated with the development of hypertrophic cardiomyopathy, but this is of uncertain physiologic significance in terms of the potential for sudden death (Harris *et al.*, 1992).

Thyroid disease

Hashimoto thyroiditis was the only significant autopsy finding in a report of a 15-year-old girl who collapsed and died suddenly. As the girl had been symptomatically hypothyroid, it was postulated that death was due to spontaneous ventricular arrhythmia associated with the hypothyroid state (Guthrie, Hunsaker & O'Connor, 1987). Fatal upper airway obstruction may occur rarely in infants with congenital hypothyroidism and macroglossia.

Multiple endocrine neoplasia

This condition can be divided into two main categories: MEN-I, or Wermer syndrome, and MEN-II, or Sipple syndrome. Both are characterized by benign and malignant tumors arising in at least two endocrine organs, with other changes in muscle, nervous, and connective tissues (Fassbender *et al.*, 2000). While MEN-I tends to manifest first in adult life, MEN-IIB syndrome represents a subgroup that is recognized in childhood by the presence of a marfanoid habitus, hypotonia, hyperlaxity of joints, kyphoscoliosis, medullary thyroid carcinoma, multiple mucosal ganglioneuromas, and pheochromocytomas (Byard *et al.*, 1990; Griffiths *et al.*, 1990). Inheritance is autosomal dominant, with a number of cases representing spontaneous mutations. The clinical manifestations are caused by activation of the RET proto-oncogene (Fassbender *et al.*, 2000). Although sudden death has not been a feature of the literature on MEN-IIB, the occurrence of pheochromocytomas could theoretically result in lethal hypertensive crises, which are a well-recognized cause of sudden death in older age groups (Bravo, 2002; Ciftci *et al.*, 2001). Unfortunately, measurement of urinary catecholamines after death cannot be used to identify functional pheochromocytomas and so is of limited use in the assessment of such cases (Tormey, Carney & FitzGerald, 1999).

REFERENCES

Al Sabri, A. M., Smith, N. & Busuttil, A. (1997). Sudden death due to auto-immune Addison's disease in a 12-year-old girl. *International Journal of Legal Medicine*, **110**, 278–80.

Allen, I. V., Swallow, M., Nevin, N. C. & McCormick, D. (1978). Clinicopathological study of Refsum's disease with particular reference to fatal complications. *Journal of Neurology, Neurosurgery and Psychiatry*, **41**, 323–32.

Allen, J. M., Thompson, G. R., Myant, N. B., Steiner, R. & Oakley, C. M. (1980). Cardiovascular complications of homozygous familial hypercholesterolaemia. *British Heart Journal*, **44**, 361–8.

Allison, F., Bennett, M. J., Variend, S. & Engel, P. C. (1988). Acyl-coenzyme A dehydrogenase deficiency in heart tissue from infants who died unexpectedly with fatty change in the liver. *British Medical Journal*, **296**, 11–12.

Almgren, B., Eriksson, I., Hemmingsson, A., Hillerdal, G., Larsson, E. & Åberg, H. (1978). Abdominal aortic aneurysm in homocystinuria. *Acta Chirurgica Scandinavica* **144**, 545–8.

Anonymous (1986). Sudden infant death and inherited disorders of fat oxidation. *Lancet*, **ii**, 1073–5.

Anonymous (1991). Medium chain CoA dehydrogenase deficiency. *Lancet*, **338**, 544–5.

Antozzi, C. & Zeviani, M. (1997). Cardiomyopathies in disorders of oxidative metabolism. *Cardiovascular Research*, **35**, 184–99.

Applegarth, D. A., Dimmick, J. E. & Toone, J. R. (1989). Laboratory detection of metabolic disease. *Pediatric Clinics of North America*, **36**, 49–65.

Arens, R., Gozal, D., Jain, K., *et al.* (1993). Prevalence of medium-chain acyl-coenzyme A dehydrogenase deficiency in the sudden infant death syndrome. *Journal of Pediatrics* **122**, 715–18.

Atluru, V. L. (1986). Spontaneous intracerebral hematomas in juvenile diabetic ketoacidosis. *Pediatric Neurology*, **2**, 167–9.

Bacon, C. J. & Hall, S. M. (1992). Haemorrhagic shock encephalopathy syndrome in the British Isles. *Archives of Disease in Childhood*, **67**, 985–93.

Batch, J. A., Montalto, J., Yong, A. B. W., Gold, H., Goss, P. & Warne, G. L. (1991). Three cases of congenital adrenal hypoplasia: a cause of salt-wasting and mortality in the neonatal period. *Journal of Paediatrics and Child Health*, **27**, 108–12.

Bennett, M. J. & Powell, S. (1994). Metabolic disease and sudden, unexpected death in infancy. *Human Pathology*, **25**, 742–6.

Bennett, M. J., Rinaldo, P., Millington, D. S., Tanaka, K., Yokota, I. & Coates, P. M. (1991). Medium-chain acyl-CoA dehydrogenase deficiency: postmortem diagnosis in a case of sudden infant death and neonatal diagnosis of an affected sibling. *Pediatric Pathology*, **11**, 889–95.

Berger, G. M. B. & Bonnici, F. (1977). Familial hyperchylomicronaemia in four families. Problems in diagnosis, management and aetiology reviewed. *South African Medical Journal*, **51**, 623–8.

Berry, C. L. (1989). Causes of sudden natural death in infancy and childhood. In *Paediatric Forensic Medicine and Pathology*, ed. J. K. Mason. London: Chapman & Hall Medical, pp. 165–77.

Boles, R. G., Martin, S. K., Blitzer, M. G. & Rinaldo, P. (1994). Biochemical diagnosis of fatty acid oxidation disorders by metabolite analysis of postmortem liver. *Human Pathology*, **25**, 735–41.

Bonnell, H. J. & Beckwith, J. B. (1986). Fatty liver in sudden childhood death. Implications for Reye's syndrome? *American Journal of Diseases of Children*, **140**, 30–33.

Botchan, A., Hauser, R., Kupfermine, M., Grisaru, D., Peyser, M. R. & Lessing, J. B. (1995). Pheochromocytoma in pregnancy: case report and review of the literature. *Obstetrical and Gynecological Survey*, **50**, 321–7.

Bratton, S. L. & Jardine, D. S. (1992). Cerebral infarction complicated hemorrhagic shock and encephalopathy syndrome. *Pediatrics*, **90**, 626–8.

Bravo, E. L. (2002). Pheochromocytoma. *Cardiology in Review*, **10**, 44–50.

Breningstall, G. N. (1990). Carnitine deficiency syndromes. *Pediatric Neurology*, **6**, 75–81.

Brosius, F. C., III & Roberts, W. C. (1981). Coronary artery disease in the Hurler syndrome. Qualitative and quantitative analysis of the extent of coronary narrowing at necropsy in six children. *American Journal of Cardiology*, **47**, 649–53.

Buchino, J. J., Corey, T. S. & Montgomery, V. (2002). Sudden unexpected death in hospitalized children. *Journal of Pediatrics*, **140**, 461–5.

Bulkley, B. H. & Hutchins, G. M. (1978). Pompe's disease presenting as hypertrophic myocardiomyopathy with Wolff–Parkinson–White syndrome. *American Heart Journal*, **92**, 246–52.

Burchell, A., Busuttil, A., Bell, J. E. & Hume, R. (1989). Hepatic microsomal glucose-6-phosphatase system and sudden infant death syndrome. *Lancet*, **ii**, 291–3.

Burton, B. K. & Wolf, B. (1987). Sudden death associated with biotinidase deficiency. *Pediatrics*, **79**, 482–3.

Byard, R. W., Thorner, P. S., Chan, H. S. L., Griffiths, A. M. & Cutz, E. (1990). Pathological features of multiple endocrine neoplasia type IIB in childhood. *Pediatric Pathology*, **10**, 581–92.

Carson, N. A. J., Dent, C. E., Field, C. M. B. & Gaull, G. E. (1965). Homocystinuria. Clinical and pathological review of ten cases. *Journal of Pediatrics*, **66**, 565–83.

Carter, N. & Variend, S. (1992). Fatty change of the pediatric myocardium. *Pediatric Pathology*, **12**, 325–31.

Casteels-Van Daele, M., Van Geet, C., Wouters, C. & Eggermont, E. (2000). Reye syndrome revisited: a descriptive term covering a group of heterogeneous disorders. *European Journal of Pediatrics*, **159**, 641–8.

Chapoy, P. R., Angelini, C., Brown, W. J., Stiff, J. E., Shug, A. L. & Cederbaum, S. D. (1980). Systemic carnitine deficiency – a treatable inherited lipid-storage disease presenting as

Reye's syndrome. *New England Journal of Medicine*, **303**, 1389–94.

Chaves-Carballo, E., Montes, J. E., Nelson, W. B. & Chrenka, B. A. (1990). Hemorrhagic shock and encephalopathy. Clinical definition of a catastrophic syndrome in infants. *American Journal of Diseases of Children*, **144**, 1079–82.

Chesney, P. J. & Chesney, R. W. (1989). Hemorrhagic shock and encephalopathy: reflections about a new devastating disorder that affects normal children. *Journal of Pediatrics*, **114**, 254–6.

Ciftci, A. O., Tanyel, F. C., Şenocak, M. E. & Büyükpamukçu, N. (2001). Pheochromocytoma in children. *Journal of Pediatric Surgery*, **36**, 447–52.

Clayton, P. T., Hyland, K., Brand, M. & Leonard, J. V. (1986). Mitochondrial phosphoenolpyruvate carboxykinase deficiency. *European Journal of Pediatrics*, **145**, 46–50.

Cleveland, W. W., Green, O. C. & Wilkins, L. (1962). Deaths in congenital adrenal hyperplasia. *Pediatrics*, **29**, 3–17.

Coltart, D. J. & Hudson, R. E. B. (1971). Primary oxalosis of the heart: a cause of heart block. *British Heart Journal*, **33**, 315–19.

Colucci, W. S., Lorell, B. H., Schoen, F. J., Warhol, M. J. & Grossman, W. (1982). Hypertrophic obstructive cardiomyopathy due to Fabry's disease. *New England Journal of Medicine*, **307**, 926–8.

Cornelio, F. & DiDonato, S. (1985). Myopathies due to enzyme deficiencies. *Journal of Neurology*, **232**, 329–40.

Dagartzikas, M. I., Sprague, K., Carter, G. & Tobias, J. D. (2002). Cerebrovascular event, dilated cardiomyopathy, and pheochromocytoma. *Pediatric Emergency Care*, **18**, 33–5.

Daniels, S. R., Bates, S., Lukin, R. R., Benton, C., Third, J. & Glueck, C. J. (1982). Cerebrovascular arteriopathy (arteriosclerosis) and ischemic childhood stroke. *Stroke*, **13**, 360–65.

Danks, D. M., Campbell, P. E., Stevens, B. J., Mayne, V. & Cartwright, E. (1972). Menkes's kinky hair syndrome. An inherited defect in copper absorption with widespread effects. *Pediatrics*, **50**, 188–201.

Dardir, M., Ferrans, V. J. & Roberts, W. C. (1989). Coronary artery disease in familial and metabolic disorders. In *Nonatherosclerotic Ischemic Heart Disease*, ed. R. Virmani & M. B. Forman. New York: Raven Press, pp. 185–235.

Demaugre, F., Bonnefont, J.-P., Colonna, M., Cepanec, C., Leroux, J.-P. & Saudubray, J.-M. (1991). Infantile form of carnitine palmitoyltransferase II deficiency with hepatomuscular symptoms and sudden death. Physiopathological approach to carnitine palmitoyltransferase II deficiencies. *Journal of Clinical Investigation*, **87**, 859–64.

Dettmeyer, R., Varchmin-Schultheiss, K. & Madea, B. (1998). Sudden death of an 18-year-old man with homocystinuria and intracranial inflammatory pseudotumor (IPT). *Forensic Science International*, **94**, 19–24.

DiMaio, V. J. M., Sturner, W. Q. & Coe, J. I. (1977). Sudden and unexpected deaths after the acute onset of diabetes mellitus. *Journal of Forensic Sciences*, **22**, 147–51.

Ding, J.-H., Roe, C. R., Iafolla, A. K. & Chen, Y.-T. (1991). Medium-chain acyl-coenzyme A dehydrogenase deficiency and sudden infant death. *New England Journal of Medicine*, **325**, 61–2.

Dionisi-Vici, C., Rizzo, C. Burlina, A. B., *et al.* (2002). Inborn errors of metabolism in the Italian pediatric population: a national retrospective survey. *Journal of Pediatrics*, **140**, 321–7.

Divry, P., Vianey-Liaud, C., Jakobs, C., Ten-Brink, H. J., Dutruge, J. & Gilly, R. (1990). Sudden infant death syndrome: organic acid profiles in cerebrospinal fluid from 47 children and the occurrence of N-acetylaspartic acid. *Journal of Inherited Metabolic Diseases*, **13**, 330–32.

Duran, M., Hofkamp, M., Rhead, W. J., Saudubray, J.-M. & Wadman, S. K. (1986). Sudden child death and "healthy" affected family members with medium-chain acyl-coenzyme A dehydrogenase deficiency. *Pediatrics*, **78**, 1052–7.

Duran, M., Wanders, R. J. A., deJager, J. P., *et al.* (1991). 3-Hydroxydicarboxylic aciduria due to long-chain 3-hydroxy-acyl-coenzyme A dehydrogenase deficiency associated with sudden neonatal death: protective effect of medium-chain triglyceride treatment. *European Journal of Pediatrics*, **150**, 190–5.

Edge, J. A., Ford-Adams, M. E. & Dunger, D. B. (1999). Causes of death in children with insulin dependent diabetes 1990–96. *Archives of Disease in Childhood*, **81**, 318–23.

Elpeleg, O. N. (1992). Sudden infant death syndrome in neonates. *American Journal of Diseases of Children*, **146**, 903–4.

Elpeleg, O. N. (1999). The molecular background of glycogen metabolism disorders. *Journal of Pediatric Endocrinology and Metabolism*, **12**, 363–79.

Emanuel, R. W. (1954). Gargoylism with cardiovascular involvement in two brothers. *British Heart Journal*, **16**, 417–22.

Emery, J. L., Chandra, S. & Gilbert-Barness, E. F. (1988). Findings in child deaths registered as sudden infant death syndrome (SIDS) in Madison, Wisconsin. *Pediatric Pathology*, **8**, 171–8.

Emery, J. L., Variend, S., Howat, A. J. & Vawter, G. F. (1988). Investigation of inborn errors of metabolism in unexpected infant deaths. *Lancet*, **i**, 29–31.

Factor, S. M., Biempica, L. & Goldfischer, S. (1978). Coronary intimal sclerosis in Morquio's syndrome. *Virchows Archiv. A, Pathological Anatomy and Histology*, **379**, 1–10.

Fassbender, W. J., Krohn-Grimberghe, B., Görtz, B., *et al.* (2000). Multiple endocrine neoplasia (MEN) – an overview and case report – patient with sporadic bilateral pheochromocytoma, hyperparathyroidism and marfanoid habitus. *Anticancer Research*, **20**, 4877–88.

Favara, B. E., Fransciosi, R. A. & Miles, V. (1972). Idiopathic adrenal hypoplasia in children. *American Journal of Clinical Pathology*, **57**, 287—96.

Ferrans, V. J. & Boyce, S. W. (1983). Metabolic and familial diseases. In *Cardiovascular Pathology*, vol. 2, ed. M. D. Silver. New York: Churchill Livingstone, pp. 945–1004.

Gibson, J. B., Carson, N. A. J. & Neill, D. W. (1964). Pathological findings in homocystinuria. *Journal of Clinical Pathology*, **17**, 427–37.

Gilbert, E. F. (1985). Carnitine deficiency. *Pathology*, **17**, 161–9.

Glaser, N., Barnett, P., McCaslin, I., *et al.* (2001). Risk factors for cerebral edema in children with diabetic ketoacidosis. *New England Journal of Medicine*, **344**, 264–9.

Glasgow, J. F. & Moore, R. (1993). Current concepts in Reye's syndrome. *British Journal of Hospital Medicine*, **50**, 599–604.

Glueck, C. J., Daniels, S. R., Bates, S., Benton, C., Tracy, T. & Third, J. L. H. C. (1982). Pediatric victims of unexplained stroke and their families: Familial lipid and lipoprotein abnormalities. *Pediatrics*, **69**, 308–16.

Goldfischer, S., Coltoff-Schiller, B., Biempica, L. & Wolinsky, H. (1975). Lysosomes and the sclerotic arterial lesion in Hurler's disease. *Human Pathology*, **6**, 633–7.

Gould, V. E., Memoli, V. A., Dardi, L. E. & Gould, N. S. (1983). Nesidiodysplasia and nesidioblastosis of infancy: structural and functional correlations with the syndrome of hyperinsulinemic hypoglycemia. *Pediatric Pathology*, **1**, 7–31.

Green, A. & Hall, S. M. (1992). Investigation of metabolic disorders resembling Reye's syndrome. *Archives of Disease in Childhood*, **67**, 1313–17.

Gregersen, N., Andresen, B. S. & Bross, P. (2000). Prevalent mutations in fatty acid oxidation disorders: diagnostic considerations. *European Journal of Pediatrics* (suppl. 3), **159**, S213–18.

Grieco, A. J. (1977). Homocystinuria: pathogenetic mechanisms. *American Journal of the Medical Sciences*, **273**, 120–32.

Griffiths, A. M., Mack, D. R., Byard, R. W., Stringer, D. A. & Shandling, B. (1990) Multiple endocrine neoplasia IIb: an unusual cause of chronic constipation. *Journal of Pediatrics*, **116**, 285–8.

Guertl, B., Noehammer, C. & Hoefler, G. (2000). Metabolic cardiomyopathies. *International Journal of Experimental Pathology*, **81**, 349–72.

Guthrie G. P., Jr, Hunsaker, J. C., III & O'Connor, W. N. (1987). Sudden death in hypothyroidism. *New England Journal of Medicine*, **317**, 1291.

Hallock, J., Morrow, G., III, Karp, L. A. & Barness, L. A. (1969). Postmortem diagnosis of metabolic disorders. The finding of maple syrup urine disease in a case of sudden and unexpected death in infancy. *American Journal of Diseases of Children*, **118**, 649–51.

Halpin, T. J., Holtzhauer, F. J., Campbell, R. J., *et al.* (1982). Reye's syndrome and medication use. *Journal of the American Medical Association*, **248**, 687–91.

Harker, L. A., Slichter, S. J., Scott, C. R. & Ross, R. (1974). Homocystinemia. Vascular injury and arterial thrombosis. *New England Journal of Medicine*, **291**, 537–43.

Harpey, J.-P., Charpentier, C., Coude, M., Divvy, P. & Paturneau-Jouas, M. (1987). Sudden infant death syndrome and multiple acyl-coenzyme A dehydrogenase defiency, ethylmalonic-adipic aciduria, or systemic carntine deficiency. *Journal of Pediatrics*, **110**, 881–4.

Harpey, J.-P., Charpentier, C. & Paturneau-Jouas, M. (1987). Erreurs inées du métabolisme et mort subite 'inexpliquée' du nourisson. *Bulletin de l'Academie Nationale de Médecine*, **2**, 261–9.

Harpey, J.-P., Charpentier, C. & Paturneau-Jouas, M. (1990). Sudden infant death syndrome and inherited disorders of fatty acid β-oxidation. *Biology of the Neonate*, **58** (Suppl 1), 70–80.

Harris, J. P., Ricker, A. T., Gray, R. S., Steed, R. D. & Gutai, J. J. P. (1992). Reversible hypertrophic cardiomyopathy associated with nesidioblastosis. *Journal of Pediatrics*, **120**, 272–5.

Hayes, T. M. & Woods, C. J. (1968). Unexpected death during treatment of uncomplicated diabetic ketoacidosis. *British Medical Journal*, **4**, 32–3.

Hayflick, S., Rowe, S., Kavanaugh-McHugh, A., Olson, J. L. & Valle, D. (1992). Acute infantile cardiomyopathy as a presenting feature of mucopolysaccharidosis VI. *Journal of Pediatrics*, **120**, 269–72.

Hirvonen, J., Jantti, M., Syrjala, H., Lautala, P. & Akerblom, H. K. (1980). Hyperplasia of islets of Langerhans and low serum insulin in cot deaths. *Forensic Science International*, **16**, 213–26.

Holton, J. B., Allen, J. T., Green, C. A., Gilbert, R. E. & Berry, P. J. (1991). Inherited metabolic diseases in the sudden infant death syndrome. *Archives of Disease in Childhood*, **66**, 1315–17.

Howat, A. J., Bennett, M. J., Variend, S., Shaw, L. & Engel, P. C. (1985). Defects of metabolism of fatty acids in the sudden infant death syndrome. *British Medical Journal*, **290**, 1771–3.

Hug, G., Bove, K. E. & Soukup, S. (1991). Lethal neonatal multiorgan deficiency of carnitine palmitoyltransferase II. *New England Journal of Medicine*, **325**, 1862–4.

Iafolla, A. K., Thompson, R. J. & Roe, C. R. (1994). Medium-chain acyl-coemzyme A dehydrogenase deficiency: clinical course in 120 affected children. *Journal of Pediatrics*, **124**, 409–15.

Inabnet, W. B., Caragliano, P. & Pertsemlidis, D. (2000). Pheochromocytoma: inherited associations, bilaterality, and cortex preservation. *Surgery*, **128**, 1007–11.

Ince, E., Kuloglu, Z. & Akinci, Z. (2000). Hemorrhagic shock and encephalopathy syndrome: neurologic features. *Pediatric Emergency Care*, **16**, 260–64.

Ino, T., Sherwood, W. G., Benson, L. N., Wilson, G. J., Freedom, R. M. & Rowe, R. D. (1988). Cardiac manifestations in disorders of fat and carnitine metabolism in infancy. *Journal of the American College of Cardiology*, **11**, 1301–8.

Irwin, J. & Cohle, S. D. (1988). Sudden death due to diabetic ketoacidosis. *American Journal of Forensic Medicine and Pathology*, **9**, 119–21.

Jaffe, R., Hashida, Y. & Yunis, E. J. (1982). The endocrine pancreas of the neonate and infant. *Perspectives in Pediatric Pathology*, **7**, 137–65.

James, T. N., Carson, N. A. J. & Froggatt, P. (1974). De subitanies mortibus. IV. Coronary vessels and conduction system in homocystinuria. *Circulation*, **49**, 367–74.

Jessurun, C. R., Adam, K., Moise, K. J., Jr. & Wilansky, S. (1993). Pheochromocytoma-induced myocardial infarction in pregnancy. A case report and literature review. *Texas Heart Institute Journal*, **20**, 120–22.

Jindrich, E. J. (1984). Adrenal hypofunction and sudden death. *Journal of Forensic Sciences*, **29**, 930–33.

Kaler, S. G. (1998). Metabolic and molecular bases of Menkes disease and occipital horn syndrome. *Pediatric and Developmental Pathology*, **1**, 85–98.

Karpati, G., Carpenter, S., Engel, A. G., *et al.* (1975). The syndrome of systemic carnitine deficiency. Clinical, morphologic, biochemical and pathophysiologic features. *Neurology*, **25**, 16–24.

Kelly, D. P., Hale, D. E., Rutledge, S. L., *et al.* (1992). Molecular basis of inherited medium-chain acyl-CoA dehydrogenase deficiency causing sudden child death. *Journal of Inherited Metabolic Diseases*, **15**, 171–80.

Kemp, P. M., Little, B. B., Bost, R. O. & Dawson, D. B. (1996). Whole blood levels of dodecanoic acid, a routinely detectable forensic marker for a genetic disease often misdiagnosed as sudden infant death syndrome (SIDS): MCAD deficiency. *American Journal of Forensic Medicine and Pathology*, **17**, 79–82.

Kerenyi, N. (1961). Congenital adrenal hypoplasia. *Archives of Pathology*, **71**, 336–43.

Knight, B. (1996). Poisoning by medicines. In *Forensic Pathology*, 2nd edn. London: Arnold Publishers, pp. 565–6.

Kodama, H., Murata, Y. & Kobayashi, M. (1999). Clinical manifestations and treatment of Menkes disease and its variants. *Pediatrics International*, **41**, 423–9.

Kohlschütter, A. & Hausdorf, G. (1986). Primary (genetic) cardiomyopathies in infancy. A survey of possible disorders and guidelines for diagnosis. *European Journal of Pediatrics*, **145**, 454–9.

Koskenvuo, K., Karvonen, M. J. & Rissanen, V. (1978). Death from ischemic heart disease in young Finns aged 15–24 years. *American Journal of Cardiology*, **42**, 114–18.

Krovetz, L. J. & Schiebler, G. L. (1972). Cardiovascular manifestations of the genetic mucopolysaccharidoses. *Birth Defects*, **8**, 192–6.

Krovetz, L. J., Lorincz, A. E. & Schiebler, G. L. (1965). Cardiovascular manifestations of the Hurler syndrome. Hemodynamic and angiocardiographic observations in 15 patients. *Circulation*, **31**, 132–41.

Larsen, S. U. (1997). Reye's syndrome. *Medicine, Science and the Law*, **37**, 235–41.

Legge, M. (1985). Systemic carnitine deficiency as the cause of a prolonged illness and sudden death in a six-year-old child. *Journal of Inherited Metabolic Disorders*, **8**, 159.

Levin, M., Kay, J. D. S., Gould, J. D., *et al.* (1983). Haemorrhagic shock and encephalopathy: a new syndrome with a high mortality in young children. *Lancet*, **ii**, 64–7.

Levin, M., Pincott, J. R., Hjelm, M., *et al.* (1989). Hemorrhagic shock and encephalopathy: clinical, pathologic, and biochemical features. *Journal of Pediatrics*, **114**, 194–203.

Lindsay, S. (1950). The cardiovascular system in gargoylism. *British Heart Journal*, **12**, 17–32.

Little, D. & Wilkins, B. (1997). Hemorrhagic shock and encephalopathy syndrome. An unusual cause of sudden death in children. *American Journal of Forensic Medicine and Pathology*, **18**, 79–83.

Losty, H. C., Lee, P., Alfaham, M., Gray, O. P. & Leonard, J. V. (1991). Fatty infiltration in the liver in medium chain acyl CoA dehydrogenase deficiency. *Archives of Disease in Childhood*, **66**, 727–8.

Mabuchi, H., Miyamoto, S., Ueda, K., *et al.* (1986). Causes of death in patients with familial hypercholesterolemia. *Atherosclerosis*, **61**, 1–6.

Makos, M. M., McComb, R. D., Hart, M. N. & Bennett, D. R. (1987). Alpha-glucosidase deficiency and basilar artery aneurysm: report of a sibship. *Annals of Neurology*, **22**, 629–33.

Marshall, W. N., Jr & Lightner, E. S. (1980). Congenital adrenal hyperplasia presenting with posterior labial fusion without clitoromegaly. *Pediatrics*, **66**, 312–14.

Martin, J. J., Flament-Durand, J., Farriaux, J. P., Buyssens, N., Ketelbant-Balasse, P. & Jansen, C. (1978). Menkes kinky-hair disease. A report on its pathology. *Acta Neuropathologica*, **42**, 25–32.

Mason, J. K. & Bain, A. D. (1982). Reye's syndrome presenting as atypical sudden infant death syndrome? *Forensic Science International*, **20**, 39–44.

Matsubara, Y., Narisawa, K. & Tada, K. (1992). Medium-chain acyl-CoA dehydrogenase deficiency: molecular aspects. *European Journal of Pediatrics*, **151**, 154–9.

McCully, K. S. & Wilson, R. B. (1975). Homocysteine theory of arteriosclerosis. *Atherosclerosis*, **22**, 215–27.

McKusick, V. A. (1990). *Mendelian Inheritance in Man. Catalogs of Autosomal Dominant, Autosomal Recessive, and X-linked Phenotypes*, 9th edn. Baltimore: Johns Hopkins University Press, pp. 1215–18.

Meier, F. A., Baron, J. A. & Greenberg, E. R. (1983). Reye's syndrome. A review from the forensic viewpoint. *American Journal of Forensic Medicine and Pathology*, **4**, 323–9.

Miller, M. E., Brooks, J. G., Forbes, N., & Insel, R. (1992). Frequency of medium-chain acyl-CoA dehydrogenase deficiency G-985 mutation in sudden infant death syndrome. *Pediatric Research*, **31**, 305–7.

Molander, N. (1982). Sudden natural death in later childhood and adolescence. *Archives of Disease in Childhood*, **57**, 572–6.

Morganroth, J., Levy, R. I. & Fredrickson, D. S. (1975). The biochemical, clinical and genetic features of type III hyperlipoproteinemia. *Annals of Internal Medicine*, **82**, 158–74.

Mudd, S. H., Skovby, F., Levy, H. L., *et al.* (1985). The natural history of homocystinuria due to cystathionine ß-synthase deficiency. *American Journal of Human Genetics*, **37**, 1–31.

Neuspiel, D. R. & Kuller, L. H. (1985). Sudden and unexpected natural death in childhood and adolescence. *Journal of the American Medical Association*, **254**, 1321–5.

New, M. I. & Levine, L. S. (1981). Congenital adrenal hyperplasia. *Clinical Biochemistry*, **14**, 258–72.

New, M. I. & Levine, L. S. (1984). Recent advances in 21-hydroxylase deficiency. *Annual Review of Medicine*, **35**, 649–63.

Norman, M. G., Taylor, G. P. & Clarke, L. A. (1990). Sudden, unexpected, natural death in childhood. *Pediatric Pathology*, **10**, 769–84.

O'Donohoe, N. V. & Holland, P. D. J. (1968). Familial congenital adrenal hypoplasia. *Archives of Disease in Childhood*, **43**, 717–23.

Palareti, G., Salardi, S., Piazzi, S., *et al.* (1986). Blood coagulation changes in homocystinuria: effects of pyridoxine and other specific therapy. *Journal of Pediatrics*, **109**, 1001–6.

Pande, S. V. (1999). Carnitine-acylcarnitine translocase deficiency. *American Journal of the Medical Sciences*, **318**, 22–7.

Partin, J. C., Schubert, W. K. & Partin, J. S. (1971). Mitochondrial ultrastructure in Reye's syndrome (encephalopathy and fatty degeneration of the viscera). *New England Journal of Medicine*, **285**, 1339–43.

Patterson, K., Donnelly, W. H. & Dehner, L. P. (1992). The cardiovascular system. In *Pediatric Pathology*, vol. 1, ed. J. T. Stocker & L. P. Dehner. Philadelphia: J. B. Lippincott, pp. 575–651.

Pavlakis, S. G., Phillips, P. C., DiMauro, S., De Vivo, D. C. & Rowland, L. P. (1984). Mitochondrial myopathy, encephalopathy, lactic acidosis and strokelike episodes: a distinctive clinical syndrome. *Annals of Neurology*, **16**, 481–8.

Pellegrino, P. A., Zanesco, L. & Battistella, P. A. (1992). Coagulopathies and vasculopathies. In *Cerebrovascular Diseases in Children*, ed. A. J., Raimondi, M. Choux & C. Di Rocco. New York: Springer-Verlag, pp. 189–204.

Pien, K., van Vlem, B., van Coster, R., Dacremont, G. & Piette, M. (2002). An inherited disorder presenting as ethylene glycol intoxication in a young adult. *American Journal of Forensic Medicine and Pathology*, **23**, 96–100.

Pollack, C. V., Jr & Pender, E. S. (1991). Hemorrhagic shock and encephalopathy syndrome. *Annals of Emergency Medicine*, **20**, 1366–70.

Pollitt, R. J. (1993). Defects in mitochondrial fatty acid oxidation: clinical presentations and their role in sudden infant death. *Paediatrica-Paedologica*, **28**, 13–17.

Potter, J. M. & Hilton, J. M. N. (1983). Type 1 hyperlipoproteinemia presenting as sudden death in infancy. *Australian and New Zealand Journal of Medicine*, **13**, 381–3.

Raben, N., Plotz, P. & Byrne, B. J. (2002). Acid α-glucosidase deficiency (glycogenosis type II, Pompe disease). *Current Molecular Medicine*, **2**, 145–66.

Rebuffat, E., Sottiaux, M., Goyens, P., *et al.* (1991). Sudden infant death syndrome, as first expression of a metabolic disorder. In *Inborn Errors of Metabolism*, vol. 24, ed. J. Schaub, F. Van Hoof & H. L. Vis. New York: Raven Press, pp. 71–80.

Reddy, V. S., O'Neill, J. A., Jr., Holcomb, G. W., 3rd, *et al.* (2000). Twenty-five-year surgical experience with pheochromocytoma in children. *American Surgeon*, **66**, 1085–91.

Rennebohm, R. M., Heubi, J. E., Daugherty, C. C. & Daniels, S. R. (1985). Reye syndrome in children receiving salicylate therapy for connective tissue disease. *Journal of Pediatrics*, **107**, 877–80.

Renteria, V. G., Ferrans, V. J. & Roberts, W. C. (1976). The heart in the Hurler syndrome. Gross, histologic and ultrastructural observations in five necropsy cases. *American Journal of Cardiology*, **38**, 487–501.

Roberts, W. C., Ferrans, V. J., Levy, R. I. & Fredrickson, D. S. (1973). Cardiovascular pathology in hyperlipoproteinemia. Anatomic observations in 42 necropsy patients with normal or abnormal serum lipoprotein patterns. *American Journal of Cardiology*, **31**, 557–70.

Roe, C. R., Millington, D. S., Maltby, D. A. & Kinnebrew, P. (1986). Recognition of medium-chain acyl-CoA dehydrogenase deficiency in asymptomatic siblings of children dying of sudden infant death or Reye-like syndromes. *Journal of Pediatrics*, **108**, 13–18.

Rozin, L., Perper, J. A., Jaffe, R. & Drash, A. (1994). Sudden unexpected death in childhood due to unsuspected diabetes mellitus. *American Journal of Forensic Medicine and Pathology*, **15**, 251–6.

Russell, M. A., Opitz, J. M., Viseskul, C., Gilbert, E. F. & Bargman, G. J. (1977). Sudden infant death due to congenital adrenal hypoplasia. *Archives of Pathology and Laboratory Medicine*, **101**, 168–9.

Sartor, G. & Dahlquist, G. (1995). Short-term mortality in childhood onset insulin-dependent diabetes mellitus: a high frequency of unexpected deaths in bed. *Diabetic Medicine*, **12**, 607–11.

Schenk, E. A. & Haggerty, J. (1964). Morquio's disease. A radiologic and morphologic study. *Pediatrics*, **34**, 839–50.

Schimke, R. N., McKusick, V. A., Huang, T. & Pollack, A. D. (1965). Homocystinuria. Studies of 20 families with 38 affected members. *Journal of the American Medical Association*, **193**, 711–19.

Schwartz, M. L., Cox, G. F., Lin, A. E., *et al.* (1996). Clinical approach to genetic cardiomyopathy in children. *Circulation*, **94**, 2021–38.

Shapiro, J., Strome, M. & Crocker, A. C. (1985). Airway obstruction and sleep apnea in Hurler and hunter syndromes. *Annals of Otology, Rhinology and Laryngology*, **94**, 458–61.

Shivelhood, E. K. (1947). Myocardial infarction in a twelve-year-old boy with diabetes. *American Heart Journal*, **35**, 655–61.

Sperling, M. A., Wolfsen, A. R. & Fisher, D. A. (1973). Congenital adrenal hypoplasia: an isolated defect of organogenesis. *Journal of Pediatrics*, **82**, 444–9.

Sprecher, D. L., Schaefer, E. J., Kent, K. M., *et al.* (1984). Cardiovascular features of homozygous familial hypercholesterolemia: analysis of 16 patients. *American Journal of Cardiology*, **54**, 20–30.

Stanley, C. A., Hale, D. E., Berry, G. T., Deleeuw, S., Boxer, J. & Bonnefont, J. -P. (1992). Brief report: a deficiency of carnitine-acylcarnitine translocase in the inner mitochondrial membrane. *New England Journal of Medicine*, **327**, 19–23.

Starko, K. M. & Mullick, F. G. (1983). Hepatic and cerebral pathology findings in children with fatal salicylate intoxication: further evidence for a causal relation between salicylate and Reye's syndrome. *Lancet*, **i**, 326–9.

Starko, K. M., Ray, C. G., Dominguez, L. B., Stromberg, W. L. & Woodall, D. F. (1980). Reye's syndrome and salicylate use. *Pediatrics*, **66**, 859–64.

Stuhrmann, M., Heilbronner, H., Reis, A., Wegner, R.-D., Fischer, P. & Schmidtke, J. (1991). Characterisation of a Xp21 microdeletion syndrome in a 2-year-old boy with muscular dystrophy, glycerol kinase deficiency and adrenal hypoplasia congenita. *Human Genetics*, **86**, 414–15.

Tattersall, R. B. & Gill, G. V. (1991). Unexplained deaths of type 1 diabetic patients. *Diabetic Medicine*, **8**, 49–58.

Taylor, D. B., Blaser, S. I., Burrows, P. E., Stringer, D. A., Clarke, J. T. R. & Thorner, P. (1991). Arteriopathy and coarctation of the abdominal aorta in children with mucopolysaccharidosis: imaging findings. *American Journal of Roentgenology*, **157**, 819–23.

Thomas, C. G., Jr, Underwood, L. E., Carney, C. N., Dolcourt, J. L. & Whitt, J. J. (1977). Neonatal and infantile hypoglycemia due to insulin excess: new aspects of diagnosis and surgical management. *Annals of Surgery*, **185**, 505–17.

Thordarson, H. & Søvik, O. (1995). Dead in bed syndrome in young diabetic patients in Norway. *Diabetic Medicine*, **12**, 782–7.

Tormey, W. P., Carney, M. & FitzGerald, R. J. (1999). Catecholamines in urine after death. *Forensic Science International*, **103**, 67–71.

Touma, E. H. & Charpentier, C. (1992). Medium chain acyl-CoA dehydrogenase deficiency. *Archives of Disease in Childhood*, **67**, 142–5.

Treem, W. R. (2000). New developments in the pathophysiology, clinical spectrum, and diagnosis of disorders of fatty acid oxidation. *Current Opinion in Pediatrics*, **12**, 463–8.

Treem, W. R., Stanley, C. A., Hale, D. E., Leopold, H. B. & Hyams, J. S. (1991). Hypoglycemia, hypotonia, and cardiomyopathy: the evolving clinical picture of long-chain acyl-CoA dehydrogenase deficiency. *Pediatrics*, **87**, 328–33.

Treem, W. R., Witzleben, C. A., Piccoli, D. A., *et al.* (1986). Medium-chain and long-chain acyl CoA dehyrdogenase deficiency: clinical, pathologic and ultrastructural differentiation from Reye's syndrome. *Hepatology*, **6**, 1270–78.

Tripathy, D., Coleman, R. A., Vidaillet, H. J., Jr, Steenbergen, C., Hirschhorn, K. & Packer, D. L. (1988). Complete heart block with myocardial membrane-bound glycogen and normal peripheral α-glucosidase activity. *Annals of Internal Medicine*, **109**, 985–7.

Tripp, M. E., Katcher, M. L., Peters, H. A., *et al.* (1981). Systemic carnitine deficiency presenting as familial endocardial fibroelastosis. A treatable cardiomyopathy. *New England Journal of Medicine*, **305**, 385–90.

Trounce, J. Q., Lowe, J., Lloyd, B. W. & Johnston, D. I. (1991). Haemorrhagic shock encephalopathy and sudden infant death. *Lancet*, **337**, 202–3.

Uno, H., Arya, S., Laxova, R. & Gilbert, E. F. (1983). Menkes' syndrome with vascular and adrenergic nerve abnormalities. *Archives of Pathology and Laboratory Medicine*, **107**, 286–9.

Vawter, G. F., McGraw, C. A., Hug, G., Kozakewich, H. P. W., McNaulty, J. & Mandell, F. (1986). An hepatic metabolic profile in sudden infant death (SIDS). *Forensic Science International*, **30**, 93–8.

Wang, S. S., Fernhoff, P. M., Hannon, W. H. & Khoury, M. J. (1999). Medium chain acyl-CoA dehydrogenase deficiency: human genome epidemiology review. *Genetics in Medicine*, **1**, 332–9.

Weibley, R. E., Pimentel, B. & Ackerman, N. B. (1989). Hemorrhagic shock and encephalopathy syndrome of infants and children. *Critical Care Medicine*, **17**, 335–8.

Wheeler, E. M. & Roberts, P. F. (1976). Menkes's steely hair syndrome. *Archives of Disease in Childhood*, **51**, 269–74.

White, P. C., New, M. I. & Dupont, B. (1987). Congenital adrenal hyperplasia (first of two parts). *New England Journal of Medicine*, **316**, 1519–24.

Wilcken, B., Carpenter, K. H. & Hammond, J. (1993). Neonatal symptoms in medium chain acyl coenzyme A dehydrogenase deficiency. *Archives of Disease in Childhood*, **69**, 292–4.

Williams, M. L. (1989). Death of a child as a result of familial hypercholesterolaemia. *Medical Journal of Australia*, **150**, 93–4.

Wolf, B., Heard, G. S., Weissbecker, K. A., McVoy, J. R. S., Grier, R. E. & Leshner, R. T. (1985). Biotinidase deficiency: initial clinical features and rapid diagnosis. *Annals of Neurology*, **18**, 614–17.

Young, T. W. (1992). Reye's syndrome. A diagnosis occasionally first made at medicolegal autopsy. *American Journal of Forensic Medicine and Pathology*, **13**, 21–7.

Zangrillo, A., Valentini, G., Casati, A. & Torri, G. (1999). Myocardial infarction and death after caesarian section in a woman with protein S deficiency and undiagnosed phaeochromocytoma. *European Journal of Anaesthesiology*, **16**, 268–70.

12

Miscellaneous conditions

Introduction

This eclectic chapter deals with a variety of unrelated conditions that have not been described specifically elsewhere. For convenience, these disorders have been grouped into the following categories: connective tissue, skeletal, dermatologic, muscular, chromosomal, and immunologic. An overview of the range of anomalies that should be looked for at the time of autopsy in children with these conditions is provided. Recent advances in molecular genetics have resulted in localization of specific mutations for many of these disorders (Phillips & Vnencak-Jones, 1993), increasing the need for accuracy of postmortem diagnosis to enable appropriate genetic counselling of family members.

Connective tissue disorders

Marfan syndrome

Overview

The characteristic features of Marfan syndrome include long arms and legs (dolichostenomelia), long fingers (arachnodactyly), pectus excavatum or carinatum, kyphoscoliosis, high arched palate, cutaneous striae, ectopia lentis, dilation of the ascending aorta, and dural ectasia (Grahame, 2000; Pyeritz, 2000). There is microscopic fragmentation of arterial collagen and elastin, with accumulation of acid mucopolysaccharides. Possible mechanisms of death include arterial dissection, aortic aneurysm rupture, and cardiac arrhythmia. Associated features include mitral valve prolapse, aortic incompetence, and coronary artery aneurysms. The incidence in the population is at least one in 10,000 (Robinson & Godfrey, 2000).

Clinical features

Marfan syndrome is characterized by cardiovascular, ocular, and skeletal abnormalities, which have quite variable degrees of clinical expression (Buntinx *et al.*, 1991; Salzberg & Kramer, 1984). Patients may have a history of joint hyperextensibility, recurrent joint dislocations, spontaneous pneumothoraces, and ocular abnormalities such as lens dislocation and retinal detachment. Cardiac arrhythmias may occur (Phornphutkul, Rosenthal & Nadas, 1973), and there may be arterial dissection or rupture precipitated by pregnancy or by strenuous exercise (Bain, Zumwalt & van der Bel-Kahn, 1987; Pyeritz, 1981).

Etiology

While most cases of Marfan syndrome are inherited in an autosomal dominant manner, 25–30% of cases are sporadic (Robinson & Godfrey, 2000). Two hundred mutations responsible for the Marfan phenotype have been found in the fibrillin-1 gene on chromosome 15q21.1 (Dietz *et al.*, 1991; Giampietro, Raggio & Davis, 2002; Francke & Furthmayr, 1994; Kainulainen *et al.*, 1990; Liu *et al.*, 2001). Fibrillin-1 is the major glycoprotein in extracellular microfibrils. It is required for elastogenesis, elasticity, and homeostasis of elastic fibers (Robinson & Booms, 2001). Such genetic heterogeneity may have significant

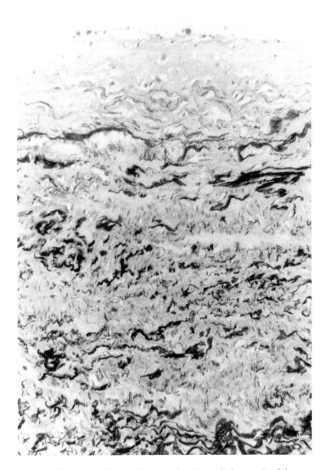

Figure 12.1 Typical features of cystic medial necrosis of the aorta in Marfan syndrome, with fragmentation of elastic lamina and accumulation of interstitial mucopolysaccharide (Movat pentachrome, ×280).

effects on ultimate phenotype and risk of sudden death (Pereira *et al.*, 1994). There may also be a second locus on chromosome 3p24.2-p25 (Collod *et al.*, 1994), although this has been disputed (Nijbroek *et al.*, 1995).

Pathological findings

At autopsy, affected children are often readily identifiable due to their increased height and excessive thinness, associated with reduced amounts of subcutaneous fat. The arms and legs are long due to a disproportionate increase in the length of the distal long bones, and typically the arm span exceeds the height.

The major internal findings involve the cardiovascular system, which may show dissection of the ascending aorta and/or ectasia of the aortic root and valve (Color Plate 27), with saccular aneurysm formation. There may be aneurysmal dilation of the sinuses of Valsalva, coronary artery aneurysms, and dilation of the mitral and tricuspid valve rings (Bruno *et al.*, 1984; Buchanan & Wyatt, 1985; Dardir, Ferrans & Roberts, 1989; Pyeritz, 1993). There is an increased incidence of mitral valve prolapse due to an increase in size of the valve leaflets, an increase in length of the chordae, and dilation of the valve annulus (Pyeritz & McKusick, 1979; Roberts & Honig, 1982). Occasionally, subpleural pulmonary cysts give rise to spontaneous pneumothoraces (Pyeritz & McKusick, 1979).

Microscopically, involved vessels demonstrate cystic medial necrosis with degeneration of elastin fibers, fragmentation of collagen, and accumulation of acid mucopolysaccharides (Takebayashi, Kubota & Takagi, 1973) (Figure 12.1). Affected cardiac valves also show interstitial mucopolysaccharide aggregation (Byard *et al.*, 1991). The aggregated material results from attempted repair of tissues that contain defectively cross-linked collagen following exposure to the stress of hemodynamic pressures (Saruk & Eisenstein, 1977). Fibrointimal and medial hyperplasia of intramural coronary arteries and of arteries supplying the sinoatrial and atrioventricular nodes have been described (James, Frame & Schatz, 1964).

Occurrence of sudden death

Individuals with Marfan syndrome are at increased risk of death at all ages due to major arterial dissection, aneurysm rupture (Crawford, 1983), arrhythmia, heart failure, or myocardial infarction (Murdoch *et al.*, 1972). While the average age of death in one series was 32 years, a significant number of children have died within the first decade of life (Murdoch *et al.*, 1972). Sudden and unexpected death may even occur prior to establishment of the diagnosis, as was the case in two infants whose first presentation was that of fatal dissecting aneurysm of a patent ductus arteriosus (Byard *et al.*, 1991; Gillan *et al.* 1984) (Color Plate 28). Dissecting aneurysms and arterial rupture have also been reported in the aorta and pulmonary artery in children (Phornphutkul, Rosenthal & Nadas, 1973; Thilenius *et al.*, 1980). Pregnancy may increase the risk of aortic dissection in affected individuals due to increased hemodynamic stresses and possibly hormonal effects (Colman *et al.*, 2000).

Associated features

While patent ductus arteriosus, pulmonary stenosis, tetralogy of Fallot, and atrial or ventricular septal defects have rarely been reported in association with Marfan syndrome (Phornphutkul, Rosenthal & Nadas, 1973), the presence of septal defects is considered coincidental (Grondin, Steinberg & Edwards, 1969). Very occasionally, supravalvular aortic stenosis may be present (Burry, 1958; Grimm & Wesselhoeft, 1980).

Ehlers–Danlos syndrome type IV

Overview

Ehlers–Danlos syndrome is a heterogeneous group of at least 10 subgroups that have different clinical manifestations, biochemical defects, and inheritance patterns (Steinmann, Royce & Superti-Furga, 1993). While the majority of cases belong to types I, II, and III, sudden and unexpected death is generally only a feature of type IV, the so-called "arterial-ecchymotic" variant. The following discussion will deal mainly with this subtype.

The characteristic features of Ehlers–Danlos syndrome type IV include easy bruisability, herniae, colonic diverticulae, and thin facies. There is variable fragmentation of arterial elastin on microscopy. Possible mechanisms of death include arterial rupture and dissection, and left ventricular, uterine, colonic, or splenic rupture. Associated features include a variety of possibly coincidental congenital cardiac defects, saccular arterial aneurysms, and pneumothoraces. Intra-abdominal aneurysms have also been reported in the occipital horn syndrome (Ehlers–Danlos syndrome type IX) (Mentzel *et al.*, 1999).

Clinical features

Individuals with Ehlers–Danlos syndrome type IV have thin, translucent skin, with premature aging of the hands and feet (acrogeria). In later childhood and adult life, the face is characteristically thin due to a lack of subcutaneous fat. Unlike the other subtypes, skin and large joint hyperextensibility are not a feature of type IV. Further manifestations of Ehlers–Danlos syndrome in general are rectal prolapse in young children, multiple bruises, and dermal scars (Hollister, 1978; Steinmann, Royce & Superti-Furga, 1993). In children, the skin manifestations may be so pronounced that non-accidental injury has been suspected (Owen & Durst, 1984; Roberts *et al.*, 1984). Other cases may appear phenotypically normal (Pope *et al.*, 1983).

Carotid-cavernous fistulae have been documented (Fox *et al.*, 1988), and saccular aneurysms of the intracranial and coronary arteries occur occasionally (Ferrans & Boyce, 1983; Kato *et al.*, 2001). Problems during pregnancy include premature and precipitate labor, vessel rupture, postpartum hemorrhage, and uterine prolapse (Hollister, 1978; Rudd *et al.*, 1983; Snyder, Gilstrap & Hauth, 1983).

Etiology

Ehlers–Danlos syndrome type IV is dominantly inherited, with approximately half of all cases representing new mutations. The phenotype has been associated with a variety of mutations within the COL3A1 locus on chromosome 2q31, which codes for the polypeptide chains of type III collagen (Burrows, 1999; Milewicz, 1998; Steinmann, Royce & Superti-Furga, 1993).

Pathological findings

The most significant complications of Ehlers–Danlos syndrome are spontaneous rupture of large arteries, aortic dissection, left ventricular rupture, and splenic and intestinal rupture (Beighton, 1968; Harris, Slater & Austin, 1985; Umlas, 1972). Death commonly results from rupture of branches of the abdominal aorta. Rupture of the gravid uterus and pneumothorax are additional serious complications (Jaffe *et al.*, 1981; Thomas & Frias, 1987).

Microscopic findings are variable and cannot be relied upon to establish the diagnosis, since there may be no abnormal features discernable even in the presence of typical macroscopic and biochemical features (Byard, Keeley & Smith, 1990). Some cases may show decreased, absent, fragmented, or disorganized elastin fibers within large arteries, thinning of the vessel wall, and an increase in interstitial acid mucopolysaccharide (Cikrit, Miles & Silver, 1987; Ferrans & Boyce, 1983; Shohet *et al.*, 1987). Other cases have not shown marked differences from controls (Lach *et al.*, 1987; Sulica *et al.*, 1979). Electron microscopy may reveal a reduction in collagen fiber diameter (Gertsch *et al.*, 1986) and prominent dilation of endoplasmic reticulum, but this is also not invariable (Byers *et al.*, 1979).

Occurrence of sudden death

Although the average age of death in Ehlers–Danlos syndrome type IV is between 35 and 40 years (Steinmann, Royce & Superti-Furga, 1993), affected individuals may die suddenly and unexpectedly in infancy from arterial rupture and dissections (Byard, Keeley & Smith, 1990). Fatal arterial rupture may be the only morphologic feature of Ehlers–Danlos syndrome present.

Diagnosis

Arterial and visceral rupture are caused by reduced amounts of type III collagen (Byers *et al.*, 1979; Pope, Martin & McKusick, 1977). Standard non-molecular diagnosis, therefore, depends on analysis of connective tissue for type III collagen and on demonstration of decreased production of type III procollagen by cultured fibroblasts (Byers, Barsh & Holbrook, 1982). DNA analysis will reveal mutations on chromosome 2q31.

Autopsy investigation

Localized hemorrhage in patients at autopsy, particularly if it is multifocal with no obvious reason for a bleeding diathesis, should prompt consideration of underlying occult Ehlers–Danlos syndrome type IV (Byard, Keeley & Smith, 1990) (Figure 12.2).

The taking of fresh and frozen skin and aorta from cases of unexplained spontaneous hemorrhage will allow collagen studies to be performed (Figure 12.3). Blood or tissue for linkage analysis may also be taken.

Associated features

Mitral valve prolapse occurs in children with type IV Ehlers–Danlos syndrome (Jaffe *et al.*, 1981), but congenital cardiovascular anomalies such as bicuspid aortic valve and tetralogy of Fallot, which have been reported in the other subtypes, may be coincidental (Becker & Anderson, 1981; Hernández *et al.*, 1979; Lees *et al.*, 1969; Leier *et al.*, 1980; Wallach & Burkhart, 1950). Aortic root dilation has been found in children with types I and III Ehlers–Danlos syndrome (Tiller *et al.*, 1998). Epilepsy may also occur in individuals with type IV Ehlers–Danlos syndrome associated with congenital or acquired central nervous system malformations (Jacome, 1999).

Pseudoxanthoma elasticum

Overview

This is a generalized connective tissue disorder characterized by calcification of elastic fibers in the arteries, eyes, and skin. Typical features include yellow-orange papular skin lesions, angioid streaks radiating out from the optic discs, and calcification of arteries (Ringpfeil, Pulkkinen & Uitto, 2001). Possible mechanisms of death include myocardial ischemia and spontaneous gastrointestinal hemorrhage. Associated features include systemic hypertension and mitral valve prolapse.

Clinical features

Skin and ocular changes include drooping skin folds, linear or aggregated yellow cutaneous papules, and angioid streaks of the retina. Vascular manifestations are quite variable and result from ischemia due to vessel narrowing (Bete *et al.*, 1975; Bowen, Boudoulas & Wooley, 1987), which may cause spontaneous hemorrhage, particularly from the gastrointestinal tract.

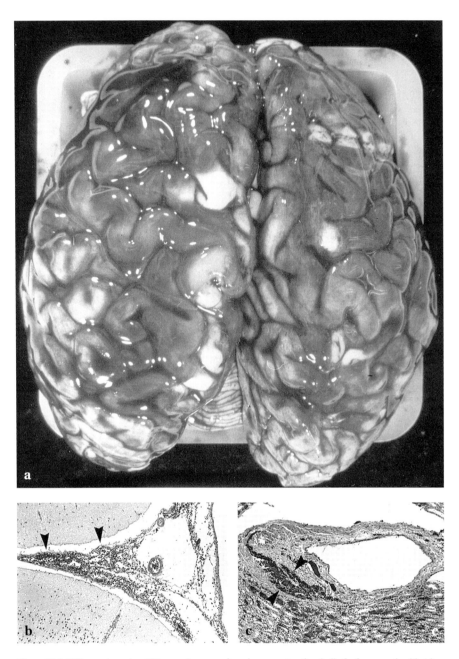

Figure 12.2 Diffuse subarachnoid hemorrhage was found on opening the skull of a five-month-old girl who was thought to have died from SIDS (a). Microscopic examination of tissues confirmed subarachnoid hemorrhage (arrowheads) (b) and also revealed periarterial hemorrrhage in the kidneys (arrowheads) (c) (hematoxylin and eosin, ×45). Although there was no family history, subsequent collagen analysis revealed absent type III collagen characteristic of Ehlers–Danlos syndrome type IV.

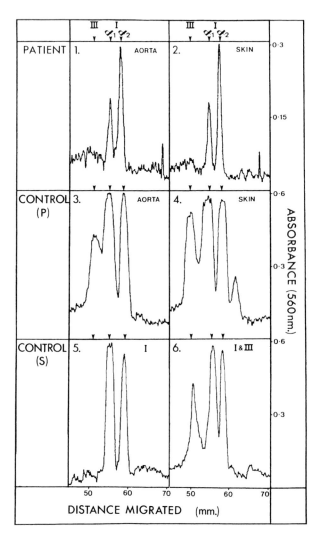

Figure 12.3 Collagen analysis from the case illustrated in Figure 12.2, a control infant, and two standard controls, revealing no type III collagen in the aorta or skin of the infant being investigated.

Etiology

The inheritance pattern is varied, with both autosomal recessive (90% of cases) and dominant forms reported (Pope, 1975; Viljoen, Pope & Beighton, 1987). Mutations have been identified within the ABCC6 gene on chromosome 16p13.1, which codes for the MRP6 protein, a member of the ATP-binding cassette (ABC) superfamily of membrane transporter proteins (Uitto, Pulkkinen & Ringpfeil, 2001). As MRP6 is found mainly in the kidneys and liver, it has been proposed that pseudoxanthoma elasticum may be primarily a metabolic disorder with only secondary involvement of connective tissue (Ringpfeil, Pulkkinen & Uitto, 2001).

Pathological features

At autopsy, "cobblestone" skin lesions, acute myocardial infarction, myocardial scarring, calcified endocardial plaques, and gastrointestinal or intracranial hemorrhage may be found.

Elastic fibers in the retina, skin, and vasculature are fragmented, disorganized, and calcified, although cutaneous lesions may not always be visible. Affected arteries show calcification of the intima and media. Rarely, cardiac conduction tracts may be surrounded by fibrous scar tissue, resulting in sudden unexpected death in adult life (Becker & Anderson, 1981; Dardir, Ferrans & Roberts, 1989; Huang *et al.*, 1967; Lebwohl *et al.*, 1987; Mendelsohn, Bulkley & Hutchins, 1978; Neldner, 1993).

Occurrence of sudden death

Sudden death is rare but may occur in adolescence in association with strenuous exercise (Wilhelm & Paver, 1972). Acute myocardial infarction has been reported in a six-week-old infant with arterial calcification and a maternal history of pseudoxanthoma elasticum (Hamilton-Gibbs, 1970), and significant vascular disease has been documented in other children (Schachner & Young, 1974). Patients may also have systemic hypertension, gastrointestinal bleeding, and mitral valve prolapse (Malcolm, 1985; Altman *et al.*, 1974), which may lead to sudden death. Restrictive cardiomyopathy with pulmonary edema was reported in one young adult due to calcified endocardial bands (Challenor, Conway & Monro, 1988). Rarely, in adults, there may be symptoms and signs from cerebral ischemia or hemorrhage from vessel rupture (Iqbal, Alter & Lee, 1978).

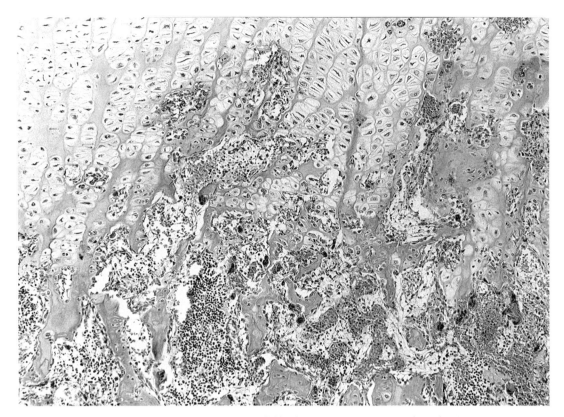

Figure 12.4 Marked disorganization of the growth plate in a child with achondroplasia (hematoxylin and eosin, ×80), contrasting with a normal growth plate (see Figure 13.5).

Arterial tortuosity syndrome

This is a rare disorder of connective tissue characterized by generalized tortuosity and elongation of major arteries associated with decreased numbers of elastic fibers. The inheritance is thought to be autosomal dominant, but the genetic locus and clinical course are, at present, uncertain. Infant and early childhood deaths have been reported in affected families (Franceschini *et al.*, 2000).

Skeletal disorders

Achondroplasia

Overview

Achondroplasia is the most common type of short-limbed dwarfism found in 0.5–1.5 of 10,000 births

(Baitner *et al.*, 2000). The characteristic features of achondroplasia include rhizomelic dwarfism, enlargement of the head, trident-shaped hands, an exaggerated lumbar lordosis, and thoracic kyphosis. There is a defect in endochondral bone formation, with microscopic disorganization of the growth plate (Figure 12.4), loss of the normal orderly columns of chondrocytes, and irregular metaphyseal ossification.

Clinical features

Affected children have shortening of the proximal limbs (rhizomelic dwarfism) with enlargement of the head. The cranial vault has a characteristic shape due to compensatory overgrowth of the membranous calvarial bones, with prominent frontal bones, maxillary hypoplasia, and mandibular prognathism

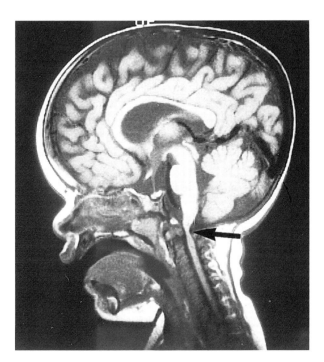

Figure 12.5 MRI scan in an achondroplastic boy demonstrating reduction in size of the foramen magnum with narrowing of the upper cervical spinal cord (arrow).

(Lemyre *et al.*, 1999). The foramen magnum and spinal canal are reduced in size due to failure of growth of the cartilagenous bones at the base of the skull, and there is hydrocephalus possibly due to obstruction of venous return at the jugular foramina (Pierre-Kahn *et al.*, 1980). Radiologic features have been described in detail elsewhere (Langer, Baumann & Gorlin, 1967).

Etiology

Inheritance is autosomal dominant, with a high rate of spontaneous mutation. The gene locus involves the fibroblast growth factor receptor-3 (FGFR3) on chromosome 4p16.3 (Baitner *et al.*, 2000; Horton, 1997).

Occurrence of sudden death

Achondroplastic infants are at increased risk of sudden death due to lower brainstem and upper spinal cord compression (Horton & Hecht, 1993; Hunter *et al.*, 1998; Pauli *et al.*, 1983). A study of 13 achondroplastic infants who manifested significant apneic episodes and sudden death demonstrated narrowing of the foramen magnum and spinal canal (Pauli *et al.*, 1984) (Figure 12.5). Other authors have also reported sudden death in apparently well achondroplastic infants (Bland & Emery, 1982; Marin-Padilla & Marin-Padilla, 1977), presumably associated with this type of compression of respiratory control centres (Fremion, Garg & Kalsbeck, 1984; Nelson *et al.*, 1988; Yang *et al.*, 1977). An exacerbating factor in these children may be arterial hypoxia caused by thoracic cage abnormalities and sleep-related upper airway obstruction (Stokes *et al.*, 1983; Waters *et al.*, 1993). There is also an increased risk of subdural hematoma formation, in the absence of a history of trauma, possibly associated with enlargement of the subarachnoid spaces (Gordon, 2000).

It is difficult to estimate the exact increase in risk of sudden death of these infants; however, the risk of dying suddenly in the first year of life was 7.5% in a study by Hecht and colleagues (1987). These investigators also found that nine of the 13 children dying before five years of age died suddenly, with brainstem compression found in three of the four children who had autopsies. It is, therefore, important to examine the cervical cord and brainstem in detail in these cases.

Craniosynostotic syndromes

Overview

Premature fusion of cranial sutures, craniosynostosis, occurs in a number of inherited conditions and has been associated with sudden death (Rabl, Tributsch & Ambach, 1990). Possible mechanisms of death are uncertain but may involve upper airway obstruction due to hypoplasia of the facial skeleton, seizures, hydrocephalus, and prolonged central apneas during sleep (Guilleminault, 1989; Katzen & McCarthy, 2000). Associated features include cerebral compression and possibly coincidental congenital cardiac defects.

Dermatologic disorders

Hypohidrotic ectodermal dysplasia

Overview
Characteristic features of this disorder include decreased sweating, anomalies of dentition, sparse hair, and characteristic facies, with frontal bossing and malar hypoplasia. Death is caused by uncontrolled hyperthermia.

Clinical features
Hypohidrosis, hypodontia, and hypotrichosis occur, with affected children having frontal bossing, low-set ears, malar hypoplasia, and flattened nasal bridges (Reed, Lopez & Landing, 1970). One of the major clinical problems related to the absence or hypoplasia of eccrine glands is a reduced capacity to tolerate heat.

Etiology
Inheritance is X-linked (Kruse *et al.*, 1989).

Occurrence of sudden death
Although the disorder is not usually life-threatening, affected children must be protected from high temperatures, as uncontrolled hyperthermia may result in sudden death (Bernstein, Hatchuel & Jenkins, 1980; Bernstein, & Weakley-Jones, 1987).

Epidermolysis bullosa

The possibility of acute airway obstruction in epidermolysis bullosa has already been considered in Chapter 7.

Muscular disorders

Malignant hyperthermia

Clinical features
This rare autosomal dominant condition is characterized by a marked increase in muscle metabolism triggered by anesthesia. Classically, this results in tachycardia, hyperthermia, and acidosis.

Etiology
There is considerable genetic heterogeneity in this condition, with more than 20 mutations being found in the ryanodine receptor locus on chromosome 19 in affected individuals, as well as loci being identified on chromosomes 1, 3, 5, and 17 (MacLennan *et al.*, 1990; McCarthy *et al.*, 1990; Robinson & Hopkins, 2001; Wappler, 2001).

Occurrence of sudden death
A number of cases have now been reported with atypical presentations, which include sudden and unexpected death in the absence of anesthetic exposure (Wingard, 1974). This has occurred in families who were not known to have this disorder (Ranklev, Fletcher & Krantz, 1985) and has mimicked the clinical presentation of SIDS (Denborough, Galloway & Hopkinson, 1982).

Pathological features
Autopsy findings are uninformative and further information may need to be derived from halothane- or caffeine-induced contraction tests performed on skeletal muscle biopsy material from other family members.

Chromosomal abnormalities

The trisomic syndromes

Overview
Infants with any one of the three common trisomies, 21, 18, and 13, may have congenital cardiac defects that predispose to early death. It is reasonably clear, however, that death in trisomies 18 and 13 is usually not particularly sudden and is certainly not unexpected, as it is assumed that most infants will succumb within the first few months of life, if not before. Children with Down syndrome are different, in that they usually survive into later childhood and adolescence. Characteristic dysmorphic features that may be detected at autopsy include prominent epicanthic folds, with slanting eyes, a flattened nasal bridge, a small mouth with protruding tongue, a small round

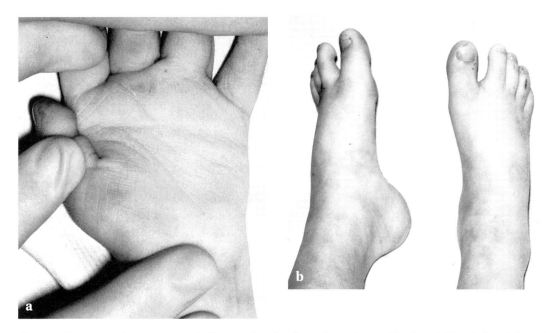

Figure 12.6 Transverse palmar crease (a) and wide separation of the first and second toes, which show clubbing (b) in an infant with trisomy 21 and cyanotic congenital heart disease.

head with flattening of the occiput, transverse palmar creases, and widely separated first and second toes (Figure 12.6).

Occurrence of sudden death

Sudden death in Down syndrome children can occur from a variety of mechanisms particularly associated with congenital cardiac defects. Structural cardiac defects are found in 40–60% of cases and consist predominantly of endocardial cushion defects resulting in hypoxia and cardiomegaly from left-to-right shunting (Tubman *et al.*, 1991). A full listing of the types of congenital cardiac defects that may be found in children with chromosomal abnormalities may be found in a review by Ferrans & Boyce (1983).

Pulmonary hypertension may be an added problem in these children, related to cardiac shunting that occurs through endocardial cushion defects; and also to sleep apnea (Loughlin, Wynne & Victorica, 1981; Stebbens *et al.*, 1991). Systemic

hypertension due to diffuse fibrointimal hyperplasia has also been reported in Down syndrome (Fleisher, Buck & Cornfeld, 1978). Down syndrome children are also at risk of hemorrhagic complications, due to an increased incidence of leukemia, and of hyperviscosity problems during infancy caused by neonatal polycythemia. Death may also occur because of spinal cord compression from atlanto-occipital instability or from airway compromise due to congenital subglottic stenosis.

Fragile X syndrome

Clinical features

Fragile X syndrome represents the most common heritable form of mental retardation, and is one of the most frequently encountered genetic syndromes. It is characterized by variable intellectual impairment and a typical morphology, which includes a prominent jaw and forehead, dysmorphic ears, macro-orchidism, hyperextensible joints, and other connective tissue abnormalities such as kyphoscoliosis and pectus excavatum (Sutherland, Mulley & Richards, 1993). The fragile site on the X chromosome at band q27.3 disrupts the FMR1 gene. The clinical and genetic features have been summarized by Sutherland & Richards (1993).

Occurrence of sudden death

Six of 68 (9%) live-born children died suddenly after one year of age in a study of eight families who had members with fragile X syndrome (Fryns *et al.*, 1988). In a follow-up study of the progeny of 86 normal obligate carriers, the mortality rate before the age of 18 months was 17/219 (8%) in males and 6/169 (4%) in females. Unfortunately, meaningful pathologic interpretation of these data is not possible because of the absence of autopsy information in all but one case.

These deaths cannot be attributed to SIDS given the age, lack of autopsy investigation, possibility of hypothalamic-pituitary abnormalities, and occurrence of transiently raised intracerebral pressure in affected children (Fryns *et al.*, 1988). They do, however, indicate a significantly increased risk of sudden death in infants with this syndrome. Cardiovascular abnormalities that may be associated with sudden death in the form of mitral valve prolapse and aortic root dilation have also been reported in older affected children and adolescents (Crabbe *et al.*, 1993).

Turner syndrome

Clinical features

Turner syndrome has a characteristic phenotype of short stature, webbing of the neck, broad chest, and delayed sexual maturation. Ovarian dysgenesis and horseshoe kidney are found.

Etiology

The Turner phenotype is associated with complete or partial absence of the short arm of the X chromosome (Xp), resulting in deficiencies that include the short stature homeobox (SHOX) gene (Ranke & Saenger, 2001; Zinn & Ross, 2001).

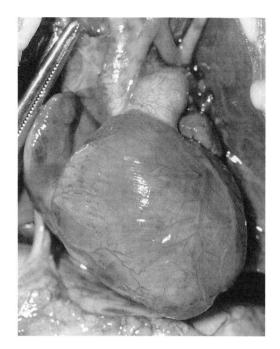

Figure 12.7 Left ventricular and aortic arch hypoplasia in a case of Turner syndrome.

Occurrence of sudden death

As well as the above features, children with Turner syndrome have a variety of cardiovascular anomalies that may result in sudden and unexpected death. These include aortic coarctation, bicuspid aortic valve, aortic stenosis, and anomalous pulmonary venous drainage (Miller *et al.*, 1983; Moore *et al.*, 1990). Aortic arch and left ventricular hypoplasia (Figure 12.7) may occur, as may rupture of a dissecting aortic aneurysm (DiGeorge, 1979).

Noonan syndrome

Noonan syndrome is an autosomal dominant condition with a similar phenotype to that of Turner syndrome (Figure 12.8), but with a normal karyotype. It is also characterized by cardiovascular abnormalities, including pulmonary stenosis, coarctation of the aorta, aortic valve dysplasia, patent ductus arteriosus, anomalous pulmonary venous drainage, and hypertrophic cardiomyopathy

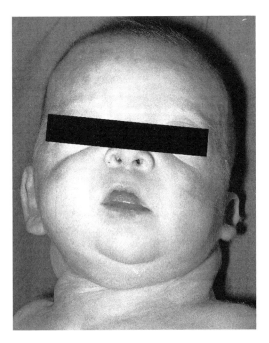

Figure 12.8 Typical facial features of Noonan syndrome in a boy who died of hypertrophic cardiomyopathy.

(Figure 12.9). It has been suggested that the Noonan phenotype results from variable expression of the neurofibromatosis type 1 gene (Küster & Happle, 1993).

Prader–Willi syndrome

Prader–Willi syndrome is a rare condition found in one in 10,000–15,000 individuals. It is characterized by hypotonia, hypogonadism, morbid obesity, and developmental delay. It is caused by deletions in chromosome 15q11-q13 (Cassidy, 2001). If weight can be controlled, then most people with the syndrome have a normal lifespan, but an increased incidence of sudden and unexpected death has been reported, possibly due to sepsis (Schrander-Stumpel *et al.*, 1998). Affected individuals are also potentially at increased risk of death from massive gastric dilation, with gastric necrosis (Wharton *et al.*, 1997), and epilepsy.

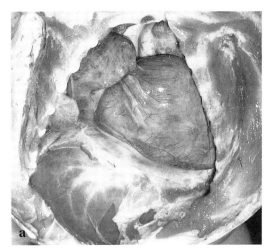

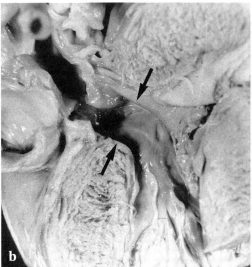

Figure 12.9 Marked enlargement of the heart in an infant with Noonan syndrome and hypertrophic cardiomyopathy (a). Further dissection revealed marked left ventricular hypertrophy, with narrowing of the aortic outflow tract (arrows) (b).

Immunologic conditions

Immunologic deficiency

Although immunologic underreactivity has been proposed as a cause of SIDS, research has not supported this contention. Children with immunologic

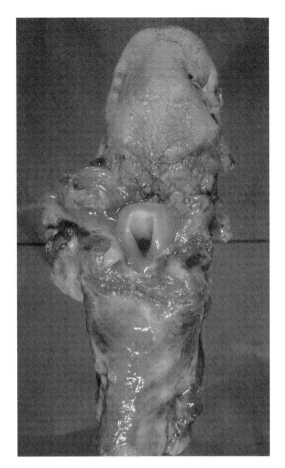

Figure 12.10 Swelling of the epiglottis in a case of fatal angioneurotic edema.

deficiencies are, however, at increased risk of developing overwhelming sepsis, which may result in rapid death (see Chapter 4). Often, but not invariably the diagnosis has been established prior to death.

Anaphylaxis

Anaphylaxis refers to a serious, potentially fatal reaction that is most often due to immunoglobulin E (IgE)-mediated sensitivity to a foreign substance. It is less common in children than in adults and is usually associated with drugs such as penicillin, food, or bee or wasp stings (Delage & Irey, 1972; Jensen, 1962; Riches, Gillis & James, 2002). In the latter cases, death may also result from asphyxia if there has been a sting involving the upper airway (Mosbech, 1983). Occasionally, angioneurotic edema may also cause critical epiglottal swelling (Figure 12.10) (Strife, 1988).

Fatal anaphylactic reactions to food in children are characterized poorly in the literature; however, these are well-recognized events, most often involving the ingestion of nuts, eggs, or milk. Young females are at highest risk (Sampson, Mendelson & Rosen, 1992). Death is caused by a combination of factors, including asphyxia from bronchospasm, upper airway obstruction due to edema, and shock (Roberts & Pumphrey, 2001). Hemorrhagic and thrombo-embolic phenomena have occurred in adults (Riches, Gillis & James, 2002). Very rarely, fatal anaphylaxis may follow rupture of an echinococcal cyst (Madariaga *et al.*, 1984).

Pathological features

Autopsy findings are often relatively non-specific and unhelpful, although cutaneous urticaria and swelling, upper airway edema, and hyperinflation of the lungs with mucus plugging may be observed.

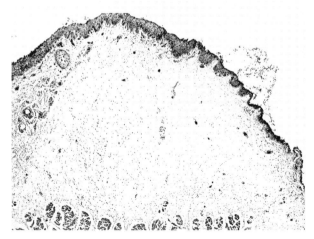

Figure 12.11 Marked edema of the upper airway may be the only finding in cases of fatal anaphylaxis (hematoxylin and eosin, ×45).

Swelling of the upper airways may be generalized or limited to the oropharynx, nasopharynx, epiglottis, larynx, or upper trachea (Pumphrey & Roberts 2000; Roberts & Pumphrey, 2001). In cases of fatal insect stings, the site of the sting may also be identified. Histologically, there may be edema of the upper airways (Figure 12.11), with an infiltrate of eosinophils and changes of asthma within the lungs. Immunohistochemical staining of sections of mucosa may reveal tryptase, a mast-cell-specific enzyme that is released after massive mast cell degranulation.

Elevated levels of allergen-specific IgE in postmortem sera indicate antemortem sensitization and support a diagnosis of anaphylaxis (Schwartz et al., 1984; Schwartz et al., 1988; Yunginger et al., 1991). However, a more specific test is measurement of tryptase within the serum (Ansari, Zamora & Lipscomb, 1993; Fisher & Baldo, 1993). A level of 10 µg/l or greater has been found to be a sensitive and specific marker for individuals suffering from anaphylaxis, and postmortem measurements correspond well with antemortem levels. While tryptase may remain stable in samples for up to four days at room temperature, freezing of samples at −20 °C is recommended if the assay cannot be performed immediately (Edston & van Hage-Hamsten, 1998; Prahlow & Barnard, 1998). Although tryptase is usually absent from normal serum, elevated levels are not absolutely specific for anaphylaxis, since it has been detected in individuals at postmortem who have died from a range of other conditions, including trauma, SIDS, and heroin overdose (Edston & van Hage-Hamsten, 1998). It has, however, been suggested that this finding might indicate that certain heroin-related deaths involve an allergic component (Fineschi et al., 2001). Serum histamine levels are of limited use due to the short half-life and possibility of artifactual postmortem leakage from basophils (Randall, Butts & Halsey, 1995).

The diagnosis of fatal anaphylaxis usually relies, therefore, on a history of exposure to a particular agent followed by dyspnea and collapse in a sensitized individual. Most deaths occur within one to two hours of exposure to the allergenic material (Prahlow & Barnard, 1998). Serum testing for allergen-specific IgE and elevated levels of tryptase can be used to support the diagnosis. As autopsy findings may be either minimal or non-specific, exclusion of other causes of death is important.

Myasthenia gravis

Myasthenia gravis is a disorder of the neuromuscular junction caused by an autoantibody to acetylcholine receptors. Although uncommon in infancy and childhood, sudden and unexpected death has been reported in young children following respiratory arrest (Baptist, Landes & Sturman, 1985), with minimal clinical evidence of the disorder preceding the terminal lethal event (Conomy, Levinsohn & Fanaroff, 1975). In older children, life-threatening myasthenic crises may follow infections. Some of these cases have a familial distribution.

Miscellaneous

Although other quite varied conditions having an immunologic basis, such as some of the vasculidites and glomerulonephritides, may result in severe illness in childhood, sudden death is not a usual or expected outcome.

REFERENCES

Altman, L. K., Fialkow, P. J., Parker, F. & Sagebiel, R. W. (1974). Pseudoxanthoma elasticum. An underdiagnosed genetically heterogeneous disorder with protean manifestations. *Archives of Internal Medicine*, **134**, 1048–54.

Ansari, M. Q., Zamora, J. L. & Lipscomb, M. F. (1993). Postmortem diagnosis of acute anaphylaxis by serum tryptase analysis. *American Journal of Clinical Pathology*, **99**, 101–3.

Bain, M. A., Zumwalt, R. E. & van der Bel-Kahn, J. (1987). Marfan syndrome presenting as aortic rupture in a young athlete: sudden unexpected death? *American Journal of Forensic Medicine and Pathology*, **8**, 334–7.

Baitner, A. C., Maurer, S. G., Gruen, M. B. & Di Cesare, P. E. (2000). The genetic basis of the osteochondrodysplasias. *Journal of Pediatric Orthopaedics*, **20**, 594–605.

Baptist, E. C., Landes, R. V. & Sturman, J. K., Jr (1985). Familial infantile myasthenia gravis: a preventable cause of sudden death. *Southern Medical Journal*, **78**, 201–2.

Becker, A. E. & Anderson, R. H. (1981). Inherited cardiovascular disease. In *Pathology of Congenital Heart Disease*. London: Butterworth, pp. 433–64.

Beighton, P. (1968). Lethal complications of the Ehlers–Danlos syndrome. *British Medical Journal*, **3**, 656–9.

Bernstein, M. L. & Weakley-Jones, B. (1987). "Sudden infant death" associated with hypohidrotic ectodermal dysplasia. *Journal of the Kentucky Medical Association*, **85**, 191–4.

Bernstein, R., Hatchuel, I. & Jenkins, T. (1980). Hypohidrotic ectodermal dysplasia and sudden infant death syndrome. *Lancet*, **ii**, 1024.

Bete, J. M., Banas, J. S., Jr, Moran, J., Pinn, V. & Levine, H. J. (1975). Coronary artery disease in an 18 year old girl with pseudoxanthoma elasticum: successful surgical therapy. *American Journal of Cardiology*, **36**, 515–20.

Bland, J. D. & Emery, J. L. (1982). Unexpected death of children with achondroplasia after the perinatal period. *Developmental Medicine and Child Neurology*, **24**, 489–92.

Bowen, J., Boudoulas, H. & Wooley, C. F. (1987). Cardiovascular disease of connective tissue origin. *American Journal of Medicine*, **82**, 481–8.

Bruno, L., Tredici, S., Mangiavacchi, M., Colombo, V., Mazzotta, G. F. & Sirtori, C. R. (1984). Cardiac, skeletal, and ocular abnormalities in patients with Marfan's syndrome and in their relatives. Comparison with the cardiac abnormalities in patients with kyphoscoliosis. *British Heart Journal*, **51**, 220–30.

Buchanan, R. & Wyatt, G. P. (1985). Marfan's syndrome presenting as an intrapartum death. *Archives of Disease in Childhood*, **60**, 1074–6.

Buntinx, I. M., Willems, P. J., Spitaels, S. E., Van Reempst, P. J., De Paepe, A. M. & Dumon, J. E. (1991). Neonatal Marfan syndrome with congenital arachnodactyly, flexion contractures, and severe cardiac valve insufficiency. *Journal of Medical Genetics*, **28**, 267–73.

Burrows, N. P. (1999). The molecular genetics of the Ehlers–Danlos syndrome. *Clinical and Experimental Dermatology*, **24**, 99–106.

Burry, A. F. (1958). Supra-aortic stenosis associated with Marfan's syndrome. *British Heart Journal*, **20**, 143–6.

Byard, R. W., Jimenez, C. L., Carpenter, B. F., Cutz, E. & Smith, C. R. (1991). Four unusual cases of sudden and unexpected cardiovascular death in infancy and childhood. *Medicine, Science and the Law*, **31**, 157–61.

Byard, R. W., Keeley, F. W. & Smith, C. R. (1990). Type IV Ehlers–Danlos syndrome presenting as sudden infant death. *American Journal of Clinical Pathology*, **93**, 579–82.

Byers, P. H., Barsh, G. S. & Holbrook, K. A. (1982). Molecular pathology in inherited disorders of collagen metabolism. *Human Pathology*, **13**, 89–95.

Byers, P. H., Holbrook, K. A., McGillivray, B., MacLeod, P. M. & Lowry, R. B. (1979). Clinical and ultrastructural heterogeneity of type IV Ehlers–Danlos syndrome. *Human Genetics*, **47**, 141–50.

Cassidy, S. B. (2001). Prader–Willi syndrome. In *Management of Genetic Syndromes*, ed. S. B. Cassidy & J. E. Allanson. New York: Wiley-Liss, pp. 301–22.

Challenor, V. F., Conway, N. & Monro, J. L. (1988). The surgical treatment of restrictive cardiomyopathy in pseudoxanthoma elasticum. *British Heart Journal*, **59**, 266–9.

Cikrit, D. F., Miles, J. H. & Silver, D. (1987). Spontaneous arterial perforation: the Ehlers–Danlos specter. *Journal of Vascular Surgery*, **5**, 248–55.

Collod, G., Babron, M.-C., Jondeau, G., *et al.* (1994). A second locus for Marfan syndrome maps to chromosome 3p24.2–p25. *Nature Genetics*, **8**, 264–8.

Colman, J. M., Sermer, M., Seaward, P. G. R. & Siu, S. C. (2000). Congenital heart disease in pregnancy. *Cardiology in Review*, **8**, 166–73.

Conomy, J. P., Levinsohn, M. & Fanaroff, A. (1975). Familial infantile myasthenia gravis: a cause of sudden death in young children. *Journal of Pediatrics*, **87**, 428–30.

Crabbe, L. S., Bensky, A. S., Hornstein, L. & Shwartz, D. C. (1993). Cardiovascular abnormalities in children with fragile X syndrome. *Pediatrics*, **91**, 714–15.

Crawford, E. S. (1983). Marfan's syndrome. Broad spectral surgical treatment of cardiovascular manifestations. *Annals of Surgery*, **198**, 487–505.

Dardir, M., Ferrans, V. J. & Roberts, W. C. (1989). Coronary artery disease in familial and metabolic disorders. In *Nonatherosclerotic Ischemic Heart Disease*, ed. R. Virmani & M. B. Forman, New York: Raven Press, pp. 185–235.

Delage, C. & Irey, N. S. (1972). Anaphylactic deaths: a clinicopathological study of 43 cases. *Journal of Forensic Sciences*, **17**, 525–40.

Denborough, M. A., Galloway, G. J. & Hopkinson, K. C. (1982). Malignant hyperpyrexia and sudden infant death. *Lancet*, **ii**, 1068–9.

Dietz, H. C., Pyeritz, R. E., Hall, B. D., *et al.* (1991). The Marfan syndrome locus: confirmation of assignment to chromosome 15 and identification of tightly linked markers at 15q15-q21.3. *Genomics*, **9**, 355–61.

DiGeorge, A. M. (1979). Endocrine system. In *Nelson Textbook of Pediatrics*, 11th edn, ed. V. C. Vaughan, III, R. J. McKay, Jr, R. E. Behrman & W. E. Nelson. Philadelphia: W. B. Saunders, pp. 1611–704.

Edston, E. & van Hage-Hamsten, M. (1998). β-Tryptase measurements post-mortem in anaphylactic deaths and in controls. *Forensic Science International*, **93**, 135–42.

Ferrans, V. J. & Boyce, S. W. (1983). Metabolic and familial diseases. In *Cardiovascular Pathology*, vol. 2, ed. M. D. Silver. New York: Churchill Livingstone, pp. 945–1004.

Fineschi, V., Cecchi, R., Centini, F., Reattelli, L. P. & Turillazzi, E. (2001). Immunohistochemical quantification of pulmonary mast-cells and post-mortem blood dosages of tryptase and eosinophil cationic protein in 48 heroin-related deaths. *Forensic Science International*, **120**, 189–94.

Fisher, M. M. & Baldo, B. A. (1993). The diagnosis of fatal anaphylactic reactions during anaesthesia: employment of immunoassays for mast cell tryptase and drug-reactive IgE antibodies. *Anaesthesia and Intensive Care*, **21**, 353–7.

Fleisher, G. R., Buck, B. E. & Cornfeld, D. (1978). Primary intimal fibroplasia in a child with Down's syndrome. *American Journal of Diseases in Children*, **132**, 700–703.

Fox, R., Pope, F. M., Narcisi, P., *et al.* (1988). Spontaneous carotid cavernous fistula in Ehlers Danlos syndrome. *Journal of Neurology, Neurosurgery and Psychiatry*, **51**, 984–6.

Franceschini, P., Guala, A., Licata, D., Di Cara, G. & Franceschini, D. (2000). Arterial tortuosity syndrome. *American Journal of Medical Genetics*, **91**, 141–3.

Francke, U. & Furthmayr, H. (1994). Marfan's syndrome and other disorders of fibrillin. *New England Journal of Medicine*, **330**, 1384–5.

Fremion, A. S., Garg, B. P. & Kalsbeck, J. (1984). Apnea as the sole manifestation of cord compression in achondroplasia. *Journal of Pediatrics*, **104**, 398–401.

Fryns, J.-P., Moerman, P., Gilis, F., d'Espallier, L. & Van den Berghe, H. (1988). Suggestively increased rate of infant death in children of FRA(X) positive mothers. *American Journal of Medical Genetics*, **30**, 73–5.

Gertsch, P., Loup, P.-W., Lochman, A. & Anani, P. (1986). Changing patterns in the vascular form of Ehlers–Danlos syndrome. *Archives of Surgery*, **121**, 1061–4.

Giampietro, P. F., Raggio, C. & Davis, J. G. (2002). Marfan syndrome: orthopedic and genetic review. *Current Opinion in Pediatrics*, **14**, 35–41.

Gillan, J. E., Costigan, D. C., Keeley, F. W. & Rose, V. (1984). Spontaneous dissecting aneurysm of the ductus arteriosus in an infant with Marfan syndrome. *Journal of Pediatrics*, **105**, 952–5.

Gordon, N. (2000). The neurological complications of achondroplasia. *Brain & Development*, **22**, 3–7.

Grahame, R. (2000). Heritable disorders of connective tissue. *Ballière's Clinical Rheumatology*, **14**, 345–61.

Grimm, T. & Wesselhoeft, H. (1980). Zur genetik des Williams–Beuren-syndromes und der isoloerten form der supravalvularen aortenstenose. Untersuchungen von 128 familien. *Zeitschrift fur Kardiologie*, **69**, 168–72.

Grondin, C. M., Steinberg, C. L. & Edwards, J. E. (1969). Dissecting aneurysm complicating Marfan's syndrome (arachnodactyly) in a mother and son. *American Heart Journal*, **77**, 301–6.

Guilleminault, C. (1989). Sleep-related respiratory function and dysfunction in postneonatal infantile apnea. In *Sudden Infant Death Syndrome. Medical Aspects and Psychological Management*, ed. J. L. Culbertson, H. F. Krous & R. D. Bendell. London: Edward Arnold, pp. 94–120.

Hamilton-Gibbs, J. S. (1970). Death from coronary calcinosis occurring in the baby of a mother presenting with pseudoxanthoma elasticum. *Australian Journal of Dermatology*, **11**, 145–8.

Harris, S. C., Slater, D. N. & Austin, C. A. (1985). Fatal splenic rupture in Ehlers–Danlos syndrome. *Postgraduate Medical Journal*, **61**, 259–60.

Hecht, J. T., Francomano, C. A., Horton, W. A. & Annegers, J. F. (1987). Mortality in achondroplasia. *American Journal of Human Genetics*, **41**, 454–64.

Hernández, A., Aguirre-Negrete, M. G., Ramírez-Soltero, *et al.* (1979). A distinct variant of the Ehlers–Danlos syndrome. *Clinical Genetics*, **16**, 335–9.

Hollister, D. W. (1978). Heritable disorders of connective tissue: Ehlers–Danlos syndrome. *Pediatric Clinics of North America*, **25**, 575–91.

Horton, W. A. (1997). Fibroblast growth factor receptor 3 and the human chondrodysplasias. *Current Opinion in Pediatrics*, **9**, 437–42.

Horton, W. A. & Hecht, J. T. (1993). The chondrodysplasias. In *Connective Tissue and Its Heritable Disorders. Molecular, Genetic and Medical Aspects*, ed. P. M. Royce & B. Steinmann. New York: Wiley-Liss, pp. 641–75.

Huang, S., Kumar, G., Steele, H. D. & Parker, J. O. (1967). Cardiac involvement in pseudoxanthoma elasticum. Report of a case. *American Heart Journal*, **74**, 680–85.

Hunter, A. G. W., Bankier, A., Rogers, J. G., Sillence, D. & Scott, C. I., Jr (1998). Medical complications of achondroplasia: a multicentre patient review. *Journal of Medical Genetics*, **35**, 705–12.

Iqbal, A., Alter, M. & Lee, S. H. (1978). Pseudoxanthoma elasticum: a review of neurological complications. *Annals of Neurology*, **4**, 18–20.

Jacome, D. E. (1999). Epilepsy in Ehlers–Danlos syndrome. *Epilepsia*, **40**, 467–73.

Jaffe, A. S., Geltman, E. M., Rodey, G. E. & Uitto, J. (1981). Mitral valve prolapse: a consistent manifestation of type IV Ehlers–Danlos syndrome. The pathogenetic role of the abnormal production of type III collagen. *Circulation*, **64**, 121–5.

James, T. N., Frame, B. & Schatz, I. J. (1964). Pathology of cardiac conduction system in Marfan's syndrome. *Archives of Internal Medicine*, **114**, 339–43.

Jensen, O. M. (1962). Sudden death due to stings from bees and wasps. *Acta Pathologica et Microbiologica Scandinavica*, **54**, 9–29.

Kainulainen, K., Pulkkinen, L., Savolainen, A., Kaitila, I. & Peltonen, L. (1990). Location on chromosome 15 of the gene defect causing Marfan syndrome. *New England Journal of Medicine*, **323**, 935–9.

Kato, T., Hattori, H., Yorifuji, T., Tashiro, Y. & Nakahata, T. (2001). Intracranial aneurysms in Ehlers–Danlos syndrome type IV in early childhood. *Pediatric Neurology*, **25**, 336–9.

Katzen, J. T. & McCarthy, J. G. (2000). Syndromes involving craniosynostoses and midface hypoplasia. *Otolaryngologic Clinics of North America*, **33**, 1257–84.

Kruse, T. A., Kolvraa, S., Bolund, L., *et al.* (1989). X-linked anhidrotic ectodermal dysplasia (EDA). Multipoint linkage analysis. *Cytogenetics and Cell Genetics*, **51**, 1026.

Küster, W. & Happle, R. (1993). Neurocutaneous disorders in children. *Current Opinion in Pediatrics*, **5**, 436–40.

Lach, B., Nair, S. G., Russell, N. A. & Benoit, B. G. (1987). Spontaneous carotid-cavernous fistula and multiple arterial dissections in type IV Ehlers–Danlos syndrome. *Journal of Neurosurgery*, **66**, 462–7.

Langer, L. O., Jr, Baumann, P. A. & Gorlin, R. J. (1967). Achondroplasia. *American Journal of Roentgenology, Radium Therapy and Nuclear Medicine*, **100**, 12–26.

Lebwohl, M., Phelps, R. G., Yannuzzi, L., Chang, S., Schwartz, I. & Fuchs, W. (1987). Diagnosis of pseudoxanthoma elasticum by scar biopsy in patients without characteristic skin lesions. *New England Journal of Medicine*, **317**, 347–50.

Lees, M. H., Menashe, V. D., Sunderland, C. O., Morgan, C. L. & Dawson, P. J. (1969). Ehlers–Danlos syndrome associated with multiple pulmonary artery stenoses and tortuous systemic arteries. *Journal of Pediatrics*, **75**, 1031–6.

Leier, C. V., Call, T. D., Fulkerson, P. K. & Wooley, C. F. (1980). The spectrum of cardiac defects in the Ehlers–Danlos syndrome, types I and III. *Annals of Internal Medicine*, **92**, 171–8.

Lemyre, E., Azouz, M., Teebi, A. S., Glanc, P. & Chen, M.-F. (1999). Achondroplasia, hypochondroplasia and thanatophoric dysplasia: review and update. *Canadian Association of Radiologists Journal*, **50**, 185–97.

Liu, W., Schrijver, I., Brenn, T., Furthmayr, H. & Franke, U. (2001). Multi-exon deletions of the FBN1 gene in Marfan syndrome. *BMC Medical Genetics*, **2**, 11–19.

Loughlin, G. M., Wynne, J. W. & Victorica, B. E. (1981). Sleep apnea as a possible cause of pulmonary hypertension in Down syndrome. *Journal of Pediatrics*, **98**, 435–7.

MacLennan, D. H., Duff, C., Zorzato, F., *et al.* (1990). Ryanodine receptor gene is a candidate for predisposition to malignant hyperthermia. *Nature*, **343**, 559–61.

Madariaga, I., de la Fuente, A., Lezaun, R., *et al.* (1984). Cardiac echinococcosis and systemic embolism. Report of a case. *Thoracic Cardiovascular Surgeon*, **32**, 57–9.

Malcolm, A. D. (1985). Mitral valve prolapse associated with other disorders. Casual coincidence, common link, or fundamental genetic disturbance? *British Heart Journal*, **53**, 353–62.

Marin-Padilla, M. & Marin-Padilla, T. M. (1977). Developmental abnormalities of the occipital bone in human chondrodystrophies. (Achondroplasia and thanatophoric dwarfism.) *Birth Defects*, **3**, 7–23.

McCarthy, T. V., Healy, J. M. S., Heffron, J. J. A., *et al.* (1990). Localization of the malignant hyperthermia susceptibility locus to human chromosome 19q12-13.2. *Nature*, **343**, 562–4.

Mendelsohn, G., Bulkley, B. H. & Hutchins, G. M. (1978). Cardiovascular manifestations of pseudoxanthoma elasticum. *Archives of Pathology and Laboratory Medicine*, **102**, 298–302.

Mentzel, H.-J., Seidel, J., Vogt, S., Vogt, L. & Kaiser, W. A. (1999). Vascular complications (splenic and hepatic artery aneurysms) in the occipital horn syndrome: report of a patient and review of the literature. *Pediatric Radiology*, **29**, 19–22.

Milewicz, D. M. (1998). Molecular genetics of Marfan syndrome and Ehlers–Danlos type IV. *Current Opinion in Cardiology*, **13**, 198–204.

Miller, M. J., Geffner, M. E., Lippe, B. M., *et al.* (1983). Echocardiography reveals a high incidence of bicuspid aortic valve in Turner syndrome. *Journal of Pediatrics*, **102**, 47–50.

Moore, J. W., Kirby, W. C., Rogers, W. M. & Poth, M. A. (1990). Partial anomalous pulmonary venous drainage associated with 45,X Turner's syndrome. *Pediatrics*, **86**, 273–76.

Mosbech, H. (1983). Death caused by wasp and bee stings in Denmark 1960–1980. *Allergy*, **38**, 195–200.

Murdoch, J. L., Walker, B. A., Halpern, B. L., Kuzma, J. W. & McKusick, V. A. (1972). Life expectancy and causes of death in the Marfan syndrome. *New England Journal of Medicine*, **286**, 804–8.

Neldner, K. H. (1993). Pseudoxanthoma elasticum. In *Connective Tissue and Its Heritable Disorders. Molecular, Genetic and Medical Aspects*, ed. P. M. Royce & B. Steinmann. New York: Wiley-Liss, pp. 425–36.

Nelson, F. W., Hecht, J. T., Horton, W. A., Butler, I. J., Goldie, W. D. & Miner, M. (1988). Neurological basis of respiratory complications in achondroplasia. *Annals of Neurology*, **24**, 89–93.

Nijbroek, G., Sood, S., McIntosh, I., *et al.* (1995). Fifteen novel FBNI mutations causing Marfan syndrome detected by heteroduplex analysis of genomic amplicons. *American Journal of Human Genetics*, **21**, 8–21.

Owen, S. M. & Durst, R. D. (1984). Ehlers–Danlos syndrome simulating child abuse. *Archives of Dermatology*, **120**, 97–101.

Pauli, R. M., Conroy, M. M., Langer, L. O., Jr, *et al.* (1983). Homozygous achondroplasia with survival beyond infancy. *American Journal of Medical Genetics*, **16**, 459–73.

Pauli, R. M., Scott, C. I., Wassman, E. R., Jr, *et al.* (1984). Apnea and sudden unexpected death in infants with achondroplasia. *Journal of Pediatrics*, **104**, 342–8.

Pereira, L., Levran, O., Ramirez, F., *et al.* (1994). A molecular approach to the stratification of cardiovascular risk in families with Marfan's syndrome. *New England Journal of Medicine*, **331** 148–53.

Phillips, J. A. & Vnencak-Jones, C. L. (1993). Molecular genetics and prenatal diagnosis. *Baillière's Clinical Pediatrics*, **1**, 505–52.

Phornphutkul, C., Rosenthal, A. & Nadas, A. S. (1973). Cardiac manifestations of Marfan syndrome in infancy and childhood. *Circulation*, **47**, 587–96.

Pierre-Kahn, A., Hirsch, J. F., Renier, D., Metzger, J. & Maroteaux, P. (1980). Hydrocephalus and achondroplasia. A study of 25 observations. *Child's Brain*, **7**, 205–19.

Pope, F. M. (1975). Historical evidence for the genetic heterogeneity of pseudoxanthoma elasticum. *British Journal of Dermatology*, **92**, 493–509.

Pope, F. M., Martin, G. R. & McKusick, V. A. (1977). Inheritance of Ehlers–Danlos type IV syndrome. *Journal of Medical Genetics*, **14**, 200–204.

Pope, F. M., Nicholls, A. C., Dorrance, D. E., Child, A. H. & Narcisi, P. (1983). Type III collagen deficiency with normal phenotype. *Journal of the Royal Society of Medicine*, **76**, 518–20.

Prahlow, J. A. & Barnard, J. J. (1998). Fatal anaphylaxis due to fire ant stings. *American Journal of Forensic Medicine and Pathology*, **19**, 137–42.

Pumphrey, R. S. & Roberts, I. S. (2000). Postmortem findings after fatal anaphylactic reactions. *Journal of Clinical Pathology*, **53**, 273–6.

Pyeritz, R. E. (1981). Maternal and fetal complications of pregnancy in the Marfan syndrome. *American Journal of Medicine*, **71**, 784–90.

Pyeritz, R. E. (1993). The Marfan syndrome. In *Connective Tissue and Its Heritable Disorders. Molecular, Genetic and Medical Aspects*, ed. P. M. Royce & B. Steinmann. New York: Wiley-Liss, pp. 437–68.

Pyeritz, R. E. (2000). The Marfan syndrome. *Annual Review of Medicine*, **51**, 481–510.

Pyeritz, R. E. & McKusick, V. A. (1979). The Marfan syndrome: diagnosis and management. *New England Journal of Medicine*, **300**, 772–7.

Rabl, V. W., Tributsch, W. & Ambach, E. (1990). Prämature Kraniosynostosis – Ursache plötzlicher todesfälle im kindes- und jungen erwachsenenalter. *Beitrage Zur Gerichtlichen Medizin*, **48**, 217–21.

Randall, B., Butts, J. & Halsey, J. F. (1995). Elevated postmortem tryptase in the absence of anaphylaxis. *Journal of Forensic Sciences*, **40**, 208–11.

Ranke, M. B. & Saenger, P. (2001). Turner's syndrome. *Lancet*, **358**, 309–14.

Ranklev, E., Fletcher, R. & Krantz, P. (1985). Malignant hyperplexia and sudden death. *American Journal of Forensic Medicine and Pathology*, **6**, 149–50.

Reed, W. B., Lopez, D. A. & Landing, B. (1970). Clinical spectrum of anhidrotic ectodermal dysplasia. *Archives of Dermatology*, **102**, 134–43.

Riches, K. J., Gillis, D. & James, R. A. (2002). An autopsy approach to bee sting-related deaths. *Pathology*, **34**, 257–62.

Ringpfeil, F., Pulkkinen, L. & Uitto, J. (2001). Molecular genetics of pseudoxanthoma elasticum. *Experimental Dermatology*, **10**, 221–8.

Roberts, W. C. & Honig, H. S. (1982). The spectrum of cardiovascular disease in the Marfan syndrome: a clinico-morphologic study of 18 necropsy patients and comparison to 151 previously reported necropsy patients. *American Heart Journal*, **104**, 115–35.

Roberts, I. S. D. & Pumphrey, R. S. H. (2001). The autopsy in fatal anaphylaxis. In *Recent Advances in Histopathology 19*, ed. D. G. Lowe & J. C. E. Underwood. Edinburgh: Churchill Livingstone, pp. 145–62.

Roberts, D. L. L., Pope, F. M., Nicholls, A. C. & Narcisi, P. (1984). Ehlers–Danlos syndrome type IV mimicking non-accidental injury in a child. *British Journal of Dermatology*, **3**, 341–5.

Robinson, P. N. & Booms, P. (2001). The molecular pathogenesis of the Marfan syndrome. *Cellular and Molecular Life Sciences*, **58**, 1698–707.

Robinson, P. N. & Godfrey, M. (2000). The molecular genetics of Marfan syndrome and related microfibrillopathies. *Journal of Medical Genetics*, **37**, 9–25.

Robinson, R. L. & Hopkins, P. M. (2001). A breakthrough in the genetic diagnosis of malignant hyperthermia. *British Journal of Anaesthesia*, **86**, 166–8.

Rudd, N. L., Holbrook, K. A., Nimrod, C. & Byers, P. H. (1983). Pregnancy complications in type IV Ehlers–Danlos syndrome. *Lancet*, **i**, 50–53.

Salzberg, M. R. & Kramer, R. J. (1984). Dissecting thoracic aortic aneurysm in a 16-year-old. *Annals of Emergency Medicine*, **13**, 191–3.

Sampson, H. A., Mendelson, L. & Rosen, J. P. (1992). Fatal and near-fatal anaphylactic reactions to food in children and adolescents. *New England Journal of Medicine*, **327**, 380–84.

Saruk, M. & Eisenstein, R. (1977). Aortic lesion in Marfan syndrome. The ultrastructure of cystic medial degeneration. *Archives of Pathology and Laboratory Medicine*, **101**, 74–7.

Schachner, L. & Young, D. (1974). Pseudoxanthoma elasticum with severe cardiovascular disease in a child. *American Journal of Diseases of Children*, **127**, 571–5.

Schrander-Stumpel, C., Sijstermans, H., Curfs., L. & Fryns, J.-P. (1998). Sudden death in children with Prader–Willy syndrome: a call for collaboration. *Genetic Counselling*, **9**, 231–2.

Schwartz, H. J., Sutheimer, C., Gauerke, M. B. & Yunginger, J. W. (1988). Hymenoptera venom-specific IgE antibodies in postmortem sera from victims of sudden, unexpected death. *Clinical Allergy*, **18**, 461–8.

Schwartz, H. J., Yunginger, J. W., Teigland, J. D., Suthmeimer, C. & Hiss, Y. (1984). Sudden death due to stinging insect hypersensitivity: postmortem demonstration of IgE antivenom antibodies in a fatal case. *American Journal of Clinical Pathology*, **81**, 794–5.

Shohet, I., Rosenbaum, I., Frand, M., Duksin, D., Engelberg, S. & Goodman, R. M. (1987). Cardiovascular complications in the Ehlers–Danlos syndrome with minimal external findings. *Clinical Genetics*, **31**, 148–52.

Snyder, R. R., Gilstrap, L. C. & Hauth, J. C. (1983). Ehlers–Danlos syndrome and pregnancy. *Obstetrics and Gynecology*, **61**, 649–51.

Stebbens, V. A., Dennis, J., Samuels, M. P., Croft, C. B. & Southall, D. P. (1991). Sleep related upper airway obstruction in a cohort with Down's syndrome. *Archives of Disease in Childhood*, **66**, 1333–8.

Steinmann, B., Royce, P. M. & Superti-Furga, A. (1993). The Ehlers–Danlos syndrome. In *Connective Tissue and Its Heritable Disorders. Molecular, Genetic and Medical Aspects*, ed. P. M. Royce & B. Steinmann. New York: Wiley-Liss, pp. 351–407.

Stokes, D. C., Phillips, J. A., Leonard, C. O., *et al.* (1983). Respiratory complications of achondroplasia. *Journal of Pediatrics*, **102**, 534–41.

Strife, J. L. (1988). Upper airway and tracheal obstruction in infants and children. *Radiologic Clinics of North America*, **26**, 309–22.

Sulica, V. I., Cooper, P. H., Pope, F. M., Hambrick, G. W., Jr, Gerson, B. M. & McKusick, V. A. (1979). Cutaneous histologic features in Ehlers–Danlos syndrome. *Archives of Dermatology*, **115**, 40–42.

Sutherland, G. R. & Richards, R. I. (1993). The fragile X syndrome. In *Baillière's Clinical Paediatrics*, ed. I. Young. London: Baillière Tindall Saunders, pp. 477–504.

Sutherland, G. R., Mulley, J. C. & Richards, R. I. (1993). Fragile X syndrome. The most common cause of familial intellectual handicap. *Medical Journal of Australia*, **158**, 482–5.

Takebayashi, S., Kubota, I. & Takagi, T. (1973). Ultrastructural and histochemical studies of vascular lesions in Marfan's syndrome, with report of 4 autopsy cases. *Acta Pathologica Japonica*, **23**, 847–66.

Thilenius, O. G., Bharati, S., Arcilla, R. A. & Lev, M. (1980). Cardiac pathology of Marfan's syndrome. Can dissection and rupture of aortic aneurysms be prevented? *Cardiology*, **65**, 193–204.

Thomas, I. T. & Frias, J. L. (1987). The cardiovascular manifestations of genetic disorders of collagen metabolism. *Annals of Clinical and Laboratory Science*, **17**, 377–82.

Tiller, G. E., Cassidy, S. B., Wensel, C. & Westrup, R. J. (1998). Aortic root dilatation in Ehlers–Danlos syndrome types I, II, and III. A report of five cases. *Clinical Genetics*, **53**, 460–65.

Tubman, T. R. J., Shields, M. D., Craig, B. G., Mulholland, H. C. & Nevin, N. C. (1991). Congenital heart disease in Down's syndrome: two year prospective early screening study. *British Medical Journal*, **302**, 1425–7.

Uitto, J., Pulkkinen, L. & Ringpfeil, F. (2001). Molecular genetics of pseudoxanthoma elasticum: a metabolic disorder at the environment-genome interface. *Trends in Molecular Medicine*, **7**, 13–17.

Umlas, J. (1972). Spontaneous rupture of the subclavian artery in the Ehlers–Danlos syndrome. *Human Pathology*, **3**, 121–6.

Viljoen, D. L., Pope, F. M. & Beighton, P. (1987). Heterogeneity of pseudoxanthoma elasticum: delineation of a new form? *Clinical Genetics*, **32**, 100–105.

Wallach, E. A. & Burkhart, E. F. (1950). Ehlers–Danlos syndrome associated with the tetralogy of Fallot. *Archives of Dermatology and Syphilology*, **61**, 750–52.

Wappler, F. (2001). Malignant hyperthermia. *European Journal of Anaesthesiology*, **18**, 632–52.

Waters, K. A., Everett, F., Sillence, D., Fagan, E. & Sullivan, C. E. (1993). Breathing abnormalities in sleep in achondroplasia. *Archives of Disease in Childhood*, **69**, 191–6.

Wharton, R. H., Wang, T., Graeme-Cook, F., Briggs, S. & Cole, R. E. (1997). Acute idiopathic gastric dilation with gastric necrosis in individuals with Prader Willi syndrome. *American Journal of Medical Genetics*, **73**, 437–41.

Wilhelm, K. & Paver, K. (1972). Sudden death in pseudoxanthoma elasticum. *Medical Journal of Australia*, **2**, 1363–5.

Wingard, D. W. (1974). Malignant hyperthermia: a human stress syndrome? *Lancet*, **ii**, 1450–51.

Yang, S. S., Corbett, D. P., Brough, A. J., Heidelberger, K. P. & Bernstein, J. (1977). Upper cervical myelopathy in achondroplasia. *American Journal of Clinical Pathology*, **68**, 68–72.

Yunginger, J. W., Nelson, D. R., Squillance, D. L., *et al.* (1991). Laboratory investigation of deaths due to anaphylaxis. *Journal of Forensic Sciences*, **36**, 857–65.

Zinn, A. R. & Ross, J. L. (2001). Molecular analysis of genes on Xp controlling Turner syndrome and premature ovarian failure (POF). *Seminars in Reproductive Medicine*, **19**, 141–6.

Part V

Sudden infant death syndrome

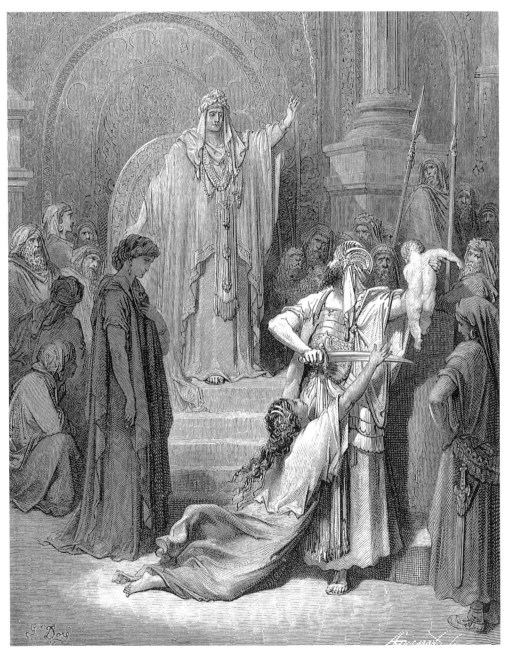

The Judgement of Solomon (1 Kings 3: 16–28), involving the first recorded case of "overlaying:" " . . . And when I arose in the morning to give my child suck, behold, it was dead . . . " (Taken from a nineteenth-century engraving by Doré.)

13

Sudden infant death syndrome

Introduction and historical background

Sudden infant death syndrome (SIDS), cot or crib death is the term that is used when a previously well infant is found unexpectedly dead after sleeping, with no cause for the death being established (Beckwith, 1970a; Byard & Krous, 2001). Since the first edition of this text, there have been dramatic changes in the profile of these cases. Following the identification of specific environmental risk factors, community awareness campaigns were undertaken that have resulted in deaths from SIDS falling precipitously in many communities (Henderson-Smart, Ponsonby & Murphy, 1998). For example, the number of SIDS deaths per year in California, USA, has fallen from 110.5/100,000 live births in 1990 to 47.2/100,000 live births in 1998 (Byard & Krous, 2003a), and the number of SIDS deaths nationally in Australia has fallen from over 500 per year in 1988 to just 134 per year in 1999 (Byard, 2001a). Research has clarified possible mechanisms of death, with the "triple risk" or "fatal triangle" models being proposed to integrate complex individual susceptibilities with developmental stages and environmental factors (Filiano & Kinney, 1994; Rognum & Saugstad, 1993). This model has, however, been challenged with suggestions that a more appropriate theoretical framework should encompass multifactorial causation involving variable probabilities for a range of risk factors (Guntheroth & Spiers, 2002).

Despite these great successes, however, problems remain. Infant deaths are still investigated poorly in many jurisdictions, with deaths being attributed to SIDS without fulfilling the requirements of recognized definitions or following accepted protocols for autopsy and death scene investigation. Cases may not even have autopsies performed (Burnell & Byard, 2002; Byard, 2001a; l'Hoir et al., 1998). Single-cause theories of SIDS continue to be expounded through the media without appropriate peer review, causing considerable parental confusion and anxiety, and research is based not infrequently on cases that simply have not been investigated sufficiently for the conclusion of SIDS to be sustainable. Infants whose deaths are now attributed to SIDS also often come from socially disadvantaged groups, who may be difficult to investigate and counsel (Willinger et al., 1998; Willinger et al., 2000). Despite standard definitions of SIDS precluding the use of the term if significant lethal disease is found at autopsy, confusion prevails, with some publications referring to "cardiovascular causes" of SIDS such as myocarditis, congenital heart disease, rhabdomyomas, myocardial infarction, and aortic stenosis (Rambaud, Guilleminault & Campbell, 1994; Valdés-Dapena & Gilbert-Barness, 2002).

Thus, although we have progressed considerably in the examination and assessment of unexpected infant deaths, SIDS appears destined to continue to be a difficult, contentious, and emotive term that can, unfortunately, be used very easily as a "diagnostic dustbin" to disguise incomplete investigations and inaccurate conclusions (Emery, 1989).

Definition

It is a rather disappointing fact that debate continues about the most appropriate definition of SIDS. In 1969 at the Second International Conference on Causes of Sudden Death in Infants, SIDS was defined as "the sudden death of any infant or young child, which is unexpected by history, and in which a thorough postmortem examination fails to demonstrate an adequate cause for death" (Beckwith, 1973).

More recently in the USA, the National Institute of Child Health and Human Development (NICHD) Group revised the definition as "the sudden death of an infant under one year of age which remains unexplained after a thorough case investigation, including performance of a complete autopsy, examination of the death scene, and review of the clinical history" (Willinger, James & Catz, 1991). The major features of the latter definition are an upper limit of one year of age and emphasis on a proper death scene investigation. Despite the usefulness of this definition, it has not been accepted universally, and a number of alternate definitions have been proposed. While these have placed different emphases on the age range, associations with sleep, death scene investigations, and history reviews, the performance of ancillary testing, and the presence or absence of minor pathologic findings, they have not advanced greatly our understanding of the term (Cordner & Willinger, 1995; Mitchell *et al.*, 1994; Rambaud, Guilleminault & Campbell, 1994; Sturner, 1998). Stratification of cases into two or three categories has been suggested to better define the requirements that have been fulfilled, or not, for diagnostic purposes. This has been proposed to separate classic SIDS cases from atypical or incompletely investigated deaths and would certainly provide a more solid basis for subsequent research (Beckwith, 1993; Beckwith, 2003).

Although one of the concerns with the NICHD definition is the cut-off point of one year of age, SIDS is a condition of early infancy, with unexpected deaths after the first year being unusual (Figure 13.1). The major contribution of the definition has been to recognize that attributing a death to SIDS requires more than just an autopsy, as many natural and unnatural diseases and conditions may cause unexpected infant death with only very subtle presenting symptoms and minimal or no postmortem signs (Byard, 1996a; Byard, 1996b; Byard, Donald & Chivell, 1999; Byard & Krous, 1999a; Moore & Byard, 1993; Whybourne *et al.*, 2001).

Historical theories

SIDS is not a new phenomenon, having been thought for many thousands of years to be caused by a sleeping parent lying over an infant in a shared bed. It is mentioned in the Bible, where the Judgement of Solomon (1 Kings 3: 19) reads " . . . and this woman's child died in the night because she overlaid it" (see frontispiece on p. 489). Much later, mention of overlaying can be found in manuscripts from the sixth and seventh centuries, with various penalties for parents found guilty of "overlaying" their children. These included a bread-and-water diet for a year, sleeping in separate beds, and abstinence from wine and meat (Norvenius, 1988; Norvenius, 1993).

The belief in overlaying, or *oppressio infantis*, continued during the Middle Ages in Europe, and a wooden device called an *arcuccio* was constructed in Florence to prevent its occurrence (Figure 13.2). So seriously was death due to overlaying taken that excommunication was a possible penalty if an infant died in bed with a mother or a wet nurse who had not used the frame (Limerick, 1992). A separate category of "overlaid and starved at nurse" as a cause of death can be found in the "Bills of Mortality for the City of London in 1632" (Peterson, 1980), and a variant of the *arcuccio* was still in use in Tuscany well into the nineteenth century (Anonymous, 1895). Given the poor level of investigation of unexpected infant deaths in the past, it is not possible to determine the epidemiology of infant deaths and the number of SIDS deaths in previous centuries with any accuracy.

Reports in the *Lancet* in the nineteenth century confirm how entrenched the belief in overlaying had become. In a case in which the dead infant's mother maintained that the child had not been sleeping near her, Fearn's (1834) initial impression was "in spite of the evidence of the mother, that the child must have

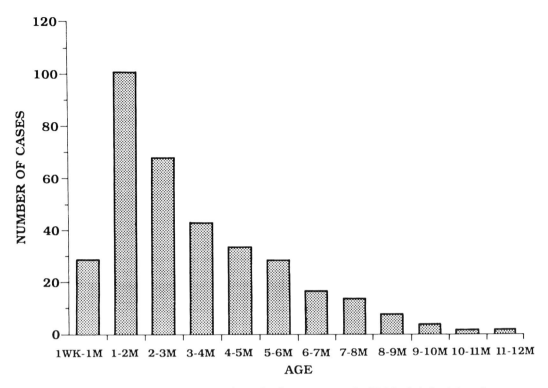

Figure 13.1 Characteristic age distribution of SIDS infants taken from 351 consecutive SIDS deaths in South Australia.

been destroyed by overlaying." This opinion was "a good deal shaken," however, when a second infant who had been in bed alone was found in similar circumstances.

W.B. Yeats in 1889 confirmed the popular perception of the cause of SIDS in "The Ballad of Moll Magee," in which he describes the treatment of a woman by her husband and others following the loss of her child (Yeats, 1962):

I lay upon my baby;
Ye little childer dear,
I looked on my cold baby
When the morn grew frosty and clear.

A weary woman sleeps so hard!
My man grew red and pale,
And gave me money, and bade me go
To my own place Kinsale.

He drove me out and shut the door,
And gave his curse to me;

I went away in silence,
No neighbour could I see.

So now, ye little childer,
Ye won't fling stones at me;
But gather with your shinin' looks
And pity Moll Magee.

Charles Templeman (1892), a Scottish police surgeon in the latter part of the nineteenth century, who was a staunch supporter of overlaying as a major cause of infant death, suggested that it should be illegal for infants and young children to sleep in bed with their parents. He also proposed that parents who had slept in an intoxicated state with their children should be prosecuted. This was the case in Australia in 1897, where a mother was convicted of manslaughter following the "overlaying" of her infant son while she was "under the influence of drink," although she was later acquitted on appeal (Bowden, 1952; R. *v.* Egan, 1897). Almost 100 years

The ARCUCCIO. *Vide Fig.* 3.

a, The Place where the Child lies.
b, The Head-board.
c, The Hollows for the Nurfes Breafts.
d, A Bar of Wood to lean on when fhe fuckles the Child.
e, A fmall Iron Arch to fupport the faid Bar.
The Length 3 Feet, 2 Inches and a half.

Every Nurfe in *Florence* is obliged to lay the Child in it, under Pain of Excommunication. The *Arcutio,* with the Child in it, may be fafely laid entirely under the Bed-cloaths in the Winter, without Danger of fmothering.

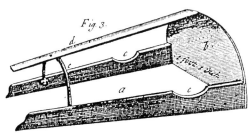

Figure 13.2 An eighteenth-century device, the *arcuccio,* designed to prevent overlaying while breastfeeding (*Philosophical Transactions of the Royal Society of London,* 1733).

later, sleeping in an intoxicated state in the same bed as an infant who was later found dead was still considered to be a criminal offence under the *Children and Young Persons Act of Great Britain* (Russell-Jones, 1985).

The disproportionately high number of infant deaths on Saturday nights in Victorian Dundee (46% of the total) gave some credence to Templeman's theories. He concluded that: "The principal causes producing this great mortality from overlaying are, 1. Ignorance and carelessness of mothers; 2, drunkenness; [and] 3, overcrowding . . ." Although overlaying is diagnosed less often today, it still may be impossible to exclude as a cause of death if an infant is found dead in bed with a sleeping adult, particularly

if the adult is obese or has taken sedatives or alcohol (Gilbert-Barness *et al.*, 1991; Thach, 1986; Thach, 1989).

One of the earliest alternate theories to suggest that sudden infant death may be caused by factors other than overlaying was *mors thymica*, described by Plater in 1614, and repopularized in 1830 by Kopp as "thymic asthma." This proposed that tracheal obstruction occurred in vulnerable infants due to pressure from an enlarged thymus gland (reported in Krous, 1989). Other authors writing in the nineteenth century also raised the possibility of either unknown or intrinsic asphyxial mechanisms as the cause of sudden death (Fearn, 1834; Ross, 1862). French investigators suggested that "suffocating catarrh" was responsible for many cases of sudden death (reported in Golding, Limerick & Macfarlane, 1985). If the prodrome could be identified, "Leeches, in large numbers, or, still better, cupping on the chest, with counter-irritation by means of blisters" were recommended forms of therapy (Laennec, 1834). Apparent life-threatening events were also known to nineteenth-century physicians, who referred to them as *asphyxia imminens* (Beal, 1992a).

Folk superstition warned against allowing a cat near an infant in a crib, as the cat may "suck the baby's breath out" and cause death. Whether this belief stemmed from the generally unsavory reputation that cats acquired in the Middle Ages, or from actual cases of smothering from sleeping cats "overlaying" infants, will probably never be known. There is, however, contemporary evidence in the literature that cats may indeed smother sleeping infants (Heaton & Sage, 1995; Kearney, Dahl & Stalsberg, 1982). Another medieval belief was that witches were able to murder children and replace them in their parents' bed without being detected (Savitt, 1979). Centuries before, the Babylonians had blamed sudden infant death on Larbatu, one of their demon gods (Russell-Jones, 1985).

In a slightly less bizarre theory, that of Paultauf's *status thymicolymphaticus*, infants who succumbed to SIDS were thought to have had grossly enlarged thymus glands associated with generalized lymphadenopathy, and arterial and adrenal hypoplasia. Death was thought to occur from airway compression, or pressure on adjacent nerves, or ill-defined metabolic imbalances (Krous, 1989). Although subsequently discredited, this theory led to the writing of 820 papers in the 34 years following its publication and can still be found in medical texts published as late as the 1950s (Bailey & Love, 1959). In quoting a paper by Greenwood & Woods from 1927, Boyd (1931) took a reasonably strong alternate stance and commented that "status thymico-lymphaticus is a good example of the growth of medical mythology, that a nucleus of truth is buried beneath a pile of intellectual rubbish, conjecture, bad observations, and rash generalization, and that it is as accurate to attribute the cause of death to 'the visitation of God' as to status lymphaticus." In spite of this assertion, the following statement was made in 1945 by Carr: "The now popular attitude that there is no such thing as Status Thymical [sic] Lymphaticus can be quickly dissipated by autopsy studies in any Coroner's office where children are studied." Old beliefs tend to linger on.

The latter part of the twentieth century saw the emergence of a plethora of alternate theories on the possible pathogenesis of SIDS (Byard, 1994a; Kendeel & Ferris, 1977b; Merritt & Valdes-Dapena, 1984; Valdes-Dapena, 1967; Valdes-Dapena, 1977; Valdes-Dapena, 1980), but it was not until 1971 that SIDS was accepted as a diagnosis on death certificates in the UK, and only after 1979 that "sudden infant death" was given a separate coding in the World Health Organization's International Classification of Diseases (coding number 798.0) (Russell-Jones, 1985).

Our understanding of the pathogenesis of SIDS is still incomplete, and this is reflected in the vast number of often contradictory papers that have been published in recent years. Froggatt's statement in 1977 that "The theories of the accredited scientist and of the quack are alike to the eyes of the gullible beholder" should be borne in mind by investigators before tackling the literature, as it still applies. This makes reviewing the literature an onerous and time-consuming task, as nearly 1500 papers on SIDS and related topics were published between the years 1960 and 1983 (Kraus, 1983), with 5612 PubMed citations for "sudden infant death syndrome" listed in March 2003.

Epidemiology

Despite calls for the abandonment of the term SIDS (Gilbert-Barness, 1993; Gilbert-Barness & Barness, 1993; Meadow, 1999), typical cases continue to occur with characteristic features that fulfil the requirements for a syndrome. Obviously not all risk factors will be present in every case (Haas *et al.*, 1993), and

SIDS still occurs in only 1% of the most vulnerable group (Shannon & Kelly, 1982a).

Incidence

The incidence of SIDS, once greater than six deaths per 1000 live births per year in certain communities, has recently dropped to less than one death per 1000 live births per year in areas where risk campaigns have been undertaken (Fleming *et al.*, 2000; Hauck, 2001; Rognum, 1995). While SIDS is an infrequent event, it remains the most common cause of unexpected death in infants aged between one week and one year of life in Western countries and has ranged from the seventh to the eighth most important cause

of death in the USA in terms of years of potential life lost (YPLL) before the age of 65 (Centers for Disease Control and Prevention, 1987; Centers for Disease Control and Prevention, 1992). Even allowing for changes in diagnostic preferences (Helweg-Larsen *et al.*, 1992), there was a genuine increase in the incidence of SIDS in several countries between the 1960s and the 1980s (Irgens, Skjaerven & Lie, 1989; Mitchell, 1990). The fall during the 1990s was also genuine and could not be attributed to changes in diagnostic preferences by pathologists (Adams *et al.*, 1998; Byard, 1997a; Byard & Beal, 1995).

Data taken from SIDS autopsies in South Australia over a 10-year period are shown in Figures 13.1, 13.3, and 13.4. These demonstrate the young age,

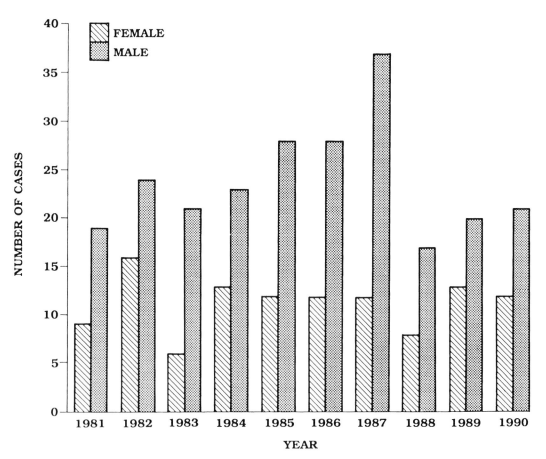

Figure 13.3 Sex distribution of SIDS cases in South Australia between 1981 and 1990, showing a male predominance.

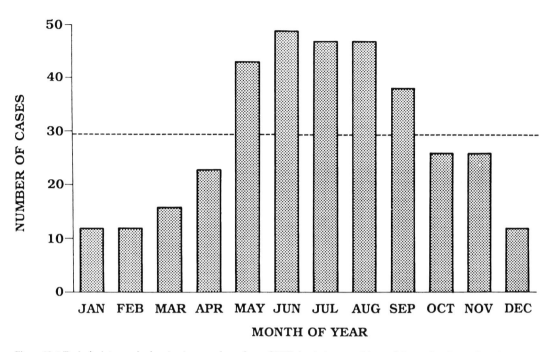

Figure 13.4 Typical winter peak, showing increased numbers of SIDS deaths between May and September (Australian winter).

male predominance, and high winter rates that are found consistently, as well as the variability in incidence from year to year (Beal & Porter, 1991; Douglas, Allan & Helms, 1996). In this population, the rate is now 0.5 per 1000 live births per year, having been as high as 2.5 per 1000 live births per year (South Australian Health Commission, 1989). The winter peak is not unique for SIDS deaths and has been documented in other conditions (Spiers & Guntheroth, 1997).

Infant characteristics

Male infants are affected more often than girls, and there may be a history of prematurity (Kraus, Greenland & Bulterys, 1989), although this has not always been demonstrated (Naeye, Ladis & Drage, 1976). Low birth weights and an extended stay in hospital have been noted, with the most frequent age at death being between two and four months. There may be a history of poor prenatal care (Hoffman & Hillman, 1992; Walker & McMillan, 1993).

Although infants are most often found dead in their cribs after sleeping (Standfast *et al.*, 1983), death due to SIDS can occur at any time of the day (Peterson, 1989). An increase in deaths has occurred at weekends (Mitchell & Stewart, 1988). Victims are often of high birth order, and there is frequently a history of minor respiratory or gastrointestinal illness in the days leading up to death (Carpenter *et al.*, 1979). The validity of suggested behavioral differences such as less movement, abnormal crying, and less response to environmental stimuli (Naeye *et al.*, 1976b) as predictors of the likelihood of SIDS is doubtful, with clinical symptoms tending to be non-specific and not predictive of SIDS (Gilbert *et al.*, 1990).

Environmental factors

Prone sleeping

The association of infant death with sleeping position was reported many years ago by Abramson (1944). He recommended that "the routine nursing practice of placing infants in the prone position be avoided except during such times as the babies are constantly attended" and that "the practice should, furthermore, be entirely done away with at night."

Beal (1986b) in South Australia and de Jonge *et al.* (1989) in the Netherlands were among the first in recent times to draw attention to the possible link between sleeping position and sudden death. De Jonge & Engelberts (1989) noted that there had been an increase in incidence of SIDS in the Netherlands since the early 1970s after policies recommending prone sleeping position for infants were introduced. Once de Jonge's initial findings were published, the incidence of prone infant sleeping fell by almost 30%, paralleled by a fall in the incidence of SIDS of 40%. A subsequent study in England demonstrated a relative risk of SIDS of 8.8 times in infants who slept prone (Fleming *et al.*, 1990). Although this study was criticized for being retrospective (Southall, Stebbens & Samuels, 1990), two later studies have shown that recall bias in this situation is not a major confounding factor (Drews, Kraus & Greenland, 1990; Dwyer *et al.*, 1991b).

While there was initial debate about the likelihood of sleeping position being related to sudden death (Golding, Limerick & Macfarlane, 1985; Guntheroth, 1989a; Guntheroth & Spiers, 1990; Hunt & Shannon, 1992; Milner & Ruggins, 1989; Naeye, 1988), many studies have since confirmed this association, with a relative risk of between 3.5 and 9.3 (Beal, 1986a; Beal, 1986b; Beal, 1988a; Beal, 1988b; Beal, 1991; Beal, 1996; Beal & Finch, 1991; Brooke *et al.*, 1997; Dwyer *et al.*, 1991a; Dwyer *et al.*, 1995; Engelberts, 1991; Engelberts & de Jonge, 1990; Guntheroth & Spiers, 1992; Hoffman *et al.*,1988; Irgens *et al.*, 1995; Markestad *et al.*, 1995; McGlashan, 1988; Mitchell, 1991; Mitchell, 1993; Mitchell *et al.*, 1992a; Mitchell *et al.*, 1997; Mitchell, Brunt & Everard, 1994; Mitchell & Milerad, 1999; Nelson, Taylor & Mackay, 1989; Nicholl & O'Cathain, 1988; Ponsonby *et al.*, 1995; Taylor, 1991; Taylor *et al.*, 1996b; Tonkin & Hassall, 1989; Wigfield *et al.*, 1992).

Infants who sleep on their sides also have an increased risk of SIDS, as they may roll on to their abdomens, and infants who sleep prone for the first time (so-called "unaccustomed prone") are in a higher-risk group (Mitchell *et al.*, 1999; Øyen *et al.*, 1997; Scragg & Mitchell, 1998). The latter has been found to be a factor in SIDS deaths in childcare centers (Moon, Patel & Shaefer, 2000).

An assumption is sometimes made simplistically that the mechanism of death with prone sleeping is simple suffocation. Suffocation certainly may occur if an infant slips between a mattress and cot side and the upper airway obstructs, but whereas all infants placed in this position for long enough will die, 99% of infants who sleep prone will survive. The mechanism of death in prone sleeping is, therefore, more complex than simple smothering and involves contributions from a number of factors.

Postulated mechanisms have included diaphragmatic splinting/fatigue, rebreathing of carbon dioxide, reflex lowering of vasomotor tone with tachycardia, blunting of arousal responses including decreased cardiac response to auditory stimulation, alteration of sleep patterns, compromise of cerebral blood flow, upper airway obstruction from distortion of nasal cartilages, posterior displacement of the mandible, soft bedding, nasopharyngeal bacterial overgrowth, and overheating. It is also possible that prone position in infants may lead to unfavorable ventilation/perfusion ratios (American Academy of Pediatrics Task Force on Infant Positioning and SIDS, 1992; Bayes, 1974; Bolton *et al.*, 1993; Chiodini & Thach, 1993; Chong, Murphy & Matthews, 2000; de Silva, Icke & Hilton, 1992; Franco *et al.*, 1996; Galland *et al.*, 1998; Galland, Taylor & Bolton, 2002; Kemp *et al.*, 1993; Kemp *et al.*, 1998; Kemp, Nelson & Thach, 1994; Kemp & Thach, 1993; Mitchell, Scragg & Clements, 1996; Morris, 1989; Myers *et al.*, 1998; Ponsonby *et al.*, 1995; Stanley & Byard, 1991; Waters *et al.*, 1996).

While upper airway obstruction due to flattening of the nose and backward displacement of the tongue from the weight of the head in the prone position (Simson & Brantley, 1977) initially appeared to be quite a plausible explanation for infant death in this position, certain difficulties exist. It has been shown in one series, for example, that only 3% of infants sleeping in the prone position had their heads face down, with most having their faces to the side (Hassall & Vandenberg, 1985). Orr *et al.* (1985) also did not show a relationship between the duration or rate of apneic episodes and sleeping posture.

Although suggestions that infants may be exposed to high levels of carbon dioxide (Gale, Redner-Carmi & Gale, 1977) were not confirmed in the earlier literature (Bolton, Cross & McKettrick, 1972), it is possible that very localized areas of atmospheric alteration may occur (e.g. under the covers or within cushions around the head) (Kemp & Thach, 1991; Kemp & Thach, 2001). Evidence suggesting that quilts increase the risk of SIDS has been contradictory (Mitchell, Williams & Taylor, 1999; Ponsonby *et al.*, 1998).

The theory of oxygen deprivation is also a time-honored one; as W.W. Hall put it so succinctly in 1869: "Many infants are found dead in bed, and it is attributed to having been overlaid by the parents; but the idea that any person could lay still for a moment on a baby, or anything else of the same size, is absurd. Death was caused by the want of pure air."

Concerns have been raised that back-sleeping may be associated with an increased risk of gastric aspiration. While it is well known that aspiration of gastric contents may cause death (Thach, 2000), studies have shown that fatal episodes due to this mechanism have not increased since sleeping practices were changed (Byard & Beal, 2000).

It has been asserted that there is an increased risk of SIDS in infants who are sleeping on a sofa with an adult (Blair *et al.*, 1999), but in the author's experience such deaths are usually due to accidental asphyxia from wedging or overlaying (Beal & Byard, 1995; Beal & Byard, 2000; Byard *et al.*, 2001; Byard, Beal & Bourne, 1994). Full death scene examinations and reconstruction of sleeping positions are required to clarify many of these events. Devices designed to prevent infants from rolling to supine unfortunately may hold infants in this position once they have turned and so cannot be recommended (Mallak, Milch & Horn, 2000).

Cigarette smoke exposure

Despite contradictory evidence, it is now accepted that infants who have been exposed to cigarette smoke toxins before and after delivery have an increased risk of SIDS of up to five times (Blair *et al.*, 1996; Haglund, Cnattingius & Otterblad-Olausson, 1995; Klonoff-Cohen *et al.*, 1995; Mitchell, 1995; Milerad & Sundell, 1993; Taylor & Sanderson, 1995). The exact mechanism is uncertain, but it has been suggested that smoking may be responsible for reduction in body and placental size in SIDS infants compared with matched controls, as a marker for adverse in utero factors (Buck *et al.*, 1989; van Belle, Hoffman & Peterson, 1988; Samet, 1991). Nicotine and cotinine levels in postmortem fluids and tissues may provide an objective way to assess the degree of cigarette smoke exposure that has occurred prior to death (Rajs *et al.*, 1997).

A recent study has shown that poor postnatal weight gain increases the risk of SIDS (Blair *et al.*, 2000), and animal experiments have shown that a smaller placenta will lead to both a reduction in body weight and a marked reduction in the weight of the lungs (Maloney *et al.*, 1983). The evidence is again contradictory, since placental weights have been reported as being similar in both control and SIDS infants (Lewak, van den Berg & Beckwith, 1979), and no evidence of growth retardation has been shown histologically or morphometrically in rib growth plates in SIDS cases (Figures 13.5 and 13.6) (Byard *et al.*, 1997a; Byard, Foster & Byers, 1993). Impaired arousal has also been demonstrated in infants exposed to tobacco smoke (Horne *et al.*, 2002).

Hyperthermia

Infants who have died of SIDS may have had a history of elevated temperatures or profuse night sweats (Nelson, 1996a; Taylor *et al.*, 1996a), and this has prompted studies into a possible role for overheating. Although an association of sudden death with overheating has been demonstrated in patients with malignant hyperpyrexia (Denborough, Galloway & Hopkinson, 1982; Peterson & Davis, 1986) and with hypohydrotic ectodermal dysplasia (Bernstein, Hatchuel & Jenkins, 1980; Bernstein

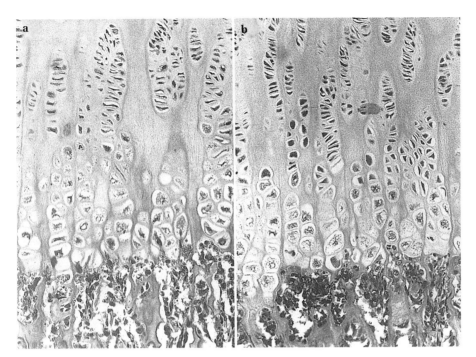

Figure 13.5 Orderly growth plate structure, showing hypertrophic chondrocytes abutting marrow spaces where new bone formation occurs. There are no obvious differences between a SIDS case (a) and an age-matched control infant (b) (hematoxylin and eosin, ×250).

Number of trabeculae/mm of growth plate versus depth

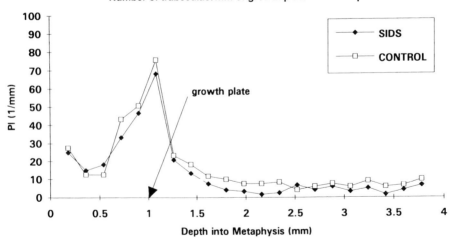

Figure 13.6 Morphometric assessment of bone growth plates from a SIDS infant and a control infant comparing the number of trabeculae per millimeter of growth plate at different points in the metaphysis. No differences could be demonstrated.

& Weakley-Jones, 1987), it appears unlikely that this could account for more than a small percentage of cases that present as SIDS. While intrathoracic petchiae reported in infants dying from environmental hyperthermia may suggest a link between SIDS and overheating (Krous *et al.*, 2001b), selection bias has been blamed for the results in the original report purporting to show an association between SIDS and malignant hyperpyrexia (Ellis, Halsall & Harriman, 1988).

Elevated temperatures in SIDS infants may be endogenous from infections or increased amounts of brown adipose tissue (Lean & Jennings, 1989) or may result from external factors such as increased room heating or excessive clothing (Kleeman *et al.*, 1996; Nelson, Taylor & Weatherall, 1989; Stanton, Scott & Downham, 1980). It has been claimed that heavy wrapping with bedclothing is an independent risk factor for SIDS, particularly in infants older than 70 days (Fleming *et al.*, 1990); in a series of 13 pairs of simultaneous SIDS deaths in twins, Bass (1989) noted possible or definite hyperthermia due to exogenous factors such as excessive heating in eight (62%) instances.

As the relatively larger head in infants radiates a considerable amount of generated heat, the wearing of a bonnet or covering the head with blankets in an infant sleeping prone with a large part of the face against the mattress interferes with normal heat exchange (Guntheroth & Spiers, 2001; Sawczenko & Fleming, 1996). This is exacerbated when the room temperature is raised, as has been reported in 41% of cases, and in 50% of cases where there is ongoing infection (Stanton, 1984).

"Overwrapping" of infants has been shown to occur when there is a minor fall in ambient temperature, with parents tending to overcompensate by adding extra clothes and blankets. Figure 13.7 shows a case where an infant had been excessively clothed and covered. This is not a new problem, as Dr William Cadogan noted in 1748: "The first great Mistake is that they think that a new-born Infant cannot be kept too warm: from this Prejudice they load it and bind it with Flannels, Wrappers, Swathes, Stays, etc." (cited in Bacon, 1983).

Wailoo *et al.* (1989) have shown that there may be an increase in thermal insulation of as much as 188% in response to falls in room temperature of as little as 4.4 °C. Parents may also add extra wrapping to infants who are febrile (Nelson & Taylor, 1989), and this is recommended treatment in certain alternate medical practices. Animal experiments have shown a considerable rise in core temperature when the head is covered by bedclothes (Galland *et al.*, 1994).

The possible role played by an increase in body temperature in causing sudden death is not well understood, and various mechanisms have been suggested. These include vagally mediated cerebral ischemia, surfactant denaturation, enhancement of the laryngeal closure reflex, unobserved convulsions, apnea, failure of respiratory control, and respiratory chemoreceptor dysfunction (Bacon, 1983; Fleming *et al.*, 1993; Fleming, Azaz & Wigfield, 1992; Gozal *et al.*, 1988; Haraguchi, Fung & Sasaki, 1983; Sunderland & Emery, 1981; Talbert, 1990). Alternately, it may be that the role of hyperthermia is mainly as a risk modifier in infants who are sleeping prone (Fleming *et al.*, 1990; Fleming *et al.*, 1996; Ponsonby *et al.*, 1992a; Ponsonby *et al.*, 1993; Williams, Taylor & Mitchell, 1996).

Bed sharing

There is increasing evidence that infants who sleep near their parents will have a reduced risk of SIDS, possibly due to increased arousals (McKenna *et al.*, 1993; McKenna *et al.*, 1994; McKenna & Mosko, 2001; Mitchell & Thompson, 1995; Mosko *et al.*, 1997; Mosko, Richard & McKenna, 1997; Scragg *et al.*, 1996). It has been shown, however, that the risk of infant death doubles if an infant shares a bed with a mother who smokes, although the mechanisms of this relationship remain unclear (Scragg *et al.*, 1993; Scragg *et al.*, 1995). While it has been stated that "there is no evidence that bed sharing is hazardous for infants of parents who do not smoke" (Blair *et al.*, 1999), this was not the finding of Scragg & Mitchell (1998), who quoted a relative risk of death of 1.42 (95% CI 1.12, 1.79) in infants of non-smoking mothers who bed-shared. Other studies have reported infant deaths due to suffocation in these circumstances.

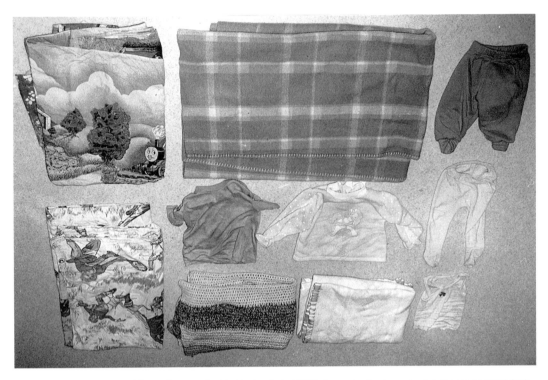

Figure 13.7 Clothing removed from a five-month-old girl who died of SIDS, demonstrating two sets of clothes and several thick quilts and blankets. Her room was also noted by police investigators to be warm.

As there are a number of communities around the world where shared sleeping is the usual practice, apparently without significantly increased infant mortality, it could be argued that certain contemporary practices are responsible for making this practice dangerous, for example placing infants between obese, sedated, or intoxicated parents on a soft mattress (Byard, 1994b; Byard & Hilton, 1997). Further cross-cultural studies will undoubtedly help to clarify these issues.

Certain infants may also be very vulnerable to apnea following transient upper airway occlusion and to oxygen desaturation when exposed to airway hypoxia (Byard & Burnell, 1995; Parkins *et al.*, 1998). Cases have occurred where infants have been taken to bed for breastfeeding and have suffocated under the maternal breast after the mother has fallen asleep. These cases have even occurred in hospital postnatal wards and were reported in the literature over a century ago (Anonymous, 1892; Byard, 1998; Byard & Hilton, 1997). Unfortunately, the pathologic findings at autopsy in these cases are entirely non-specific and do not help in distinguishing SIDS from this type of asphyxia (Mitchell, Krous & Byard, 2002). It is, therefore, difficult to know what the precise mechanisms of death are in the increasing numbers of infants who are dying in parental beds (Bourne, Beal & Byard, 1994), but it cannot be denied that accidental smothering must account for a certain percentage.

Given that extra stimulation may reduce deep sleep, alter breathing patterns, and enhance neurologic maturation (McKenna & Mosko, 1993; McKenna & Mosko, 1994; Richard, Mosko & McKenna, 1998), and thus alter the risk of SIDS, proximity to parents would appear desirable. It would seem reasonable, therefore, to place an infant in a cot beside the parental bed. In this way, the infant is protected in a safe environment but is still able to interact closely with parents and be available for breastfeeding (McKenna, Mosko & Richard, 1997). A balance has to be achieved between increasing the possiblity of smothering and reducing the risks of SIDS, and until we can more accurately predict vulnerable infants and identify situations of high risk, this is probably the safest option.

Maternal characteristics

Mothers of SIDS infants tend to be young (under 20 years of age), to be of lower socioeconomic status, and to have had a number of children over a relatively short period of time (Arntzen *et al.*, 1995; Babson & Clarke, 1983; Byard, 1991a; Daltveit *et al.*,1998; Ford & Nelson, 1995; Kraus *et al.*, 1988; Peterson, van Belle & Chinn, 1982). Young paternal age is also considered a risk factor (Jørgensen, Biering-Sørensen & Hilden, 1979).

Maternal marital status was not found to be associated with SIDS in a study by Kraus, Greenland & Bulterys (1989) once family income had been adjusted. This contrasts with the finding of Mehl & Malcolm (1990) that single marital status was one of the three major risk factors for SIDS in New Zealand, the other two factors being low birth weight and mothers of Maori descent. A second New Zealand study has also implicated single maternal marital status in the etiology of SIDS (Nelson *et al.*, 1990), as have a number of previous studies reviewed by Golding (1989).

The proposal that different maternal blood groups (O and B) are associated with SIDS (Arsenault, 1980; Naeye, Ladis & Drage, 1976) remains unproven due to a failure to control for racial origin in the original studies (Kelly & Shannon, 1982).

Role of breastfeeding

The likely protective role of breastfeeding has been debated vigorously, with studies demonstrating a lower incidence of SIDS in breastfed infants (Biering-Sørensen, Jorgensen & Hilden, 1978) being challenged over a failure to control for social class and smoking habits (Golding, 1989). The finding of lower levels of docosohexanoic acid (DHA) in the brain tissue of formula-fed infants compared with breastfed controls offered a potential mechanism to explain the increased rates of SIDS in this group, since DHA is required for neural maturation (Figure 13.8) (Byard *et al.*, 1995). However, despite further studies favoring formula feeding as a risk factor (Mitchell *et al.*, 1992b), this is no longer generally accepted (British Paediatric Association, Standing Committee on Nutrition, 1994; Fleming *et al.*, 2000; Gilbert *et al.*, 1995).

Maternal drug use

As noted earlier, maternal smoking during and after pregnancy is associated with an increased risk of SIDS (Haglund & Cnattingius, 1990; Malloy *et al.*, 1988; McGlashan, 1989). Determining the possible role of other drugs is often complicated by the abuse of multiple illicit and prescription medications. For example, it is difficult to separate cocaine usage from other associated environmental risk factors, and reports have again produced contradictory results (Bauchner *et al.*, 1988; Davidson Ward *et al.*, 1990). However, infants of mothers who have used cocaine appear to have abnormal cardiorespiratory and electrocardiographic patterns, with a higher risk of sudden death (Chasnoff *et al.*, 1989; Davidson Ward & Keens, 1992; Durand, Espinoza & Nickerson, 1990; Mehta *et al.*, 1993; Roland & Volpe, 1989).

Maternal abuse of opiates also increases the risk of infant death (Chavez *et al.*, 1979; Kandall *et al.*, 1993; Rosen & Johnson, 1988), and breastfed infants exposed to opioids in breast milk have increased risks of apnea (Naumburg & Meny, 1988). Maternally ingested amphetamines may also contaminate breast milk.

There has been no association demonstrated between increased maternal caffeine consumption during pregnancy and subsequent SIDS (Bergman & Wiesner, 1976; Kandall & Gaines, 1991), with one study showing lower coffee consumption during pregnancy in mothers of SIDS infants compared with mothers of infants with "near-miss" episodes (Kahn

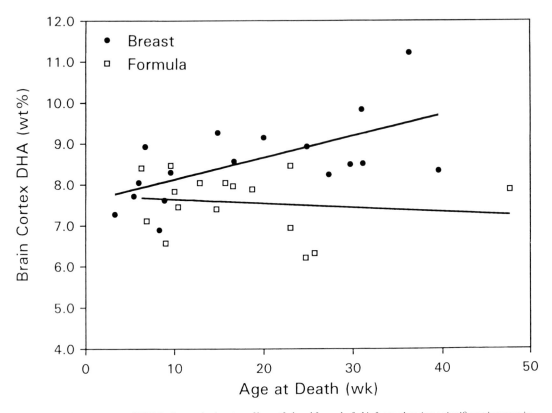

Figure 13.8 Measurements of DHA in the cerebral cortex of breastfed and formula-fed infants, showing a significant increase in levels in infants who had been breastfed.

et al., 1984). Heavy postnatal intake of alcohol has, however, been associated with an increased risk of infant death (Alm *et al.*, 1999).

Although Smialek & Monforte (1977) failed to find drugs on postmortem screening of 103 SIDS infants, Hickson *et al.* (1989) have described nine infants with anoxic episodes and who were suffering from drug overdosage. Kahn & Blum (1982) noted a significantly higher usage rate of phenothiazine-containing medications prior to death in SIDS infants compared with controls, but this has been challenged due to "severe flaws in methodology" by Shannon & Bergman (1991). Other workers noted a lower incidence of drug isolation in a series of 715 SIDS infants when compared with controls (Finkle *et al.*, 1979). The drugs found in this study were those expected

for the age group, and none was present in significant amounts. Assessment of these variable results is difficult, and it may be that they were influenced heavily by the drug-using profile of the different population groups studied.

Interpretation of results in individual cases is also often difficult as therapeutic ranges for a variety of drugs have not been established for infants, and infant responses to therapeutic levels of drugs may be different to those of older age groups. In addition, the effect of low levels of drugs on infants predisposed to SIDS is also unknown. It may be that sedative drugs that are quite safe in some infants may further exacerbate respiratory depression in others. Rare organic toxins are not likely to be included in routine screening panels and may be difficult to exclude

Table 13.1. Variation in the incidence of SIDS among different countries and geographic areas over time

Country	Rate before RTR (/1000 live births/years)	Rate after RTR (/1000 live births/year)
New Zealand	2.4–7.3	1.04
US	1.7–3.06	0.77
UK	2.06–2.78	0.45
France	2.71	0.49
Eire	2.67	0.9
Norway	2.34	0.6
Scotland	2.3	0.6
Belgium	1.72	0.6
Canada	1.5	0.45
Japan	1.2	0.3
Sweden	0.44–1.0	0.45
Denmark	0.92	0.3
Finland	0.31–0.51	0.25
Israel	0.31	0.2
Hong Kong	0.3	0.1

RTR = Reduce the Risks campaign.

Arneil *et al.* (1985); Biering-Sørensen *et al.* (1978); Bloch (1973); Fitzgerald (2001); Froggatt, Lynas & MacKenzie (1971); Hilton & Turner (1976); Irgens, Skjaerven & Lie (1989); Kahn *et al.* (1990b); Lee *et al.* (1989); Matthews & O'Brien (1985); Nelson & Taylor (1988); Newman (1986); Norvenius (1987); Rintahaka & Hirvonen (1986); Shiono *et al.* (1988); Wagner, Samson-Dollfus & Menard (1984); Wennergren *et al.* (1987); Williams (1990).

even when searched for specifically (Byard, James & Felgate, 2002).

Geographic differences

The incidence of SIDS varies between different geographic areas, being generally more common in colder northern and southern climates (Dwyer & Ponsonby, 1992; Vege, Rognum & Opdal, 1998). Israel and Hong Kong have had a rate of 0.3 per 1000 live births (Williams, 1990), compared with the South Island of New Zealand, where rates as high as 7.3 per 1000 live births have been reported previously (Nelson & Taylor, 1988).

The contribution of SIDS to overall infant mortality may be influenced by other diseases. A study comparing the rate of sudden infant death in two European countries (Germany and Finland) showed a higher percentage of SIDS cases in Finland due to the lower number of deaths from respiratory infec-

tions (Lignitz & Hirvonen, 1989). A list of reported rates from various countries is given in Table 13.1.

Climatic factors

SIDS has a winter predominance and an association with low temperatures (Beal & Porter, 1991; Campbell *et al.*, 1991; Ponsonby, Dwyer & Jones, 1992). The regional variations in the incidence of SIDS in Australia have been shown to be due mostly to differences in climatic temperatures (Ponsonby *et al.*, 1992b). The association with colder months of the year led to the suggestion that hypothermia may be a factor in some SIDS deaths (Bonser, Knight & West, 1978). No consistent relationship with barometric pressure has been identified (Heaney & McIntire, 1979). The winter peak in SIDS deaths is still present but has reduced since the fall in numbers of cases following the risks campaigns (Beal, Need & Byard, 1994). For ill-understood reasons, neither Alaska nor Sweden demonstrated a winter peak in SIDS deaths during the 1970s (Dwyer & Ponsonby, 1992).

Racial differences

Differences in SIDS rates among different racial groups have been well documented (Davies, 1994; Mitchell & Scragg, 1994) and may be related to differences in childcare practices, although this has not been confirmed (Nelson, 1996b; Nelson, Schiefenhoevel & Haimerl, 2000; Petersen & Wailoo, 1994). A number of studies have demonstrated a low incidence of SIDS in oriental groups (Grether, Schulman & Croen, 1990), but this may be due partly to local diagnostic practices, with deaths being attributed to suffocation rather than to SIDS (Knöbel, Yang & Chen, 1996). The higher incidence that was reported in black American infants was not found in a study by Kraus, Greenland & Bulterys (1989) once socioeconomic factors such as income and level of education had been controlled for. Similarly, Kaplan, Bauman & Krous (1984) failed to show a significant increase in SIDS deaths among a native American population, as had been reported previously (Blok, 1978). This finding was supported by Irwin, Mannino & Daling (1992), who found that the high rate of SIDS deaths in native American mothers in Washington state was due to the presence of increased risk factors, such as young maternal age and high parity, rather than to a genetic predisposition.

Despite these contradictions, certain indigenous populations and African-American groups do have high rates of infant death (Alessandri *et al.*, 1995; Alessandri *et al.*, 1996; Mitchell *et al.*, 1993a; Øyen *et al.*, 1990; Read, 2002; Tipene-Leach, Everard & Haretuku, 2001). Determining the precise causes of these deaths may be difficult, particularly in isolated groups, as adequate death scene examinations and postmortem examinations are not always performed (Byard, 2001a). For example, infant deaths in northern Queensland, Australia, continue to be labeled as SIDS without autopsies being performed (Panaretto *et al.*, 2002). Attributing deaths to SIDS under these circumstances may confuse health issues in these communities.

Table 13.2. Variation in the incidence of SIDS among different racial groups

Racial group	Rate (/1000 live births/year)
Native Americans	1.4–6.56
New Zealand Maori	5.0–6.47
Native Alaskans and Inuit	2.17–6.28
British Afro-Caribbeans	5.25
New Zealand Europeans	1.8–3.86
New Zealand South Pacific Islanders	1.2–1.86
Californian Asians	0.51–1.5
British Asians	1.18
Hong Kong (98% Chinese)	0.04–0.3

Adams (1985); Blok (1978); Borman, Fraser & de Boer (1988); Bulterys (1990); Davies (1985); Fleshman & Peterson (1977); Grether, Schulman & Croen (1990); Kraus & Borhani (1972); Kyle *et al.* (1990); Lee *et al.* (1989); Tonkin (1986).

Infants of Asian descent living in California have a higher rate of SIDS compared with Asian infants living in their country of ethnic origin, suggesting that different environmental or social factors have come into play following family migration (Grether, Schulman & Croen, 1990). These factors may explain the differences in incidence noted among various racial and ethnic groups, as demonstrated in Table 13.2.

Sibling deaths

Although it has been alleged that some families have had as many as five deaths attributed to SIDS (Diamond, 1986), the reported increased incidence of SIDS of between two and 10 times in infants who have had a sibling or twin death (Beal, 1983; Beal, 1989; Beal & Blundell, 1988; Oren, Kelly & Shannon, 1987) has been questioned once maternal age and birth order have been controlled for and environmental risk factors managed (Beal, 2001a; Peterson, Sabotta & Daling, 1986). Also, repeated infant deaths in the same family must raise serious concerns of inflicted injury. While it is generally accepted that any increase in incidence is due most probably to exposure to the same environmental risk factors rather than to heritability (Beal, 1992b;

Peterson, Chinn & Fisher, 1980), Peterson (1988) has not completely excluded a genetic component in the etiology of SIDS. This includes the possibility of an inherited metabolic disorder in some cases (Roe *et al.*, 1986). The demonstration of inherited substitutions in the first hypervariable region of the displacement loop of mitochondrial DNA in a small group of SIDS infants does raise the possibility of inherited predisposition in a certain number of victims (Arnestad *et al.*, 2002). However, there is no "SIDS gene," as has been claimed in recent media reports.

As noted, parentally imposed upper airway obstruction must be considered when there has been a history of repeated medical attendance or of previous unexpected infant deaths in the family (Alexander, Smith & Stevenson, 1990; Byard & Beal, 1993; Meadow, 1990; Poets & Southall, 1991). Unfortunately, the autopsy findings of asphyxia in infants are often identical to those present in SIDS infants (Cashell, 1987; Smialek & Lambros, 1988; Valdes-Dapena, 1982), making it impossible to exclude homicide on purely morphologic grounds (Bass, 1989; Berry & Keeling, 1989; Hilton, 1989).

Although non-accidental injury is a possibility in some cases of unexpected infant death, and while Di Maio & Di Maio (1989) caution that "a third case, in our opinion, is not possible and is a case of homicide," the quoted incidence of "gentle battering" by some authors of around 10% of all "SIDS" deaths (Emery, 1985) does not appear to be representative of general experience (Di Maio & Di Maio, 1989; Southall, Samuels & Stebbens, 1989). The author does not agree with the philosophphy of "three strikes and you are out" and feels that multiple deaths within the same family should equally raise concerns about possible inhertited conditions such as prolonged QT interval.

Features that should be considered in the event of simultaneous SIDS deaths in siblings are carbon monoxide exposure, poisoning, overheating, and mechanical obstruction of the airways (Koehler *et al.*, 2001; Ladham *et al.*, 2001; Ramos, Hernández & Villanueva, 1997).

Table 13.3. Features commonly associated with SIDS

Age 2–4 months
Male
Premature
Low birth weight
High birth order
Multiple birth
Short inter-pregnancy interval
Prone sleeper
Lower socioeconomic family
Young (<20 years) parents
Previous premature deliveries
Cigarette smoke exposure
Maternal drug abuse
Infection during pregnancy
Low level of maternal education

Current trends

Following the fall in the number of SIDS deaths, there has been a change in the socioeconomic profile of affected families. Families where SIDS deaths tend to occur now have been termed "chaotic" due to significant social problems, including substandard housing, domestic violence, unemployment, and illicit drug use (Davies, 1999; Mitchell *et al.*, 2000a). Multiple partners and an itinerant lifestyle are also found. This makes assessment of such deaths difficult, as childcare may have been suboptimal and relevant information may be unobtainable, resulting in the cause of death being left as undetermined. Although it has been suggested that SIDS and unexplained intrauterine deaths represent a continuum, this appears unlikely as risk factors for each have been shown to be different (Frøen *et al.*, 2002).

Summary

The epidemiologic characteristics of SIDS described above are summarized in Table 13.3.

Diagnosis

The diagnosis of SIDS can be considered only after other causes of sudden death have been sought scrupulously, and if abnormal autopsy findings have been interpreted correctly, given that the accepted current definition of SIDS is one of exclusion. There are, therefore, a number of difficulties that may confront a pathologist when dealing with a "typical" case of SIDS, particularly as the presenting history and autopsy findings are often characteristic but are in no way diagnostic of the entity (Sturner, 1995).

Lack of an adequate control population with which autopsy findings may be compared has been a major problem for pathologists and researchers for over 100 years. Accidental deaths in early infancy that could be used as controls are distinctly uncommon. A sobering reminder of the problems that may occur in SIDS research if appropriate control groups are not obtained occurred when the size of the normal thymus gland was misinterpreted as being markedly enlarged. This led to the apparently plausible theory of "thymic asthma" or "*status thymico lymphaticus.*" Unfortunately, the conclusion that the thymus was enlarged in SIDS infants was based on an erroneous comparison with infants with markedly involuted thymic glands who had died from debilitating diseases such as generalized infection. In spite of this obvious flaw, the theory persisted for decades. This problem continues, with postmortem findings in SIDS infants continually being given undue weight without comparison being made with age-matched control populations.

In some countries, an infant death may be attributed to SIDS without the performance of a postmortem examination. For example, in the Netherlands, in the past only 50–60% of children dying within the first year of life were autopsied (Engelberts, de Jonge & Kostense, 1991), and in Belgium the autopsy rate was less than 25% (Kahn *et al.*, 1990b). Attributing death to SIDS is still occurring in parts of Australasia either without autopsies or where autopsies are performed by non-pathologists (Byard, 2001a). Not every case of sudden infant death in Australia has had the cranial cavity routinely opened (Armstrong & Wood, 1991). Infant autopsy rates vary in other countries from 0 to 100% (Fitzgerald, 2001).

Previously, an alternate diagnosis to SIDS could be made in 8–18% of cases of sudden infant death following an autopsy (Byard, Carmichael & Beal, 1994;

Emery, Chandra & Gilbert-Barness, 1988; Fleming *et al.*, 1991); with the fall in numbers of SIDS deaths and the relative increase in the percentage of other causes of infant death, this has risen to 25% (Mitchell *et al.*, 2000b). It is important, therefore, that epidemiologic and tissue research results from regions where autopsies are not a mandatory part of the diagnostic process are interpreted with caution. This is of particular significance when reviewing etiologic theories or conclusions that have been based on small series of children, as these are very vulnerable to the potential confounding influence of even a very low number of non-SIDS cases. A further point to consider is that an autopsy may be far from "thorough" due to variation in local practices.

The diagnosis of SIDS does not depend on the demonstration of any particular pathognomonic features in the same way, for example, that the diagnosis of myocarditis depends on the finding of an inflammatory infiltrate with tissue necrosis. There is a very real possibility, therefore, that the label "SIDS" may be used uncritically to shelve all cases of poorly investigated sudden infant death. Emery (1983, 1989) has pointed out the dangers of adopting the diagnosis too readily and missing other types of sudden natural death, and also the occasional case of accidental death or of infanticide. Of course, this may even be the case after a careful postmortem examination has been performed, given the difficulties that exist in attempting to extrapolate back from autopsy material to the living infant.

Steps in the performance of the autopsy

Death scene investigation

The importance of an adequate death scene investigation in all cases of sudden death in both infancy and childhood cannot be emphasized enough, and the revised definition proposed by the National Institute of Health group underscores this point with the statement that "a complete postmortem examination must include an investigation of the scene of death" (Willinger, James & Catz, 1991).

It can be argued strongly that the diagnosis of SIDS cannot be made or defended if there has not been an examination of the death scene by experienced personnel who are capable of dealing sensitively with bereaved parents while at the same time checking for evidence of accidental or non-accidental injury (Byard *et al.*, 1996; Hanzlick, 2001a). Given the lack of autopsy findings in cases of infantile asphyxia, the death scene findings may provide the only evidence of accidental death due to wedging (Figure 13.9), overlaying, or plastic-bag suffocation (Bass, Kravath & Glass, 1986; Byard & Hilton, 1997). Particular types of bedding that have been implicated in suffocation of infants include waterbeds, soft pillows, sheepskin rugs, and polystyrene-filled cushions (Emery & Thornton, 1968; Gilbert-Barness & Barness, 1992; Gilbert-Barness *et al.*, 1991; Kemp & Thach, 1991). Broken or poorly constructed cribs are also potential causes of asphyxiation. Other information that may be collected includes the time the infant was last seen alive, the time of discovery, sleeping position, quantity and quality of bedding, and other pertinent epidemiologic facts being collated for local SIDS data bases (Jones & Weston, 1976) (see Table 13.4).

The Sudden Unexplained Infant Death Investigation Report Form (SUIDIRF) devised by the Centers for Disease Control outlines standard steps that should be undertaken in the investigation of unexpected infant death (Centers for Disease Control, 1996) (see Appendix III).

Medical history review

Review of the deceased infant's medical history is a mandatory part of the autopsy. This may provide clues to the possibility of a potentially lethal medical condition that should be checked for specifically, such as a congenital cardiac defect. Also, the immediate antemortem history may be significant. Although it is very common for infants who die of SIDS to have had a minor upper respiratory tract infection or a gastrointestinal upset prior to death, the presence of a fever over several days may be a clue to the presence of fatal sepsis.

Table 13.4. Important information to be obtained at the time of the death scene investigation in SIDS

Age of infant
Previous medical history
Family medical history, including previous infant/child
    deaths
Details of sleeping arrangements, e.g. shared or not
Full details concerning household activity over the preceding
    24 hours
Time and circumstances of death
Type of crib/bed
Type of mattress, e.g. size relative to crib
Presence of plastic coverings
Type of clothing and bedding
Type of room heating
Position of body
Full details concerning discovery of the body and
    subsequent resuscitation attempts
Evidence of injury to body
Any unusual features at death scene

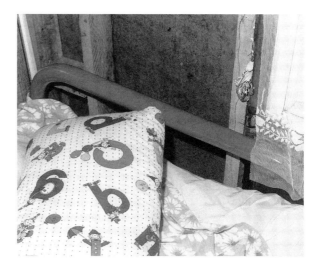

Figure 13.9 The initial autopsy diagnosis of SIDS had to be changed when it was revealed that the infant who died in this bed was found wedged so firmly between the bed and the wall cavity that the bed had to be partially dismantled to enable the body to be removed. The value of an adequate history and investigation of the death scene is clearly reinforced by such a case, in which death was due to wedging and positional asphyxia and not to SIDS.

Table 13.5. Important features to be noted on review of the medical history in cases of SIDS

Details of pregnancy and delivery
Growth and development parameters
Type of feeding
Immunization status
Previous illnesses
Recent fevers, respiratory infections,
   gastrointestinal upsets
Recent medications
Family history of sudden death
   (particularly infants and young children)

Included in the infant's history should be a relatively detailed description of the pregnancy, delivery, type of feeding, and immunization status (Table 13.5). The family history should also provide information on major parental illnesses and addictions, including smoking habits, particularly of the mother during pregnancy. Details of significant sibling illnesses, including any previous deaths, are pertinent, as these may raise the possibility of an inherited disease such as one of the inborn errors of metabolism or of non-accidental injury. There is, however, often minimal difference in the history elicited from cases of SIDS compared with infants who die suddenly from subsequently identifiable causes (Bartholomew, MacArthur & Bain, 1987).

Pathological features

In addition to death scene examination and medical history review, the autopsy in cases of unexpected infant death must be carried out in as comprehensive a manner as possible, utilizing accepted protocols (Byard, Mackenzie & Beal, 1997a; Mitchell *et al.*, 2000b). The International Standardized Autopsy Protocol (ISAP) (see Appendix IV) was developed for this purpose by SIDS International and the NICHD (Krous, 1995).

All stages of the autopsy that are specified in protocols, including external examination, radi-

ology, internal examination, histology, microbiology, toxicology, electrolyte/metabolic studies, and molecular/genetic studies, have been shown to have diagnostic yields (Figure 13.10). Use of protocols has significantly increased the accuracy of diagnosis, with more infant deaths due to dangerous sleeping environments and drug effects now being identified (Figure 13.11) (Arnestad, 2002; Arnestad, Vege & Rognum, 2002; Berry *et al.*, 2000; Langlois *et al.*, 2002; Mitchell *et al.*, 2000b). Protocols also help to standardize variations in practice that have been documented to occur even among pathologists within the same institution (Ballenden, Laster & Lawrence, 1993).

Macroscopic autopsy findings

The morphologic findings in infants who are subsequently considered to have died of SIDS are not specific (Figure 13.12), although there are a number of features that are characteristically present (Table 13.6) (Berry, 1992; Rognum, 2001; Valdes-Dapena, 1992a; Valdes-Dapena, 1992b). Generally the infant is well-nourished, with no evidence of injury except for occasional cases where there may be signs of iatrogenic trauma from attempted resuscitation. Examples of this include oozing venepuncture wounds around the wrists, elbows, and feet, with impressions over the precordium from electrocardiography (ECG) pads and around the nares from endotracheal tubes. The hands are often clenched and the fingers may be holding fibers from bedding. Postmortem blanching and folding of the skin of the neck with impressions left by clothing should not be mistaken for ligature marks (Figure 13.13).

Pulmonary edema fluid may be observed as frothy white fluid exuding from the nares or mouth (Figure 13.14); it may, on occasion, be blood-tinged or fill the trachea (Figure 13.15) (Byard & Krous, 2003b). It most likely represents terminal left ventricular failure. Purulent mucus in this fluid may attest to the presence of antemortem upper respiratory tract infection. Frank blood around the mouth and nares is a concern and raises the possibility of asphyxia if cardiopulmonary resuscitation has not been attempted

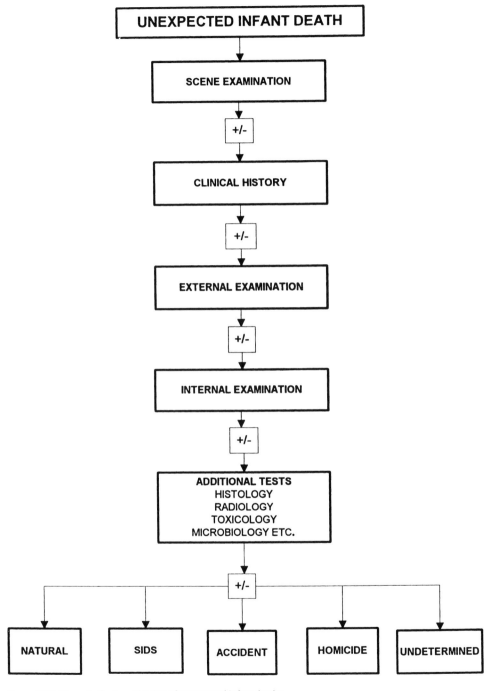

Figure 13.10 Stages in the investigation of unexpected infant deaths.

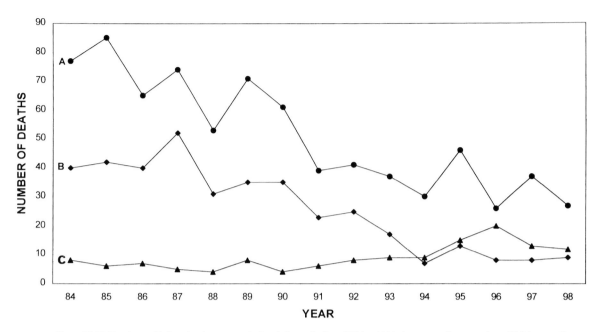

Figure 13.11 Numbers of infant deaths per year in South Australia from 1984 to 1998, demonstrating a continued fall in overall deaths in children under one year of age (A) and in SIDS deaths (B). Line (C) represents all other causes of unexpected infant deaths and shows an increase after 1994 due to more cases of accidental asphyxia being found and more cases being classified as "undetermined."

(Becroft, Thompson & Mitchell, 2001; Krous *et al.*, 2001a). Given the difficulties that may arise in the interpretation of the degree of blood staining in upper airway secretions, examination of stained bedding at the scene or in the morgue should be undertaken if this is an issue.

On opening the pleural cavity, the lungs are usually bulky, edematous, and congested. Intrathoracic petechial hemorrhages are often found in abundance in the thymus, over the epicardium, and over the pleural surfaces of the lungs (Figure 13.16), and have been reported in 68–95% of SIDS victims (Beckwith, 1989). The distribution of petechiae is not influenced by the infant's final sleeping position (Byard, Stewart & Beal, 1996). Although in some infants these pinpoint hemorrhages can be found over the root of the aortic arch and on the pleural surface of the domes of the diaphragms, there is a paucity in the dorsal portions of the cervical lobes of the thymus (Beckwith, 1988). The etiology of thymic petechiae

remains unclear as they are certainly not specific for SIDS deaths.

The presence of petechiae on the skin of the face, neck, or conjunctivae suggests asphyxia from chest or neck compression, unless there is evidence of generalized petechiae from other conditions, such as meningococcal disease, hematological disease, or a history of forceful vomiting or coughing from pertussis (Byard & Krous, 1999b; Hilton, 1989; Knight, 1983; Oemichen, Gerling & Meissner, 2000). Interpretation is usually not difficult if there are numerous petechiae but becomes more difficult in the presence of only one or two. The author would personally err on the side of conservatism and not attribute death to asphyxia based solely on the presence of several small skin hemorrhages. Other typical findings are of liquid blood within the heart and no urine within the bladder (Valdes-Dapena, 1983).

Dysmorphic lesions, such as pectus excavatum, polydactyly, and talipes, and lesions such as

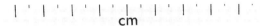

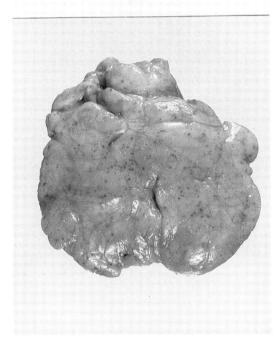

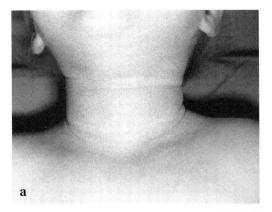

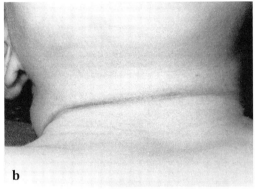

Figure 13.12 Readily identifiable thymic petechiae in an infant dying unexpectedly from pneumococcal sepsis, not from SIDS.

Table 13.6. Typical gross autopsy findings in SIDS

Morphologically normal infant
Good nutritional status
Marks of attempted resuscitation
Mucoid fluid at nares
Perianal fecal soiling
Petechial hemorrhages in thymus and thoracic cavity viscera
Bulky, congested, edematous lungs
Liquid blood within the heart
Clenched hands
Empty bladder

Figure 13.13 Typical skin folds around the neck of a SIDS infant (a) compared with a characteristic centrally placed ligature mark in an infant who died from hanging (b).

association with certain dysmorphic features has been reported in SIDS infants as suggestive of an intrauterine or genetic basis for the syndrome (Kozakewich *et al.*, 1992), this is also most likely a purely coincidental association.

Microscopic autopsy findings

Histologic sections from intrathoracic organs, in particular the thymus and lungs, will confirm the presence of petechial hemorrhages (Figures 13.17 and 13.18). Petechiae tend to be found in greater numbers in infants dying of SIDS than in infants dying of asphyxia, drowning, or recognizable diseases (Figure 13.19) (Byard & Moore, 1993a). The lungs usually show congestion and edema, with filling of

hemangiomas and nevi may occur in SIDS infants (Biering-Sørensen, Jorgensen & Hilden, 1979; Molz & Hartmann, 1984; Molz *et al.*, 1992; Vawter & Kozakewich, 1983) but are in no way specific to this group of infants and are usually absent. Although a differing frequency of dermatoglyph patterns in

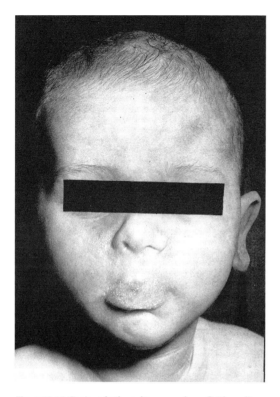

Figure 13.14 Copious frothy pulmonary edema fluid exuding from the mouth in a SIDS infant.

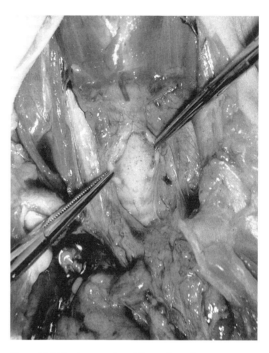

Figure 13.15 In situ opening of the trachea, demonstrating unusually abundant amounts of pulmonary edema fluid in a SIDS infant.

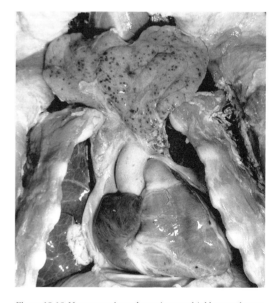

Figure 13.16 Numerous intrathoracic petechial hemorrhages, with petechiae present within the thymus and over the epicardium and aortic root in a SIDS infant.

alveoli with eosinophilic proteinaceous fluid, extravasated erythrocytes, and scattered macrophages (Figure 13.20). Intra-alveolar hemorrhage has been proposed as a marker of airway obstruction from overlaying or smothering (Yukawa *et al.*, 1999), but it has been pointed out that intra-alveolar hemorrhage is a common finding in infants that may be influenced by prolonged postmortem intervals, attempts at resuscitation, and the position of the infant's body after death (Hanzlick, 2001b). Tissue sampling from dependent areas may also introduce bias.

Subpleural aggregates of hemosiderin-containing macrophages representing areas of previous interstitial hemorrhage have been proposed as histologic markers of previous anoxia (Stewart, Fawcett & Jacobson, 1985), although it should be noted that their demonstration in 54% of cases would reflect an extremely high incidence of previous hypoxic episodes. Hemosiderin within intra-alveolar

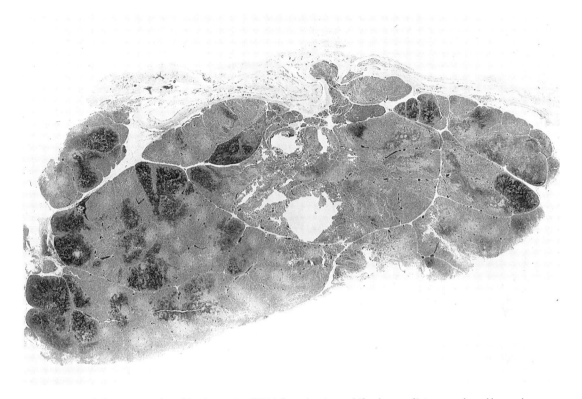

Figure 13.17 A whole-mount section of the thymus in a SIDS infant, showing multifocal areas of intraparenchymal hemorrhage corresponding to macroscopic petechiae.

macrophages has also been put forward as a marker for previous trauma or asphyxial episodes (Becroft & Lockett, 1997; Milroy, 1999). The author has, however, found this in occasional cases that have otherwise typical clinical, historic, and autopsy features of SIDS, suggesting that this finding is not specific. While interstitial pulmonary hemosiderin was found in a significantly greater number of SIDS infants who had histories of apparent life-threatening events (ALTEs) compared with controls, it was also found in 18% of unremarkable SIDS cases (Byard *et al.*, 1997b).

Focal aggregates of submucosal chronic inflammatory cells are often found within the upper airways, extending on occasion to the alveolar septae (Emery & Dinsdale, 1974; Williams, 1980). Proposals have been made that these minor inflammatory infiltrates indicate significant underlying lethal sepsis (Rambaud *et al.*, 1992; Shatz, Hiss & Arensburg,

1997), but there has been no verification of this hypothesis and it is difficult to perceive how death could occur with negative microbiologic screening and no organ disruption, hemorrhage, necrosis, or vascular compromise (Byard & Krous, 1995). While it is possible that cytokines associated with these foci of inflammation may contribute to the terminal episode, this remains conjectural (Blackwell *et al.*, 1995; Blackwell, Weir & Busuttil, 2001; Guntheroth, 1989c; Summers *et al.*, 2000). Such infiltrates are very common in infants who die from a variety of non-infectious causes, and a recent study found similar respiratory symptoms and inflammation in infants who had died of SIDS, accidents, and homicides (Krous *et al.*, 2003). Typical microscopic findings are listed in Table 13.7.

No significance is attached to a variety of other reported histologic changes, such as fibrinoid necrosis of the vocal cords (Cullity & Emery, 1975; Pinkham &

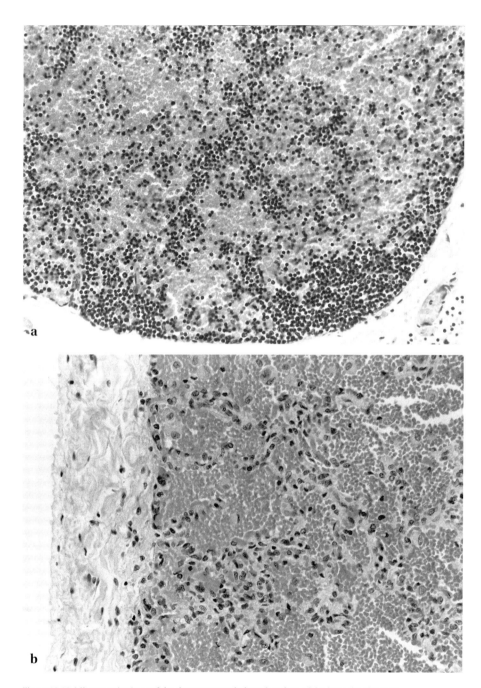

Figure 13.18 Microscopic views of the thymus (a) and pleural surface of the lung (b), showing intraparenchymal and subpleural intra-alveolar hemorrhage corresponding to macroscopically noted petechiae (hematoxylin and eosin, ×280).

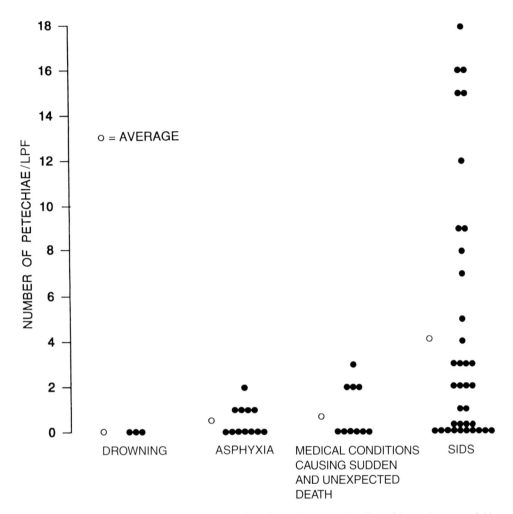

Figure 13.19 Results from a study of thymic petechiae where the maximum number of petechiae per low-power field were recorded for a variety of conditions. Although overlap occurred, infants whose deaths were attributed to SIDS generally had greater numbers of petechiae.

Beckwith, 1970), cardiac myocytolysis (Kariks, 1988), and pulmonary lymphatic dilation (Ogbuihi & Zink, 1988), although it was hypothesized that the vocal cord changes may be a marker of gastric reflux (Herbst, Book & Bray, 1978). Laryngeal basement membrane thickening, once proposed as a marker for SIDS deaths (Shatz *et al.*, 1994), has been found in many non-SIDS infants (Castro & Peres, 1999; Krous *et al.*, 1999).

The microscopic identification of minor dysmorphic and dysplastic lesions in a minority of SIDS infants led to the speculation that these lesions may be markers of adverse intrauterine conditions that contribute to later sudden death (Valdes-Dapena, 1988a), but this is not proven or likely. Adverse prenatal influences on the developing brainstem have also been postulated but again not proven (Henderson-Smart, Pettigrew & Campbell, 1983).

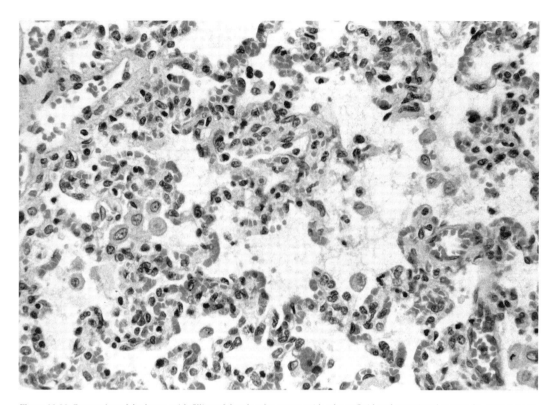

Figure 13.20 Congestion of the lungs, with filling of the alveolar spaces with edema fluid and occasional macrophages in a SIDS infant (hematoxylin and eosin, ×280).

Table 13.7. Typical microscopic findings in SIDS

Petechial hemorrhages in thymus and thoracic cavity viscera
Submucosal chronic inflammatory infiltrate of upper airways
Edema and congestion of lungs

Other studies have failed to confirm that increased numbers of sclerosed or immature glomeruli are found in SIDS cases (Hirvonen, Autio-Harmainen & Nyblom, 1982; Suzuki, Kashimura & Umetsu, 1980; Valdes-Dapena *et al.*, 1990). The frequency and functional significance of diaphragmatic muscle fiber necrosis is also unclear (Kariks, 1989), particularly given normal manometric studies of diaphragm strength in infants who have survived anoxic episodes (Scott *et al.*, 1982).

Possible mechanisms responsible for SIDS

"A diagnosis in search of a disease"

Given the vast amount of conflicting information on the causation of SIDS, the following summary attempts to cover the available evidence for and against the major current theories, with mention of as many of the less well-established hypotheses as is possible given the constraints of space (and, it must be admitted, sometimes of credibility). Thirty years ago Luke, Blackbourne & Donovan (1974) commented that "SIDS may well represent the final common pathway of various etiological factors," and the author would concur with this. It would appear unlikely that SIDS is a single disease entity with one cause. Rather, it is the common endpoint for a variety of mechanisms that represent a complicated mix of predisposing factors, environmental stresses, and underlying vulnerabilities. It is also possible that different factors affect infants in particular ways, so that the population of SIDS infants may be quite heterogeneous, being composed of subgroups with unique predispositions and characteristics (Byard, 1995; Byard & Krous, 2001).

Aesop (c. 550 BC) provided sensible advice for those who persist in hunting for an elusive single "cause" of SIDS: "Beware that you do not lose the substance by grasping at the shadow."

Respiratory theories

The apparent plausibility of airway obstruction, underlying defects in respiratory control, and failure of arousal in early infancy has generated a number of hypotheses implicating respiratory failure in the causation of SIDS (Keens & Davidson Ward, 2001). These theories have been placed into the categories of obstructive, central, mixed, and expiratory apneas (Baba et al., 1983; Southall, 1988a).

Ever since Steinschneider reported two homicides as SIDS deaths in 1972 in infants who had documented antemortem apneic episodes, there has been considerable research into infant respiratory physiology, often with apparently conflicting results (Southall et al., 1986b). The occasional occurrence of death due to SIDS in infants being investigated for apnea has, however, reinforced this association (Guilleminault et al., 1979; Shannon, Kelly & O'Connell, 1977). Part of the difficulty in interpreting conflicting reports has been in working out the normal range for infantile breathing patterns and determining whether SIDS infants differ significantly from this (Glotzbach et al., 1989; Kahn et al., 1988a; Weese-Mayer et al., 1990).

Apparent life-threatening events

The situation was partially clarified by the US National Institutes of Health Consensus Statement on infantile apnea (Little et al., 1987). This stated that apnea may be a risk factor for SIDS if it takes the form of an apparent life-threatening event (ALTE) in which an unexpected episode occurs, and that

is frightening to an observer, in which the infant is apneic for 20 seconds or longer or where the cessation of respiration is shorter but is associated with cyanosis, pallor, or bradycardia (Brooks, 1982; Brooks, 1992). Difficulties remain, however, as infants who have had these characteristic types of episodes make up only a very small percentage of SIDS victims (<7%) (Little et al., 1987), which compares with a general population frequency of 2–3% (Brooks, 1988). These figures may not be exact, however, due to inaccurate reporting of these events. ALTEs may also result from a wide variety of definable processes, including tracheomalacia, sepsis, brainstem neoplasia, epilepsy, hyperekplexia, gastroesophageal reflux, hypoglycemic episodes, respiratory syncytial virus infection, and inflicted suffocation (Table 13.8) (Brooks, 1998; Kahn et al., 1993). Multichannel monitoring, including oximetry, electroencephalography, and electrocardiography, during hypoxic episodes can be used to identify treatable causes of ALTEs (Southall et al., 1993).

The debate has continued, fuelled partly by cases of ALTEs and SIDS that have subsequently been shown to be homicides (Byard & Burnell, 1994; Pinholster, 1994; Reece, 1993). Although repeated ALTEs must raise the possibility of parentally-induced suffocation, it would seem reasonable to accept that an infant with defective autonomic control who is at increased risk of SIDS might suffer ALTEs when exposed to particular environmental stresses. While this is supported by documentation of cases in hospital nurseries, the level of supervision by hospital staff at the time of the episodes is often not specified (Burchfield & Rawlings, 1991). Investigations must consider all of the possible causes of ALTEs, including inflicted injury.

Monitoring of infants considered to be at increased risk of SIDS has been undertaken in homes for many years, despite there being no evidence that morbidity or mortality has been reduced (Burnell & Beal, 1994; Byard, 2001b). One of the most obvious benefits reported by parents has been the increase in support and symptom recording that occurs with monitoring programs (Emery et al., 1985). This is not always the case as some parents have found that monitoring

Table 13.8. Possible causes of an ALTE

Cardiovascular
  Arrhythmia
  Cardiomyopathy
  Congenital malformation
  Myocarditis
  Vascular rings
Respiratory
  Infection
  Airway stenosis
  Tracheomalacia
  Congenital alveolar hypoventilation
  Vocal cord paralysis
Neurologic
  Epilepsy
  Hyperekplexia
  Subdural hematoma
  Brain tumor
  Congenital malformation
  Cerebral infection
Infectious
  Septicemia
Gastrointestinal
  Gastroesophageal reflux/aspiration
  Pyloric stenosis
Metabolic and endocrine
  Hypoglycemia
  Hypocalcemia
  Hypothyroidism
  Hyponatremia
  Reye syndrome
  Carnitine deficiency
  Fructosemia
  Leigh syndrome
Mechanical
  Accidental asphyxia
  Munchausen syndrome by proxy
  Shaken infant syndrome
Miscellaneous
  Anemia
  Hypothermia
Idiopathic

From Brooks (1998); Kahn *et al.* (1988b); Kelly & Shannon (1988); Rahilly (1991).

increased feelings of anxiety (Grögaard, 1993). Monitors have been recommended in situations where an infant has had an unexplained ALTE, or where there has been more than one previous SIDS death in the family, but this is for diagnostic and not therapeutic purposes. Monitoring is not considered necessary for twins or where there has been only one previous SIDS death (Poets, 2001).

Obstructive apnea

Obstructive apnea is characterized by failure of inspiratory airflow despite continued respiratory efforts. A typical example occurs with foreign body impaction in a major airway; however, there are numerous other conditions and situations in which obstructive apnea may occur, acting at all levels of the respiratory tract. It has been suggested that infants who die of SIDS are predisposed to obstructive episodes during feeding (Steinschneider, Weinstein & Diamond, 1982).

Anatomical abnormalities

Anatomical abnormalities that have been reported in SIDS infants include narrowed nasal passages, shallow temporomandibular joints, retroposition of the maxillae, short mandibular rami, and close proximity of the soft palate to pharyngeal walls (Rees *et al.*, 1998; Tonkin 1975; Tonkin, Davis & Gunn, 1994). A high position of the larynx in infants with relatively short necks also predisposes to airway blockage when the tongue and mandible displace backwards (Beckwith, 1975). The finding of small upper airways in five families with obstructive sleep apnea, ALTEs and SIDS raises the possibility of a familial anatomical defect that predisposes to obstructive apnea (Guilleminault *et al.*, 1986). However, structural abnormalities are not usually observed radiographically in SIDS infants (French *et al.*, 1972).

At autopsy, the narrowness of the normal infant upper aerodigestive tract is striking (Figure 13.21), and it is easy to appreciate how further narrowing might occur with sleep-related pharyngeal hypotonia (Cozzi, Albani & Cardi, 1979). This could be exacerbated by increased secretions and submucosal edema from nasopharyngitis (Steinschneider, 1977)

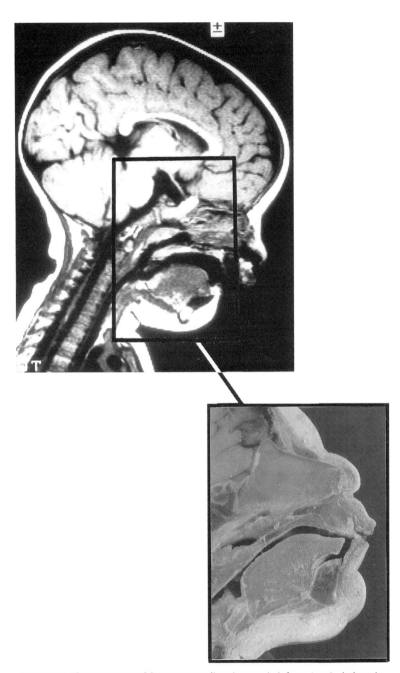

Figure 13.21 The narrowness of the upper aerodigestive tract in infancy (particularly at the junction of the oral and nasal cavities with the pharynx) can be appreciated in this MRI image and sagittal section, which show the oropharynx and nose from two non-SIDS infants with normal anatomy.

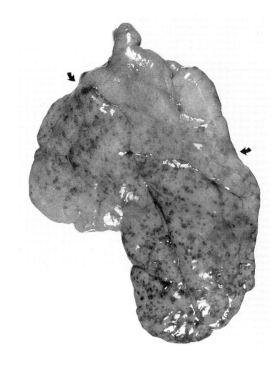

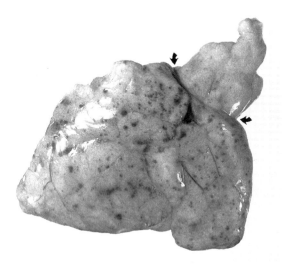

Figure 13.22 Beckwith's sign, showing decreased numbers of petechiae in the posterior cervical portion of the thymus gland, superior to the course of the left innominate vein (marked by arrows) in two SIDS cases.

or by tonsillar and adenoidal hyperplasia. Improvement in the clinical condition of four children with obstructive sleep apnea and ALTEs in infancy following adenoidectomy was in keeping with this possibility (Guilleminault *et al.*, 1984). An increase in laryngeal mucus glands may result in either a critical narrowing of the airway or excessive secretions (Fink & Beckwith, 1980; Harrison, 1991a; Harrison, 1991b), but again this is not a usual finding at autopsy.

Greater compliance of the nasal cartilages in infancy (Harding, 1986) has been blamed for nasal obstruction due to downward pressure from the head in infants who are sleeping prone (Thach, Davies & Koenig, 1988). However, other factors must also be involved if this is to be linked causally to death, as it has been demonstrated that infants are capable of initiating mouth breathing following nasal occlusion (Rodenstein, Perlmutter & Stanescu, 1985). It has also been proposed that the tongue is anatomically larger in SIDS infants, possibly predisposing to upper airway obstruction (Siebert & Haas, 1991). In contrast, other authors have suggested that obstruction occurs more peripherally, involving the intrapulmonary airways rather than the larger air passages (Martinez, 1991). Proliferation of dendritic cells within bronchioles of victims of SIDS has been proposed as a marker for peripheral airway narrowing, with subsequent reduction in airflow (Haque & Mancuso, 1993).

Microscopic thymic petechiae were found in 45% of SIDS cases compared with 25% of controls in an NICHD study (Willinger, James & Catz, 1991). Similarities in the distribution of petechial hemorrhages in infants dying of SIDS and lethal upper airway obstruction have suggested a common pathophysiologic basis to some authors (Krous, 1984a; Krous & Jordan, 1984; Krous & Jordan, 1988; Krous *et al.*, 2001c). Beckwith (1988, 1989) noted lower numbers of petechiae above the left innominate (brachiocephalic) vein in SIDS infants, in keeping with localized protection from the effects of increased negative intrathoracic pressure caused by upper airway obstruction (Figure 13.22). Animal studies have not, however, confirmed that petechiae necessarily follow sudden major airway occlusion (Guntheroth, Breazeale & McGough, 1973). Winn (1986) demonstrated that large numbers of thoracic petechial hemorrhages occurred in rats who survived an episode of anoxic anoxia (95% nitrogen exposure) in the absence of airway occlusion. Another study could induce petechiae in rats subjected to hypoxic asphyxia only if there was a concomitant viral infection (Guntheroth et al., 1980). It is probable, therefore, that petechiae result from the interaction of a variety of factors, including severe hypoxia with continued blood flow, terminal left ventricular failure, and unsuccessful gasping respiratory efforts, and that this may be exacerbated by the presence of infection (Byard & Krous, 1999b; Farber, Catron & Krous, 1983; Poets et al., 1999). It has also been proposed that environmental factors, including known risk factors, may also influence the distribution and frequency of petechiae (Becroft, Thompson & Mitchell, 1998).

Several studies have shown an apparent protective effect against SIDS from pacifiers (dummies), possibly by keeping the airway open; however, consensus has not yet been reached on their possible role in maintaining airway patency (Arnestad, Anderson & Rognum, 1997; Fleming et al., 1999; Mitchell et al., 1993b; Righard, 1998).

Neurologic abnormalities

Functional immaturity in autonomic control of the larynx has been put forward as a possible cause of fatal laryngospasm in infancy based partly on the results of animal experiments (Taylor et al., 1976). Patients with defective neural control of airways and rabbits with denervated airway musculature are known to have potential for obstruction (Brouillette & Thach, 1979). The observation of unusual crying during sleep in infants who subsequently died of SIDS (Golub & Corwin, 1982) has also been cited as evidence of abnormal neural control of upper airway musculature, which may result in airway obstruction (Shannon & Kelly, 1982b). Infants at risk of SIDS may also show reduced autonomic reponses to airway obstruction during sleep (Franco et al., 1999).

Two other neurologic mechanisms that could cause upper airway obstruction are worth considering, although little supportive evidence is available for either. Naeye, Olsson & Combs (1989) have suggested that a deficiency of neurons within the hypoglossal nucleus may contribute to upper aerodigestive tract obstruction by causing impaired movement of the tongue. However, a later study has failed to confirm this, demonstrating instead a reduction in the size, but not in the number, of neurons in the hypoglossal and vagal nuclei in SIDS infants (Konrat et al., 1992). There is also hypothesis that fatal laryngospasm due to compression of the left recurrent laryngeal nerve by the pulmonary artery may occur in SIDS due to left-to-right shunting of blood (Vesselinova-Jenkins, 1980); however, as SIDS infants do not have a persistent fetal circulation, this is most unlikely.

Physiologic mechanisms

Reduction in postpalatal pressure causing suction of the tongue into the pharynx has been demonstrated in infants with partial nasal occlusion (Tonkin et al., 1979). This may combine with an absence of positive distending pressures within the infantile pharynx preventing reopening of the airway once blockage has occurred and exacerbated by mucosal adhesive forces (Thach, 1983; Tonkin & Beach, 1988). As relaxation of the pharyngeal musculature is known to occur during rapid eye movement (REM) sleep, this may represent a particularly vulnerable time for obstruction (Franco et al., 1999; Kahn et al., 1992a; Tonkin, Stewart & Withey, 1980). The continuation of respiratory efforts in a series of term infants following complete upper airway occlusion does suggest, however, that other mechanisms must also be involved in the generation of apnea (Milner, Saunders & Hopkin, 1977). Certain infants may also show inadequate arousal patterns when confronted with an increase in upper airway resistance (Guilleminault et al., 1993).

Central apnea

Central apnea is characterized by failure of both airflow and respiratory efforts. Susceptible infants demonstrate breathing abnormalities that are also found in premature infants, in patients with seizures, and normally during REM sleep. Mixed apnea is characterized by central apnea that is followed by respiratory efforts without airflow. It is hypothesized that central apnea is caused by an abnormality in the neural control of respiration that is influenced by sleep state (Guilleminault & Coons, 1983). While certain authors consider that obstructive apnea is a more likely mode of sudden death than central apnea (Davies *et al.*, 1990), not all investigators would agree (Southall, 1988b).

Influence of sleep state
A particularly vulnerable time for central apnea occurs during REM sleep (Read & Jeffery, 1983), when lowered hypercapnic respiratory drive in combination with reduced intercostal muscle tone and relative underinflation of the lungs predisposes to hypoxemia (Read, 1978). Sleep deprivation has also been shown to have an effect similar to REM sleep in kittens, associated with a reduced arousal response to apnea (reported in Hasselmeyer & Hunter, 1975). It may also be that infants who have significant apneic episodes have a reduced respiratory response to carbon dioxide breathing (Shannon & Kelly, 1977) and to hypoxia (Brady *et al.*, 1978), although this finding may represent a secondary response to hypoxia rather than being a primary abnormality. The interaction of sleep, arousal states, and cardiorespiratory instability is likely to be highly complex and involve both thermoregulation and autonomic feedback (Ariagno & Mirmiran, 2001). The occurrence of SIDS in infants known to have been awake immediately prior to the terminal episode does imply that non-sleep-related mechanisms may be involved in a very small number of cases (Weinstein, Steinschneider & Diamond, 1983).

Possible defects
Suggested sites for underlying respiratory defects have ranged from brainstem nuclei to peripheral airway stretch receptors, and to chemoreceptors such as the carotid body (Becker, 1983). Suprapontine cerebral defects may also be implicated in the pathogenesis of this type of apnea (Harper & Frysinger, 1988), supported by observations of similar episodes occurring in epileptic patients during seizures and the demonstration of ictal apneas in a small percentage of infants with previous ALTEs (Clancy & Spitzer, 1985).

Goyco & Beckerman (1990) have listed possible defects that may be responsible for central apneas in infants. All, except for the first group, may be involved in the pathogenesis of SIDS:
- Respiratory center failure due to underlying pathology such as structural malformation, sepsis, trauma, or brain tumor.
- Defective chemoreceptor function, resulting in reduced ventilatory response to changes in arterial oxygen and carbon dioxide levels.
- Increased C-fiber reactivity, causing vocal cord adduction and arrested inspiration.
- Unusual stretch receptor sensitivity or increased Hering–Breuer reflex, resulting in inhibition of inspiration.
- Defective upper airway chemoreceptors, causing laryngospasm.
- Increased limbic system activation.

Expiratory apnea
The final group of infants who have demonstrated abnormal respiratory patterns have shown marked hypoxemia with continued expiratory efforts and no inspiratory flow, the so-called "apnea braking syndrome" (Southall & Talbert, 1987). The basis for this expiratory apnea is not understood well, although it has been suggested that sudden alveolar collapse with intrapulmonary shunting of venous blood may be implicated (Southall, Samuels & Talbert, 1990). The possibility of apnea being caused by definable organic lesions such as central nervous system tumors (Byard, 1991b; Kelly, Krishnamoorthy & Shannon, 1980; Southall *et al.*, 1987b) or epilepsy (Amir *et al.*, 1983; Southall *et al.*, 1987c) must, however, always be borne in mind.

Surfactant abnormality
A contributing factor to alveolar collapse may be qualitative or quantitative abnormalities of

surfactant (Milner, 1987; Talbert & Southall, 1985). This is a complex phospholipid produced by type II pneumocytes, which normally reduces surface tension within alveoli and thus assists in lung inflation by decreasing compliance (Gibson & McMurchie, 1988b). Although it has been suggested that SIDS infants have abnormalities of surfactant similar to those of infants with hyaline membrane disease (Morley, Hill & Brown, 1988), research has produced variable results.

The finding of a reduction in absolute levels of surfactant phospholipid by some workers (Hill *et al.*, 1988; Morley *et al.*, 1982) has not been confirmed by others, who have instead reported lower levels of only the biologically active component, disaturated phosphatidylcholine (Gibson & McMurchie, 1986; Gibson & McMurchie, 1988a). Surfactant may also be altered secondarily, and it has been postulated that both phospholipase-A2-producing bacteria (James *et al.*, 1990) and denaturation of surfactant due to overheating may reduce the levels of active phospholipid in SIDS cases (Talbert, 1990). Two children with recurrent cyanotic episodes have been reported who had abnormalities in the amount and activity of their surfactant (Hills, Masters & O'Duffy, 1992).

On the other hand, postmortem pulmonary inflation studies have not confirmed a difference in compliance in the lungs of SIDS infants, as would be anticipated if the amount of biological activity of surfactant was altered significantly (Fagan & Milner, 1985). The negative findings in this study may have been due to the use of non-physiologic distending pressures or to postmortem changes in surfactant (Southall & Talbert, 1988). The significance of altered surface tension characteristics of surfactant (hysteresis inversion) in SIDS infants is uncertain, since the criteria that were used to arrive at the diagnosis of SIDS were not specified and the study also included children up to the age of two years (Hills *et al.*, 1997).

Evidence for chronic hypoxia

It is logical to suppose that infants who have suffered significant antemortem hypoxia might have characteristic histologic changes that can be detected at postmortem examination, but evidence for this is quite variable.

In support of antemortem hypoxia, Naeye (1973, 1974, 1976, 1978, 1980) has claimed that there are a number of subtle morphologic changes in infants who have died of SIDS. These include pulmonary arteriolar thickening, right ventricular hypertrophy, altered carotid body volume, bone marrow erythroid hyperplasia, increased extramedullary hematopoiesis in the liver, increased amounts of periadrenal brown fat, and brainstem gliosis. In addition, Rognum and colleagues (Rognum *et al.*, 1988, Rognum & Saugstad, 1991) have demonstrated increased levels of hypoxanthine in the vitreous humor, and Giulian, Gilbert & Moss (1987) have reported elevated fetal hemoglobin levels in SIDS, features that may be associated with chronic hypoxia (Poulsen *et al.*, 1993; Rognum & Saugstad, 1991; Rognum & Saugstad, 1993). Impaired postnatal growth in infants destined to die of SIDS may be another manifestation of underlying sustained hypoxia (Peterson *et al.*, 1974).

While there has been some support for Naeye's work (Kinney *et al.*, 1983; Mason *et al.*, 1975; Valdes-Dapena *et al.*, 1980b; Weiler & de Haardt, 1983; Williams, Vawter & Reid, 1979), none of the markers has been confirmed definitely, due to the presence of considerable overlap with controls, contradictory findings, and the highly subjective nature of histologic assessment of these parameters (Emery & Dinsdale, 1978; Kendeel & Ferris, 1977a; Krous, 1984b; Krous, 1988; Krous *et al.*, 2002; Singer & Tilly, 1988; Valdes-Dapena *et al.*, 1979; Valdes-Dapena *et al.*, 1980a; Valdes-Dapena, Gillane & Catherman, 1976). Confirmation of elevated fetal hemoglobin levels in SIDS has not occurred (Zielke *et al.*, 1989), and no elevation in serum erythropoietin was found by Kozakewich *et al.* (1986), as would be anticipated if an infant had been exposed to prolonged hypoxia.

It can be concluded, therefore, that most of these findings have not been reproducible, and that while some may be of statistical significance (Beckwith, 1983; Kinney *et al.*, 1983), they are of little practical or diagnostic help.

Other morphologic features that are characteristic of hypoxia, such as renal glomerular enlargement and lipid-containing macrophages in the cerebrospinal fluid and brain (Gadson & Emery, 1976), are not found in SIDS autopsies (Esiri, Urry & Keeling, 1990; Variend & Howat, 1986).

Bronchopulmonary dysplasia

Bronchopulmonary dysplasia is a chronic lung disease found in premature infants who have been treated with prolonged assisted ventilation for hyaline membrane disease. It is characterized pathologically by emphysema and interstitial fibrosis, with squamous metaplasia and smooth muscle hypertrophy of bronchioles (Northway, 1990). It has been claimed that there is a sevenfold increase in the risk of SIDS in infants who leave hospital with this condition (Werthammer *et al.*, 1982). Although there appears to be no doubt that infants with bronchopulmonary dysplasia are at increased risk of sudden and unexpected death, a diagnosis of SIDS cannot be made in an infant who demonstrates obvious chronic lung damage with a wide range of developmental, physiologic, biochemical, and metabolic defects. Certain infants with bronchopulmonary dysplasia may appear clinically well with normal growth parameters and yet still have obvious interstitial lung scarring, with a significant reduction in pulmonary gas exchange area on lung morphometry.

Miscellaneous

While there is no evidence to suggest that infants who have suffered ALTEs have impaired diaphragmatic function (Scott *et al.*, 1982), studies have shown a reduction in the number and increase in the size of type 1 fibers in the diaphragms of SIDS infants (de Silva, Icke & Hilton, 1992; Tennyson, Pereyra & Becker, 1994). This might render the diaphragm susceptible to early fatigue, particularly in the prone position; however, not all SIDS infants have shown abnormalities of diaphragmatic nerves (Weis *et al.*, 1998). The finding of higher levels of asbestos bodies in 10 SIDS infants (Haque, Hernandez & Dillard, 1985) may indicate an impaired pulmonary clearing mechanism; however, unrelated environmental exposure would be more probable.

Conclusion

Thus, although it appears that several respiratory mechanisms may be involved in the etiology of SIDS, the percentage of cases having an underlying respiratory defect remains uncertain.

Cardiovascular theories

Defective brainstem cardiac control centers, autonomic imbalance, and aberrant conduction pathways have all been implicated as causes of SIDS (Bharati, Krongrad & Lev, 1985; Schwartz, 1976; Schwartz, 1987; Schwartz, 1989), with the suggested terminal event being arrhythmia rather than apnea. In support of this, there are a number of entities such as the prolonged QT interval syndromes, congenital heart block, and Wolff–Parkinson–White syndrome in which abnormalities of cardiac conduction have been associated with an increased risk of sudden infant death. Cardiac arrhythmias have also been documented in infants with a history of ALTEs associated with mixed apneas (Guilleminault *et al.*, 1985).

Pathological evidence

Problems arising in attempting to prove a cardiac cause of SIDS include lack of antemortem ECG tracings in the majority of infants who die of SIDS, the relative insensitivity of routine light microscopy in assessing central cardiac control pathways, and the difficulty in relating mechanisms of death to morphologic findings (Thiene, 1988). Studies of conduction pathways have not been able to differentiate SIDS infants from controls (Anderson *et al.*, 1974; Ho & Anderson, 1988; Lie, Rosenberg & Erickson, 1976), and extensive remodeling of the atrioventricular node and bundle of His in SIDS infants now appears to be part of normal early infantile development (James, 1968; James, 1976). Also, trying to explain retrospectively an event as kinetic as sudden death from examination of fixed tissues is fraught with difficulty, as the absence of morphologic abnormalities does not preclude serious antemortem physiologic and biochemical derangements.

In addition, it must be borne in mind that the finding of an apparent anatomic abnormality in the heart, such as intimal thickening of the nodal arteries (Anderson & Hill, 1982; Kozakewich, McManus & Vawter, 1982), lymphocytic infiltrates (Jankus, 1976), or accessory pathways (Marino & Kane, 1985), may be quite coincidental to the cause of death. This was well demonstrated in a study of 30 young people who died of trauma or other non-cardiac disease, a significant number of whom showed histologic abnormalities of the conduction pathways, including fibrosis, degenerative changes, accessory pathways, and focal myocarditis (Cohle & Lie, 1990).

Although hearts from SIDS infants often show septal fiber disarray (Figure 13.23) reminiscent of hypertrophic cardiomyopathy, the absence of septal and individual myocyte hypertrophy indicates that this is part of normal postnatal development (Maron & Fisher, 1977). As endocardial fibroelastosis is known to be associated with sudden death (Valdes-Dapena, 1985), the finding of significant amounts precludes the diagnosis of SIDS. Focal anoxic changes and intimal hyperplasia reported by Kariks (1988) most likely represent secondary phenomena.

Prolonged QT syndromes

A number of physiologic studies have demonstrated apparent cardiac abnormalities, such as prolongation of the QT interval, in infants who later die of SIDS or in relatives of SIDS infants (Maron *et al.*, 1976; Southall *et al.*, 1979). However, normal QT intervals have been shown in other studies (Kelly, Shannon & Liberthson, 1977; Southall *et al.*, 1983a; Southall *et al.*, 1983b; Southall *et al.*, 1986a; Weinstein & Steinschneider, 1985), and no prolongation of the QT interval was found in a study of siblings and parents of SIDS infants by Steinschneider (1978).

Part of the problem may have been that certain study populations have been biased by a high number of families with prolonged QT intervals as an inherited disorder (Guntheroth, 1989b). It is also difficult to reconcile the shortened QT intervals in seven

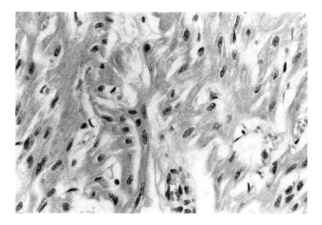

Figure 13.23 Section from the interventricular septum of a heart from a typical SIDS case, showing the considerable degree of myofiber disarray that may normally be found at this site (hematoxylin and eosin, ×440).

infants with ALTEs reported by Haddad *et al.* (1979) with these studies. Problems with differing methods of data collection and analysis, and significant variability in inter- and intraobserver ECG interpretation, may have contributed to these contradictory and confusing data (Guntheroth, 1989a; Guntheroth & Spiers, 1998).

More recent work by Schwartz and colleagues has, however, shown prolongation of QT intervals in certain infants whose deaths were attributed to SIDS, suggesting that some infants may indeed be at increased risk of lethal arrhythmias (Schwartz, 2001; Schwartz *et al.*, 1998; Schwartz *et al.*, 2001). Molecular studies have also confirmed this link, with a 44-day-old boy presenting in cardiac arrest who was found to have a prolonged QT interval and mutation of SCN5A, the cardiac sodium channel gene responsible for the LQT3 subtype (Schwartz *et al.*, 2000). In another study, cardiac tissue from 93 SIDS infants revealed two cases with cardiac sodium channel mutations associated with prolonged QT interval (see Chapter 5), with none in the 400 controls (Ackerman *et al.*, 2001). The role of clinical screening for this defect remains uncertain (Towbin & Friedman, 1998).

Other rhythm disturbances

Other abnormalities reported in infants who subsequently die of SIDS, or who have been resuscitated following an ALTE, include elevation and variation in mean heart rate, reduced heart rate variability in the waking state, and reduced variation in cardiac rate during REM and quiet sleep (Pincus, Cummins & Haddad, 1993; Schechtman *et al.*, 1988; Schechtman *et al.*, 1989; Schechtman *et al.*, 1992b; Southall *et al.*, 1988). There have also been sporadic reports of possible associations with heart block with junctional escape, and with Wolff–Parkinson–White syndrome (Keeton *et al.*, 1977; Lipsitt *et al.*, 1979). The increase in heart rate in siblings of SIDS infants reported by Harper *et al.* (1982) was not verified in a subsequent study (Southall *et al.*, 1987a). No relationship between RT intervals and heart rate has been established (Wynn & Southall, 1992).

Diving reflex activation

The major abnormality noted in three infants who were monitored during a terminal episode was severe bradycardia, both with and without apnea (Kelly, Pathak & Meny, 1991). Inappropriate activation of the diving reflex has, therefore, been put forward as a possible physiologic process linking bradycardia with apnea (Lobban, 1991). Other possible mechanisms include intrinsic vagal dysfunction as a cause of bradycardia in certain infants at increased risk of sudden death (Coryllos, 1982) and sleep-associated arrhythmias (Verrier & Kirby, 1988).

Mechanical theories

Theories in which lethal mechanical compromise of the heart, brainstem, or vessels occurs, such as compression of the cardiac ventricles by the thymus in the prone position (Hori, 1987), and compression or stretching of the medulla and vertebral arteries during head rotation/extension (Deeg, Alderath & Bettendorf, 1998; Gilles, Bina & Sotrel, 1979; Maslowski, 1996; Pamphlett, Raisanen & Kum-Jew, 1999; Saternus, Koebke & Von Tamaska, 1986), have not been substantiated (Byard & Krous, 2001; Krous

et al., 2001d). For example, cerebral blood flow was not found to change with alterations in head position using in vivo radiographic studies (Lawson *et al.*, 1987). The significance of a possible variation in the size of the vertebral artery diameters in SIDS infants (Hebold, Saternus & Schleicher, 1986) is also uncertain, given the usual lack of neuropathologic findings.

Conclusion

Although many of these findings suggest that defective cardiac conduction may be implicated in some SIDS deaths, the data are contradictory. This may merely be a reflection of the heterogeneity in underlying pathophysiologic defects that exists within this group of infants. Again, as with respiratory theories of SIDS, it is difficult to determine the exact percentage of deaths that have been caused by cardiac abnormalities; however, conditions such as prolonged QT interval have accounted for approximately 2% of cases in some studies (Ackerman *et al.*, 2001).

Central and peripheral nervous system theories

Central and peripheral nervous system dysfunction is thought to be the basis for a number of the above cardiorespiratory abnormalities observed in infants who have subsequently died of SIDS (Hunt, 1992; Matthews, 1992). Unfortunately, however, our understanding of the complexities of neurophysiologic mechanisms is far from complete, and in some cases even knowledge of neuroanatomic pathways and connections is lacking. This makes assessment of postmortem findings difficult, particularly given the rapid deterioration that occurs in nervous tissue after death. As always, paucity of normal controls also complicates interpretation of apparent pathologic findings, and judgments must be made as to whether a certain feature is a primary, secondary, or even an unrelated phenomenon. This assumes particular significance in infants who may have an array of changes due to attempted resuscitation. These problems may explain some of the contradictions present in the neuropathologic SIDS literature.

Brainstem gliosis

Brainstem gliosis has been reported in several studies (Summers & Parker, 1981; Takashima *et al.*, 1978a) and is found most prominently in the tegmental region of the medulla, involving the dorsal nucleus of the vagus, the inferior olivary nucleus, the solitary nucleus, and the reticular nuclei.

Postmortem angiographic studies have demonstrated that this area is relatively underperfused compared with the adjacent brainstem, implying that gliosis may be a reaction to previous ischemic damage (Becker, 1990). A case report has documented ischemic necrosis in this region (Atkinson *et al.*, 1984), and Becker (1990) has pointed out that the more significant abnormality may be neuronal loss rather than gliotic scarring.

The similarity in the pattern of gliosis in patients with various types of myopathy or Ondine's curse (central hypoventilation syndrome) to the pattern in infants with SIDS has led to the speculation that the underlying mechanism in these cases is similar and involves chronic hypoventilation (Becker & Takashima, 1985; Faigel, 1974).

Not all studies have detected these abnormalities (Pearson & Brandeis, 1983), and even when present there appears to be so much overlap with controls (Ambler, Neave & Sturner, 1981) that the findings are of minimal diagnostic usefulness. The etiology and significance of brainstem gliosis in SIDS infants is, therefore, uncertain (Kinney & Filiano, 1988).

Neuronal changes

Increased numbers of dendritic spines in brainstem reticular neurons have been described in SIDS infants (Quattrochi, McBride & Yates, 1985; Takashima & Becker, 1991; Takashima, Yamanouchi & Becker, 1993). This may be due to maturational delay in neuronal function (Quattrochi *et al.*, 1980; Takashima & Becker, 1985), with the possibility of subsequent effects on control of cardiorespiratory function. Further evidence for maturational delay in SIDS infants has been provided by Schechtman *et al.* (1990), who showed an immature pattern in the integration of cardiorespiratory functions. An alternate explanation has been that increased dendritic spines result

from loss of afferent connecting neurons (Kinney, Filiano & Harper, 1992).

It has also been hypothesized that reduced numbers of neurons in the hypoglossal nucleus (cranial nerve XII) may contribute to upper airway obstruction by impairing normal tongue movements (Naeye, Olsson & Combs, 1989), although dendritic spine density has been reported as normal or increased in the hypoglossal nucleus in other studies (O'Kusky & Norman, 1992; Takashima, Mito & Becker, 1990).

A further finding that reflects more disordered than delayed maturation of neurons is the demonstration of increased neuronal degeneration in SIDS infants based on increased staining of neurons using the monoclonal antibody ALZ-50. This antibody was raised against extracts from brains of patients with Alzheimer's disease (Sparks & Hunsaker, 1991). Hypoplasia of the arcuate nucleus has been found in a small number of SIDS infants. This may be another cause of disturbed central respiratory control (Filiano & Kinney, 1992; Filiano, 1994).

The significance of possible functional brainstem changes in infants who have suffered an ALTE in the form of abnormal auditory evoked potentials (Orlowski, Nodar & Lonsdale, 1979) is unclear given the failure of subsequent studies to demonstrate the anticipated abnormal responses (Gupta, Guilleminault & Dorfman, 1981; Marx, 1981). It is also possible that the observed changes were merely a secondary effect of prolonged hypoxia. Infants with hyperekplexia (exaggeration of the startle reflex possibly due to abnormal cortical-brainstem interaction) are also known to have episodes of ALTEs (Nigro & Lim, 1992).

White matter changes

Changes have been described in the white matter of SIDS infants, consisting of leukomalacia in the periventricular and subcortical regions (Takashima *et al.*, 1978b). The presence of similar findings in approximately the same percentage of infants dying of congenital heart disease again suggests that this is a secondary phenomenon due to anoxia rather than a primary abnormality involved directly in the pathogenesis of SIDS (Kalnins, 1986). Also, not all studies have confirmed similarities between SIDS and hypoxically damaged brains (Esiri, Urry & Keeling, 1990). It has been suggested that an apparent delay in central nervous system myelination in SIDS infants may be an expression of an associated developmental disorder (Kinney *et al.*, 1991).

Neurotransmitter abnormalities

Another theory proposes that an increase in brain endorphin levels may cause respiratory depression and bradycardia in at-risk infants (Kuich & Zimmerman, 1981). Elevated β-endorphin levels have also been found in the cerebrospinal fluid (CSF) of infants who have suffered significant apneas (Myer *et al.*, 1987; Orlowski, 1986). This hypothesis gains support from animal studies that have demonstrated respiratory depression following addition of β-endorphin to the CSF (Sitsen, Van Ree & de Jong, 1982). Elevated CSF β-endorphin levels have also been correlated with increased hypoxanthine levels in vitreous humor and brainstem gliosis, suggesting previous hypoxic episodes (Storm *et al.*, 1994).

However, assessments of neurotransmitter and enzyme levels have shown variable results. Reduced levels of dopamine-β-hydroxylase, normal levels of L-dopa decarboxylase with increased levels of substance P, tyrosine hydroxylase, and possibly brainstem opioids have all been reported (Bergstrom, Largercrantz & Terenius, 1984; Denoroy *et al.*, 1987; Frankfater & Wilcockson, 1983; Kalaria *et al.*, 1993; Kopp *et al.*, 1994; Ozand & Tildon, 1983; Pasi *et al.*, 1983). Phenylethanolamine-*N*-methyl transferase, an enzyme involved in catecholamine production, has been reported as being both reduced and normal in amount in the brainstem, and met-enkephalin levels have been found to be elevated, equivocally elevated, and normal (Becker, 1990; Denoroy *et al.*, 1987; Kopp *et al.*, 1993).

These inconsistent findings may be partly the result of combining analyses from a number of anatomically and functionally different areas of the brain, and it has been suggested that clarification of results may be achieved only by combining microdissection and autoradiographic techniques with biochemical analysis (Becker, 1990).

More recently, abnormalities have been detected within the arcuate nucleus of the ventral medulla in SIDS victims. Kinney *et al.* (1995, 1998) have shown defects in the medullary serotonergic network, including the arcuate nucleus, with reduced muscarinic, kainate, and serotonergic receptor binding. These receptors are involved in responses to carbon dioxide and may play a crucial role in hypoxic or hypercapneic states. An underlying defect in this region may result in failure of an infant to rouse or respond to airway obstruction or asphyxial rebreathing (Kinney & Filiano, 2001; Panigrahy *et al.*, 1997; Panigrahy *et al.*, 2000). Abnormalities in the promotor region of the serotonin transporter (5-HTT) gene may provide a basis for some of these abnormalities and thus possibly a marker for certain at risk infants (Weese-Mayer *et al.*, 2003). Reduction in nicotinic receptor binding in this area of the brainstem has also been found in infants with a history of maternal smoking during pregnancy (Nachmanoff *et al.*, 1998). On the other hand, despite these specific defects, brainstem changes in SIDS infants have been attributed to the non-specific effects of hypoxia by other researchers (Guntheroth & Spiers, 2002).

Axonal changes

Deranged vagal function could cause respiratory abnormalities due to hypoventilation, with loss of the usual response to hypercarbia, Hering–Breuer, or cough reflexes (Kelly & Shannon, 1982). Vagal dysfunction is also one of the reasons proposed for an exaggerated oculocardiac reflex in infants who have suffered ALTEs, manifested by prolonged asystolic episodes following ocular compression (Kahn, Riazi & Blum, 1983). The possibility of bradycardia secondary to vagal dysfunction as a cause of sudden death in infancy has, therefore, raised the prospect of atropine therapy in certain at-risk infants (Coryllos, 1982; Schey *et al.*, 1981b). This therapy has not been adopted.

Some studies have demonstrated abnormalities in the structure of the vagus. Although the mean number of myelinated fibers in the vagus nerve appears normal, a significant decrease has been noted in the number of fibers of less than 2 μm in diameter in

SIDS infants (Sachis *et al.*, 1981). This was interpreted as being due either to maturational delay or to abnormal development of the vagus (Becker, Zhang & Pereyra, 1993). Similar findings were present in an infant with a long history of alveolar hypoventilation secondary to deranged respiratory control (Armstrong, *et al.*, 1982). No delay in myelination of nerve axons has been found in a study of the phrenic nerve (Sachis *et al.*, 1981).

Chemoreceptor changes

The integral homeostatic role played by the carotid body and peripheral chemoreceptors in monitoring blood pH and oxygen levels with direct feedback to brainstem autonomic centers makes them attractive candidates in the search for defective mechanisms in SIDS infants (Heath, 1991; Heath, Khan & Smith, 1990). Interpretation of the possible role of the carotid body is, however, very difficult, as studies have demonstrated a full spectrum of conflicting results, with normal, increased, and reduced carotid body size, normal and reduced numbers of neurosecretory granules, and normal and elevated levels of transmitters (Cole *et al.*, 1979; Dinsdale, Emery & Gadsdon, 1977; Lack, Perez-Atayde & Young, 1986; Naeye *et al.*, 1976a; Perrin *et al.*, 1984a; Perrin *et al.*, 1984b).

Although the finding of increased numbers of bombesin-containing pulmonary neuroendocrine cells may be a marker of peripheral chemoreceptor immaturity or developmental delay, it may also occur secondary to chronic hypoxia (Cutz, Chan & Perrin, 1988; Cutz & Jackson, 2001; Gillan *et al.*, 1989; Perrin, McDonald & Cutz, 1991).

Influence of sleep states

It is possible that sleep states on their own may increase susceptibility to sudden death (Gould, 1983) by altering the interaction between suprapontine structures and cardiorespiratory control centers in vulnerable infants or by acting through the brainstem reticular formation (McGinty & Hoppenbrouwers, 1983). In support of this, it has been shown that siblings of SIDS infants have a reduced arousal response to partial nasal obstruction during quiet

sleep (Newman *et al.*, 1986). Other workers have demonstrated decreased waking time during the early morning in infants who have subsequently died of SIDS (Schechtman *et al.*, 1992a).

Abnormalities noted in the organization, structure, and level of maturation of sleep in a group of "near-miss" SIDS infants have also been attributed to both a maturational delay and a defect in brain functioning (Guilleminault & Coons, 1983).

The report of episodic hypothermia associated with ALTEs in several infants (Dunne & Matthews, 1988), along with the well-known phenomenon of hyperhidrosis during sleep in infants who later die of SIDS, gives added support to a possible role for disturbance in autonomic function, (Kahn *et al.*, 1987).

Miscellaneous

Morphometric assessment of autonomic and sensory ganglia has shown variable features, with no discernible differences found between SIDS infants and controls in one study (Pearson & Brandeis, 1983), compared with increased numbers of dendrites in the superior cervical ganglion reported by Read *et al.* (1988). One of the conclusions drawn from the latter study was that the reported changes may be evidence of accelerated rather than delayed neural maturation. This was also the conclusion of another group of workers, who suggested that accelerated maturation of neural substrates might create a higher arousal threshold in susceptible infants (Sterman & Hodgman, 1988).

Reports claiming a role for the pineal gland in SIDS have not been confirmed (Kocsard-Varo, 1991; Pearson & Greenaway, 1990; Sparks & Hunsaker, 1988). Similarly, the significance of an apparent increase in the weight of the brain in SIDS infants is uncertain (Aranda, Teixeira & Becker, 1990).

Conclusion

In spite of the inconsistencies in the literature, it is quite plausible that neural maturational imbalance in certain infants, in combination with a general arousal deficit (McCulloch *et al.*, 1982; Newman *et al.*, 1989; Schechtman *et al.*, 1990), renders them susceptible to cardiorespiratory compromise. This is particularly so around the age of two to four months, when marked changes in the neural control of cardiac and respiratory function and sleep cycles occur (Gould, Lee & Morelock, 1988; Kinney, 1988).

Gastrointestinal theories

Aspiration of gastric contents

Cases of death due to massive aspiration of gastric material into the lungs are quite rare in infants, and the most likely reason for stomach contents to be found in the peripheral airways is agonal aspiration secondary to the terminal event or merely to postmortem drainage of fluid following movement of the body. This was demonstrated in a study of adult cadavers following postmortem instillation of barium into the stomach, in which 70% were subsequently found to have barium in their lungs (Gardner, 1958). (Interestingly, the author was unable to replicate this effect in a small unpublished study using infant cadavers.) Knight (1975) has also reported the presence of gastric contents in the airways unrelated to the cause of death in 25% of adult autopsies and in a similar percentage in SIDS cases. Thus, the presence of gastric contents within the airways, and even within the alveoli, must always be interpreted with caution, particularly if resuscitation has been attempted. In a study of 196 infants and children under the age of three years, only three had significant filling of the airways with gastric contents (Figures 13.24 and 13.25). All three had been sleeping face down, with the face in a pool of vomitus in at least one case (Byard & Beal, 2000). If required, the extent of aspiration of milk can be further assessed histologically by immunohistochemical staining (Iwadate *et al.*, 1997).

Reflux

Reflux of gastric contents into the upper aerodigestive tract has also been implicated as a cause of SIDS, with a variety of different mechanisms being proposed. It is well recognized that infants who suffer from significant gastroesophageal reflux manifest a wide range of respiratory problems, including stridor, wheezing, cough, choking, ALTE, and respiratory

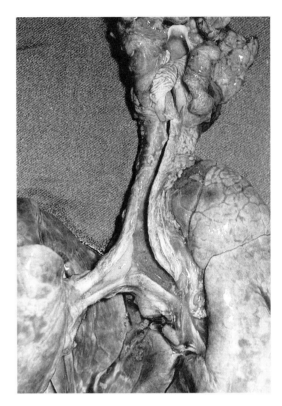

Figure 13.24 Plugging of bronchi by aspirated gastric contents.

arrest (Jolley *et al.*, 1991; Leape *et al.*, 1977). The increased incidence of reflux reported during active sleep (Paton, MacFadyen & Simpson, 1989) would be in keeping with the occurrence of SIDS in sleeping infants, and elevation of the head of the cot associated with a reduced rate of SIDS may also be supportive of reflux being a factor in some cases (Mitchell, Scragg & Clements, 1997).

Mechanisms by which reflux could cause sudden death other than filling of peripheral airways with gastric contents involve stimulation of peripheral esophageal receptors by acid stomach contents, resulting in vagally mediated fatal apnea or bradycardia (de Bethmann *et al.*, 1993). Apnea and bradycardia have been reported in infants and young animals following intraesophageal manipulation and introduction of saline and dilute acid (Baccino *et al.*, 1988; Herbst, Minton & Book, 1979; Kenigsberg *et al.*,

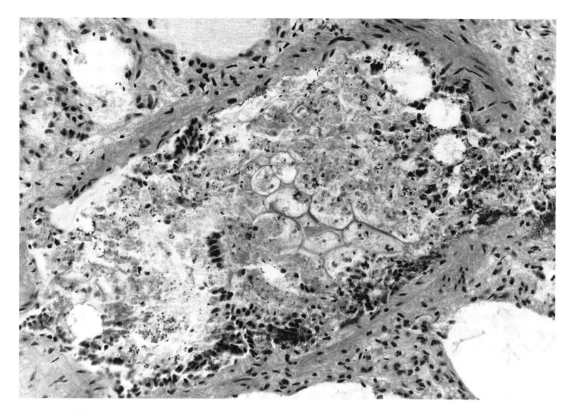

Figure 13.25 Filling of smaller airways in a case of fatal gastric aspiration.

1983; Rimell, Goding & Johnson, 1993; Schey *et al.*, 1981a). However, other studies utilizing continuous intraesophageal, respiratory and cardiac monitors have not demonstrated a convincing temporal relationship between apnea and reflux (Ariagno *et al.*, 1982; Kahn *et al.*, 1990a; Kahn *et al.*, 1992b).

Certain infants who are at risk of SIDS may be unusually responsive to laryngeal stimulation (Gomes *et al.*, 1986). It is possible, therefore, that laryngeal receptors are more sensitive to the effects of acid than are those within the esophagus, and a number of animal experiments have demonstrated hypoventilation and apnea following instillation of fluid into the upper airways (Gaultier, 1990).

It has also been suggested that reflux of cow's milk protein into the airways may result in fatal anaphylaxis (Coombs & McLaughlan, 1982) and that acid damage to type II pneumocytes may compromise

surfactant production resulting in alveolar collapse (Southall, 1988b).

Pathological findings

In a study of 38 infants who died of SIDS, only eight had diagnostic histologic changes of reflux (Figure 13.26) (Byard & Moore, 1993b). While this may reflect the insensitivity of standard light microscopy or suggest that reflux may occur without producing histologically detectable changes, it may also mean that chronic reflux is absent in a significant number of SIDS infants. Thus, although it appears that some infants who have gastroesophageal reflux are at greater risk of sudden death (Jolley *et al.*, 1991) it must be remembered that reflux is a common finding in early infancy and that in the majority of cases reflux and apnea may be independent manifestations of a more generalized developmental

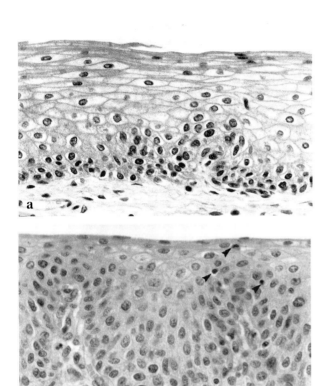

Figure 13.26 A normal segment of esophagus (a) compared with a segment showing evidence of gastroesophageal reflux, with thickening of the basal layer and a scattered background infiltrate of esosinophils (arrowheads) (b) (hematoxylin and eosin, ×400).

delay having a purely coincidental relationship to each other. (Walsh *et al.*, 1981).

Microbiological theories

Several factors give plausibility to a possible microbiological etiology in SIDS. These include increased incidence in winter (Newman, 1986), the presence of upper respiratory infections in many infants dying of SIDS (Naeye, 1983), the association of obstructive apnea with upper respiratory infections (Abreu *et al.*, 1986), histories of antemortem fever, and the known occurrence of sudden infant death

in a wide variety of infectious diseases. However, no single infectious agent has been isolated consistently, and research has shown repeatedly that there is little evidence of significant ongoing sepsis in SIDS victims (Carmichael, Goldwater & Byard, 1996). Moreover, if evidence of a serious infection is found at autopsy, then the diagnosis of SIDS cannot be applied. Thus, cases of sudden infant death due to myocarditis, pneumonia, epiglottis, or meningitis are due to precisely those entities, and not to SIDS.

A variety of viruses and bacteria have been implicated as possible agents responsible for SIDS, including respiratory syncytial virus (RSV), cytomegalovirus (CMV), and *Bordetella pertussis* (Anonymous, 1989; Variend, 1990; Williams, Uren & Bretherton, 1984). Occasionally, routine postmortem bacteriology identifies a previously unsuspected infectious agent, but this occurs relatively rarely and normal C-reactive protein levels in the sera of SIDS infants suggests that significant bacterial sepsis is unlikely in most cases (Benjamin & Siebert, 1990).

The increased incidence of chorioamnionitis that was reported in the placentas of infants who died of SIDS (Naeye, 1977) was not verified in a later study, which suggested that the discrepancy between the two reports was due to a failure to control for prematurity in the initial work (Denmead *et al.*, 1987). It is unlikely that chlamydial inclusions found in otherwise unremarkable lung sections in 19.4% of SIDS infants in one report are significant (Lundemose *et al.*, 1990). A study that suggested a link between SIDS and *Helicobacter pylori* infection failed to control for a number of factors, including socioeconomic status (Kerr *et al.*, 2000).

Respiratory syncytial virus

The occurrence of apnea in hospitalized infants with RSV appeared to add weight to the suggested association with SIDS (Abreu *et al.*, 1982; Anas *et al.*, 1982; Colditz, Henry & de Silva, 1982; Lindgren, 1993). However, lack of obvious postmortem symptomatology, normal interferon levels, and other studies that have shown that patients with RSV do not generally

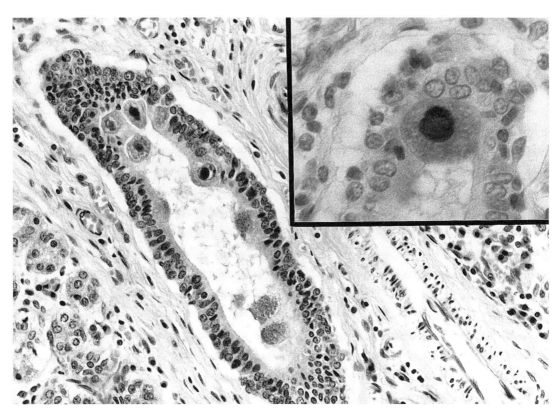

Figure 13.27 A section from the submandibular gland, demonstrating ducts that are lined by occasional cells containing large "owl's eye" intranuclear cytomegalovirus (CMV) inclusions (hematoxylin and eosin, ×280). Inset shows positive immunoperoxidase staining for intranuclear CMV antigens (×1100).

have significant episodes of apnea appear to mitigate against a possible causal role (Southall *et al.*, 1986c). A study in Bristol has also demonstrated that infants dying of SIDS have a similar viral load to neighboring age-matched controls (Gilbert *et al.*, 1992).

Cytomegalovirus

It has been reported that SIDS infants have a higher rate of infection with CMV than controls (Huff & Carpenter, 1987) and that this is associated with residual brainstem microglial knots, reflecting previous encephalitis (Variend & Pearse, 1986). However, no difference has been demonstrated in the presence of salivary-gland CMV inclusions (Figure 13.27) or brainstem microglial nodules between SIDS

infants and controls taken from the general autopsy population, casting some doubt on the purported association (Smith, Telfer & Byard, 1992). DNA hybridization studies have also not shown evidence of CMV viremia around the time of death (Coumbe *et al.*, 1990).

Toxin-producing bacteria

While toxin-producing clostridia have been implicated in the pathogenesis of SIDS, possibly associated with the ingestion of honey and lack of breast-feeding (Arnon, 1983; Arnon, Damus & Chin, 1981; Murrell *et al.*, 1993; Sonnabend *et al.*, 1985), several reports have failed to substantiate this association (Hilton, 1989; Smialek & Lambros, 1988; Williams,

1990). Significantly, a study that prospectively analyzed small and large bowel contents from 258 SIDS infants over a 10-year period failed to find a single isolate of *Clostridium botulinum* (Byard *et al.*, 1992). In addition, the isolation of these organisms in feces from asymptomatic infants (Kahn, Demol & Blum, 1985; Thompson *et al.*, 1980) raises the possibility of a purely coincidental association. The evidence linking SIDS with *Clostridium difficile* is even more tenuous (Cooperstock *et al.*, 1982; Laughon *et al.*, 1983).

Toxigenic *Escherichia coli* has been reported in SIDS infants as being both absent (Gurwith, Langston & Citron, 1981) and increased (Bettelheim *et al.*, 1990; Bettiol *et al.*, 1994; Goldwater, 1992). However, as toxin has not yet been identified consistently in serum or tissues, the possibility of a coincidental association in the latter instance has not been excluded. This gains support from the finding of toxigenic *E. coli* in the feces of similar numbers of SIDS infants and controls (16.8% *v.* 16.5%) (Bettelheim *et al.*, 1993). The isolation of *E. coli* expressing a Shiga-like toxin from the feces of a purported SIDS infant (Paton *et al.*, 1992) raises the possibility of a systemic thrombotic microangiopathy, such as hemolytic uremic syndrome, rather than SIDS.

Other workers have proposed that toxins from commonly occurring bacteria may be involved in SIDS pathogenesis in infants at the time between waning of maternal immunoglobulin levels and the development of acquired immunity (Malam *et al.*, 1992; McKendrick *et al.*, 1992). This may be predisposed to by elevated nasopharyngeal temperatures in children, leading to colonization by *Staphylococci* that produce pyrogenic toxins (Molony *et al.*, 1996). Other researchers have, however, failed to demonstrate endotoxin in blood from SIDS infants (Platt *et al.*, 1994). It appears unlikely, therefore, that a bacterial toxin or virus in isolation could account for the majority of cases of SIDS given the apparently heterogeneous nature of the entity.

Possible pathophysiology
Although SIDS infants and controls appear microbiologically similar, it is still possible that mild infections may contribute to lethal episodes in infants who are not fully equipped to deal with additional stresses, a feature that would certainly accord with the seasonal pattern of SIDS. Also, it has been demonstrated in animal studies that the effect of a bacterial toxin may be exacerbated by a concomitant viral infection (Jakeman *et al.*, 1991) and that the presence of several bacterial species may be significantly more damaging than a single bacterial species in isolation (Lee *et al.*, 1987). Thus, the possibility remains that synergistic and additive activity among several bacterial or viral strains, compounded by environmental and other risk factors, contributes to infant death (Blackwell *et al.*, 1992; Blackwell *et al.*, 1994; Blackwell, Weir & Busuttil, 1995; Blackwell, Weir & Busuttil, 1997; Fleming, 1992; Kleeman, Hiller & Troger, 1995; Murrell, Murrell & Lindsay, 1994; Sayers *et al.*, 1995).

Establishing the diagnosis of infection
In certain cases, it may be difficult to decide whether an infection was of sufficient severity to be responsible for death. This has often led to problems in certification, for example when minor pulmonary inflammation is designated as fatal bronchiolitis (Byard & Krous, 1995). Beckwith (1970b) provided guidelines for assisting the classification of infant deaths based on the degree and type of histologic changes present in the lungs and airways. In occasional cases, precise determination of the cause of death may simply not be possible, and the term "sudden death cause undetermined" may be the least confusing solution. A comment can be appended to the diagnosis, in which the possible role of infection in the causation of death is discussed, along with the difficulty in excluding mechanisms responsible for SIDS.

Immunologic theories

The higher incidence of SIDS in premature infants has prompted investigation into the immune status of infants considered to be at increased risk.

Immunodeficiency
The finding of lower immunoglobulin levels in premature infants and in infants of mothers who have

smoked during pregnancy has led to the suggestion that these infants are immunologically incompetent. It has also been proposed that mothers with short inter-pregnancy intervals may be protein-deficient. This has been shown to cause immunodeficiencies in offspring in animal experiments (Golding, Limerick & Macfarlane, 1985). Research results have not, however, confirmed this hypothesis, and there is no evidence of increased antemortem infections in infants who die of SIDS. Similarly, serum complement and cell-mediated immunity in infants aged between two and four months are usually normal (Huang, 1983).

Increased immunoreactivity

An alternate approach suggests that SIDS infants are in fact immunologically "too" competent, and that allergic responses to a wide variety of materials are responsible for their unexpected deaths. Many substances have been proposed, including a variety of intrauterine pathogens, fungal organisms, house dust mite (*Dermatophagoides pteronyssinus*), and cow's milk protein (Coombs & McLaughlan, 1983; Turner, Baldo & Hilton, 1975). The latter is in keeping with the suggestion that significant gastro-esophageal reflux of milk may occur into the airways in SIDS infants.

Further evidence of possible cow's milk sensitivity has been provided by reports that showed elevated specific anti-cow's milk protein antibodies in the sera of some SIDS infants. Milk has also been found in the lungs of 40% of SIDS cases, and animal studies have demonstrated anaphylaxis in milk-sensitized guinea-pigs after the instillation of milk into the trachea (Devey *et al.*, 1976). However, although it was initially considered that formula feeding may increase the risk of SIDS (Mitchell *et al.*, 1991), this is no longer so (Fleming *et al.*, 2000; Golding, Limerick & Macfarlane, 1985; Kelly & Shannon, 1982). Moreover, SIDS does occur in breastfed infants, raised levels of anti-cow's milk IgE have not been a consistent finding, and serum complement levels are often normal in SIDS infants (Boulloche *et al.*, 1986; Golding, Limerick & Macfarlane, 1985; Huang, 1983). This casts considerable doubt on the cow's milk anaphylaxis hypothesis.

At autopsy, lack of mast cell degranulation in tissues (Seto, Uemura & Hokama, 1983) is not characteristic of an allergic episode, and while increased eosinophils have been reported in lung sections (Howat *et al.*, 1994; Roche, 1992) this is not a usual finding. As for other possible inciting antigens, neither elevated levels of serum IgE nor specific antibodies to house dust and house dust mite have been consistently demonstrated (Mirchandani, Mirchandani & House, 1984).

Increased levels of IgG, IgM, and IgA have been reported in pulmonary lavage fluid taken from a series of SIDS victims, along with an increase in immunohistochemical staining for immunoglobulins in lung sections (Forsyth *et al.*, 1989). The same group previously reported a difference in cellular phenotype of pulmonary lavage fluid cells, with markedly reduced expression of macrophage antigenic sites that mark with CD14A antibodies (Forsyth *et al.*, 1988). The significance of these findings is uncertain, and the reason for the increase in pulmonary immunoglobulins is unclear, although CD14 is involved in the binding of bacterial endotoxins to macrophages (Rietschel & Brade, 1992). Levels of IgG and IgM in bronchial washings are not always abnormal, although mucosal secretory component may be reduced (Ogra, Ogra & Coppola, 1975). Other workers have shown elevated numbers of mucosal IgM-containing cells in the trachea and IgA-containing cells in the duodenum in SIDS infants compared with controls, suggesting that there is stimulation of the mucosal immune system in SIDS infants (Stoltenberg, Saugstad & Rognum, 1992).

Elevated levels of interleukin-6 in cerebrospinal fluid in SIDS infants have been proposed as a marker of immune activation that may cause respiratory depression (Vege, 1998; Vege *et al.*, 1995).

Immunization

The possibility that diphtheria–tetanus–polio (DTP) vaccine was causally related to SIDS was first postulated following the deaths in Tennessee in 1979 of four infants from SIDS within 24 hours of vaccination (Centers for Disease Control and Prevention,

1979). A later report of six SIDS deaths within a day of immunization seemed to add support to this theory (Baraff, Ablon & Weiss, 1983), although this was subsequently criticized on methodologic grounds (Mortimer, Jones & Adelson, 1983). The occurrence of significant fever ($\geq$38 °C) in over 67% of infants following vaccination (Verschoor *et al.*, 1991) provides some plausibility to this hypothesis, given that hyperthermia may increase the risk of SIDS (Sunderland & Emery, 1981). However, all other works, including several large multicenter studies from different countries, have failed to demonstrate anything but a coincidental association between immunization and SIDS (Bernier *et al.*, 1982; Byard *et al.*, 1991; Byard, Mackenzie & Beal, 1995; Cherry *et al.*, 1988; Flahault *et al.*, 1988; Jonville-Bera *et al.*, 2001; Jonville-Bera, Autret & Laugier, 1995; Mortimer, 1987; Walker *et al.*, 1987).

In the USA, data from 757 SIDS infants and matched controls taken from the NICHD Cooperative Epidemiological Study of Sudden Infant Death Syndrome Risk Factors found no causal link (Hoffman *et al.*, 1987), and an English study of 10,028 infants (Pollock *et al.*, 1984), followed by a cohort study of 129,834 infants in Tennessee, USA, reported similar findings (Griffin *et al.*, 1988). SIDS actually appears to be less common in infants who have received triple immunization (Fleming *et al.*, 2001; Mitchell *et al.*, 1995; Roberts, 1987; Taylor & Emery, 1982; Valdes-Dapena, 1988b), although this may be a reflection of access to medical care rather than a direct protective effect (Damus *et al.*, 1988).

Significantly, Beal (1990) noted in South Australia that there was no fall in the median or average age of SIDS infants after the age of first immunization was reduced from three to two months, as would be expected if the two events were related causally. An additional study from South Australia of 115 consecutive SIDS deaths found that only 53 (46%) had been immunized (Byard, Mackenzie & Beal, 1997b). Steinschneider *et al.* (1991) confirmed the earlier work of Keens *et al.* (1985) and showed no increase in frequency or severity in prolonged apnea in 100 siblings of SIDS infants following DTP immunization. Thus, it has been demonstrated convincingly that immunization is not related causally to SIDS.

Metabolic theories

In recent years, a wide variety of inborn errors of metabolism have been identified that may result in sudden and unexpected death (Allison *et al.*, 1988; Anonymous, 1986; Emery, Chandra & Gilbert-Barness, 1988). The most commonly identified abnormality is a deficiency of medium-chain acyl-coenzyme A dehydrogenase (MCAD). This enzyme catalyzes the breakdown of C16–20 fatty acids in one of the major energy-producing pathways in humans, the beta-oxidation pathway. Interruption to the pathway renders an individual susceptible to hypoglycemia, as alternative glycogen reserves are much smaller than fat stores. The possibility of a metabolic defect should be considered particularly in infants presenting with SIDS who have a family history of sudden infant or childhood death.

Frequency

Estimates of the percentage of cases presenting initially as SIDS that are due to a metabolic defect have varied considerably. Although some reports have suggested that as many as 5–20% of SIDS cases are due to occult biochemical derangements (Chace *et al.*, 2001; Emery, Chandra & Gilbert-Barness, 1988; Vawter *et al.*, 1986), and metabolic disorders are associated with ALTEs (Arens *et al.*, 1993b), the figure is probably more in the order of 2–3% or less (Arens *et al.*, 1993a; Bonham & Downing, 1992; Divry *et al.*, 1990; Dundar, Lanyon & Connor, 1993; Green, 1993; Holton *et al.*, 1991; Lemieux *et al.*, 1993; Penzien *et al.*, 1994; Rebuffat *et al.*, 1991). Studies have failed to find evidence of significant hypoglycemia in SIDS infants (Sturner & Susa, 1980; Sumbilla *et al.*, 1983; Tildon & Roeder, 1983), and a study of DNA extracted from paraffin-embedded tissues taken from SIDS infants concluded that MCAD deficiency was not involved in the etiology of SIDS in a significant way (Miller *et al.*, 1992). Normal levels of vitreous free amino acids would seem to exclude aminoacidopathy as a factor in SIDS deaths (Patrick & Logan, 1988).

Pathological features

Features at the time of autopsy that may give a clue to the presence of a metabolic defect are subtle dysmorphism, enlargement or pallor of the liver, splenomegaly, cardiomegaly, and pallor and flabbiness of skeletal muscles (Bennett *et al.*, 1991; Goyco & Beckerman, 1990). Although the presence of mild fatty change in the liver is found occasionally in SIDS autopsies, the finding of lipid droplets within cardiac myocytes, skeletal muscle, and renal tubular cells is more suggestive of an underlying metabolic abnormality (Howat *et al.*, 1985). (Further details are available in Chapter 11.)

Electrolyte derangements

A variety of controversial biochemical changes have been described in infants dying of SIDS. While Richards, Fukumoto & Clardy (1983) found significant differences in vitreous levels of potassium, calcium, phosphorus, and a variety of enzymes in SIDS infants, they qualify their findings by acknowledging that their control group was composed mainly of hospital-treated patients, making the significance of their findings "far from clear." The detection of elevated levels of vitreous sodium has been attributed to the effects of overconcentrated foods (Emery, Swift & Worthy, 1974). Another possible contributing factor may be high levels of sodium in the water supply (Robertson & Parker, 1978). On the other hand, Blumenfeld *et al.* (1979) showed no elevations in postmortem vitreous levels of sodium, potassium, calcium, creatinine, or total protein in SIDS infants. Based on this and other studies that have failed to demonstrate elevated levels of electrolytes, it is extremely unlikely that such biochemical derangements play any role in SIDS deaths.

Endocrine theories

Abnormalities of endocrine function involving the hypothalamic-pituitary axis (Tildon, Chacon & Blair, 1983) and adrenal, parathyroid, and thyroid glands have, at various stages, been proposed as occult causes of sudden death in infancy (Geertinger, 1967).

It appears likely, however, that their contribution to the total number of cases of SIDS is minimal.

Thyroid abnormalities

While raised serum levels of tri-iodothyronine in SIDS infants suggests thyroid dysfunction (Chacon & Tildon, 1981; Peterson, Green & van Belle, 1983), the problem remains of determining the role of this finding in the mechanism of death. It is quite possible that these results may be either coincidental or due to postmortem artifact (Golding, Limerick & Macfarlane, 1985). Although elevation of thyroid hormone levels in an infant who was investigated following an ALTE and who allegedly died of SIDS does mitigate against postmortem artifact in perhaps one case (Ross, Moffat & Reid, 1983), it has been shown convincingly in both human and animal studies that tri-iodothyronine levels increase in serum with increasing postmortem interval (Lee, Strzelecki & Root, 1983; Wellby, Farror & Pannall, 1987).

Miscellaneous

Cortisol and growth hormone levels in SIDS infants are comparable with those in controls (Naeye *et al.*, 1980), and reports of pancreatic pathology in the form of nesidioblastosis in infants dying (or almost dying) suddenly (Aynsley-Green *et al.*, 1978; Polak & Wigglesworth, 1976) must be evaluated critically, given the lack of evidence of significant hypoglycemia in the majority of tested SIDS infants. Subsequent reports have also documented "nesidioblastosis" as part of the normal maturational process (Figure 13.28) (Ariel *et al.*, 1988; Jaffe, Hashida & Yunis, 1982). Histologic and immunohistochemical studies of the pituitary gland have failed to demonstrate specific abnormalities (Reuss, Saeger & Bajanowski, 1994).

Nutritional theories

Trace metal deficiencies

Lack of normal levels of trace metals, in particular magnesium, has been proposed as a cause of SIDS (Caddell, 1972). However, no consistent deficiencies in serum or hepatic levels of zinc, calcium, copper, or

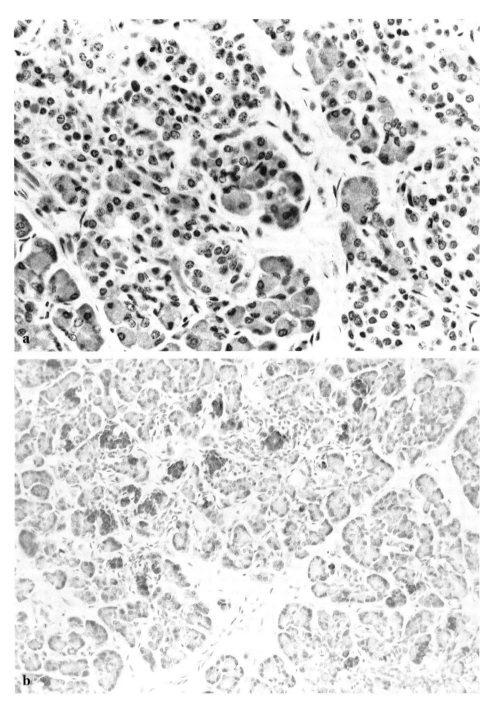

Figure 13.28 Scattered distribution of islet cells throughout the parenchyma of the pancreas (a) (hematoxylin and eosin, ×200), demonstrated more clearly on immunoperoxidase staining for insulin (b) (×110) taken from a two-month-old infant with otherwise typical features of SIDS.

magnesium have been demonstrated subsequently (Hillman, Erickson & Haddad, 1980; Erickson *et al.*, 1983b; Lapin *et al.*, 1976). Vitreous levels of magnesium were even shown to be elevated in one study (Blumenfeld *et al.*, 1979). A possible role for copper deficiency in SIDS (Reid, 1987) is unlikely, since serum levels have been reported as normal (Hillman, Erickson & Haddad, 1980).

Following the observation that selenium deficiency causes sudden death in pigs (Money, 1970) and cardiac damage of the type found in Chinese children with Keshan disease, it was postulated that it may also be involved in the causation of SIDS. However, this connection has not been substantiated (Lapin *et al.*, 1976; McGlashan, 1991; Rhead, 1977; Rhead *et al.*, 1972).

Vitamin deficiencies

A variety of vitamin deficiencies have been implicated in the etiology of SIDS, including a lack of vitamins A, C, D, and E, biotin, and thiamine, but none appears significant. No evidence was found in a subsequent investigation by the Australian College of Pediatrics (Phelan, 1979) to support the suggestion that sudden death in infants was due to vitamin C deficiency (Kalokerinos & Dettman, 1976). Vitamin D deficiency (Kraus *et al.*, 1971) has also not been confirmed as a significant factor in a subsequent study (Hillman, Erickson & Haddad, 1980). There is no evidence to suggest that deficiencies of vitamins A or E play a role in sudden death in humans, despite suggestions that vitamin A deficiency may cause mandibular hypoplasia or pressure on nerves passing through narrowed jugular foramena (Skinner, 1995).

Low levels of hepatic biotin have been reported in SIDS infants (Johnson, Hood & Emery, 1980), but it is difficult to accept that this finding has functional significance given that death in biotin deficiency occurs through hypoglycemia and this has not been a feature of SIDS deaths.

The occurence of apnea in patients with Leigh disease (subacute necrotizing encephalomyelopathy) in association with abnormal thiamine-dependent brainstem function led to the hypothesis that thiamine deficiency could be associated with SIDS (Tildon & Roeder, 1983). Subsequent research results are difficult to interpret, even for the SIDS literature, as deficiencies (Jeffrey, Rahilly & Read, 1983; Jeffrey *et al.*, 1985), normal levels (Peterson *et al.*, 1981), and elevated levels (Davis, Icke & Hilton, 1982; Davis, Icke & Hilton, 1983; Hilton, 1986) of thiamine and associated enzymes have been reported in SIDS victims, their siblings, and infants who have suffered ALTEs. The validity of increased postmortem levels of thiamine must be questioned given that elevation in levels has been demonstrated as a postmortem artifact in deaths from a variety of causes (Wyatt *et al.*, 1984).

Environmental theories

Toxin exposure

The possibility of accumulated toxins causing sudden death in infancy has been investigated extensively. One study demonstrated that lung lead concentrations were elevated (Erickson *et al.*, 1983a), and a further study reported elevated levels of lead in serum from SIDS cases (Drasch, Kretschmer & Lochner, 1988). This was not confirmed in a subsequent study, which could find no difference between SIDS infants and controls in the levels of lead and also in levels of cadmium and chlorohydrocarbons, such as dieldrin and DDT (Kleeman *et al.*, 1991).

The possibility of carbon monoxide poisoning due to faulty domestic heating and ventilation (Cleary, 1984) should also be considered in multiple home deaths, but it is not a factor in the pathogenesis of SIDS (Variend & Forrest, 1987).

Mattress toxins

Richardson (1990, 1994, 1995a, 1995b) hypothesized that a fungus, *Scopulariopsis brevicaulis*, metabolizes antimony-, arsenic-, and phosphorous-based fire-retardant chemicals within mattresses and/or their PVC coverings, producing lethal amounts of highly toxic trihydride gases, stibine, arsine, and phosphine. He then proposed that sleeping infants exposed to these gases die. Despite a number of subsequent investigations, however, this theory has not been proven (Anonymous, 1991; Blair *et al.*, 1995; Cullen *et al.*, 2000; Fleming *et al.*, 1994; Warnock *et al.*, 1995). Specifically, *Scopulariopsis brevicaulis* is not always found within mattresses and is not present in higher concentrations in mattresses of SIDS infants. Under optimum laboratory conditions, the fungus fails to generate trihydride gases, and SIDS infants show no evidence of poisoning by toxic gas. Difficulties may also arise in the interpretation of tissue levels, as small quantities of antimony are routinely ingested in the diet and environmental contamination of reagents and tissues is possible (Beal, 2001b; Byard, Palmer & Towsty, 1995; Cullen *et al.*, 1998; Howatson *et al.*, 1995; Kelley, Allsopp & Hawksworth, 1992). Similarly, there has been no support for Tyler's (1983) theory that SIDS is caused by exposure to ammonia generated from urine.

Homicide

While homicides due to bashing, stabbing, and shooting are not difficult to diagnose because of obvious injuries at autopsy, deliberate suffocation or poisoning of an infant may not be identified as readily (Krous *et al.*, 2002c). Most pathologists have experienced cases where the initial conclusion of SIDS has been changed to homicide when additional information has become available (Byard & Burnell, 1994), and several widely publicized cases have drawn considerable attention to this problem (Firstman & Talan, 1997; Firstman & Talan, 2001). For example, it is now known that two of the infants in Steinschneider's (1972) original paper linking SIDS with ALTEs were victims of homicide (Pinholster, 1994).

The exact number of occult homicides that have been misdiagnosed as SIDS in the past will never be known, but the total number in different jurisdictions is probably inversely proportional to the extent and quality of the investigations. Meadow (1999) reported 42 cases of infant homicide that had been misdiagnosed as SIDS in the UK, raising the probability that the initial investigations and autopsy procedures were of suboptimal quality. Other authors have commented that "investigations into

the pathology and circumstances of sudden infant death are often scanty and inexpert," with significant omissions such as failing to take routine lung histology being documented when cases were audited (Anonymous, 1999; Bacon, 1997). Use of more extensive protocols with special training for police officers and other investigators involved in infant deaths must occur to improve this situation.

Conclusion

One of the aims of this text is to assist in the separation of cases of sudden infant death in which a cause is found from cases in which no adequate explanation for death can be determined. It is the latter group that represents those physiologically compromised infants who truly warrant the label of SIDS. It is apparent, however, that there are several distinct subgroups present.

In one category are found those entities in which the clinical presentation may be identical to SIDS, in that a previously supposedly well infant was found dead in his or her crib. However, at autopsy, a lesion or disease is found that has caused death. It seems most likely that specific conditions in this group, such as overwhelming sepsis, inherited metabolic disorders, and accidental asphyxia, each account for a small subset of cases of sudden and unexpected non-SIDS infant death rather than representing a mysterious "single cause" of SIDS that has previously eluded detection.

In the next category are found those infants with no diseases or lesions found at autopsy to whom the term SIDS can truly be applied. Table 13.9 gives an overview of postulated defects that have been found in infants within this group.

In the final group are those infants in whom the autopsy reveals an abnormality that appears to be significant but whose precise role in the terminal episode is difficult to determine. A lesion may be worthy of note and yet may be secondary or entirely coincidental to the underlying mechanism of death (Byard, 1997b). For example, if an anatomic abnormality such as a high take-off coronary artery is found

Table 13.9. Summary of postulated causal mechanisms responsible for SIDS

Respiratory
    Defective brainstem respiratory control centers
    Defective peripheral pulmonary receptors
    Abnormal surfactant
    Pulmonary immunologic abnormalities
    Intrinsic upper airway obstruction
    Laryngomalacia
    Laryngospasm
    Extrinsic upper airway obstruction
    Rebreathing/toxic gas inhalation
    Overlaying
    Positional asphyxia
    Smothering
Cardiovascular
    Defective brainstem cardiac control centers
    Aberrant conduction pathways
    Prolongation of the QT interval
    Intrapulmonary venous shunting
    Vertebral artery compression
    Cardiac chamber compression
Central and peripheral nervous system
    Defective autonomic control
    Abnormal brainstem nuclei
    Vagal dysfunction
    Chemoreceptor dysfunction
    Arousal/sleep state disturbance
    Hyperpyrexia
    Abnormality of neurotransmitters
    Maturational imbalance
    Increased neuronal degeneration
    Pineal gland abnormalities
    Activation of diving reflex
Gastrointestinal
    Gastric aspiration
    Gastroesophageal reflux
Microbiologic
    Viral infections
    Bacterial sepsis
    Toxigenic bacteria
    Phospholipase A-2-producing bacteria
Immunologic
    Anaphylaxis
    Immunologic incompetence
    Sequel to immunization

Table 13.9. (*cont.*)

Metabolic
    Congenital enzyme deficiencies
Endocrine
    Adrenal insufficiency
    Disturbed calcium metabolism
    Hyperthyroidism
Nutritional
    Vitamin deficiencies
    Deficiencies in trace metals
Environmental
    Toxin exposure
    Hyperthermia
    Sleeping position
Miscellaneous

in an infant with an otherwise typical story of SIDS, then it may still be impossible to exclude SIDS as the cause of death if there is no histologic evidence of myocardial ischemia. The presence of a potentially significant abnormality, however, by definition precludes the diagnosis of SIDS. It is preferable for certification purposes to assign such an infant to a "gray area" and to document the cause of death as "undetermined" or as "sudden unexpected death" in an infant with a certain pathologic lesion. This acknowledges that those mechanisms responsible for SIDS are still a possibility but flags the case as being more complex than usual.

As can be gathered from this chapter, there has been considerable ongoing and often acerbic disagreement in the research literature regarding the contribution of various abnormalities to the mechanism of death in SIDS infants. This not only reflects variability in the quality of different research techniques but also suggests that there is quite probably considerable heterogeneity in pathophysiologic abnormalities present in SIDS infants who do not all exhibit the same kinds of functional impairments or developmental delays. The interrelation of the various predisposing factors may be extremely complex, with great individual variability in the susceptibility of different organ systems to a variety of stresses.

This may mean that the system that is compromised to the point of initiating a lethal episode varies from infant to infant, resulting in variability in the mechanisms responsible for death. This hypothesis may partly explain the tangle of contradictory data in the literature that has built up around that enigmatic "non-diagnosis" that we have chosen to call "SIDS."

REFERENCES

Abramson, H. (1944). Accidental mechanical suffocation in infants. *Journal of Pediatrics*, **25**, 404–13.

Abreu, E., Silva, F. A., Brezinova, V. & Simpson, H. (1982). Sleep apnoea in acute bronchiolitis. *Archives of Disease in Childhood*, **57**, 467–72.

Abreu, E., Silva, F. A., MacFadyen, U. M., Williams, A. & Simpson, H. (1986). Sleep apnoea during upper respiratory infection and metabolic alkalosis in infancy. *Archives of Disease in Childhood*, **61**, 1056–62.

Ackerman, M. J., Siu, B. L., Sturner, W. Q., *et al.* (2001). Postmortem molecular analysis of *SCN5A* defects in sudden infant death syndrome. *Journal of the American Medical Association*, **286**, 2264–9.

Adams, E. J., Chavez, G. F., Steen, D., Shah, R., Iyasu, S. & Krous, H. F. (1998). Changes in the epidemiologic profile of sudden infant death syndrome as rates decline among California infants: 1990–1995. *Pediatrics*, **102**, 1445–51.

Adams, M. M. (1985). The descriptive epidemiology of sudden infant deaths among natives and whites in Alaska. *American Journal of Epidemiology*, **122**, 637–43.

Alessandri, L. M., Read, A. W., Burton, P. R. & Stanley, F. J. (1996). An analysis of sudden infant death syndrome in aboriginal infants. *Early Human Development*, **45**, 235–44.

Alessandri, L. M., Read, A. W., Dawes, V. P., Cooke, C. T., Margolius, K. A. & Cadden, G. A. (1995). Pathology review of sudden and unexpected death in Aboriginal and non-Aboriginal infants. *Paediatric and Perinatal Epidemiology*, **9**, 406–19.

Alexander, R., Smith, W. & Stevenson, R. (1990). Serial Munchausen syndrome by proxy. *Pediatrics*, **86**, 581–5.

Allison, F., Bennett, M. J., Variend, S. & Engel, P. C. (1988). Acyl-coenzyme A dehydrogenase deficiency in heart tissue from infants who died unexpectedly with fatty change in the liver. *British Medical Journal*, **296**, 11–12.

Alm, B., Wennergren, G., Norvenius, G., *et al.* (1999). Caffeine and alcohol as risk factors for sudden infant death syndrome. *Archives of Disease in Childhood*, **81**, 107–11.

Ambler, M. W., Neave, C. & Sturner, W. Q. (1981). Sudden and unexpected death in infancy and childhood. Neuropathological findings. *American Journal of Forensic Medicine and Pathology*, **2**, 23–30.

American Academy of Pediatrics Task Force on Infant Positioning and SIDS (1992). Positioning and SIDS. *Pediatrics*, **89**, 1120–66.

Amir, J., Ashkenazi, S., Schonfeld, T., Weitz, R. & Nitzan, M. (1983). Laryngospasm as a single manifestation of epilepsy. *Archives of Disease in Childhood*, **58**, 151–3.

Anas, N., Boettrich, C., Hall, C. B. & Brooks, J. G. (1982). The association of apnea and respiratory syncytial virus infection in infants. *Journal of Pediatrics*, **101**, 65–8.

Anderson, K. R. & Hill, R. W. (1982). Occlusive lesions of cardiac conducting tissue arteries in sudden infant death syndrome. *Pediatrics*, **69**, 50–52.

Anderson, R. H., Bouton, J., Burrow, C. T. & Smith, A. (1974). Sudden death in infancy: a study of cardiac specialized tissue. *British Medical Journal*, **ii**, 135–9.

Anonymous. (1892). The prevention of overlaying. *Lancet*, **i**, 45.

Anonymous. (1895). The Arcuccio. *British Medical Journal*, **i**, 380.

Anonymous. (1986). Sudden infant death and inherited disorders of fat oxidation. *Lancet*, **ii**, 1073–5.

Anonymous. (1989). Respiratory infection and sudden infant death. *Lancet*, **ii**, 1191–2.

Anonymous. (1991). Mattresses and sudden infant death. *Lancet*, **i**, 1537.

Anonymous. (1999). Unexplained deaths in infancy. *Lancet*, **353**, 161.

Aranda, F. J., Teixeira, F. & Becker, L. E. (1990). Assessment of growth in cases of sudden infant death syndrome. *Neuroepidemiology*, **9**, 95–105.

Arens, R., Gozal, D., Jain, K., *et al.* (1993a). Prevalence of medium-chain acyl-coenzyme A dehydrogenase deficiency in the sudden infant death syndrome. *Journal of Pediatrics*, **122**, 715–18.

Arens, R., Gozal, D., Williams, J. C., Davidson Ward, S. L. & Keens, T. G. (1993b). Recurrent apparent life-threatening events during infancy: a manifestation of inborn errors of metabolism. *Journal of Pediatrics*, **123**, 415–18.

Ariagno, R. L. & Mirmiran, M. (2001). Arousal and brain homeostatic control. In *Sudden Infant Death Syndrome. Problems, Progress and Possibilities*, ed. R. W. Byard & H. F. Krous. London: Arnold, pp. 96–117.

Ariagno, R. L., Guilleminault, C., Baldwin, R. & Owen-Boeddiker, M. (1982). Movement and gastroesophageal reflux in awake term infants with "near-miss" SIDS, unrelated to apnea. *Journal of Pediatrics*, **100**, 894–7.

Ariel, I., Kerem, E., Schwartz-Arad, D., *et al.* (1988). Nesidiodysplasia – a histologic entity? *Human Pathology*, **19**, 1215–18.

Armstrong, D., Sachis, P., Bryan, C. & Becker, L. (1982). Pathological features of persistent infantile sleep apnea with reference to the pathology of sudden infant death syndrome. *Annals of Neurology*, **12**, 169–74.

Armstrong, K. L. & Wood, D. (1991). Can infant death from child abuse be prevented? *Medical Journal of Australia*, **155**, 593–6.

Arneil, G. C., Gibson, A. A. M., McIntosh, H., Brooke, H., Harvie, A. & Patrick, W. J. A. (1985). National post-perinatal infant mortality and cot death study, Scotland 1981–82. *Lancet*, **i**, 740–43.

Arnestad, M. (2002). *Sudden Unexpected Death in Intrauterine Life, Infancy and Early Childhood in Southeast Norway 1984–1999*. Oslo: University of Oslo Press.

Arnestad, M., Andersen, M. & Rognum, T. O. (1997). Is the use of dummy or carry-cot of importance for sudden infant death? *European Journal of Pediatrics*, **156**, 968–70.

Arnestad, M., Opdal, S. H., Musse, M. A., Vege, Å. & Rognum, T. O. (2002). Are substitutions in the first hypervariable region of the mitochondrial DNA displacement-loop in SIDS due to maternal inheritance? *Acta Paediatrica*, **91**, 1060–64.

Arnestad, M., Vege, Å. & Rognum, T. O. (2002). Evaluation of diagnostic tools applied in the examination of sudden unexpected deaths in infancy and early childhood. *Forensic Science International*, **125**, 262–8.

Arnon, S. S. (1983). Breast-feeding and toxigenic intestinal infections: missing links in SIDS? In *Sudden Infant Death Syndrome*, ed. J. A. Tildon, L. M. Roeder & A. Steinschneider. New York: Academic Press, pp. 539–55.

Arnon, S. S., Damus, K. & Chin, J. (1981). Infant botulism: epidemiology and relation to sudden infant death syndrome. *Epidemiologic Review*s, **3**, 45–66.

Arntzen, A., Moum, T., Magnus, P. & Bakketeig, L. S. (1995). Is the higher postneonatal mortality in lower social status groups due to SIDS? *Acta Paediatrica*, **84**, 188–92.

Arsenault, P. S. (1980). Maternal and antenatal factors in the risk of sudden infant death syndrome. *American Journal of Epidemiology*, **111**, 279–84.

Atkinson, J. B., Evans, O. B., Ellison, R. S. & Netsky, M. G. (1984). Ischemia of the brain stem as a cause of sudden infant death syndrome. *Archives of Pathology and Laboratory Medicine*, **108**, 341–2.

Aynsley-Green, A., Polak, J. M., Keeling, J., Gough, M. H. & Baum, J. D. (1978). Averted sudden neonatal death due to pancreatic nesidioblastosis. *Lancet*, **i**, 550–51.

Baba, N., Quattrochi, J. J., Reiner, C. B., Adrion, W., McBride, P. T. & Yates, A. J. (1983). Possible role of the brain stem in sudden infant death syndrome. *Journal of the American Medical Association*, **249**, 2789–91.

Babson, S. G. & Clarke, N. G. (1983). Relationship between infant death and maternal age. Comparison of sudden infant death incidence with other causes of infant mortality. *Journal of Pediatrics*, **103**, 391–3.

Baccino, E., Le Goff, D., Lancien, G., Le Guillou, M., Alix, D. & Mottier, D. (1988). Exploration of acid gastroesophageal reflux by 24-H pH metry in infants at risk of sudden infant death syndrome: a study of 50 cases. *Forensic Science International*, **36**, 255–60.

Bacon, C. J. (1983). Over heating in infancy. *Archives of Disease in Childhood*, **58**, 673–4.

Bacon, C. J. (1997). Cot death after CESDI. *Archives of Disease in Childhood*, **76**, 171–3.

Bailey, H. & Love, M. (1959). *A Short Practice of Surgery*, 11th edn. London: H. K. Lewis & Co., p. 252.

Ballenden, N. R., Laster, K. & Lawrence, J. A. (1993). Pathologist as gatekeeper: discretionary decision-making in cases of sudden infant death. *Australian Journal of Social Issues*, **28**, 124–39.

Baraff, L. J., Ablon, W. J. & Weiss, R. C. (1983). Possible temporal association between diphtheria-tetanus toxoid-pertussis vaccination and sudden infant death syndrome. *Pediatric Infectious Disease*, **2**, 7–11.

Bartholomew, S. E. M., MacArthur, B. A. & Bain, A. D. (1987). Sudden infant death syndrome in south east Scotland. *Archives of Disease in Childhood*, **62**, 951–6.

Bass, M. (1989). The fallacy of the simultaneous sudden infant death syndrome in twins. *American Journal of Forensic Medicine and Pathology*, **10**, 200–205.

Bass, M., Kravath, R. E. & Glass, L. (1986). Death-scene investigation in sudden infant death. *New England Journal of Medicine*, **315**, 100–105.

Bauchner, H., Zuckerman, B., McClain, M., Frank, D., Fried, L. E. & Kayne, H. (1988). Risk of sudden infant death syndrome among infants with *in utero* exposure to cocaine. *Journal of Pediatrics*, **113**, 831–4.

Bayes, B. J. (1974). Prone infants and SIDS. *New England Journal of Medicine*, **290**, 693–4.

Beal, S. M. (1983). Some epidemiological factors about sudden infant death syndrome (SIDS) in South Australia. In *Sudden Infant Death Syndrome*, ed. J. A. Tildon, L. M. Roeder & A. Steinschneider. New York: Academic Press, pp. 15–28.

Beal, S. (1986a). Sudden infant death syndrome. MD thesis, Flinders University of South Australia, Australia.

Beal, S. M. (1986b). Sudden infant death syndrome: epidemiological comparisons between South Australia and communities with a different incidence. *Australian Paediatric Journal*, **22** (Suppl), 13–16.

Beal, S. (1988a). Sleeping position and SIDS. *Lancet*, **ii**, 512.

Beal, S. (1988b). Sleeping position and sudden infant death syndrome. *Medical Journal of Australia*, 149, 562.

Beal, S. (1989). Sudden infant death syndrome in twins. *Pediatrics*, 84, 1038–44.

Beal, S. M. (1990). SIDS and immunization. *Medical Journal of Australia*, 153, 117.

Beal, S. (1991). Sudden infant death syndrome related to sleeping position and bedding. *Medical Journal of Australia,* 155, 507–8.

Beal, S. (1992a). Apparent life threatening events with serious sequelae in infants and young children. *Journal of Paediatrics and Child Health*, 28, 151–5.

Beal, S. M. (1992b). Siblings of sudden infant death syndrome victims. *Clinics in Perinatology*, 19, 839–48.

Beal, S. M. (1996). Sudden infant death syndrome. *Medical Journal of Australia*, 165, 179–80.

Beal, S. M. (2001a). Recurrence of sudden unexpected infant death in a family. In *Sudden Infant Death Syndrome. Problems, Progress and Possibilities*, ed. R. W. Byard & H. F. Krous. London: Arnold, pp. 283–90.

Beal, S. M. (2001b). The rise and fall of several theories. In *Sudden Infant Death Syndrome. Problems, Progress and Possibilities*, ed. R. W. Byard & H. F. Krous. London: Arnold, pp. 236–42.

Beal, S. M. & Blundell H. K. (1988). Recurrence incidence of sudden infant death syndrome. *Archives of Disease in Childhood*, 63, 924–30.

Beal, S. M. & Byard, R. W. (1995). Accidental death or sudden infant death syndrome? *Journal of Paediatrics and Child Health*, 31, 269–71.

Beal, S. M. & Byard, R. W. (2000). Sudden infant death syndrome in South Australia 1968–1997. Part 3: is bed-sharing safer for infants? *Journal of Paediatrics and Child Health*, 36, 552–4.

Beal, S. M. & Finch, C. F. (1991). An overview of retrospective case–control studies investigating the relationship between prone sleeping position and SIDS. *Journal of Paediatrics and Child Health*, 27, 334–9.

Beal, S. & Porter, C. (1991). Sudden infant death syndrome related to climate. *Acta Paediatrica Scandinavica*, 80, 278–87.

Beal, S., Need, M. & Byard, R. W. (1994). Which infants are no longer dying because of avoidance of prone sleeping? *Medical Journal of Australia*, 160, 660.

Becker, L. E. (1983). Neuropathological basis for respiratory dysfunction in sudden infant death syndrome. In *Sudden Infant Death Syndrome*, ed. J. A. Tildon, L. M. Roeder & A. Steinschneider. New York: Academic Press, pp. 99–114.

Becker, L. E. (1990). Neural maturational delay as a link in the chain of events leading to SIDS. *Canadian Journal of Neurological Sciences*, 17, 361–71.

Becker, L. E. & Takashima, S. (1985). Chronic hypoventilation and development of brain stem gliosis. *Neuropediatrics*, 16, 19–23.

Becker, L. E., Zhang, W. & Pereyra, P. M. (1993). Delayed maturation of the vagus nerve in sudden infant death syndrome. *Acta Neuropathologica*, 86, 617–22.

Beckwith, J. B. (1970a). Discussion of terminology and definition of the sudden infant death syndrome. In *Sudden Infant Death Syndrome*, ed. A. B. Bergman, J. B. Beckwith & C. G. Ray. Seattle: University of Washington Press, pp. 14–22.

Beckwith, J. B. (1970b). Observations on the pathological anatomy of the sudden infant death syndrome. In *Sudden Infant Death Syndrome*, ed. A. B. Bergman, J. B. Beckwith & C. G. Ray. Seattle: University of Washington Press, pp. 83–103.

Beckwith, J. B. (1973). The sudden infant death syndrome. *Current Problems in Pediatrics*, 3, 1–36.

Beckwith, J. B. (1975). The sudden infant death syndrome: a new theory. *Pediatrics*, 55, 583–4.

Beckwith, J. B. (1983). Chronic hypoxemia in the sudden infant death syndrome: a critical review of the data base. In *Sudden Infant Death Syndrome*, ed. J. A. Tildon, L. M. Roeder & A. Steinschneider. New York: Academic Press, pp. 145–59.

Beckwith, J. B. (1988). Intrathoracic petechial hemorrhages: a clue to the mechanism of death in sudden infant death syndrome? *Annals of New York Academy of Sciences*, 533, 37–47.

Beckwith, J. B. (1989). The mechanism of death in sudden infant death syndrome. In *Sudden Infant Death Syndrome. Medical Aspects and Psychological Management*, ed. J. L. Culbertson, H. F. Krous & R. D. Bendell. London: Edward Arnold, pp. 48–61.

Beckwith, J. B. (1993). A proposed new definition of sudden infant death syndrome. In *Second SIDS International Conference*, ed. A. M. Walker & C. McMillen. Ithaca: Perinatology Press, pp. 421–4.

Beckwith, J. B. (2003). Defining the sudden infant death syndrome. *Archives of Pediatric and Adolescent Medicine*, 157, 286–90.

Becroft, D. M. & Lockett, B. K. (1997). Intra-alveolar pulmonary siderophages in sudden infant death: a marker for previous imposed suffocation. *Pathology*, 29, 60–63.

Becroft, D. M. O., Thompson, J. M. D. & Mitchell, E. A. (1998). Epidemiology of intrathoracic petechial hemorrhages in sudden infant death syndrome. *Pediatric and Developmental Pathology*, 1, 200–209.

Becroft, D. M., Thompson, J. M. & Mitchell, E. A. (2001). Nasal and intrapulmonary haemorrhage in sudden infant death syndrome. *Archives of Disease in Childhood*, 85, 116–20.

Benjamin, D. R. & Siebert, J. R. (1990). C-reactive protein and prealbumin in suspected sudden infant death syndrome. *Pediatric Pathology*, 10, 503–7.

Bennett, M. J., Hale, D. E., Coates, P. M. & Stanley, C. A. (1991). Postmortem recognition of fatty acid oxidation disorders. *Pediatric Pathology*, **11**, 365–70.

Bergman, A. B. & Wiesner, L. A. (1976). Relationship of passive cigarette-smoking to sudden infant death syndrome. *Pediatrics*, **58**, 665–8.

Bergstrom, L., Lagercrantz, H. & Terenius, L. (1984). Postmortem analyses of neuropeptides in brains from sudden infant death victims. *Brain Research*, **323**, 279–85.

Bernier, R. H., Frank, J. A., Jr, Dondero, T. J., Jr & Turner, P. (1982). Diphtheria-tetanus toxoids-pertussis vaccination and sudden infant deaths in Tennessee. *Journal of Pediatrics*, **101**, 419–21.

Bernstein, M. L. & Weakley-Jones, B. (1987). "Sudden infant death" associated with hypohidrotic ectodermal dysplasia. *Journal of the Kentucky Medical Association*, **85**, 191–4.

Bernstein, R., Hatchuel, I. & Jenkins, T. (1980). Hypohidrotic ectodermal dysplasia and sudden infant death syndrome. *Lancet*, **i**, 1024.

Berry, J., Allibone, E., McKeever, P., Moore, I., Wright, C. & Fleming, P. (2000). The pathology study: the contribution of ancillary pathology tests to the investigation of unexpected infant death. In *Sudden Unexpected Deaths in Infancy. The CESDI SUDI Studies 1993–1996*, ed. P. Fleming, P. Blair, C. Bacon & J. Berry. London: The Stationary Office, pp. 97–112.

Berry, P. J. (1992). Pathological findings in SIDS. *Journal of Clinical Pathology*, **45** (Suppl), 11–16.

Berry, P. J. & Keeling, J. W. (1989). The investigation of sudden unexpected death in infancy. In *Recent Advances in Histopathology*, vol. 14, ed. P. P. Anthony & R. N. M. MacSween. Edinburgh: Churchill Livingstone, pp. 251–79.

Bettelheim, K. A., Evangelidis, H., Pearce, J. L., Goldwater, P. N. & Luke, R. K. J. (1993). The isolation of cytotoxic necrotizing factor (CNF)-producing *Escherichia coli* from the intestinal contents of babies who died of sudden infant death syndrome (SIDS) and other causes as well as from the faeces of healthy babies. *Comparative Immunology, Microbiology and Infectious Diseases*, **16**, 87–90.

Bettelheim, K. A., Goldwater, P. N., Dwyer, B. W., Bourne, A. J. & Smith, D. L. (1990). Toxigenic *Escherichia coli* associated with sudden infant death syndrome. *Scandinavian Journal of Infectious Diseases*, **22**, 467–76.

Bettiol, S. S., Radcliff, F. J., Hunt, A. L. C. & Goldsmid, J. M. (1994). Bacterial flora of Tasmanian SIDS infants with special reference to pathogenic strains of *Escherichia coli*. *Epidemiology of Infection*, **112**, 275–84.

Bharati, S., Krongrad, E. & Lev, M. (1985). Study of the conduction system in a population of patients with sudden infant death syndrome. *Pediatric Cardiology*, **6**, 29–40.

Biering-Sørensen, F., Jorgensen, T. & Hilden, J. (1978). Sudden infant death in Copenhagen 1956–71. I. Infant feeding. *Acta Paediatrica Scandinavica*, **67**, 129–37.

Biering-Sørensen, F., Jorgensen, T. & Hilden, J. (1979). Sudden infant death in Copenhagen 1956–71. II. Social factors and morbidity. *Acta Paediatrica Scandinavica*, **68**, 1–9.

Blackwell, C. C., Saadi, A. T., Raza, M. W., Stewart, J. & Weir, D. M. (1992). Susceptibility to infection in relation to SIDS. *Journal of Clinical Pathology*, **45** (Suppl), 20–24.

Blackwell, C. C., Weir, D. M., Busuttil, A., *et al.* (1994). The role of infectious agents in sudden infant death syndrome. *FEMS Immunology and Medical Microbiology*, **9**, 91–100.

Blackwell, C. C., Weir, D. M. & Busuttil, A. (1995). Infectious agents, the inflammatory responses of infants and sudden infant death syndrome (SIDS). *Molecular Medicine Today*, **1**, 72–8.

Blackwell, C. C., Weir, D. M., Busuttil, A., *et al.* (1995). Infection, inflammation, and the developmental stage of infants: a new hypothesis for the aetiology of SIDS. In *Sudden Infant Death Syndrome. New Trends in the Nineties*, ed. T. O. Rognum. Oslo: Scandinavian University Press, pp. 189–98.

Blackwell, C. C., Weir, D. M. & Busuttil, A. (1997). Infectious agents and SIDS: analysis of risk factors and preventative measures. *Journal of Sudden Infant Death Syndrome and Infant Mortality*, **2**, 61–76.

Blackwell, C. C., Weir, D. M. & Busuttil, A. (2001). A microbiological perspective. In *Sudden Infant Death Syndrome. Problems, Progress and Possibilities*, ed. R. W. Byard & H. F. Krous. London: Arnold, pp. 182–208.

Blair, P., Fleming, P., Bensley, D., Smith, I., Bacon, C. & Taylor, E. (1995). Plastic mattresses and sudden infant death syndrome. *Lancet*, **345**, 720.

Blair, P. S., Fleming, P. J., Bensley, D., *et al.* (1996). Smoking and the sudden infant death syndrome: results from 1993–5 case–control study for confidential inquiry into stillbirths and deaths in infancy. *British Medical Journal*, **313**, 195–8.

Blair, P. S., Fleming, P. J., Smith, I. J., *et al.* (1999). Babies sleeping with parents: case–control study of factors influencing the risk of the sudden infant death syndrome. *British Medical Journal*, **319**, 1457–62.

Blair, P. S., Nadin, P., Cole, T. J., *et al.* (2000). Weight gain and sudden infant death syndrome: changes in weight z scores may identify infants at increased risk. *Archives of Disease in Childhood*, **82**, 462–9.

Bloch, A. (1973). Sudden infant death syndrome in the Ashkelon district. A 10–year survey. *Israeli Journal of Medical Science*, **9**, 452–8.

Blok, J. H. (1978). The incidence of sudden infant death syndrome in North Carolina's cities and counties: 1972–1974. *American Journal of Public Health*, **68**, 367–72.

Blumenfeld, T. A., Mantell, C. H., Catherman, R. L. & Blanc, W. A. (1979). Postmortem vitreous humor chemistry in sudden infant death syndrome and in other causes of death in childhood. *American Journal of Clinical Pathology*, **71**, 219–23.

Bolton, D. P. G., Cross, K. W. & McKettrick, A. C. (1972). Are babies in carry cots at risk from CO_2 accumulation? *British Medical Journal*, **4**, 80–81.

Bolton, D. P. G., Taylor, B. J., Campbell, A. J., Galland, B. C. & Cresswell, C. (1993). Rebreathing expired gases from bedding: a cause of cot death? *Archives of Disease in Childhood*, **69**, 187–90.

Bonham, J. R. & Downing, M. (1992). Metabolic deficiencies and SIDS. *Journal of Clinical Pathology*, **45** (Suppl), 33–8.

Bonser, R. S. A., Knight, B. H. & West, R. R. (1978). Sudden infant death syndrome in Cardiff, association with epidemic influenza and with temperature – 1955–1974. *International Journal of Epidemiology*, **7**, 335–40.

Borman, B., Fraser, J. & de Boer, G. (1988). A national study of sudden infant death syndrome in New Zealand. *New Zealand Medical Journal*, **101**, 413–15.

Boulloche, J., Mallet, E., Basuyau, J. P., Tayot, P. & Samson-Dollfus, D. (1986). The value of serum IgE assay in milk aspiration and the sudden infant death syndrome. *Acta Paediatrica Scandinavica*, **75**, 530–33.

Bourne, A. J., Beal, S. M. & Byard, R. W. (1994). Bed sharing and sudden infant death syndrome. *British Medical Journal*, **308**, 537–8.

Bowden, K. M. (1952). Overlaying of infants. *Medical Journal of Australia*, **ii**, 609–11.

Boyd, W. (1931). *The Pathology of Internal Diseases*. Philadelphia: Lea & Febiger, pp. 675–6.

Brady, J. P., Ariagno, R. L., Watts, J. L., Goldman, S. L. & Dumpit, F. M. (1978). Apnea, hypoxemia and aborted sudden infant death syndrome. *Pediatrics*, **62**, 686–91.

British Paediatric Association, Standing Committee on Nutrition. (1994). Is breast feeding beneficial in the UK? *Archives of Disease in Childhood*, **71**, 376–80.

Brooke, H., Gibson, A., Tappin, D. & Brown, H. (1997). Case–control study of sudden infant death syndrome in Scotland, 1992–5. *British Medical Journal*, **314**, 1516–20.

Brooks, J. G. (1982). Apnea of infancy and sudden infant death syndrome. *American Journal of Diseases of Children*, **136**, 1012–23.

Brooks, J. G. (1988). Infantile apnea and home monitoring. *Pediatrician*, **15**, 212–16.

Brooks, J. G. (1992). Apparent life-threatening events and apnea of infancy. *Clinics in Perinatology*, **19**, 809–38.

Brooks, J. G. (1998). SIDS and ALTE. In *Kendig's Disorders of the Respiratory Tract in Children*, 6th edn, ed. V. Chernick & T. F. Boat. Philadelphia: W. B. Saunders Co., pp. 1166–72.

Brouillette, R. T. & Thach, B. T. (1979). A neuromuscular mechanism maintaining extrathoracic airway patency. *Journal of Applied Physiology*, **46**, 772–9.

Buck, G. M., Cookfair, D. L., Michaelek, A. M., *et al.* (1989). Intrauterine growth retardation and risk of sudden infant death syndrome (SIDS). *American Journal of Epidemiology*, **129**, 874–84.

Bulterys, M. (1990). High incidence of sudden infant death syndrome among northern Indians and Alaska Natives compared with southwestern Indians: possible role of smoking. *Journal of Community Health*, **15**, 185–94.

Burchfield, D. J. & Rawlings, D. J. (1991). Sudden deaths and apparent life-threatening events in hospitalized neonates presumed to be healthy. *American Journal of Diseases of Children*, **145**, 1319–22.

Burnell, R. H. & Beal, S. M. (1994). Monitoring and sudden infant death. *Journal of Paediatrics and Child Health*, **30,** 461–2.

Burnell, R. H. & Byard, R. W. (2002). Are these really SIDS deaths? – Not by definition. *Journal of Paediatrics and Child Health*, **38**, 623–4.

Byard, R. W. (1991a). Possible mechanisms responsible for the sudden infant death syndrome. *Journal of Paediatrics and Child Health*, **27**, 147–57.

Byard, R. W. (1991b). Recurrent cyanotic episodes with severe arterial hypoxaemia and intrapulmonary shunting: a mechanism for sudden death. *Archives of Disease in Childhood*, **66**, 369.

Byard, R. W. (1994a). Sudden infant death syndrome: historical background, possible mechanisms and diagnostic problems. *Journal of Law and Medicine*, **2**, 18–26.

Byard, R. W. (1994b). Is co-sleeping in infancy a desirable or dangerous practice? *Journal of Paediatrics and Child Health*, **30**, 198–9.

Byard, R. W. (1995). Sudden infant death syndrome – a 'diagnosis' in search of a disease. *Journal of Clinical Forensic Medicine*, **2**, 121–8.

Byard, R. W. (1996a). Sudden infant death syndrome: the mystery continues. *Australian Family Physician*, **25,** 210–15.

Byard, R. W. (1996b). Hazardous infant and early childhood sleeping environments and death scene examination. *Journal of Clinical Forensic Medicine*, **3**, 115–22.

Byard, R. W. (1997a). Issues in diagnosis following the sudden infant death syndrome intervention campaigns. *Journal of Paediatrics and Child Health*, **33**, 467–8.

Byard, R. W. (1997b). Significant coincidental findings at autopsy in accidental childhood death. *Medicine, Science and the Law*, **37**, 259–62.

Byard, R. W. (1998). Is breast feeding in bed always a safe practice? *Journal of Paediatrics and Child Health*, **34**, 418–19.

Byard, R. W. (2001a). Inaccurate classification of infant deaths in Australia: a persistent and pervasive problem. *Medical Journal of Australia*, **175**, 5–7.

Byard, R. W. (2001b). SIDS families. *Australian Doctor*, November 9, 1–8.

Byard, R. W. & Beal, S. M. (1993). Munchausen syndrome by proxy: repetitive infantile apnoea and homicide. *Journal of Paediatrics and Child Health*, **29**, 77–9.

Byard, R. W. & Beal, S. M. (1995). Has changing diagnostic preference been responsible for the recent fall in incidence of sudden infant death syndrome in South Australia? *Journal of Paediatrics and Child Health*, **31**, 197–9.

Byard, R. W. & Beal, S. M. (2000). Gastric aspiration and sleeping position in infancy and early childhood. *Journal of Paediatrics and Child Health*, **36**, 403–5.

Byard, R. W. & Burnell, R. H. (1994). Covert video surveillance in Munchausen syndrome by proxy. Ethical compromise or essential technique? *Medical Journal of Australia*, **160**, 352–6.

Byard, R. W. & Burnell, R. H. (1995). Apparent life threatening events and infant holding practices. *Archives of Disease in Childhood*, **73**, 502–4.

Byard, R. W. & Hilton, J. (1997). Overlaying, accidental suffocation, and sudden infant death. *Journal of Sudden Infant Death Syndrome and Infant Mortality*, **2**, 161–5.

Byard, R. W. & Krous, H. F. (1995). Minor inflammatory lesions and sudden infant death: cause, coincidence or epiphenomena? *Pediatric Pathology*, **15**, 649–54.

Byard, R. W. & Krous, H. F. (1999a). Suffocation, shaking and sudden infant death syndrome: can we tell the difference? *Journal of Paediatrics and Child Health*, **35**, 432–3.

Byard, R. W. & Krous, H. F. (1999b). Petechial hemorrhages and unexpected infant death. *Legal Medicine*, **1**, 193–7.

Byard, R. W. & Krous, H. F. (2001). *Sudden Infant Death Syndrome. Problems, Progress and Possibilities*. London: Arnold.

Byard, R. W. & Krous, H. F. (2003a). Sudden infant death syndrome – an overview and update. *Pediatric and Developmental Pathology*, **6**, 112–27.

Byard, R. W. & Krous, H. F. (2003b). Sudden infant death syndrome – definition and diagnostic trends. *Journal of the Japanese SIDS Research Society*, **3**, 11–16.

Byard, R. W. & Moore, L. (1993a). Can thymic petechiae be used to separate SIDS infants from controls? *Pathology*, **28**, (Suppl 7).

Byard, R. W. & Moore, L. (1993b). Gastroesophageal reflux and sudden infant death syndrome. *Pediatric Pathology*, **13**, 53–7.

Byard, R. W., Beal, S., Blackbourne, B., Nadeau, J. M. & Krous, H. F. (2001). Specific dangers associated with infants sleeping on sofas. *Journal of Paediatrics and Child Health*, **37**, 476–78.

Byard, R. W., Beal, S. M. & Bourne, A. J. (1994). Potentially dangerous sleeping environments and accidental asphyxia in infancy and early childhood. *Archives of Disease in Childhood*, **71**, 497–500.

Byard, R. W., Becker, L. E., Berry, P. J., *et al.* (1996). The pathological approach to sudden infant death – consensus or confusion? Recommendations from the 2nd SIDS Global Strategy Meeting, Stavangar, Norway, August 1994, and the 3rd Australasian SIDS Global Strategy Meeting, Gold Coast, Australia, May 1995. *American Journal of Forensic Medicine and Pathology*, **17**, 103–5.

Byard, R. W., Bourne, A. J., Burnell, R. H. & Roberton, D. M. (1991). No association between DTP vaccination and SIDS. *Medical Journal of Australia* **155**, 135–6.

Byard, R. W., Byers, S., Moore, A., Leppard, P. & Fazzalari, N. (1997a). Morphometric assessment of bone and growth plate in sudden infant death syndrome. *Journal of Sudden Infant Death Syndrome and Infant Mortality*, **2**, 151–60.

Byard, R. W., Carmichael, E. & Beal, S. (1994). How useful is postmortem examination in sudden infant death syndrome? *Pediatric Pathology*, **14**, 817–22.

Byard, R. W., Donald, T. & Chivell, W. (1999). Non-lethal and subtle inflicted injury and unexpected infant death. *Journal of Law and Medicine*, **7,** 47–52.

Byard, R. W., Foster, B. K. & Byers, S. (1993). Immunohistochemical characterisation of the costochondral junction in SIDS. *Journal of Clinical Pathology*, **46**, 108–12.

Byard, R. W., James, R. A. & Felgate, P. (2002). Detecting organic toxins in possible fatal poisonings – a diagnostic problem. *Journal of Clinical Forensic Medicine*, **9**, 85–8.

Byard, R. W., Mackenzie, J. & Beal, S. M. (1995). Vaccination and SIDS: information from the South Australian SIDS Database. *Medical Journal of Australia*, **163**, 443–4.

Byard, R. W., Mackenzie, J. & Beal, S. M. (1997a). Formal retrospective case review and sudden infant death. *Acta Paediatrica*, **86**, 1011–12.

Byard, R. W., Mackenzie, J. & Beal, S. M. (1997b). Immunization and sudden infant death syndrome in South Australia – report from the South Australian SIDS database. In *Current Topics in Forensic Science*, vol. 3. Ottawa: Shunderson Communications, pp. 278–9.

Byard, R. W., Makrides, M., Need, M., Neumann, M. A. & Gibson, R. A. (1995). Sudden infant death syndrome: effect of breast and formula feeding on frontal cortex and brainstem lipid levels. *Journal of Paediatrics and Child Health*, **31**, 14–16.

Byard, R. W., Moore, L., Bourne, A. J., Lawrence, A. J. & Goldwater, P. N. (1992). *Clostridium botulinum* and sudden infant death syndrome: a 10 year prospective study. *Journal of Pediatrics and Child Health*, **28**, 156–7.

Byard, R. W., Palmer, L. & Towsty A. (1995). Antimony detected in necropsy tissues may derive from contaminated formalin. *Lancet*, **346**, 1633–4.

Byard, R. W., Stewart, W. A. & Beal, S. M. (1996). Pathological findings in SIDS infants found in the supine position compared to the prone. *Journal of Sudden Infant Death Syndrome and Infant Mortality*, **1**, 45–50.

Byard, R. W., Stewart, W. A., Telfer, S. & Beal S. M. (1997b). Assessment of pulmonary and intrathymic hemosiderin deposition in sudden infant death syndrome. *Pediatric Pathology and Laboratory Medicine*, **17**, 275–82.

Caddell, J. L. (1972). Magnesium deprivation in sudden unexpected infant death. *Lancet*, **ii**, 258–62.

Campbell, M. J., Rodrigues, L., Macfarlane, A. J. & Murphy, M. F. G. (1991). Sudden infant deaths and cold weather: was the rise in infant mortality in 1986 in England and Wales due to the weather? *Paediatric and Perinatal Epidemiology*, **5**, 93–100.

Carmichael, E. M., Goldwater, P. N. & Byard, R. W. (1996). Routine microbiological testing in sudden and unexpected infant death. *Journal of Paediatrics and Child Health*, **32**, 412–15.

Carpenter, R. G., Gardner, A., Pursall, E., McWeeny, P. M. & Emery, J. L. (1979). Identification of some infants at immediate risk of dying unexpectedly and justifying intensive study. *Lancet*, **ii**, 343–6.

Carr, J. L. (1945). Status thymico-lymphaticus. *Journal of Pediatrics*, **27**, 1–43.

Cashell, A. W. (1987). Homicide as a cause of the sudden infant death syndrome. *American Journal of Forensic Medicine and Pathology*, **8**, 256–8.

Castro, E. C. C. & Peres, L. C. (1999). Vocal cord basement membrane in non-sudden infant death syndrome cases. *Pediatric and Developmental Pathology*, **2**, 440–45.

Centers for Disease Control and Prevention (1979). DTP vaccination and sudden infant deaths – Tennessee. *Morbidity and Mortality Weekly Report*, **28**, 131–2.

Centers for Disease Control and Prevention (1987). Premature mortality due to sudden infant death syndrome – United States, 1980–1986. *Morbidity and Mortality Weekly Report*, **36**, 236–9.

Centers for Disease Control and Prevention (1992). Sudden infant death syndrome – United States, 1980–1988. *Morbidity and Mortality Weekly Report*, **41**, 515–17.

Centers for Disease Control and Prevention. (1996). Guidelines for death scene investigation of sudden unexplained infant deaths: recommendations of the Interagency Panel on Sudden Infant Death Syndrome. *Morbidity and Mortality Weekly Report*, **45**, 1–22.

Chace, D. H., DiPerna, J. C., Mitchell, B. L., Sgroi, B., Hofman, L. F. & Naylor, E. W. (2001). Electrospray tandem mass spectrometry for analysis of acylcarnitines in dried postmortem blood specimens collected at autopsy from infants with unexplained cause of death. *Clinical Chemistry*, **47**, 1166–82.

Chacon, M. A. & Tildon, J. T. (1981). Elevated levels of triiodothyronine in victims of sudden death syndrome. *Journal of Pediatrics*, **99**, 758–60.

Chasnoff, I. J., Hunt, C. E., Kletter, R. & Kaplan, D. (1989). Prenatal cocaine exposure is associated with respiratory pattern abnormalities. *American Journal of Diseases of Children*, **143**, 583–7.

Chavez, C. J., Ostrea, E. M., Jr, Stryker, J. C. & Smialek, Z. (1979). Sudden infant death syndrome among infants of drug-dependent mothers. *Journal of Pediatrics*, **95**, 407–9.

Cherry, J. D., Brunell, P. A., Golden, G. S. & Karzon, D. T. (1988). Report of the task force on pertussis and pertussis immunization – 1988. *Pediatrics*, **81** (Suppl), 939–84.

Chiodini, B. A. & Thach, B. T. (1993). Impaired ventilation in infants sleeping facedown: potential significance for sudden infant death syndrome. *Journal of Pediatrics*, **123**, 686–92.

Chong, A., Murphy, N. & Matthews, T. (2000). Effect of prone sleeping on circulatory control in infants. *Archives of Disease in Childhood*. **82**, 253–6.

Clancy, R. R. & Spitzer, A. R. (1985). Cerebral cortical function in infants at risk for sudden infant death syndrome. *Annals of Neurology*, **18**, 41–7.

Cleary, J. (1984). Carbon monoxide and cot death. *Lancet*, **ii**, 1403.

Cohle, S. D. & Lie, J. T. (1990). Cardiac conduction system in young adults. Paper presented at the 12th World Triennial Meeting of the International Association of Forensic Sciences, Adelaide, Australia, 25–27 October, 1990.

Colditz, P. B., Henry, R. L. & de Silva, L. M. (1982). Apnoea and bronchiolitis due to respiratory syncytial virus. *Australian Paediatric Journal*, **18**, 53–4.

Cole, S., Lindenberg, L. B., Galioto, F. M., Jr, *et al.* (1979). Ultrastructural abnormalities of the carotid body in sudden infant death syndrome. *Pediatrics*, **63**, 13–17.

Coombs, R. R. A. & McLaughlan, P. (1982). The enigma of cot death: is the modified-anaphylaxis hypothesis an explanation for some cases? *Lancet*, **i**, 1388–9.

Coombs, R. R. A. & McLaughlan, P. (1983). The modified anaphylactic hypothesis for sudden infant death syndrome. In

Sudden Infant Death Syndrome, ed. J. A. Tildon, L. M. Roeder & A. Steinschneider. New York: Academic Press, pp. 531–8.

Cooperstock, M. S., Steffen, E., Yolken, R. & Onderdonk, A. (1982). *Clostridium difficile* in normal infants and sudden infant death syndrome: an association with infant formula feeding. *Pediatrics*, **70**, 91–5.

Cordner, S. M. & Willinger, M. (1995). The definition of the sudden infant death syndrome. In *Sudden Infant Death Syndrome. New Trends in the Nineties*, ed. T. O. Rognum. Oslo: Scandinavian University Press, pp. 17–20.

Coryllos, E. (1982). Vagal dysfunction and sudden infant death syndrome. One possible cause and its management. *New York State Journal of Medicine*, **82**, 731–5.

Coumbe, A., Fox, J. D., Briggs, M., Tedder, R. S. & Berry, C. L. (1990). Cytomegalovirus and human herpesvirus-6 in sudden infant death syndrome: an *in situ* hybridization study. *Pediatric Pathology*, **10**, 483–90.

Cozzi, F., Albani, R. & Cardi, E. (1979). A common pathophysiology for sudden cot death and sleep apnoea. "The vacuum-glossoptosis syndrome." *Medical Hypotheses*, **5**, 329–38.

Cullen, A., Kiberd, B., Devaney, D., *et al.* (2000). Concentrations of antimony in infants dying from SIDS and infants dying from other causes. *Archives of Disease in Childhood*. **82**, 244–7.

Cullen, A., Kiberd, B., Matthews, T., Mayne, P., Delves, H. T. & O'Regan, M. (1998). Antimony in blood and urine of infants. *Journal of Clinical Pathology*, **51**, 238–40.

Cullity, G. J. & Emery, J. L. (1975). Ulceration and necrosis of vocal cords in hospital and unexpected child deaths. *Journal of Pathology*, **115**, 27–31.

Cutz, E. & Jackson, A. (2001). Airway inflammation and peripheral chemoreceptors. In *Sudden Infant Death Syndrome. Problems, Progress and Possibilities*, ed. R. W. Byard & H. F. Krous. London: Arnold, pp. 156–81.

Cutz, E., Chan, W. & Perrin, D. G. (1988). Pulmonary neuroendocrine cells in SIDS. An immunohistochemical and quantitative study. *Annals of New York Academy of Sciences*, **533**, 461–3.

Daltveit, A. K., Irgens, L. M., Øyen, N., *et al.* (1998). Sociodemographic risk factors for sudden infant death syndrome: associations with other risk factors. The Nordic Epidemiologic SIDS Study. *Acta Paediatrica*, **87**, 284–90.

Damus, K., Pakter, J. Krongrad, E., Standfast, S. J. & Hoffman, H. J. (1988). Postnatal medical and epidemiological risk factors for the sudden infant death syndrome. In *Sudden Infant Death Syndrome. Risk Factors and Basic Mechanisms*, ed. R. M. Harper & H. J. Hoffman. New York: PMA Publishing, pp. 187–201.

Davidson Ward, S. L., Bautista, D., Chan, L., *et al.* (1990). Sudden infant death syndrome in infants of substance-abusing mothers. *Journal of Pediatrics*, **117**, 876–81.

Davidson Ward, S. L. & Keens, T. G. (1992). Prenatal substance abuse. *Clinics in Perinatology*, **19**, 849–60.

Davies, D. P. (1985). Cot death in Hong Kong: a rare problem? *Lancet*, **ii**, 1346–9.

Davies, D. P. (1994). Ethnicity and the sudden infant death syndrome: an introduction. *Early Human Development*, **38**, 139–41.

Davies, D. P. (1999). Short QTc interval as an important factor in sudden infant death syndrome. *Archives of Disease in Childhood*, **80**, 105–9.

Davies, P. A., Milner, A. D., Silverman, M. & Simpson, H. (1990). Monitoring and sudden infant death syndrome: an update. Report from the Foundation for the Study of Infant Deaths and the British Paediatric Respiratory Group. *Archives of Disease in Childhood*, **65**, 238–40.

Davis, R. E., Icke, G. C. & Hilton, J. M. (1982). High serum thiamine and the sudden infant death syndrome. *Clinica Chimica Acta*, **123**, 321–8.

Davis, R. E., Icke, G. C. & Hilton, J. M. (1983). Sudden infant death and abnormal thiamin metabolism. In *Sudden Infant Death Syndrome*, ed. J. A. Tildon, L. M. Roeder & A. Steinschneider. New York: Academic Press, pp. 201–10.

De Bethmann, O., Couchard, M., de Ajuriaguerra, M., *et al.* (1993). Role of gastro-oesophageal reflux and vagal overactivity in apparent life-threatening events: 160 cases. *Acta Paediatrica*, **389** (Suppl), 102–4.

Deeg, K. H., Alderath, W. & Bettendorf, U. (1998). Basilar artery insufficiency – a possible cause of sudden infant death? Results of a Doppler ultrasound study of 39 children with apparent life-threatening events. *Ultraschall in der Medizen*, **19**, 250–58.

De Jonge, G. A. & Engelberts, A. C. (1989). Cot deaths and sleeping position. *Lancet*, **ii**, 1149–50.

De Jonge, G. A., Engelberts, A. C., Koomen-Liefting, A. J. M. & Kostense, P. J. (1989). Cot death and prone sleeping position in the Netherlands. *British Medical Journal*, **298**, 722.

Denborough, M. A., Galloway, G. J. & Hopkinson, K. C. (1982) Malignant hyperpyrexia and sudden infant death. *Lancet*, **ii**, 1068–9.

Denmead, D. T., Ariagno, R. L., Carson, S. H. & Benirschke, K. B. (1987). Placental pathology is not predictive for sudden infant death syndrome (SIDS). *American Journal of Perinatology*, **4**, 308–12.

Denoroy, L., Gay, N., Gilly, R., Tayot J., Pasquier B. & Kopp N. (1987). Catecholamine synthesizing enzyme activity in brainstem areas from victims of sudden infant death syndrome. *Neuropediatrics*, **18**, 187–90.

De Silva, R. E., Icke, G. C. & Hilton, J. M. (1992). Diaphragm fibre types in the sudden infant death syndrome. *Medical Journal of Australia*, **156**, 886–8.

Devey, M. E., Anderson, K. J., Coombs, R. R. A., Henschel, M. J. & Coates, M. E. (1976). The modified anaphylaxis hypothesis for cot death. Anaphylactic sensitization in guinea-pigs fed cow's milk. *Clinical and Experimental Immunology*, **26**, 542–8.

Diamond, E. F. (1986). Sudden infant death in five consecutive siblings. *Illinois Medical Journal*, **170**, 33–4.

Di Maio, D. J. & Di Maio, V. J. M. (1989). Sudden infant death syndrome. In *Forensic Pathology*. New York: Elsevier, pp. 291.

Dinsdale, F., Emery, J. L. & Gadsdon, D. R. (1977). The carotid body – a quantitative assessment in children. *Histopathology*, **1**, 179–87.

Divry, P., Vianey-Liaud, C., Jakobs, C., Ten-Brink, H. J., Dutruge, J. & Gilly, R. (1990). Sudden infant death syndrome: organic acid profiles in cerebrospinal fluid from 47 children and the occurrence of N-acetylaspartic acid. *Journal of Inherited and Metabolic Disease*, **13**, 330–32.

Douglas, A. S., Allan, T. M. & Helms, P. J. (1996). Seasonality and the sudden infant death syndrome during 1987–9 and 1991–3 in Australia and Britain. *British Medical Journal*, **312**, 1381–3.

Drasch, G. A., Kretschmer, E. & Lochner, C. (1988). Lead and sudden infant death. Investigations on blood samples of SID babies. *European Journal of Pediatrics*, **147**, 79–84.

Drews, C. D., Kraus, J. F. & Greenland, S. (1990). Recall bias in a case–control study of sudden infant death syndrome. *International Journal of Epidemiology*, **19**, 405–11.

Dundar, M., Lanyon, W. G. & Connor, J. M. (1993). Scottish frequency of the common G985 mutation in the medium-chain acyl-coA dehydrogenase (MCAD) gene and the role of MCAD deficiency in sudden infant death syndrome (SIDS). *Journal of Inherited and Metabolic Disease*, **16**, 991–3.

Dunne, K. P. & Matthews, T. G. (1988). Hypothermia and sudden infant death syndrome. *Archives of Disease in Childhood*, **63**, 438–40.

Durand, D. J., Espinoza, A. M. & Nickerson, B. G. (1990). Association between prenatal cocaine exposure and sudden infant death syndrome. *Journal of Pediatrics,* **117**, 909–11.

Dwyer, T. & Ponsonby, A.-L. (1992). Sudden infant death syndrome – insights from epidemiological research. *Journal of Epidemiology and Community Health*, **46**, 98–102.

Dwyer, T., Ponsonby, A.-L., Blizzard, L., Newman, N. M. & Cochrane, J. A. (1995). The contribution of changes in the prevalence of prone sleeping position to the decline in sudden infant death syndrome in Tasmania. *Journal of the American Medical Association*, **273**, 783–9.

Dwyer, T., Ponsonby, A.-L., Gibbons, L. E. & Newman, N. M. (1991a). Prone sleeping position and SIDS: evidence from recent case–control and cohort studies in Tasmania. *Journal of Paediatrics and Child Health*, **27**, 340–43.

Dwyer, T., Ponsonby, A.-L., Newman, N. M. & Gibbons, L. E. (1991b). Prospective cohort study of prone sleeping position and sudden infant death syndrome. *Lancet*, **337**, 1244–7.

Ellis, F. R., Halsall, P. J. & Harriman, D. G. F. (1988). Malignant hyperpyrexia and sudden infant death syndrome. *British Journal of Anaesthesia*, **60**, 28–30.

Emery, J. L. (1983). The necropsy and cot death. *British Medical Journal*, **287**, 77–8.

Emery, J. L. (1985). Infanticide, filicide, and cot death. *Archives of Disease in Childhood*, **60**, 505–7.

Emery, J. L. (1989). Is sudden infant death syndrome a diagnosis? Or is it just a diagnostic dustbin? *British Medical Journal*, **299**, 1240.

Emery, J. L. & Dinsdale, F. (1974). Increased incidence of lymphoreticular aggregates in lungs of children found unexpectedly dead. *Archives of Disease in Childhood*, **49**, 107–11.

Emery, J. L. & Dinsdale, F. (1978). Structure of periadrenal brown fat in childhood in both expected and cot deaths. *Archives of Disease in Childhood*, **53**, 154–8.

Emery, J. L. & Thornton, J. A. (1968). Effects of obstruction to respiration in infants, with particular reference to mattresses, pillows, and their coverings. *British Medical Journal*, **3**, 209–13.

Emery, J. L., Chandra, S. & Gilbert-Barness, E. F. (1988). Findings in child deaths registered as sudden infant death syndrome (SIDS) in Madison, Wisconsin. *Pediatric Pathology*, **8**, 171–8.

Emery, J. L., Swift, P. G. F. & Worthy, E. (1974). Hypernatraemia and uraemia in unexpected death in infancy. *Archives of Disease in Childhood,* **49**, 686–92.

Emery, J. L., Waite, A. J., Carpenter, R. G., Limerick, S. R. & Blake, D. (1985). Apnoea monitors compared with weighing scales for siblings after cot death. *Archives of Disease in Childhood*, **60**, 1055–60.

Engelberts, A. C. (1991). *Cot Death in the Netherlands. An Epidemiological Study*. Amsterdam: VU University Press, pp. 119–22.

Engelberts, A. C. & de Jonge, G. A. (1990). Choice of sleeping position for infants: possible association with cot death. *Archives of Disease in Childhood*, **65**, 462–7.

Engelberts, A. C., de Jonge, G. A. & Kostense, P. J. (1991). An analysis of trends in the incidence of sudden infant death in The Netherlands 1969–89. *Journal of Paediatrics and Child Health*, **27**, 329–33.

Erickson, M. M., Poklis, A., Gantner, G. E., Dickinson, A. W. & Hillman, L. S. (1983a). Tissue mineral levels in victims of sudden infant death syndrome: I. Toxic metals – lead and cadmium. *Pediatric Research*, **17**, 779–83.

Erikson, M. M., Poklis, A., Gantner, G. E., Dickinson, A. W. & Hillman, L. S. (1983b). Tissue mineral levels in victims of sudden infant death syndrome II. Essential minerals: copper, zinc, calcium, and magnesium. *Pediatric Research*, **17**, 784–7.

Esiri, M. M., Urry, P. & Keeling, J. (1990). Lipid-containing cells in the brain in sudden infant death syndrome. *Developmental Medicine and Child Neurology*, **32**, 319–24.

Fagan, D. G. & Milner, A. D. (1985). Pressure volume characteristics of the lungs in sudden infant death syndrome. *Archives of Disease in Childhood*, **60**, 471–85.

Faigel, H. C. (1974). Ondine's curse and sudden infant death syndrome: teetering on the brink. *Clinical Pediatrics*, **7**, 567–8.

Farber, J. P., Catron, A. C. & Krous, H. F. (1983). Pulmonary petechiae: ventilatory-circulatory interactions. *Pediatric Research*, **17**, 230–33.

Fearn, S. W. (1834). Sudden and unexplained death of children. *Lancet*, **ii**, 246.

Filiano, J. J. (1994). Arcuate nucleus hypoplasia in sudden infant death syndrome: a review. *Biology of the Neonate*, **65**, 156–9.

Filiano, J. J. & Kinney, H. C. (1992). Arcuate nucleus hypoplasia in the sudden infant death syndrome. *Journal of Neuropathology and Experimental Neurology*, **51**, 394–403.

Filiano, J. J. & Kinney, H. C. (1994). A perspective on neuropathologic findings in victims of the sudden infant death syndrome: the triple risk model. *Biology of the Neonate*, **65**, 194–7.

Fink, B. R. & Beckwith, J. B. (1980). Laryngeal mucous gland excess in victims of sudden infant death. *American Journal of Diseases of Children*, **134**, 144–6.

Finkle, B. S., McCloskey, K. L., Kopjak, L. & Carroll, J. M. (1979). Toxicological analyses in cases of sudden infant death: a national feasibility study. *Journal of Forensic Sciences*, **24**, 775–89.

Firstman, R. & Talan, J. (1997). *The Death of Innocents*. New York: Bantam Books.

Firstman, R. & Talan, J. (2001). SIDS and infanticide. In *Sudden Infant Death Syndrome. Problems, Progress and Possibilities*, ed. R. W. Byard & H. F. Krous. London: Arnold, pp. 291–300.

Fitzgerald, K. (2001). The 'Reduce the Risks' campaign, SIDS International, the Global Strategy Task Force and the European Society for the Study and Prevention of Infant Death. In *Sudden Infant Death Syndrome. Problems, Progress and Possibilities*, ed. R. W. Byard & H. F. Krous. London: Arnold, pp. 310–18.

Flahault, A., Messiah, A., Jougla, E., Bouvet, E., Perin, J. & Hatton, F. (1988). Sudden infant death syndrome and diphtheria/tetanus toxoid/pertussis/poliomyelitis immunisation. *Lancet*, **i**, 582–3.

Fleming, K. A. (1992). Viral respiratory infection and SIDS. *Journal of Clinical Pathology*, **45** (Suppl), 29–32.

Fleming, P., Bacon, C., Blair, P. & Berry, P. J. (2000). *Sudden Unexpected deaths in Infancy. The CESDI SUDI Studies 1993–1996*. London: The Stationary Office.

Fleming, P. J., Azaz, Y. & Wigfield, R. (1992). Development of thermoregulation in infancy: possible implications for SIDS. *Journal of Clinical Pathology*, **45** (Suppl), 17–19.

Fleming, P. J., Berry, P. J., Gilbert, R., *et al.* (1991). Categories of preventable unexpected infant deaths. *Archives of Disease in Childhood*, **66**, 171–2.

Fleming, P. J., Blair, P. S., Bacon, C., *et al.* (1996). Environment of infants during sleep and the risk of sudden infant death syndrome: results of 1993–5 case–control study for confidential inquiry into stillbirths and deaths in infancy. *British Medical Journal*, **313**, 191–5.

Fleming, P. J., Blair, P. S., Platt, M. W., *et al.* (2001). The UK accelerated immunisation programme and sudden unexpected death in infancy: case–control study. *British Medical Journal*, **322**, 822–5.

Fleming, P. J., Blair, P. S., Pollard, K., *et al.* (1999). Pacifier use and sudden infant death syndrome: results from the CESDI/SUDI case control study. *Archives of Disease in Childhood*, **81,** 112–16.

Fleming, P. J., Cooke, M., Chantler, S. M. & Golding, J. (1994). Fire retardants, biocides, plasticisers, and sudden infant deaths. *British Medical Journal*, **309**, 1594–6.

Fleming, P. J., Gilbert, R., Azaz, Y., *et al.* (1990). Interaction between bedding and sleeping position in the sudden infant death syndrome: a population based case–control study. *British Medical Journal*, **301**, 85–9.

Fleming, P. J., Levine, M. R., Azaz, Y., Wigfield, R. & Stewart, A. J. (1993). Interactions between thermoregulation and the control of respiration in infants: possible relationship to sudden infant death. *Acta Paediatrica*, **389** (Suppl), 57–9.

Fleshman, J. K. & Peterson, D. R. (1977). The sudden infant death syndrome among Alaskan natives. *American Journal of Epidemiology*, **105**, 555–8.

Ford, R. P. K. & Nelson, K. P. (1995). Higher rates of SIDS persist in low income groups. *Journal of Paediatrics and Child Health*, **31**, 408–11.

Forsyth, K. D., Bradley, J., Weeks, S. C., Smith, M. D., Skinner, J. & Zola, H. (1988). Immunocytologic characterization using monoclonal antibodies of lung lavage cell phenotype in infants who have died from sudden infant death syndrome. *Pediatric Research*, **23**, 187–90.

Forsyth, K. D., Weeks, S. C., Koh, L., Skinner, J. & Bradley, J. (1989). Lung immunoglobulins in the sudden infant death syndrome. *British Medical Journal*, **298**, 23–6.

Franco, P., Groswasser, J., Sottiaux, M., Broadfield, E. & Kahn, A. (1996). Decreased cardiac responses to auditory stimulation during prone sleep. *Pediatrics*, **97**, 174–8.

Franco, P., Szliwowski, H., Dramaix, M. & Kahn, A. (1999). Decreased autonomic responses to obstructive sleep events in future victims of sudden infant death syndrome. *Pediatric Research*, **46**, 33–9.

Frankfater, A. & Wilcockson, D. (1983). Tissue levels of L-dopa decarboxylase and other putative markers of autonomic nervous control in SIDS. In *Sudden Infant Death Syndrome*, ed. J. A. Tildon, L. M. Roeder & A. Steinschneider. New York: Academic Press, pp. 223–31.

French, J. W., Beckwith, J. B., Graham, C. B. & Guntheroth, W. G. (1972). Lack of postmortem radiographic evidence of nasopharyngeal obstruction in the sudden infant death syndrome. *Journal of Pediatrics*, **81**, 1145–8.

Frøen, J. F., Arnestad, M., Vege Å., *et al.* (2002). Comparative epidemiology of sudden infant death syndrome and sudden intra-uterine unexplained death. *Archives of Disease in Childhood*, **87**, F118–22.

Froggatt, P. (1977). A cardiac cause in cot death: a discarded hypothesis? *Journal of the Irish Medical Association*, **70**, 408–14.

Froggatt, P., Lynas, M. A. & MacKenzie, G. (1971). Epidemiology of sudden unexpected death in infants ('cot death') in Northern Ireland. *British Journal of Preventative and Social Medicine*, **25**, 119–34.

Gadsdon, D. R. & Emery, J. L. (1976). Fatty change in the brain in perinatal and unexpected death. *Archives of Disease in Childhood*, **51**, 42–8.

Gale, R., Redner-Carmi, R. & Gale, J. (1977). Accumulation of carbon dioxide in oxygen hoods, infant cots and incubators. *Pediatrics*, **60**, 453–6.

Galland, B. C., Peebles, C. M., Bolton, D. P. G. & Taylor, B. J. (1994). The micro-environment of the sleeping newborn piglet covered by bedclothes: gas exchange and temperature. *Journal of Paediatrics and Child Health*, **30**, 144–50.

Galland, B. C., Reeves, G., Taylor, B. J. & Bolton, D. P. G. (1998). Sleep position, autonomic function and arousal. *Archives of Disease in Childhood*, **78**, F186–94.

Galland, B. C., Taylor, B. J. & Bolton, D. P. G. (2002). Prone verses supine sleep position: a review of physiological studies in SIDS research. *Journal of Paediatrics and Child Health*, **38**, 332–8.

Gardner, A. M. N. (1958). Aspiration of food and vomit. *Quarterly Journal of Medicine*, **27**, 227–42.

Gaultier, C. L. (1990). Interference between gastroesophageal reflux and sleep in near miss SIDS. *Clinical Reviews in Allergy*, **8**, 395–401.

Geertinger, P. (1967). Sudden, unexpected death in infancy, with special reference to the parathyroids. *Pediatrics*, **39**, 43–8.

Gibson, R. A. & McMurchie, E. J. (1986). Changes in lung surfactant lipids associated with the sudden infant death syndrome. *Australian Paediatric Journal*, **22** (Suppl), 77–80.

Gibson, R. A. & McMurchie, E. J. (1988a). Decreased lung surfactant disaturated phosphatidylcholine in sudden infant death syndrome. *Early Human Development*, **17**, 145–55.

Gibson, R. A. & McMurchie, E. J. (1988b). The role of pulmonary surfactant in SIDS. *Annals of New York Academy of Sciences*, **533**, 296–300.

Gilbert, R. E., Fleming, P. J., Azaz, Y. & Rudd, P. T. (1990). Signs of illness preceding sudden unexpected death in infants. *British Medical Journal*, **300**, 1237–9.

Gilbert, R., Rudd, P., Berry, P. J., *et al.* (1992). Combined effect of infection and heavy wrapping on the risk of sudden unexpected infant death. *Archives of Disease in Childhood*, **67**, 171–7.

Gilbert, R. E., Wigfield, R. E., Fleming, P. J., Berry, P. J. & Rudd, P. T. (1995). Bottle feeding and the sudden infant death syndrome. *British Medical Journal*, **310**, 88–90.

Gilbert-Barness, E. (1993). Is sudden infant death syndrome a cause of death? *American Journal of Diseases of Children*, **147**, 25–6.

Gilbert-Barness, E. & Barness, L. A. (1992). Cause of death: SIDS or something else? *Contemporary Pediatrics*, **9**, 13–29.

Gilbert-Barness, E. F. & Barness, L. A. (1993). Sudden infant death syndrome. Is it a cause of death? *Archives of Pathology and Laboratory Medicine*, **117**, 1246–8.

Gilbert-Barness, E., Hegstrand, L., Chandra, S., *et al.* (1991). Hazards of mattresses, beds and bedding in deaths of infants. *American Journal of Forensic Medicine and Pathology*, **12**, 27–32.

Gillan, J. E., Curran, C., O'Reilly, E., Cahalane, S. F. & Unwin, A. R. (1989). Abnormal patterns of pulmonary neuroendocrine cells in victims of sudden infant death syndrome. *Pediatrics*, **84**, 828–34.

Gilles, F. H., Bina, M. & Sotrel, A. (1979). Infantile atlantooccipital instability. The potential danger of extreme extension. *American Journal of Diseases of Children*, **133**, 30–37.

Giulian, G. G., Gilbert, E. F. & Moss, R. L. (1987). Elevated fetal hemoglobin levels in sudden infant death syndrome. *New England Journal of Medicine*, **316**, 1122–6.

Glotzbach, S. F., Baldwin, R. B., Lederer, N. E., Tansey, P. A. & Ariagno, R. L. (1989). Periodic breathing in preterm infants: incidence and characteristics. *Pediatrics*, **84**, 785–92.

Golding, J. (1989). The epidemiology and sociology of the sudden infant death syndrome. In *Paediatric Forensic Medicine and Pathology*, ed. J. K. Mason. London: Chapman & Hall, pp. 141–55.

Golding, J., Limerick, S. & Macfarlane, A. (1985). *Sudden Infant Death. Patterns, Puzzles and Problems*. Shepton Mallet: Open Books.

Goldwater, P. N. (1992). Reappraisal of the SIDS enigma: an epidemiological and clinicopathological approach. *Journal of Paediatrics and Child Health*, **28** (Suppl 1), S21–5.

Golub, H. L. & Corwin, M. J. (1982). Infant cry: a clue to diagnosis. *Pediatrics*, **69**, 197–201.

Gomes, H., Menanteau, B., Motte, J. & Cymbalista, M. (1986). Laryngospasm and sudden unexpected death syndrome. *Annals of Radiology*, **29**, 313–20.

Gould, J. B. (1983). SIDS – a sleep hypothesis. In *Sudden Infant Death Syndrome*, ed. J. A. Tildon, L. M. Roeder & A. Steinschneider. New York: Academic Press, pp. 443–52.

Gould, J. B., Lee, A. F. S. & Morelock, S. (1988). The relationship between sleep and sudden death. *Annals of New York Academy of Sciences*, **533**, 62–77.

Goyco, P. G. & Beckerman, R. C. (1990). Sudden infant death syndrome. *Current Problems in Pediatrics*, **20**, 299–346.

Gozal, D., Colin, A. A., Daskalovic, Y. I. & Jaffe, M. (1988). Environmental overheating as a cause of transient respiratory chemoreceptor dysfunction in an infant. *Pediatrics*, **82**, 738–40.

Green, A. (1993). Biochemical screening in newborn siblings of cases of SIDS. *Archives of Disease in Childhood*, **68**, 793–6.

Greenwood, M. & Woods, H. M. (1927). "Status thymicolymphaticus" considered in the light of recent work on the thymus. *Journal of Hygiene*, **26**, 305–26.

Grether, J. K., Schulman, J. & Croen, L. A. (1990). Sudden infant death syndrome among Asians in California. *Journal of Pediatrics*, **116**, 525–8.

Griffin, M. R., Ray, W. A., Livengood, J. R. & Schaffner, W. (1988). Risk of sudden infant death syndrome after immunization with the diphtheria-tetanus-pertussis vaccine. *New England Journal of Medicine*, **319**, 618–23.

Grögaard, J. B. (1993). Apnea monitors. *Acta Paediatrica*, **389** (Suppl), 111–13.

Guilleminault, C. & Coons, S. (1983). Sleep states and maturation of sleep: a comparative study between full-term normal controls and near-miss SIDS infants. In *Sudden Infant Death Syndrome*, ed. J. A. Tildon, L. M. Roeder & A. Steinschneider. New York: Academic Press, pp. 401–11.

Guilleminault, C., Ariagno, R., Coons, S., *et al.* (1985). Near-miss sudden infant death syndrome in eight infants with sleep apnea-related cardiac arrhythmias. *Pediatrics*, **76**, 236–42.

Guilleminault, C., Ariagno, R. L., Forno, L. S., Nagel, L., Baldwin, R. & Owen, M. (1979). Obstructive sleep apnea and near miss for SIDS: 1. Report of an infant with sudden death. *Pediatrics*, **63**, 837–43.

Guilleminault, C., Heldt, G., Powell, N. & Riley, R. (1986). Small upper airway in near-miss sudden infant death syndrome infants and their families. *Lancet*, **i**, 402–7.

Guilleminault, C., Souquet, M., Ariagno, R. L., Korobkin, R. & Simmons, F. B. (1984). Five cases of near-miss sudden infant death syndrome and development of obstructive sleep apnea syndrome. *Pediatrics*, **73**, 71–8.

Guilleminault, C., Stoohs, R., Skrobal, A., Labanowski, M. & Simmons, J. (1993). Upper airway resistance in infants at risk for sudden infant death syndrome. *Journal of Pediatrics*, **122**, 881–6.

Guntheroth, W. G. (1989a). Final pathways: theories of cardiovascular causes of SIDS. In *Crib death. Sudden Infant Death Syndrome*, 2nd edn. New York: Futura, pp. 165–94.

Guntheroth, W. G. (1989b). Theories of cardiovascular causes in sudden infant death syndrome. *Journal of American College of Cardiology*, **14**, 443–7.

Guntheroth, W. G. (1989c). Interleukin-1 as intermediary causing prolonged sleep apnea and SIDS during respiratory infections. *Medical Hypotheses*, **28**, 121–3.

Guntheroth, W. G. & Spiers, P. S. (1990). Bedding and sleep position in the sudden infant death syndrome. *British Medical Journal*, **301**, 494.

Guntheroth, W. G. & Spiers, P. S. (1992). Sleeping prone and the risk of sudden infant death syndrome. *Journal of the American Medical Association*, **267**, 2359–62.

Guntheroth, W. G. & Spiers, P. S. (1998). Prolongation of the QT interval and the sudden infant death syndrome. *New England Journal of Medicine*, **339**, 1161.

Guntheroth, W. G. & Spiers, P. S. (2001). Thermal stress in sudden infant death: is there an ambiguity with the rebreathing hypothesis? *Pediatrics*, **107**, 693–8.

Guntheroth, W. G. & Spiers, P. S. (2002). The triple risk hypothesis in sudden infant death syndrome. *Pediatrics*, http://www.pediatrics.org/cgi/content/full/110/5/e64.

Guntheroth, W. G., Breazeale, D. & McGough, G. A. (1973). The significance of pulmonary petechiae in crib death. *Pediatrics*, **52**, 601–3.

Guntheroth, W. G., Kawabori, I., Breazeale, D. G., Garlinghouse, L. E., Jr & Van Hoosier, G. L., Jr (1980). The role of respiratory infection in intrathoracic petechiae. Implications for sudden infant death. *American Journal of Diseases of Children*, **134**, 364–6.

Gupta, P. R., Guilleminault, C. & Dorfman, L. J. (1981). Brainstem auditory evoked potentials in near-miss sudden infant death syndrome. *Journal of Pediatrics*, **98**, 791–4.

Gurwith, M. J., Langston, C. & Citron, D. M. (1981). Toxin-producing bacteria in infants. Lack of an association with sudden infant death syndrome. *American Journal of Diseases of Children*, **135**, 1104–6.

Haas, J. E., Taylor, J. A., Bergman, A. B., *et al.* (1993). Relationship between epidemiologic risk factors and clinicopathologic findings in the sudden infant death syndrome. *Pediatrics*, **91**, 106–12.

Haddad, G. G., Epstein, M. A. F., Epstein, R. A., Mazza N. M., Mellins R. B. & Krongrad E. (1979). The QT interval in aborted sudden infant death syndrome infants. *Pediatric Research*, **13**, 136–8.

Haglund, B. & Cnattingius, S. (1990). Cigarette smoking as a risk factor for sudden infant death syndrome: a population-based study. *American Journal of Public Health*, **80**, 29–32.

Haglund, B., Cnattingius, S. & Otterblad-Olausson, P. (1995). Sudden infant death syndrome in Sweden, 1983–1990: season at death, age at death, and maternal smoking. *American Journal of Epidemiology*, **142**, 619–24.

Hall, W. W. (1869). *The Guide-board to Health, Peace and Competence; or, the Road to Happy Old Age*. Springfield, Mass.: D. E. Fisk & Co., p. 400.

Hanzlick, R. (2001a). Death scene investigation. In *Sudden Infant Death Syndrome. Problems, Progress and Possibilities*, ed. R. W. Byard & H. F. Krous. London: Arnold, pp. 58–65.

Hanzlick, R. (2001b). Pulmonary hemorrhage in deceased infants. Baseline data for further study of infant mortality. *American Journal of Forensic Medicine and Pathology*, **22**, 188–92.

Haque, A. K. & Mancuso, M. G. (1993). Proliferation of dendritic cells in the bronchioles of sudden infant death syndrome victims. *Modern Pathology*, **6**, 360–70.

Haque, A. K., Hernandez, J. C. & Dillard, E. A., III (1985). Asbestos bodies found in infant lungs. *Archives of Pathology and Laboratory Medicine*, **109**, 212.

Haraguchi, S., Fung, R. Q. & Sasaki, C. T. (1983). Effect of hyperthermia on the laryngeal closure reflex. Implications in the sudden infant death syndrome. *Annals of Otology, Rhinology and Laryngology*, **92**, 24–8.

Harding, R. (1986). Nasal obstruction in infancy. *Australian Paediatric Journal*, **22** (Suppl), 59–61.

Harper, R. M. & Frysinger, R. C. (1988). Suprapontine mechanisms underlying cardiorespiratory regulation: implications for the sudden infant death syndrome. In *Sudden Infant Death Syndrome. Risk Factors and Basic Mechanisms*, ed. R. M. Harper & H. J. Hoffman. New York: PMA Publishing, pp. 399–414.

Harper, R. M., Leake, B., Hodgman, J. E. & Hoppenbrouwers, T. (1982). Developmental patterns of heart rate and heart rate variability during sleep and waking in normal infants and infants at risk for the sudden infant death syndrome. *Sleep*, **5**, 28–38.

Harrison, D. F. N. (1991a). Histologic evaluation of the larynx in sudden infant death syndrome. *Annals of Otology, Rhinology and Laryngology*, **100**, 173–5.

Harrison, D. F. N. (1991b). Laryngeal morphology in sudden unexpected death in infants. *Journal of Laryngology and Otology*, **105**, 646–50.

Hassall, I. B. & Vandenberg, M. (1985). Infant sleep position: a New Zealand survey. *New Zealand Medical Journal*, **98**, 97–9.

Hasselmeyer, E. G. & Hunter, J. C. (1975). The sudden infant death syndrome. *Obstetric and Gynecology Annual*, **4**, 213–36.

Hauck, F. R. (2001). Changing epidemiology. In *Sudden Infant Death Syndrome. Problems, Progress and Possibilities*, ed. R. W. Byard & H. F. Krous. London: Arnold, pp. 31–57.

Heaney, S. & McIntire, M. S. (1979). Sudden infant death syndrome and barometric pressure. *Journal of Pediatrics*, **94**, 433–5.

Heath, D. (1991). The human carotid body in health and disease. *Journal of Pathology*, **164**, 1–8.

Heath, D., Khan, Q. & Smith, P. (1990). Histopathology of the carotid bodies in neonates and infants. *Histopathology*, **17**, 511–20.

Heaton, P. A. J. & Sage, M. D. (1995). Fatal smothering by a domestic cat. *New Zealand Medical Journal*, **108**, 62–3.

Hebold, K., Saternus, K.-S. & Schleicher, A. (1986) Morphometric studies on the vertebral arteries in infants. *Zeitschrift fur Rechsmedizin*, **97**, 41–8.

Helweg-Larsen, K., Knudsen, L. B., Gregersen, M. & Simonsen, J. (1992). Sudden infant death syndrome (SIDS) in Denmark: evaluation of the increasing incidence of registered SIDS in the period 1972 to 1983 and results of a prospective study in 1987 through 1988. *Pediatrics*, **89**, 855–9.

Henderson-Smart, D. J., Pettigrew, A. G. & Campbell, D. J. (1983). Prenatal stress, brain stem neural maturation and apnea in preterm infants. In *Sudden Infant Death Syndrome*, ed. J. A. Tildon, L. M. Roeder & A. Steinschneider. New York: Academic Press, pp. 293–304.

Henderson-Smart, D. J., Ponsonby, A.-L. & Murphy, E. (1998). Reducing the risk of sudden infant death syndrome: a review of the scientific literature. *Journal of Paediatrics and Child Health*, **34**, 213–19.

Herbst, J. J., Book, L. S. & Bray, P. F. (1978). Gastroesophageal reflux in the "near miss" sudden infant death syndrome. *Journal of Pediatrics*, **92**, 73–5.

Herbst, J. J., Minton, S. D. & Book, L. S. (1979). Gastroesophageal reflux causing respiratory distress and apnea in newborn infants. *Journal of Pediatrics*, **95**, 763–8.

Hickson, G. B., Altemeier, W. A., Martin, E. D. & Campbell, P. W. (1989). Parental administration of chemical agents: a cause of apparent life-threatening events. *Pediatrics*, **83**, 772–6.

Hill, C. M., Brown, B. D., Morley, C. J., Davis, J. A. & Barson, A. J. (1988). Pulmonary surfactant. II. In sudden infant death syndrome. *Early Human Development*, **16**, 153–62.

Hillman, L. S., Erickson, M. & Haddad, J. G., Jr (1980). Serum 25-hydroxyvitamin D concentrations in sudden infant death syndrome. *Pediatrics*, **65**, 1137–9.

Hills, B. A., Masters, I. B. & O'Duffy, J. F. (1992). Abnormalities of surfactant in children with recurrent cyanotic episodes. *Lancet*, **339**, 1323–4.

Hills, B. A., Masters, I. B., Vance, J. C. & Hills, Y. C. (1997). Abnormalities in surfactant in sudden infant death syndrome as a postmortem marker and possible test of risk. *Journal of Paediatrics and Child Health*, **33**, 61–6.

Hilton, J. M. N. (1986). Pathology of the sudden infant death syndrome in Western Australia: a review of 50 cases. *Australian Paediatric Journal*, **22** (Suppl 1), 5–6.

Hilton, J. M. N. (1989). The pathology of the sudden infant death syndrome. In *Paediatric Forensic Medicine and Pathology*, ed. J. K. Mason. London: Chapman & Hall, pp. 156–64.

Hilton, J. M. N. & Turner, K. J. (1976). Sudden death in infancy syndrome in Western Australia. *Medical Journal of Australia*, **i**, 427–30.

Hirvonen, J., Autio-Harmainen, H. & Nyblom, O. (1982). Immature glomeruli in cot death kidneys. *Forensic Science International*, **20**, 117–20.

Ho, S. Y. & Anderson, R. H. (1988). Conduction tissue and SIDS. *Annals of New York Academy of Sciences*, **533**, 176–90.

Hoffman, H. J. & Hillman, L. S. (1992). Epidemiology of the sudden infant death syndrome: maternal, neonatal and postneonatal risk factors. *Clinics in Perinatology*, **19**, 717–37.

Hoffman, H. J., Damus, K., Hillman, L. & Krongrad, E. (1988). Risk factors for SIDS. Results of the National Institute of Child Health and Human Development SIDS Cooperative Epidemiological Study. *Annals of New York Academy of Science*, **533**, 13–30.

Hoffman, H. J., Hunter, J. C., Damus, K., *et al.* (1987). Diphtheria-tetanus-pertussis immunization and sudden infant death: results of the National Institute of Child Health and Human Development Cooperative epidemiological study of sudden infant death syndrome risk factors. *Pediatrics*, **79**, 598–611.

Holton, J. B., Allen, J. T., Green, C. A., Partington, S., Gilbert, R. E. & Berry, P. J. (1991). Inherited metabolic diseases in the sudden infant death syndrome. *Archives of Disease in Childhood*, **66**, 1315–17.

Hori, C. G. (1987). Pathology of sudden infant death syndrome. *American Journal of Forensic Medicine and Pathology*, **8**, 93–6.

Horne, R. S. C., Ferens, D., Watts, A.-M., *et al.* (2002). Effects of maternal tobacco smoking, sleeping position, and sleep state on arousal in healthy term infants. *Archives of Disease in Childhood*, **87**, F100–105.

Howat, A. J., Bennett, M. J., Variend, S., Shaw, L. & Engel, P. C. (1985). Defects of metabolism of fatty acids in the sudden infant death syndrome. *British Medical Journal*, **290**, 1771–3.

Howat, W. J., Moore, I. E., Judd, M. & Roche, W. R. (1994). Pulmonary immunopathology of sudden infant death syndrome. *Lancet*, **343**, 1390–92.

Howatson, A. G., Patrick, W. J. A., Fell, G. S., Lyon, T. D. B. & Gibson, A. A. M. (1995). Cot mattresses and sudden infant death syndrome. *Lancet*, **345**, 1044–5.

Huang, S. W. (1983). Infectious diseases, immunology and SIDS: an overview. In *Sudden Infant Death Syndrome*, ed. J. A. Tildon, L. M. Roeder & A. Steinschneider. New York: Academic Press, pp. 593–606.

Huff, D. S. & Carpenter, J. T. (1987). Cytomegalovirus inclusions in 401 consecutive autopsies on infants aged 2 weeks to 2 years: a high incidence in patients with sudden infant death syndrome. *Pediatric Pathology*, **7**, 225.

Hunt, C. E. (1992). The cardiorespiratory control hypothesis for sudden infant death syndrome. *Clinics in Perinatology*, **19**, 757–71.

Hunt, C. E. & Shannon, D. C. (1992). Sudden infant death syndrome and sleeping position. *Pediatrics*, **90**, 115–18.

Irgens, L. M., Markestad, T., Baste, V., Schreuder, P., Skjaerven, R. & Øyen, N. (1995). Sleeping position and sudden infant death syndrome in Norway 1967–91. *Archives of Disease in Childhood*, **72**, 478–82.

Irgens, L. M., Skjaerven, R. & Lie, R. T. (1989). Secular trends of sudden infant death syndrome and other causes of post perinatal mortality in Norwegian birth cohorts 1967–1984. *Acta Paediatrica Scandinavica*, **78**, 228–32.

Irwin, K. L., Mannino, S. & Daling, J. (1992). Sudden infant death syndrome in Washington state: why are Native American infants at greater risk than white infants? *Journal of Pediatrics*, **121**, 242–7.

Iwadate, K., Sakamoto, N., Park, S. H., *et al.* (1997). Immunohistochemical detection of human milk components aspirated in lungs of an infant. *Forensic Science International*, **90**, 77–84.

Jaffe, R., Hashida, Y. & Yunis, E. J. (1982). The endocrine pancreas of the neonate and infant. *Perspectives in Pediatric Pathology*, **7**, 137–65.

Jakeman, K. J., Rushton, D. I., Smith, H. & Sweet, C. (1991). Exacerbation of bacterial toxicity to infant ferrets by influenza virus: possible role in sudden infant death syndrome. *Journal of Infectious Diseases*, **163**, 35–40.

James, D., Berry, P. J., Fleming, P. & Hathaway, M. (1990). Surfactant abnormality and the sudden infant death syndrome – a primary or secondary phenomenon? *Archives of Disease in Childhood*, **65**, 774–8.

James, T. N. (1968). Sudden death in babies: new observations in the heart. *American Journal of Cardiology*, **22**, 479–506.

James, T. N. (1976). Sudden death of babies. *Circulation*, **53**, 1–2.

Jankus, A. (1976). The cardiac conduction system in sudden infant death syndrome: a report on three cases. *Pathology*, **8**, 275–80.

Jeffrey, H. E., McCleary, B. V., Hensley, W. J. & Read, D. J. C. (1985). Thiamine deficiency – a neglected problem of infants and mothers – possible relationships to sudden infant death syndrome. *Australian and New Zealand Journal of Obstetrics and Gynaecology*, **25**, 198–202.

Jeffrey, H. E., Rahilly, P. & Read, D. J. C. (1983). Multiple causes of asphyxia in infants at high risk for sudden infant death. *Archives of Disease in Childhood*, **58**, 92–100.

Johnson, A. R., Hood, R. L. & Emery, J. L. (1980). Biotin and the sudden infant death syndrome. *Nature*, **285**, 159–60.

Jolley, S. G., Halpern, L. M., Tunell, W. P., Johnson, D. G. & Sterling, C. E. (1991). The risk of sudden infant death from gastroesophageal reflux. *Journal of Pediatric Surgery*, **26**, 691–6.

Jones, A. M. & Weston, J. T. (1976). The examination of the sudden infant death syndrome infant: investigative and autopsy protocols. *Journal of Forensic Sciences*, **21**, 833–41.

Jonville-Bera, A. P., Autret, E. & Laugier, J. (1995). Sudden infant death syndrome and diphtheria-tetanus-pertussis-poliomyelitis vaccination status. *Fundamentals of Clinical Pharmacology*, **9**, 263–70.

Jonville-Bera, A. P., Autret-Leca, E., Barbeillon, F. & Paris-Llado, J. (2001). Sudden unexpected death in infants under 3 months of age and vaccination status – a case–control study. *British Journal of Clinical Pharmacology*, **51**, 271–6.

Jørgensen, T., Biering-Sørensen, F. & Hilden, J. (1979). Sudden infant death in Copenhagen 1956–1971. III. Perinatal and perimortal factors. *Acta Paediatrica Scandinavica*, **68**, 11–22.

Kahn, A. & Blum, D. (1982). Phenothiazines and sudden infant death syndrome. *Pediatrics*, **70**, 75–8.

Kahn, A., Blum, D., Hennart, P., *et al.* (1984). A critical comparison of the history of sudden-death infants and infants hospitalised for near-miss for SIDS. *European Journal of Pediatrics*, **143**, 103–7.

Kahn, A., Blum, D., Rebuffat, E., *et al.* (1988a). Polysomnographic studies of infants who subsequently died of sudden infant death syndrome. *Pediatrics*, **82**, 721–7.

Kahn, A., Demol, P. & Blum, D. (1985). *Clostridium botulinum* and near-miss SIDS. *Lancet*, **i**, 707–8.

Kahn. A., Groswasser, J., Rebuffat, E., *et al.* (1992a). Sleep and cardiorespiratory characteristics of infant victims of sudden death: a prospective case–control study. *Sleep*, **15**, 287–92.

Kahn, A., Groswasser, J., Sottiaux, M., Rebuffat, E. & Franco, P. (1993). Clinical problems in relation to apparent life-threatening events in infants. *Acta Paediatrica*, **389** (Suppl), 107–10.

Kahn, A., Rebuffat, E., Sottiaux, M. & Blum, D. (1988b). Management of an infant with an apparent life-threatening event. *Pediatrician*, **15**, 204–11.

Kahn, A., Rebuffat, E., Sottiaux, M., Blum, D. & Yasik, E. A. (1990a). Sleep apneas and acid esophageal reflux in control infants and in infants with an apparent life-threatening event. *Biology of the Neonate*, **57**, 144–9.

Kahn, A., Rebuffat, E., Sottiaux, M., Dufour, D., Cadranel, S. & Reiterer, F. (1992b). Lack of temporal relation between acid reflux in the proximal oesophagus and cardiorespiratory events in sleeping infants. *European Journal of Pediatrics*, **151**, 208–12.

Kahn, A., Riazi, J. & Blum, D. (1983). Oculocardiac reflex in near miss for sudden infant death syndrome infants. *Pediatrics*, **71**, 49–52.

Kahn, A., Van de Merckt, C., Dramaix, M., *et al.* (1987). Transepidermal water loss during sleep in infants at risk for sudden death. *Pediatrics*, **80**, 245–50.

Kahn, A., Wachholder, A., Winkler, M. & Rebuffat, E. (1990b). Prospective study on the prevalence of sudden infant death and possible risk factors in Brussels: preliminary results (1987–1988). *European Journal of Pediatrics*, **149**, 284–6.

Kalaria, R. N., Fiedler, C., Hunsaker, J. C., III & Sparks, D. L. (1993). Synaptic neurochemistry of human striatum during development: changes in sudden infant death syndrome. *Journal of Neurochemistry*, **60**, 2098–105.

Kalnins, R. (1986). Neuropathological observations in the sudden infant death syndrome: a brief survey of the literature. *Australian Paediatric Journal*, **22** (Suppl), 7–8.

Kalokerinos, A. & Dettman, G. (1976). Sudden death in infancy syndrome in Western Australia. *Medical Journal of Australia*, **2**, 31–2.

Kandall, S. R. & Gaines, J. (1991). Maternal substance use and subsequent sudden infant death syndrome (SIDS) in offspring. *Neurotoxicology and Teratology*, **13**, 235–40.

Kandall, S. R., Gaines, J., Habel, L., Davidson, G. & Jessop, D. (1993). Relationship of maternal substance abuse to subsequent sudden infant death syndrome in offspring. *Journal of Pediatrics*, **123**, 120–66.

Kaplan, D. W., Bauman, A. E. & Krous, H. F. (1984). Epidemiology of sudden infant death syndrome in American Indians. *Pediatrics*, **74**, 1041–6.

Kariks, J. (1988). Cardiac lesions in sudden infant death syndrome. *Forensic Science International*, **39**, 211–25.

Kariks, J. (1989). Diaphragmatic muscle fibre necrosis in SIDS. *Forensic Science International*, **43**, 281–91.

Kearney, M. S., Dahl, L. B. & Stalsberg, H. (1982). Can a cat smother and kill a baby? *British Medical Journal*, **285**, 777.

Keens, T. G. & Davidson Ward, S. L. (2001). Respiratory mechanisms and hypoxia. In *Sudden Infant Death Syndrome. Problems, Progress and Possibilities*, ed. R. W. Byard & H. F. Krous. London: Arnold, pp. 66–82.

Keens, T. G., Davidson Ward, S. L., Gates, E. P., Andree, D. I. & Hart, L. D. (1985). Ventilatory pattern following diphtheria-tetanus-pertussis immunization in infants at risk for sudden infant death syndrome. *American Journal of Diseases of Children*, **139**, 991–4.

Keeton, B. R., Southall, E., Rutter, N., Anderson, R. H., Shinebourne, E. A. & Southall, D. P. (1977). Cardiac conduction disorders in six infants with "near-miss" sudden infant deaths. *British Medical Journal*, **ii**, 600–601.

Kelley, J., Allsopp, D. & Hawksworth, D. L. (1992). Sudden infant death syndrome (SIDS) and the toxic gas hypothesis: microbiological studies of cot mattresses. *Human and Experimental Toxicology*, **11**, 347–55.

Kelly, D. H. & Shannon, D. C. (1982). Sudden infant death syndrome and near sudden infant death syndrome: a review of the literature, 1964 to 1982. *Pediatric Clinics of North America*, **29**, 1241–61.

Kelly, D. H. & Shannon, D. C. (1988). The medical management of cardiorespiratory monitoring in infantile apnea. In *Sudden Infant Death Syndrome. Medical Aspects and Psychological Management*, ed. J. L. Culbertson, H. F. Krous & R. D. Bendell. London: Edward Arnold, pp. 139–261.

Kelly, D. H., Krishnamoorthy, K. S. & Shannon, D. C. (1980). Astrocytoma in an infant with prolonged apnea. *Pediatrics*, **66**, 429–31.

Kelly, D. H., Pathak, A. & Meny, R. (1991). Sudden severe bradycardia in infancy. *Pediatric Pulmonology*, **10**, 199–204.

Kelly, D. H., Shannon, D. C. & Liberthson, R. R. (1977). The role of the QT interval in the sudden infant death syndrome. *Circulation*, **55**, 633–5.

Kemp, J. S. & Thach, B. T. (1991). Sudden death in infants sleeping on polystyrene-filled cushions. *New England Journal of Medicine*, 324, 1858–64.

Kemp, J. S. & Thach, B. T. (1993). A sleep position-dependent mechanism for infant death on sheepskins. *American Journal of Diseases of Children*, **147**, 642–6.

Kemp, J. S. & Thach, B. T. (2001). Rebreathing of exhaled air. In *Sudden Infant Death Syndrome. Problems, Progress and Possibilities*, ed. R. W. Byard & H. F. Krous. London: Arnold, pp. 138–55.

Kemp, J. S., Kowalski, R. M., Burch, P. M., Graham, M. A. & Thach, B. T. (1993). Unintentional suffocation by rebreathing: a death scene and physiologic investigation of a possible cause of sudden infant death. *Journal of Pediatrics*, **122**, 874–80.

Kemp, J. S., Livne, M., White, D. K. & Arfken, C. L. (1998). Softness and potential to cause rebreathing: differences in bedding used by infants at high and low risk for sudden infant death syndrome. *Journal of Pediatrics*, **132**, 234–9.

Kemp, J. S., Nelson, V. E. & Thach, B. T. (1994). Physical properties of bedding that may increase risk of sudden infant death syndrome in prone-sleeping infants. *Pediatric Research*, **36**, 7–11.

Kendeel, S. R. & Ferris, J. A. J. (1977a). Apparent hypoxic changes in pulmonary arterioles and small arteries in infancy. *Journal of Clinical Pathology*, **30**, 481–5.

Kendeel, S. R. M. & Ferris, J. A. J. (1977b). Sudden infant death syndrome. A review of literature. *Journal of the Forensic Science Society*, **17**, 223–55.

Kenigsberg, K., Griswold, P. G., Buckley, B. J., Gootman, N. & Gootman, P. M. (1983). Cardiac effects of esophageal stimulation: possible relationship between gastroesophageal reflux (GER) and sudden infant death syndrome (SIDS). *Journal of Pediatric Surgery*, **18**, 542–5.

Kerr, J. R., Al-Khattaf, A., Barson, A. J. & Burnie, J. P. (2000). An association between sudden infant death syndrome (SIDS) and *Helicobacter pylori* infection. *Archives of Disease in Childhood*, **83**, 429–34.

Kinney, H. C. (1988). The brainstem in the sudden infant death syndrome: a review. In *Sudden Infant Death Syndrome. Risk Factors and Basic Mechanisms*, ed. R. M. Harper & H. J. Hoffman. New York: PMA Publishing, pp. 115–34.

Kinney, H. C. & Filiano, J. J. (1988). Brainstem research in sudden infant death syndrome. *Pediatrician*, **15**, 240–50.

Kinney, H. C. & Filiano, J. J. (2001). Brain research in sudden infant death syndrome. In *Sudden Infant Death Syndrome. Problems, Progress and Possibilities*, ed. R. W. Byard & H. F. Krous. London: Arnold, pp. 118–37.

Kinney, H. C., Brody, B. A., Finkelstein, D. M., Vawter, G. F., Mandell, F. & Gilles, F. H. (1991). Delayed central nervous system myelination in the sudden infant death syndrome. *Journal of Neuropathology and Experimental Neurology*, **50**, 29–48.

Kinney, H. C., Burger, P. C., Harrell, F. E., Jr & Hudson, R. P., Jr (1983). 'Reactive gliosis' in the medulla oblongata of victims of the sudden infant death syndrome. *Pediatrics*, **72**, 181–7.

Kinney, H. C., Filiano, J. J., Assmann, S. F., *et al.* (1998). Tritiated-naloxone binding to brainstem opioid receptors in the sudden infant death syndrome. *Journal of the Autonomic Nervous System*, **69**, 156–63.

Kinney, H. C., Filiano, J. J. & Harper, R. M. (1992). The neuropathology of the sudden infant death syndrome. A review. *Journal of Neuropathology and Experimental Neurology*, **51**, 115–26.

Kinney, H. C., Filiano, J. J., Sleeper, L. A., Mandell, F., Valdes-Dapena, M. & White, W. F. (1995). Decreased muscarinic receptor binding in the arcuate nucleus in sudden infant death syndrome. *Science*, **269**, 1446–50.

Kleemann, W. J., Hiller, A. S. & Troger, H. D. (1995). Infections of the upper respiratory tract in cases of sudden infant death. *International Journal of Legal Medicine*, **108**, 85–9.

Kleemann, W. J., Schlaud, M., Poets, C. F., Rothamel, T. & Troger, H. D. (1996). Hyperthermia in sudden infant death. *International Journal of Legal Medicine*, **109**, 139–42.

Kleemann, W. J., Weller, J.-P., Wolf, M., Troger, H. D., Bluthgen, A. & Heeschen, W. (1991). Heavy metals, chlorinated pesticides and polychlorinated biphenyls in sudden infant death syndrome (SIDS). *International Journal of Legal Medicine*, **104**, 71–5.

Klonoff-Cohen, H. S., Edelstein, S. L., Lefkowitz, E. S., *et al.* (1995). The effect of passive smoking and tobacco exposure through breast milk on sudden infant death syndrome. *Journal of the American Medical Association*, **273**, 795–8.

Knight, B. H. (1975). The significance of the postmortem discovery of gastric contents in the air passages. *Forensic Science*, **6**, 229–34.

Knight, B. (1983). *The Coroner's Autopsy. A Guide to Non-criminal Autopsies for the General Pathologist*. Edinburgh: Churchill Livingstone, p. 139.

Knöbel, H. H., Yang, W.-S. & Chen, C.-J. (1996). Risk factors of sudden infant death in Chinese babies. *American Journal of Epidemiology*, **144**, 1070–73.

Kocsard-Varo, G. (1991). The physiological role of the pineal gland as the masterswitch of life, turning on at birth breathing and geared to it the function of the autonomic nervous system. The cause of SIDS examined in this context. *Medical Hypotheses*, **34**, 122–6.

Koehler, S. A., Ladham, S., Shakir, A. & Wecht, C. H. (2001). Simultaneous sudden infant death syndrome. A proposed definition and worldwide review of cases. *American Journal of Forensic Medicine and Pathology*, **22**, 23–32.

Konrat, G., Halliday, G., Sullivan, C. & Harper, C. (1992). Preliminary evidence suggesting delayed development in the hypoglossal and vagal nuclei of SIDS infants: a necropsy study. *Journal of Child Neurology*, **7**, 44–9.

Kopp, N., Chigr, F., Denoroy, L., Gilly, R. & Jordan, D. (1993). Absence of adrenergic neurons in nucleus tractus solitarius in sudden infant death syndrome. *Neuropediatrics*, **24**, 25–9.

Kopp, N., Denoroy, L., Eymin, C., *et al.* (1994). Studies of neuroregulators in the brain stem of SIDS. *Biology of the Neonate*, **65**, 189–93.

Kozakewich, H., Fox, K., Plato, C. C., Cronk, C., Mandell, F. & Vawter, G. F. (1992). Dermatoglyphics in sudden infant death syndrome. *Pediatric Pathology*, **12**, 637–51.

Kozakewich, H. P. W., McManus, B. M. & Vawter, G. F. (1982). The sinus node in sudden infant death syndrome. *Circulation*, **65**, 1242–6.

Kozakewich, H., Sytkowski, A., Fisher, J., Vawter, G. & Mandell, F. (1986). Serum erythropoietin in infants with emphasis on sudden infant death syndrome. *Laboratory Investigation*, **54**, 5.

Kraus, A. S., Steele, R., Thompson, M. G. & De Grosbois, P. (1971). Further epidemiologic observations on sudden, unexpected death in infancy in Ontario. *Canadian Journal of Public Health*, **62**, 210–19.

Kraus, J. F. (1983). Methodologic considerations in the search for risk factors unique to sudden infant death syndrome. In *Sudden Infant Death Syndrome*, ed. J. A. Tildon, L. M. Roeder & A. Steinschneider. New York: Academic Press, pp. 43–58.

Kraus, J. F. & Borhani, N. O. (1972). Post-neonatal sudden unexplained death in California: a cohort study. *American Journal of Epidemiology*, **95**, 497–510.

Kraus, J. F., Greenland, S. & Bulterys M. (1989). Risk factors for sudden infant death syndrome in the US collaborative perinatal project. *International Journal of Epidemiology*, **18**, 113–20.

Kraus, J. F., Peterson, D. R., Standfast, S. J., van Belle, G. & Hoffman, H. J. (1988). The relationship of socio-economic status and sudden infant death syndrome: confounding or effect modification? In *Sudden Infant Death Syndrome. Risk Factors and Basic Mechanisms*, eds. R. M. Harper & H. J. Hoffman. New York: PMA Publishing, pp. 221–9.

Krous, H. F. (1984a). The microscopic distribution of intrathoracic petechiae in sudden infant death syndrome. *Archives of Pathology and Laboratory Medicine*, **108**, 77–9.

Krous, H. F. (1984b). Sudden infant death syndrome: pathology and pathophysiology. *Pathology Annual*, **19** (part 1), 1–14.

Krous, H. F. (1988). Pathological considerations of sudden infant death syndrome. *Pediatrician*, **15**, 231–9.

Krous, H. F. (1989). The pathology of sudden infant death syndrome: an overview. In *Sudden Infant Death Syndrome. Medical Aspects and Psychological Management*, ed. J. L. Culbertson, H. F. Krous & R. D. Bendell. London: Edward Arnold, pp. 18–47.

Krous, H. F. (1995). The International Standardised Autopsy Protocol for sudden unexpected infant death. In *Sudden Infant*

Death Syndrome. New Trends in the Nineties, ed. T. O. Rognum. Oslo: Scandinavian University Press, pp. 81–95.

Krous, H. F. & Jordan, J. (1984). A necropsy study of distribution of petechiae in non-sudden infant death syndrome. *Archives of Pathology and Laboratory Medicine*, **108**, 75–6.

Krous, H. F. & Jordan, J. (1988). A comparison of the distribution of petechiae and their significance in sudden infant death syndrome (SIDS), lethal upper airway obstruction and non-SIDS. In *Sudden Infant Death Syndrome. Risk Factors and Basic Mechanisms*, ed. R. M. Harper & H. J. Hoffman. New York: PMA Publishing, pp. 91–113.

Krous, H. F., Hauck, F. R., Herman, S. M., *et al.* (1999). Laryngeal basement membrane thickening is not a reliable postmortem marker for SIDS. Results from the Chicago Infant Mortality Study. *American Journal of Forensic Medicine and Pathology*, **20**, 221–7.

Krous, H. F., Floyd, C. W., Nadeau, J. M., Silva, P. D., Blackbourne, B. D. & Langston, C. (2002). Medial smooth muscle thickness in small pulmonary arteries in sudden infant death syndrome revisited. *Pediatric and Developmental Pathology*, **5**, 375–85.

Krous, H. F., Nadeau, J. M., Byard, R. W. & Blackbourne, B. D. (2001a). Oronasal blood in sudden infant death. *American Journal of Forensic Medicine and Pathology*, **22**, 346–51.

Krous, H. F., Nadeau, J. M., Fukumoto, R. I., Blackbourne, B. D. & Byard, R. W. (2001b). Environmental hyperthermic infant and early childhood death. Circumstances, pathologic changes, and manner of death. *American Journal of Forensic Medicine and Pathology*, **22**, 374–82.

Krous, H. F., Nadeau, J. M., Silva, P. D. & Blackbourne, B. D. (2001c). Intrathoracic petechiae in sudden infant death syndrome: relationship to face position when found. *Pediatric and Developmental Pathology*, **4**, 160–66.

Krous, H. F., Nadeau, J. M., Silva, P. D. & Blackbourne, B. D. (2001d). Neck extension and rotation in sudden infant death syndrome and other natural infant deaths. *Pediatric and Developmental Pathology*, **4**, 154–9.

Krous, H. F., Nadeau, J. M., Silva, P. D. & Blackbourne, B. D. (2003). A comparison of respiratory symptoms and inflammation in sudden infant death syndrome and in accidental or inflicted infant death. *American Journal of Forensic Medicine and Pathology*, **24**, 1–8.

Krous, H. F., Nadeau, J. M., Silva, P. D. & Byard, R. W. (2002c). Infanticide: is its incidence among postneonatal infant deaths increasing? An 18–year population-based analysis in California. *American Journal of Forensic Medicine and Pathology*, **23**, 127–31.

Kuich, T. E. & Zimmerman, D. (1981). Endorphins, ventilatory control and sudden infant death syndrome – a review and synthesis. *Medical Hypotheses*, **7**, 1231–40.

Kyle, D., Sunderland, R., Stonehouse, M., Cummins, C. & Ross, O. (1990). Ethnic differences in incidence of sudden infant death syndrome in Birmingham. *Archives of Disease in Childhood*, **65**, 830–33.

Lack, E. E., Perez-Atayde, A. R. & Young, J. B. (1986). Carotid bodies in sudden infant death syndrome: a combined light microscopic, ultrastructural and biochemical study. *Pediatric Pathology*, **6**, 335–50.

Ladham, S., Koehler, S. A., Shakir, A. & Wecht, C. H. (2001). Simultaneous sudden infant death syndrome. A case report. *American Journal of Forensic Medicine and Pathology*, **22**, 33–7.

Laennec, R. T. H. (1834). *A Treatise on the Diseases of the Chest and on Mediate Auscultation*, 4th edn. London: Longman, Rees, Orme, Brown, Green & Longman; Whittaker and Co.; Simpkin and Marshall; J. Chidley; E. Portwine; and Henry Renshaw, pp. 81–2.

Langlois, N. E. I., Ellis, P. S., Little, D. L. & Hulewicz, B. (2002). Toxicologic analysis in cases of possible sudden infant death syndrome. A worthwhile exercise? *American Journal of Forensic Medicine and Pathology*, **23**, 162–6.

Lapin, C. A., Morrow, G., III, Chvapil, M., Belke, D. P. & Fisher, R. S. (1976). Hepatic trace elements in the sudden infant death syndrome. *Journal of Pediatrics*, **89**, 607–8.

Laughon, B., Bartlett, J. G., Kozakewich, H., Vawter, G. F. & Yolken, R. (1983). Role of *Clostridium difficile* in sudden infant death syndrome. In *Sudden Infant Death Syndrome*, ed. J. A. Tildon, L. M. Roeder & A. Steinschneider. New York: Academic Press, pp. 557–66.

Lawson, B., Anday, E., Guillet, R., Wagerle, L. C., Chance, B. & Delivoria-Papadopoulos, M. (1987). Brain oxidative phosphorylation following alteration in head position in preterm and term neonates. *Pediatric Research*, **22**, 302–5.

Lean, M. E. J. & Jennings, G. (1989). Brown adipose tissue activity in pyrexial cases of cot death. *Journal of Clinical Pathology*, **42**, 1153–6.

Leape, L. L., Holder, T. M., Franklin, J. D., Amoury, R. A. & Ashcraft, K. W. (1977). Respiratory arrest in infants secondary to gastro-esophageal reflux. *Pediatrics*, **60**, 924–8.

Lee, S., Barson, A. J., Drucker, D. B., Morris, J. A. & Telford, D. R. (1987). Lethal challenge of gnotobiotic weanling rats with bacterial isolates from cases of sudden infant death syndrome (SIDS). *Journal of Clinical Pathology*, **40**, 1393–6.

Lee, N. N. Y., Chan, Y. F., Davies, D. P., Lau, E. & Yip, D. C. P. (1989). Sudden infant death syndrome in Hong Kong: confirmation of low incidence. *British Medical Journal*, **298**, 721.

Lee, W. K., Strzelecki, J. & Root, A. W. (1983). Postmortem changes in serum concentrations of triiodothyronine in rats. *Journal of Pediatrics*, **102**, 257–9.

Lemieux, B., Giguere, R., Cyr, D., Shapcott, D., McCann, M. & Tuchman, M. (1993). Screening urine of 3-week-old newborns: lack of association between sudden infant death syndrome and some metabolic disorders. *Pediatrics*, **91**, 986–8.

Lewak, N., van den Berg, B. J. & Beckwith, J. B. (1979). Sudden infant death syndrome risk factors. Prospective data review. *Clinical Pediatrics*, **18**, 404–11.

L'Hoir, M. P., Engelberts, A. C., van Well, G. T. J., *et al.* (1998). Case–control study of current validity of previously described risk factors for SIDS in the Netherlands. *Archives of Disease in Childhood*, **79**, 386–93.

Lie, J. T., Rosenberg, H. S. & Erickson, E. E. (1976). Histopathology of the conduction system in the sudden infant death syndrome. *Circulation*, **53**, 3–8.

Lignitz, E. & Hirvonen, J. (1989). Inflammation in the lungs of infants dying suddenly. A comparative study from two countries. *Forensic Science International*, **42**, 85–94.

Limerick, S. R. (1992). Sudden infant death in historical perspective. *Journal of Clinical Pathology*, **45** (Suppl), 3–6.

Lindgren, C. (1993). Respiratory syncytial virus and the sudden infant death syndrome. *Acta Paediatrica*, **389** (Suppl), 67–9.

Lipsitt, L. P., Sturner, W. Q., Oh, W., Barrett, J. & Truex, R. C. (1979). Wolff–Parkinson–White and sudden-infant-death syndromes. *New England Journal of Medicine*, **300**, 1111.

Little, G. A., Ballard, R. A., Brooks, J. G., *et al.* (1987). Consensus statement. National Institutes of Health consensus development conference on infantile apnea and home monitoring, Sept 29 to Oct 1, 1986. *Pediatrics*, **79**, 292–9.

Lobban, C. D. R. (1991). The human dive reflex as a primary cause of SIDS. A review of the literature. *Medical Journal of Australia*, **155**, 561–3.

Luke, J. L., Blackbourne, B. D. & Donovan, J. W. (1974). Bedsharing deaths among victims of sudden infant death syndrome: a riddle within a conundrum. *Forensic Science Gazette*, **5**, 3–4.

Lundemose, J. B., Lundemose, A. G., Gregersen, M., Helweg-Larsen, K. & Simonsen, J. (1990). *Chlamydia* and sudden infant death syndrome. Study of 166 SIDS and 30 control cases. Paper presented at the 12th World Triennial Meeting of the International Association of Forensic Sciences, Adelaide, Australia, 25–27 October, 1990.

Malam, J. E., Carrick, G. F., Telford, D. R., Morris, J. A. (1992). Staphylococcal toxins and sudden infant death syndrome. *Journal of Clinical Pathology*, **45**, 716–21.

Mallak, C. T., Milch, K. S. & Horn, D. F. (2000). A deadly anti-SIDS device. *American Journal of Forensic Medicine and Pathology*, **21**, 79–82.

Malloy, M. H., Kleinman, J. C., Land, G. H. & Schramm, W. F. (1988). The association of maternal smoking with age and cause of infant death. *American Journal of Epidemiology*, **128**, 46–55.

Maloney, J. E., Brodecky, V., Wilkinson, M., Walker, A. M. & Bennett, K. (1983). Placental insufficiency and the development of the respiratory system "*in utero*". In *Sudden Infant Death Syndrome*, ed. J. A. Tildon, L. M. Roeder & A. Steinschneider. New York: Academic Press, pp. 305–18.

Marino, T. A. & Kane, B. M. (1985). Cardiac atrioventricular junctional tissues in hearts from infants who died suddenly. *Journal of American College of Cardiology*, **5**, 1178–84.

Markestad, T., Skadberg, B., Hordvik, E., Morild, I. & Irgens, L. M. (1995). Sleeping position and sudden infant death syndrome (SIDS): effect of an intervention programme to avoid prone sleeping. *Acta Paediatrica*, **84**, 375–8.

Maron, B. J. & Fisher, R. S. (1977). Sudden infant death syndrome (SIDS): cardiac pathologic observations in infants with SIDS. *American Heart Journal*, **93**, 762–6.

Maron, B. J., Clark, C. E., Goldstein, R. E. & Epstein, S. E. (1976). Potential role of QT interval prolongation in sudden infant death syndrome. *Circulation*, **54**, 423–30.

Martinez, F. D. (1991). Sudden infant death syndrome and small airway occlusion: facts and a hypothesis. *Pediatrics*, **87**, 190–98.

Marx, J. L. (1981). Question marks for SIDS test. *Science*, **213**, 323.

Maslowski, H. A. (1996). A new hypothesis for sudden infant death syndrome: the occlusion of vertebral arteries as a major cause. *Journal of Clinical Forensic Medicine*, **3**, 93–8.

Mason, J. M., Mason, L. H., Jackson, M., Bell, J. S., Francisco, J. T. & Jennings, B. R. (1975). Pulmonary vessels in SIDS. *New England Journal of Medicine*, **292**, 479.

Matthews, T. G. (1992). The autonomic nervous system – a role in sudden infant death syndrome. *Archives of Disease in Childhood*, **67**, 654–6.

Matthews, T. G. & O'Brien, S. J. (1985). Perinatal epidemiological characteristics of the sudden infant death syndrome in an Irish population. *Irish Medical Journal*, **78**, 251–3.

McCulloch, K., Brouillette, R. T., Guzzetta, A. J. & Hunt, C. E. (1982). Arousal responses in near-miss sudden infant death syndrome and in normal infants. *Journal of Pediatrics*, **101**, 911–17.

McGinty, D. J. & Hoppenbrouwers, T. (1983). The reticular formation, breathing disorders during sleep, and SIDS. In *Sudden Infant Death Syndrome*, ed. J. A. Tildon, L. M. Roeder & A. Steinschneider. New York: Academic Press, pp. 375–400.

McGlashan, N. D. (1988). Sleeping position and SIDS. *Lancet*, **ii**, 106.

McGlashan, N. D. (1989). Sudden infant deaths in Tasmania, 1980–1986: a seven year prospective study. *Social Sciences and Medicine*, **29**, 1015–26.

McGlashan, N. D. (1991). Low selenium status and cot deaths. *Medical Hypotheses*, **35**, 311–14.

McKendrick, N., Drucker, D. B., Morris, J. A., *et al.* (1992). Bacterial toxins: a possible cause of cot death. *Journal of Clinical Pathology*, **45**, 49–53.

McKenna, J. J. & Mosko, S. (1993). Evolution and infant sleep: an experimental study of infant-parent co-sleeping and its implications for SIDS. *Acta Paediatrica*, **389** (Suppl), 31–6.

McKenna, J. J. & Mosko, S. S. (1994). Sleep and arousal, synchrony and independence, among mothers and infants sleeping apart and together (same bed): an experiment in evolutionary medicine. *Acta Paediatrica*, **397** (Suppl), 94–102.

McKenna, J. J. & Mosko, S. (2001). Mother-infant cosleeping: toward a new scientific beginning. In *Sudden Infant Death Syndrome. Problems, Progress and Possibilities*, ed. R. W. Byard & H. F. Krous. London: Arnold, pp. 258–74.

McKenna, J. J., Mosko, S., Richard, C., *et al.* (1994). Experimental studies of infant–parent co-sleeping: mutual physiologic and behavioral influences and their relevance to SIDS (sudden infant death syndrome). *Early Human Development*, **38**, 187–201.

McKenna, J. J., Mosko, S. S. & Richard, C. A. (1997). Bedsharing promotes breastfeeding. *Pediatrics*, **100**, 214–19.

McKenna, J. J., Thoman, E. B., Anders, T. F., Sadeh, A., Schechtman, V. L. & Glotzbach, S. F. (1993). Infant-parent co-sleeping in an evolutionary perspective: implications for understanding infant sleep development and the sudden infant death syndrome. *Sleep*, **16**, 263–82.

Meadow, R. (1990). Suffocation, recurrent apnea, and sudden infant death. *Journal of Pediatrics*, **117**, 351–7.

Meadow, R. (1999). Unnatural sudden infant death. *Archives of Disease in Childhood*, **80**, 7–14.

Mehl, A. J. & Malcolm, L. A. (1990). Epidemiological factors in postneonatal mortality in New Zealand. *New Zealand Medical Journal*, **103**, 127–9.

Mehta, S. K., Finkelhor, R. S., Anderson, R. L., Harcar-Sevcik, R. A., Wasser, T. E. & Bahler, R. C. (1993). Transient myocardial ischemia in infants prenatally exposed to cocaine. *Journal of Pediatrics*, **122**, 945–9.

Merritt, T. A. & Valdes-Dapena, M. (1984). SIDS research update. *Pediatric Annals*, **13**, 193–207.

Milerad, J. & Sundell, H. (1993). Nicotine exposure and the risk of SIDS. *Acta Paediatrica*, **389** (Suppl), 70–72.

Miller, M. E., Brooks, J. G., Forbes, N. & Insel, R. (1992). Frequency of medium-chain acyl-CoA dehydrogenase deficiency G-985 mutation in sudden infant death syndrome. *Pediatric Research*, **31**, 305–7.

Milner, A. D. (1987). Recent theories on the cause of cot death. *British Medical Journal*, **295**, 1366–8.

Milner, A. D. & Ruggins, N. (1989). Sudden infant death syndrome. Recent focus on the respiratory system. *British Medical Journal*, **298**, 689–90.

Milner, A. D., Saunders, R. A. & Hopkin, I. E. (1977). Apnoea induced by airflow obstruction. *Archives of Disease in Childhood*, **52**, 379–82.

Milroy, C. M. (1999). Munchausen syndrome by proxy and intra-alveolar haemosiderin. *International Journal of Legal Medicine*, **112**, 309–12.

Mirchandani, H. G., Mirchandani, I. H. & House, D. (1984). Sudden infant death syndrome: measurement of total and specific serum immunoglobulin E (IgE). *Journal of Forensic Sciences*, **29**, 425–9.

Mitchell, E. A. (1990). International trends in postneonatal mortality. *Archives of Disease in Childhood*, **65**, 607–9.

Mitchell, F. A. (1991). Cot death: should the prone sleeping position be discouraged? *Journal of Paediatrics and Child Health*, **27**, 319–21.

Mitchell, E. A. (1993). Sleeping position of infants and the sudden infant death syndrome. *Acta Paediatrica*, **389** (Suppl), 26–30.

Mitchell, E. A. (1995). Smoking: the next major and modifiable risk factor. In *Sudden Infant Death Syndrome. New Trends in the Nineties*, ed. T. O. Rognum. Oslo: Scandinavian University Press, pp. 114–18.

Mitchell, E. A. & Milerad, J. (1999). Smoking and sudden infant death syndrome. In *International Consultation on Environmental Tobacco Smoke (ETS) and Child Health*. Geneva: World Health Organization, pp.105–29.

Mitchell, E. A. & Scragg, R. (1994). Observations on ethnic differences in SIDS mortality in New Zealand. *Early Human Development*, **38**, 151–7.

Mitchell, E. A. & Stewart, A. W. (1988). Deaths from sudden infant death syndrome on public holidays and weekends. *Australian and New Zealand Journal of Medicine*, **18**, 861–3.

Mitchell, E. A. & Thompson, J. M. D. (1995). Co-sleeping increases the risk of SIDS, but sleeping in the parents' bedroom lowers it. In *Sudden Infant Death Syndrome. New Trends in the Nineties*, ed. T. O. Rognum. Oslo: Scandinavian University Press, pp. 266–9.

Mitchell, E. A., Becroft, D. M. P., Byard, R. W., *et al.* (1994). Definition of the sudden infant death syndrome. *British Medical Journal*, **309**, 607.

Mitchell, E. A., Brunt, J. M. & Everard, C. (1994). Reduction in mortality from sudden infant death syndrome in New Zealand: 1986–92. *Archives of Disease in Childhood*, **70**, 291–4.

Mitchell, E. A., Ford, R. P. K., Taylor, B. J., *et al.* (1992a). Further evidence supporting a causal relationship between prone position and SIDS. *Journal of Paediatrics and Child Health*, **28** (Suppl 1), S9–12.

Mitchell, E., Krous, H. F. & Byard, R. W. (2002). Pathological findings in overlaying. *Journal of Clinical Forensic Medicine, 9*, 133–5.

Mitchell, E., Krous, H. F., Donald, T. & Byard, R. W. (2000a). Changing trends in the diagnosis of sudden infant death. *American Journal of Forensic Medicine and Pathology*, **21**, 311–14.

Mitchell, E., Krous, H. F., Donald, T. & Byard, R. W. (2000b). An analysis of the usefulness of specific stages in the pathological investigation of sudden infant death. *American Journal of Forensic Medicine and Pathology*, **21**, 395–400.

Mitchell, E. A., Scragg, L. & Clements, M. (1996). Soft cot mattresses and the sudden infant death syndrome. *New Zealand Medical Journal*, **109**, 206–7.

Mitchell, E. A., Scragg, L. & Clements, M. (1997). Elevation of the head of the cot and sudden infant death syndrome. *Journal of Sudden Infant Death Syndrome and Infant Mortality*, **2**, 167–73.

Mitchell, E. A., Scragg, R., Stewart, A. W., *et al.* (1991). Results from the first year of the New Zealand cot death study. *New Zealand Medical Journal*, **104**, 71–6.

Mitchell, E. A., Stewart, A. W., Clements, M. & Ford, R. P. K. (1995). Immunisation and the sudden infant death syndrome. *Archives of Disease in Childhood*, **73**, 498–501.

Mitchell, E. A., Stewart, A. W., Scragg, R., *et al.* (1993a). Ethnic differences in mortality from sudden infant death syndrome in New Zealand. *British Medical Journal*, **306**, 13–16.

Mitchell, E. A., Taylor, B. J., Ford, R. P. K., *et al.* (1992b). Four modifiable and other major risk factors for cot death: the New Zealand study. *Journal of Paediatrics and Child Health*, **28**, (Suppl 1), S3–8.

Mitchell, E. A., Taylor, B. J., Ford, R. P. K., *et al.* (1993b). Dummies and the sudden infant death syndrome. *Archives of Disease in Childhood*, **68**, 501–4.

Mitchell, E. A., Thach, B. T., Thompson, J. M. & Williams, S. (1999). Changing infants' sleep position increases risk of sudden infant death syndrome. *Archives of Pediatric and Adolescent Medicine*, **153**, 1136–41.

Mitchell, E. A., Tuohy, P. G., Brunt, J. M., *et al.* (1997). Risk factors for sudden infant death syndrome following the prevention campaign in New Zealand: a prospective study. *Pediatrics*, **100**, 835–40.

Mitchell, E. A., Williams, S. M. & Taylor, B. J. (1999). Use of duvets and the risk of sudden infant death syndrome. *Archives of Disease in Childhood*, **81**, 117–19.

Molony, N. C., Kerr, A. I. G., Blackwell, C. C. & Busuttil, A. (1996). Is the nasopharynx warmer in children than in adults? *Journal of Clinical Forensic Medicine*, **3**, 157–60.

Molz, G. & Hartmann, H. (1984). Dysmorphism, dysplasia, and anomaly in sudden infant death. *New England Journal of Medicine*, **311**, 259.

Molz, G., Brodzinowski, A., Bar, W. & Vonlanthen, B. (1992). Morphologic variations in 180 cases of sudden infant death and 180 controls. *American Journal of Forensic Medicine and Pathology*, **13**, 186–90.

Money, D. F. L. (1970). Vitamin E and selenium deficiencies and their possible etiological role in the sudden death in infants syndrome. *Journal of Pediatrics, 77*, 165–6.

Moon, R. Y., Patel, K. M. & Shaefer, S. J. M. (2000). Sudden infant death syndrome in child care settings. *Pediatrics*, **106**, 295–300.

Moore, L. & Byard, R. W. (1993). Pathological findings in hanging and wedging deaths in infants and young children. *American Journal of Forensic Medicine and Pathology*, **14**, 296–302.

Morley, C., Hill, C. & Brown, B. (1988). Lung surfactant and sudden infant death syndrome. *Annals of New York Academy of Sciences*, **533**, 289–95.

Morley, C. J., Hill, C. M., Brown, B. D., Barson, A. J. & Davis, J. A. (1982). Surfactant abnormalities in babies dying from sudden infant death syndrome. *Lancet*, **i**, 1320–22.

Morris, J. A. (1989). Sudden infant death syndrome. *British Medical Journal*, **298**, 958.

Mortimer, E. A., Jr (1987). DTP and SIDS: when data differ. *American Journal of Public Health*, **77**, 925–6.

Mortimer, E. A., Jr, Jones, P. K. & Adelson, L. (1983). DTP and SIDS. *Pediatric Infectious Disease*, **2**, 492–3.

Mosko, S., Richard, C. & McKenna, J. (1997). Infant arousals during mother–infant bed sharing: implications for infant sleep and sudden infant death syndrome research. *Pediatrics*, **100**, 841–9.

Mosko, S., Richard, C., McKenna, J., Drummond, S. & Mukai, D. (1997). Maternal proximity and infant CO_2 environment during bedsharing and possible implications for SIDS research. *American Journal of Physical Anthropology*, **103**, 315–28.

Murrell, T. G. C., Murrell, W. G. & Lindsay J. A. (1994). Sudden infant death syndrome (SIDS): are common bacterial toxins responsible, and do they have a vaccine potential? *Vaccine*, **12**, 365–8.

Murrell, W. G., Stewart, B. J., O'Neill, C., Siarakas, S. & Kariks, S. (1993). Enterotoxigenic bacteria in the sudden infant death syndrome. *Journal of Medical Microbiology*, **39**, 114–27.

Myer, E. C., Morris, D. L., Adams, M. L., Brase, D. A. & Dewey, W. L. (1987). Increased cerebrospinal fluid β-endorphin immunoreactivity in infants with apnea and in siblings of victims of sudden infant death syndrome. *Journal of Paediatrics*, **111**, 660–66.

Myers, M. M., Fifer, W. P., Schaeffer, L., *et al.* (1998). Effects of sleeping position and time after feeding on the organization of sleep/wake states in prematurely born infants. *Sleep*, **21**, 343–9.

Nachmanoff, D. B., Panigrahy, A., Filiano, J. J., *et al.* (1998). Brain-stem 3H-nicotine receptor binding in the sudden infant death syndrome. *Journal of Neuropathology and Experimental Neurology*, **57**, 1018–25.

Naeye, R. L. (1973). Pulmonary arterial abnormalities in the sudden-infant-death syndrome. *New England Journal of Medicine*, **289**, 1167–70.

Naeye, R. L. (1974). Hypoxemia and the sudden infant death syndrome. *Science*, **186**, 837–8.

Naeye, R. L. (1976). Brain-stem and adrenal abnormalities in the sudden-infant-death syndrome. *American Journal of Clinical Pathology*, **66**, 526–30.

Naeye, R. L. (1977). Placental abnormalities in victims of the sudden infant death syndrome. *Biology of the Neonate*, **32**, 189–92.

Naeye, R. L. (1978). The sudden infant death syndrome. In *The Lung: Structure, Function and Disease*, ed. W. M. Thurlbeck & M. R. Abell. Baltimore: Williams & Wilkins, pp. 262–70.

Naeye, R. L. (1980). Sudden infant death. *Scientific American*, **242**, 52–8.

Naeye, R. L. (1983). Origins of the sudden infant death syndrome. In *Sudden Infant Death Syndrome*, ed. J. A. Tildon, L. M. Roeder & A. Steinschneider. New York: Academic Press, pp. 77–83.

Naeye, R. L. (1988). Sudden infant death syndrome, is the confusion ending? *Modern Pathology*, **1**, 169–74.

Naeye, R. L., Fisher, R., Rubin, H. R. & Demers, L. M. (1980). Selected hormone levels in victims of the sudden infant death syndrome. *Pediatrics*, **65**, 1134–6.

Naeye, R. L., Fisher, R., Ryser M. & Whalen, P. (1976a). Carotid body in the sudden infant death syndrome. *Science*, **191**, 567–9.

Naeye, R. L., Ladis, B. & Drage, J. S. (1976). Sudden infant death syndrome. A prospective study. *American Journal of Diseases of Children*, **130**, 1207–10.

Naeye, R. L., Messmer, J., III, Specht, T. & Merritt, T. A. (1976b). Sudden infant death syndrome temperament before death. *Journal of Pediatrics*, **88**, 511–15.

Naeye, R. L., Olsson, J. M. & Combs, J. W. (1989). New brain stem and bone marrow abnormalities in victims of sudden infant death syndrome. *Journal of Perinatology*, **9**, 180–83.

Naumberg, E. G. & Meny, R. G. (1988). Breast milk opioids and neonatal apnea. *American Journal of Diseases of Children*, **142**, 11–12.

Nelson, E. A. S. (1996a). *Sudden Infant Death Syndrome and Child Care Practices*. Hong Kong: E. A. S. Nelson.

Nelson, E. A. S. (1996b). Child care practices and cot death in Hong Kong. *New Zealand Medical Journal*, **109**, 144–6.

Nelson, E. A. S. & Taylor, B. J. (1988). Climatic and social associations with postneonatal mortality rates within New Zealand. *New Zealand Medical Journal*, **101**, 443–6.

Nelson, E. A. S. & Taylor, B. J. (1989). Infant clothing, bedding and room heating in an area of high postneonatal mortality. *Paediatric and Perinatal Epidemiology*, **3**, 146–56.

Nelson, E. A. S., Schiefenhoevel, W. & Haimerl, F. (2000). Child care practices in nonindustrialized societies. *Pediatrics*, **105**, E75.

Nelson, E. A. S., Taylor, B. J. & Mackay, S. C. (1989). Child care practices and the sudden infant death syndrome. *Australian Paediatric Journal*, **25**, 202–4.

Nelson, E. A. S., Taylor, B. J. & Weatherall, I. L. (1989). Sleeping position and infant bedding may predispose to hyperthermia and the sudden infant death syndrome. *Lancet*, **i**, 199–201.

Nelson, E. A. S., Williams, S. M., Taylor, B. J., *et al.* (1990). Prediction of possibly preventable death: a case–control study of postneonatal mortality in southern New Zealand. *Paediatric and Perinatal Epidemiology*, **4**, 39–52.

Newman, N. M. (1986). Sudden infant death syndrome in Tasmania, 1975–81. *Australian Paediatric Journal*, **22** (Suppl), 17–19.

Newman, N. M., Frost, J. K., Bury, L., Jordan, K. & Phillips, K. (1986). Responses to partial nasal obstruction in sleeping infants. *Australian Paediatric Journal*, **22**, 111–16.

Newman, N. M., Trinder, J. A., Phillips, K. A., Jordan, K. & Cruickshank, J. (1989). Arousal deficit: mechanism of the sudden infant death syndrome? *Australian Paediatric Journal*, **25**, 196–201.

Nicholl, J. P. & O'Cathain, A. (1988). Sleeping position and SIDS. *Lancet*, **ii**, 106.

Nigro, M. A. & Lim, H. C. N. (1992). Hyperekplexia and sudden neonatal death. *Pediatric Neurology*, **8**, 221–5.

Northway, W. H., Jr (1990). Bronchopulmonary dysplasia: then and now. *Archives of Disease in Childhood*, **65**, 1076–81.

Norvenius, S. G. (1987). Sudden infant death syndrome in Sweden in 1973–1977 and 1979. *Acta Paediatrica Scandinavica*, **333** (Suppl), 5–119.

Norvenius, S. G. (1988). The contribution of SIDS to infant mortality trends in Sweden. In *Sudden Infant Death Syndrome. Risk Factors and Basic Mechanisms*, ed. R. M. Harper & H. J. Hoffman. New York: PMA Publishing, pp. 27–52.

Norvenius, S. G. (1993). Some medico-historic remarks on SIDS. *Acta Paediatrica*, **389** (Suppl), 3–9.

Oehmichen, M., Gerling, I. & Meissner, C. (2000). Petechiae of the baby's skin as differentiation symptom of infanticide versus SIDS. *Journal of Forensic Sciences*, **45**, 602–7.

Ogbuihi, S. & Zink, P. (1988). Pulmonary lymphatics in SIDS – a comparative morphometric study. *Forensic Science International*, **39**, 197–206.

Ogra, P. L., Ogra, S. S. & Coppola, P. R. (1975). Secretory component and sudden-infant-death syndrome. *Lancet*, **ii**, 387–90.

O'Kusky, J. R. & Norman, M. G. (1992). Sudden infant death syndrome: postnatal changes in the numerical density and total number of neurons in the hypoglossal nucleus. *Journal of Neuropathology and Experimental Neurology*, **51**, 577–84.

Oren, J., Kelly, D. H. & Shannon, D. C. (1987). Familial occurrence of sudden infant death syndrome and apnea of infancy. *Pediatrics*, **80**, 355–8.

Orlowski, J. P. (1986). Cerebrospinal fluid endorphins and the infant apnea syndrome. *Pediatrics*, **78**, 233–7.

Orlowski, J. P., Nodar, R. H. & Lonsdale, D. (1979). Abnormal brainstem auditory evoked potentials in infants with threatened sudden infant death syndrome. *Cleveland Clinic Quarterly*, **46**, 77–81.

Orr, W. C., Stahl, M. L., Duke, J., *et al.* (1985). Effect of sleep state and position on the incidence of obstructive and central apnea in infants. *Pediatrics*, **75**, 832–5.

Øyen, N., Bulterys, M., Welty, T. K. & Kraus, J. F. (1990). Sudden unexplained infant deaths among American Indians and whites in North and South Dakota. *Paediatric and Perinatal Epidemiology*, **4**, 175–83.

Øyen, N., Markestad, T., Skjaerven, R., Irgens, L. M., *et al.* (1997). Combined effects of sleeping position and prenatal risk factors in sudden infant death syndrome: the Nordic Epidemiological SIDS Study. *Pediatrics*, **100**, 613–21.

Ozand, P. T. & Tildon, J. T. (1983). Alterations of catecholamine enzymes in several brain regions of victims of sudden infant death syndrome. *Life Sciences*, **32**, 1765–70.

Pamphlett, R., Raisanen, J. & Kum-Jew, S. (1999). Vertebral artery compression resulting from head movement: a possible cause of the sudden infant death syndrome. *Pediatrics*, **103**, 460–68.

Panaretto, K. S., Whitehall, J. F., McBride, G., Patole, S. K. & Whitehall, J. S. (2002). Sudden infant death syndrome in Indigenous and non-Indigenous infants in north Queensland: 1990–1998. *Journal of Paediatrics and Child Health*, **38**, 135–9.

Panigrahy, A., Filiano, J., Sleeper, L. A., *et al.* (2000). Decreased serotonergic receptor binding in rhombic lip-derived regions of the medulla oblongata in the sudden infant death syndrome. *Journal of Neuropathology and Experimental Neurology*, **59**, 377–84.

Panigrahy, A., Filiano, J. J., Sleeper, L. A., *et al.* (1997). Decreased kainate receptor binding in the arcuate nucleus of the sudden infant death syndrome. *Journal of Neuropathology and Experimental Neurology*, **56**, 1253–61.

Parkins, K. J., Poets, C. F., O'Brien, L. M., Stebbens, V. A. & Southall, D. P. (1998). Effect of exposure to 15% oxygen on breathing patterns and oxygen saturation in infants: interventional study. *British Medical Journal*, **316**, 887–91.

Pasi, A., Foletta, D., Molz, G., *et al.* (1983). Regional levels of β-lipotropin and β-endorphin in the brain and the hypophysis of victims of sudden infant death syndrome. *Archives of Pathology and Laboratory Medicine*, **107**, 336–7.

Paton, J. Y., MacFadyen, U. M. & Simpson, H. (1989). Sleep phase and gastro-oesophageal reflux in infants at possible risk of SIDS. *Archives of Disease in Childhood*, **64**, 264–9.

Paton, A. W., Paton, J. C., Heuzenroeder, M. W., Goldwater, P. N. & Manning, P. A. (1992). Cloning and nucleotide sequence of a variant Shiga-like toxin II gene from *Escherichia coli* OX3:H21 isolated from a case of sudden infant death syndrome. *Microbial Pathogenesis*, **13**, 225–36.

Patrick, W. J. A. & Logan, R. W. (1988). Free amino acid content of the vitreous humour in cot deaths. *Archives of Disease in Childhood*, **63**, 660–62.

Pearson, J. & Brandeis, L. (1983). Normal aspects of morphometry of brain stem astrocytes, carotid bodies and ganglia in SIDS. In *Sudden Infant Death Syndrome*, ed. J. A. Tildon, L. M. Roeder & A. Steinschneider. New York: Academic Press, pp. 115–21.

Pearson, R. D. & Greenaway, A. C. (1990). Sudden infant death syndrome and hibernation: is there a link? *Medical Hypotheses*, **31**, 131–4.

Penzien, J. M., Molz, G., Wiesmann, U. N., Colombo, J.-P., Bühlmann, R. & Wermuth, B. (1994). Medium-chain acyl-CoA dehydrogenase deficiency does not correlate with apparent life-threatening events and the sudden infant death syndrome: results from phenylpropionate loading tests and DNA analysis. *European Journal of Pediatrics*, **153**, 352–7.

Perrin, D. G., Becker, L. E., Madapallimatum, A., Cutz, E., Bryan, A. C. & Sole, M. J. (1984a). Sudden infant death syndrome: increased carotid-body dopamine and noradrenaline content. *Lancet*, **ii**, 535–7.

Perrin, D. G., Cutz, E., Becker, L. E. & Bryan, A. C. (1984b). Ultrastructure of carotid bodies in sudden infant death syndrome. *Pediatrics*, **73**, 646–51.

Perrin, D. G., McDonald, T. J. & Cutz, E. (1991). Hyperplasia of bombesin-immunoreactive pulmonary neuroendocrine cells and neuroepithelial bodies in sudden infant death syndrome. *Pediatric Pathology*, **11**, 431–47.

Peterson, D. R. (1980). Evolution of the epidemiology of sudden infant death syndrome. *Epidemiologic Reviews*, **2**, 97–112.

Peterson, D. R. (1988). Clinical implications of sudden infant death syndrome epidemiology. *Pediatrician*, **15**, 198–203.

Peterson, D. R. (1989). The epidemiology of sudden infant death syndrome. In *Sudden Infant Death Syndrome. Medical Aspects and Psychological Management*, ed. J. L. Culbertson, H. F. Krous & R. D. Bendell. London: Edward Arnold, pp. 3–16.

Peterson, D. R. & Davis, N. (1986). Sudden infant death syndrome and malignant hyperthermia diathesis. *Australian Pediatric Journal*, **22** (Suppl), 33–5.

Petersen, S. A. & Wailoo, M. P. (1994). Interactions between infant care practices and physiological development in Asian infants. *Early Human Development*, **38**, 181–6.

Peterson, D. R., Benson, E. A., Fisher, L. D., Chinn, N. M. & Beckwith, J. B. (1974). Postnatal growth and the sudden infant death syndrome. *American Journal of Epidemiology*, **99**, 389–94.

Peterson, D. R., Chinn, N. M. & Fisher, L. D. (1980). The sudden infant death syndrome: repetitions in families. *Journal of Pediatrics*, **97**, 265–7.

Peterson, D. R., Green, W. L. & van Belle, G. (1983). Sudden infant death syndrome and hypertriiodothyroninemia: comparison of neonatal and postmortem measurements. *Journal of Pediatrics*, **102**, 206–9.

Peterson, D. R., Labbe, R. F., van Belle, G. & Chinn, N. M. (1981). Erythrocyte transketolase activity and sudden infant death. *American Journal of Clinical Nutrition*, **34**, 65–7.

Peterson, D. R., Sabotta, E. E. & Daling, J. R. (1986). Infant mortality among subsequent siblings of infants who died of sudden infant death syndrome. *Journal of Pediatrics*, **108**, 911–14.

Peterson, D. R., van Belle, G. & Chinn, N. M. (1982). Sudden infant death syndrome and maternal age: etiologic implications. *Journal of the American Medical Association*, **247**, 2250–52.

Phelan, P. (1979). Vitamin C and sudden infant death syndrome. *Medical Journal of Australia*, **ii**, 696.

Pincus, S. M., Cummins, T. R. & Haddad, G. G. (1993). Heart rate control in normal and aborted-SIDS infants. *American Journal of Physiology*, **264**, R638–46.

Pinholster, G. (1994). SIDS paper triggers a murder charge. *Science*, **264**, 197–8.

Pinkham, J. R. & Beckwith, J. B. (1970). Vocal cord lesions in the sudden infant death syndrome. In *Sudden Infant Death Syndrome*, ed. A. B. Bergman, J. B. Beckwith & C. G. Ray. Seattle: University of Washington Press, pp. 104–7.

Platt, M. S., Elin, R. J., Hosseini, J. M. & Smialek, J. E. (1994). Endotoxemia in sudden infant death syndrome. *American Journal of Forensic Medicine and Pathology*, **15**, 261–5.

Poets, C. F. (2001). The role of monitoring. In *Sudden Infant Death Syndrome. Problems, Progress and Possibilities*. ed. R. W. Byard & H. F. Krous. London: Arnold, pp. 243–57.

Poets, C. F. & Southall, D. P. (1991). Control of breathing, apnea, and sudden infant death. *Current Opinion in Pediatrics*, **3**, 413–17.

Poets, C. F., Meny, R. G., Chobanian, M. R. & Bonofiglo, R. E. (1999). Gasping and other cardiorespiratory patterns during sudden infant deaths. *Pediatric Research*, **45**, 350–54.

Polak, J. M. & Wigglesworth, J. S. (1976). Islet-cell hyperplasia and sudden infant death. *Lancet*, **ii**, 570–71.

Pollock, T. M., Miller, E., Mortimer, J. Y. & Smith, G. (1984). Symptoms after primary immunisation with DTP and with DT vaccine. *Lancet*, **ii**, 146–9.

Ponsonby, A.-L., Dwyer, T., Couper, D. & Cochrane, J. (1998). Association between use of a quilt and sudden infant death syndrome: case–control study. *British Medical Journal*, **316**, 195–6.

Ponsonby, A.-L., Dwyer, T., Gibbons, L. E., Cochrane, J. A., Jones, M. E. & McCall, M. J. (1992a). Thermal environment and sudden infant death syndrome: case control study. *British Medical Journal*, **304**, 277–82.

Ponsonby, A.-L., Dwyer, T., Gibbons, L. E., Cochrane, J. A. & Wang, Y. G. (1993). Factors potentiating the risk of sudden infant death syndrome associated with the prone position. *New England Journal of Medicine*, **329**, 377–82.

Ponsonby, A.-L., Dwyer, T. & Jones, M. E. (1992). Sudden infant death syndrome: seasonality and a biphasic model of pathogenesis. *Journal of Epidemiology and Community Health*, **46**, 33–7.

Ponsonby, A.-L., Dwyer, T., Kasl, S. V. & Cochrane, J. A. (1995). The Tasmanian SIDS Case–Control Study: univariable and multivariable risk factor analysis. *Paediatric and Perinatal Epidemiology*, **9**, 256–72.

Ponsonby, A.-L., Jones, M. E., Lumley, J., Dwyer, T. & Gilbert, N. (1992b). Climatic temperature and variation in the incidence of sudden infant death syndrome between the Australian States. *Medical Journal of Australia*, **156**, 246–51.

Poulsen, J. P., Rognum, T. O., Hauge, S., Øyasaeter, S. & Saugstad, O. D. (1993). Post-mortem concentrations of hypoxanthine in the vitreous humor – a comparison between babies with severe respiratory failure, congenital abnormalities of the heart, and victims of sudden infant death syndrome. *Journal of Perinatal Medicine*, **21**, 153–63.

Quattrochi, J. J., Baba, N., Liss, L. & Adrion, W. (1980). Sudden infant death syndrome (SIDS): a preliminary study of reticular dendritic spines in infants with SIDS. *Brain Research*, **181**, 245–9.

Quattrochi, J. J., McBride, P. T. & Yates, A. J. (1985). Brainstem immaturity in sudden infant death syndrome: a quantitative rapid Golgi. Study of dendritic spines in 95 infants. *Brain Research*, **325**, 39–48.

R. *v.* Egan (1897). *Australian Law Times*, **XVIII**, 271.

Rahilly, P. M. (1991). The pneumographic and medical investigation of infants suffering apparent life threatening episodes. *Journal of Paediatrics and Child Health*, **27**, 349–53.

Rajs, J., Råsten-Almqvist, P., Falck, G., Eksborg, S. & Andersson, B. S. (1997). Sudden infant death syndrome: postmortem findings of nicotine and cotinine in pericardial fluid of infants in relation to morphological changes and position at death. *Pediatric Pathology and Laboratory Medicine*, **17**, 83–97.

Rambaud, C., Cieuta, C., Canioni, D., *et al.* (1992). Cot death and myocarditis. *Cardiology of the Young*, **2**, 266–71.

Rambaud, C., Guilleminault, C. & Campbell, P. E. (1994). Definition of the sudden infant death syndrome. *British Medical Journal*, **308**, 1439.

Ramos, V., Hernández, A. F. & Villanueva, E. (1997). Simultaneous death of twins. An environmental hazard or SIDS? *American Journal of Forensic Medicine and Pathology*, **18**, 75–8.

Read, A. W. (2002). What are the national rates for sudden infant death syndrome for Aboriginal and Torres Strait Islander infants? *Journal of Paediatrics and Child Health*, **38**, 122–3.

Read, D. J. C. (1978). The aetiology of the sudden infant death syndrome: current ideas on breathing and sleep and possible links to deranged thiamine neurochemistry. *Australian and New Zealand Journal of Medicine*, **8**, 322–36.

Read, D. J. C. & Jeffery, H. E. (1983). Many paths to asphyxial death in SIDS – a search for underlying neurochemical defects. In *Sudden Infant Death Syndrome*, ed. J. A. Tildon, L. M. Roeder & A. Steinschneider. New York: Academic Press, pp. 183–200.

Read, D. J. C., Gray, V. F., Zacharatos, D. T., Oliver, J. R. & Kariks, J. (1988). Immunohistochemical staining reveals an increased count of dendrites in the superior cervical ganglion cells of SIDS infants: an etiological clue, artifact, or epiphenomenon? In *Sudden Infant Death Syndrome. Risk Factors and Basic Mechanisms*, ed. R. M. Harper & H. J. Hoffman. New York: PMA Publishing, pp. 265–77.

Rebuffat, E., Sottiaux, M., Goyens, P., *et al.* (1991). Sudden infant death syndrome, as first expression of a metabolic disorder. In *Inborn Errors of Metabolism*, ed. J. Schaub, F. Van Hoof & H. L. Vis. New York: Raven Press, pp. 71–80.

Reece, R. M. (1993). Fatal child abuse and sudden infant death syndrome: a critical diagnostic decision. *Pediatrics*, **91**, 423–9.

Rees, K., Wright, A., Keeling, J. W. & Douglas, N. J. (1998). Facial structure in the sudden infant death syndrome: case–control study. *British Medical Journal*, **317**, 179–80.

Reid, G. M. (1987). Sudden infant death syndrome: congenital copper deficiency. *Medical Hypotheses*, **24**, 167–75.

Reuss, W., Saeger, W. & Bajanowski, T. (1994). Morphological and immunohistochemical studies of the pituitary in sudden infant death syndrome (SIDS). *International Journal of Legal Medicine*, **106**, 249–53.

Rhead, W. J. (1977). A final note on the lack of relationship of selenium, other trace elements, and vitamin E in the causation of SIDS. *Journal of Pediatrics*, **90**, 500.

Rhead, W. J., Cary, E. E., Allaway, W. H., Saltzstein, S. L. & Schrauzer, G. N. (1972). The vitamin E and selenium status of infants and the sudden infant death syndrome. *Bioinorganic Chemistry*, **1**, 289–94.

Richard, C. A., Mosko, S. S. & McKenna, J. J. (1998). Apnea and periodic breathing in bed-sharing and solitary sleeping. *American Journal of Applied Physiology*, **84**, 1374–80.

Richards, R. G., Fukumoto, R. I. & Clardy, D. O. (1983). Sudden infant death syndrome: a biochemical profile of postmortem vitreous humor. *Journal of Forensic Sciences*, **28**, 404–14.

Richardson, B. A. (1990). Cot mattress biodeterioration and SIDS. *Lancet*, **335**, 670.

Richardson, B. A. (1994). Sudden infant death syndrome: a possible primary cause. *Journal of the Forensic Science Society*, **34**, 199–204.

Richardson, B. A. (1995a). Cot death and cot mattresses. *New Zealand Medical Journal*, **108**, 370.

Richardson, B. A. (1995b). Cot mattresses and the sudden infant death syndrome. *British Medical Journal*, **310**, 1071.

Rietschel, E. T. & Brade, H. (1992). Bacterial endotoxins. *Scientific American*, **267**, 26–33.

Righard, L. (1998). Sudden infant death syndrome and pacifiers: a proposed connection could be a bias. *Birth*, **25**, 128–9.

Rimell, F., Goding, G. S., Jr & Johnson, K. (1993). Cholinergic agents in the laryngeal chemoreflex model of sudden infant death syndrome. *Laryngoscope*, **103**, 623–30.

Rintahaka, P. J. & Hirvonen, J. (1986). The epidemiology of sudden infant death syndrome in Finland in 1969–1980. *Forensic Science International*, **30**, 219–33.

Roberts, S. C. (1987). Vaccination and cot deaths in perspective. *Archives of Disease in Childhood*, **62**, 754–9.

Robertson, J. S. & Parker, V. (1978). Cot deaths and water-sodium. *Lancet*, **ii**, 1012–14.

Roche, W. R. (1992). Immunopathology of SIDS. *Journal of Clinical Pathology*, **45** (Suppl), 46–8.

Rodenstein, D. O., Perlmutter, N. & Stanescu, D. C. (1985). Infants are not obligatory nasal breathers. *American Review of Respiratory Diseases*, **131**, 343–7.

Roe, C. R., Millington, D. S., Maltby, D. A. & Kinnebrew, P. (1986). Recognition of medium-chain acyl-CoA dehydrogenase deficiency in asymptomatic siblings of children dying of sudden infant death or Reye-like syndromes. *Journal of Pediatrics*, **108**, 13–18.

Rognum, T. O. (1995). *Sudden Infant Death Syndrome. New Trends in the Nineties*. Oslo: Scandinavian University Press.

Rognum, T. O. (2001). Definition and pathologic features. In *Sudden Infant Death Syndrome. Problems, Progress and Possibilities*, eds. R. W. Byard & H. F. Krous. London: Arnold, pp. 4–30.

Rognum, T. O. & Saugstad, O. D. (1991). Hypoxanthine levels in vitreous humor: evidence of hypoxia in most infants who died of sudden infant death syndrome. *Pediatrics*, **87**, 306–10.

Rognum, T. O. & Saugstad, O. D. (1993). Biochemical and immunological studies in SIDS victims. Clues to understanding the death mechanism. *Acta Paediatrica*, **389** (Suppl), 82–5.

Rognum, T. O., Saugstad, O. D., Øyasaeter, S. & Olaisen, B. (1988). Elevated levels of hypoxanthine in vitreous humor indicate prolonged cerebral hypoxia in victims of sudden infant death syndrome. *Pediatrics*, **82**, 615–8.

Roland, E. H. & Volpe, J. J. (1989). Effect of maternal cocaine use on the fetus and newborn: review of the literature. *Pediatric Neuroscience*, **15**, 88–94.

Rosen, T. S. & Johnson, H. L. (1988). Drug-addicted mothers, their infants, and SIDS. *Annals of New York Academy of Science*, **553**, 89–95.

Ross, F. D. (1862). Sudden death of a child. *Lancet*, **1**, 54–5.

Ross, I. S., Moffat, M. A. & Reid, I. W. (1983). Thyroid hormones in the sudden infant death syndrome (SIDS). *Clinica Chimica Acta*, **129**, 151–5.

Russell-Jones, D. L. (1985). Sudden infant death in history and literature. *Archives of Disease in Childhood*, **60**, 278–81.

Sachis, P. N., Armstrong, D. L., Becker, L. E. & Bryan, A. C. (1981). The vagus nerve and sudden infant death syndrome: a morphometric study. *Journal of Pediatrics*, **98**, 278–80.

Samet, J. M. (1991). New effects of active and passive smoking on reproduction? *American Journal of Epidemiology*, **133**, 348–50.

Saternus, K. S., Koebke, J. & Von Tamaska, L. (1986). Neck extension as a cause of SIDS. *Forensic Science International*, **31**, 167–74.

Savitt, T. L. (1979). The social and medical history of crib death. *Journal of the Florida Medical Association*, **66**, 853–9.

Sawczenko, A. & Fleming, P. J. (1996). Thermal stress, sleeping position, and the sudden infant death syndrome. *Sleep*, **19**, S267–70.

Sayers, N. M., Drucker, D. B., Morris, J. A. & Telford, D. R. (1995). Lethal synergy between toxins of staphylococci and enterobacteria: implications for sudden infant death syndrome. *Journal of Clinical Pathology*, **48**, 929–32.

Schechtman, V. L., Harper, R. M., Kluge, K. A., Wilson, A. J., Hoffman, H. J. & Southall, D. P. (1988). Cardiac and respiratory patterns in normal infants and victims of the sudden infant death syndrome. *Sleep*, **11**, 413–24.

Schechtman, V. L., Harper, R. M., Kluge, K. A., Wilson, A. J., Hoffman, H. J. & Southall, D. P. (1989). Heart rate variation in normal infants and victims of the sudden infant death syndrome. *Early Human Development*, **19**, 167–81.

Schechtman, V. L., Harper, R. M., Kluge, K. A., Wilson, A. J. & Southall, D. P. (1990). Correlations between cardiorespiratory measures in normal infants and victims of sudden infant death syndrome. *Sleep*, **13**, 304–17.

Schechtman, V. L., Harper, R. M., Wilson, A. J., Hoffman, H. J. & Southall, D. P. (1992a). Sleep state organization in normal infants and victims of sudden infant death syndrome. *Pediatrics*, **89**, 865–70.

Schechtman, V. L., Raetz, S. L., Harper, R. K., *et al.* (1992b). Dynamic analysis of cardiac R-R intervals in normal infants and in infants who subsequently succumbed to the sudden infant death syndrome. *Pediatric Research*, **31**, 606–12.

Schey, W. L., Meus, P., Levinsky, R. A., Campbell, C. & Replogle, R. (1981a). Esophageal dysmotility and the sudden infant death syndrome. Experimental observations of neonatal puppies. *Radiology*, **140**, 73–7.

Schey, W. L., Replogle, R., Campbell, C., Meus, P. & Levinsky, R. A. (1981b). Esophageal dysmotility and the sudden infant death syndrome. Clinical experience. *Radiology*, **140**, 67–71.

Schwartz, P. J. (1976). Cardiac sympathetic innervation and the sudden infant death syndrome. A possible pathogenetic link. *American Journal of Medicine*, **60**, 167–72.

Schwartz, P. J. (1987). The quest for the mechanisms of the sudden infant death syndrome: doubts and progress. *Circulation*, **75**, 677–83.

Schwartz, P. J. (1989). The cardiac theory and sudden infant death syndrome. In *Sudden Infant Death Syndrome. Medical Aspects and Psychological Management*, ed. J. L. Culbertson, H. F. Krous & R. D. Bendell. London: Edward Arnold, pp. 121–38.

Schwartz, P. J. (2001). QT prolongation – from theory to evidence. In *Sudden Infant Death Syndrome. Problems, Progress and Possibilities*, ed. R. W. Byard & H. F. Krous. London: Arnold, pp. 83–95.

Schwartz, P. J., Priori, S. G., Bloise, R., *et al.* (2001). Molecular diagnosis in a child with sudden infant death syndrome. *Lancet*, **358**, 1342–3.

Schwartz, P. J., Priori, S. G., Dumaine, R., *et al.* (2000). A molecular link between the sudden infant death syndrome and the long-QT syndrome. *New England Journal of Medicine*, **343**, 262–7.

Schwartz, P. J., Stramba-Badiale, M., Segantini, A., *et al.* (1998). Prolongation of the QT interval and the sudden infant death syndrome. *New England Journal of Medicine*, **338**, 1709–14.

Scott, C. B., Nickerson, B. G., Sargent, C. W., Dennies, P. C., Platzker, A. C. G. & Keens, T. G. (1982). Diaphragm strength in near-miss sudden infant death syndrome. *Pediatrics*, **69**, 782–4.

Scragg, R. K. R. & Mitchell, E. A. (1998). Side sleeping position and bed sharing in the sudden infant death syndrome. *Annals of Medicine*, **30**, 345–9.

Scragg, R. K. R., Mitchell, E. A., Stewart, A. W., *et al.* (1996). Infant room-sharing and prone sleep position in sudden infant death syndrome. *Lancet*, **347**, 7–12.

Scragg, R., Mitchell, E. A., Taylor, B. J., *et al.* (1993). Bed sharing, smoking, and alcohol in the sudden infant death syndrome. *British Medical Journal*, **307**, 1312–8.

Scragg, R., Stewart, A. W., Mitchell, E. A., Ford, R. P. K. & Thompson, J. M. D. (1995). Public health policy on bed sharing and smoking in the sudden infant death syndrome. *New Zealand Medical Journal*, **108**, 218–22.

Seto, D. S. Y., Uemura, H. & Hokama, Y. (1983). Viral hypersensitivity in sudden infant death syndrome. In *Sudden Infant Death Syndrome*, ed. J. A. Tildon, L. M. Roeder & A. Steinschneider. New York: Academic Press, pp. 579–613.

Shannon, D. C. & Bergman, A. (1991). Nosedrops and SIDS. *Pediatrics*, **88**, 418–19.

Shannon, D. C. & Kelly, D. (1977). Impaired regulation of alveolar ventilation and the sudden infant death syndrome. *Science*, **197**, 367–8.

Shannon, D. C. & Kelly, D. H. (1982a). SIDS and near-SIDS (first of two parts). *New England Journal of Medicine*, **306**, 959–65.

Shannon, D. C. & Kelly, D. H. (1982b). SIDS and near-SIDS (second of two parts). *New England Journal of Medicine*, **306**, 1022–8.

Shannon, D. C., Kelly, D. H. & O'Connell, K. (1977). Abnormal regulation of ventilation in infants at risk for sudden-infant-death syndrome. *New England Journal of Medicine*, **297**, 747–50.

Shatz, A., Hiss, J. & Arensburg, B. (1997). Myocarditis misdiagnosed as sudden infant death syndrome (SIDS). *Medicine, Science and the Law*, **37**, 16–18.

Shatz, A., Hiss, Y., Hammel, I., Arensburg, B. & Variend, S. (1994). Age-related basement membrane thickening of the vocal cords in sudden infant death syndrome (SIDS). *Laryngoscope*, **104**, 865–8.

Shiono, H., Tabata, N., Fujiwara, M., Azumi, J.-I. & Morita, M. (1988). Sudden infant death syndrome in Japan. *American Journal of Forensic Medicine and Pathology*, **9**, 5–8.

Siebert, J. R. & Haas, J. E. (1991). Enlargement of the tongue in sudden infant death syndrome. *Pediatric Pathology*, **11**, 813–26.

Simson, L. R., Jr & Brantley, R. E. (1977). Postural asphyxia as a cause of death in sudden infant death syndrome. *Journal of Forensic Sciences*, **22**, 178–87.

Singer, D. B. & Tilly, E. (1988). Pulmonary arteries and arterioles: normal in the sudden infant death syndrome. In *Sudden Infant Death Syndrome. Risk Factors and Basic Mechanisms*, ed. R. M. Harper & H. J. Hoffman. New York: PMA Publishing, pp. 101–13.

Sitsen, J. M. A., Van Ree, J. M. & De Jong, W. (1982). Cardiovascular and respiratory effects of β-endorphin in anesthetized and conscious rats. *Journal of Cardiovascular Pharmacology*, **4**, 883–8.

Skinner, M. (1995). Hypovitaminosis A: a model for sudden infant death syndrome. *American Journal of Human Biology*, **7**, 381–99.

Smialek, J. E. & Lambros, Z. (1988). Investigation of sudden infant deaths. *Pediatrician*, **15**, 191–7.

Smialek, J. E. & Monforte, J. R. (1977). Toxicology and sudden infant death. *Journal of Forensic Sciences*, **22**, 757–62.

Smith, N. M., Telfer, S. M. & Byard, R. W. (1992). A comparison of the incidence of cytomegalovirus inclusion bodies in submandibular and tracheobronchial glands in SIDS and non-SIDS autopsies. *Pediatric Pathology*, **12**, 185–90.

Sonnabend, O. A. R., Sonnabend, W. F. F., Krech, U., Molz, G. & Sigrist, T. (1985). Continuous microbiological and pathological study of 70 sudden and unexpected infant deaths: toxigenic intestinal *Clostridium botulinum* infection in 9 cases of sudden infant death syndrome. *Lancet*, **i**, 237–41.

South Australian Health Commission (1989). *Third Report of the Maternal, Perinatal and Infant Mortality Committee on Maternal, Perinatal and Post-neonatal Deaths in 1988*. Adelaide, South Australia.

Southall, D. P. (1988a). Can we predict or prevent sudden unexpected deaths during infancy? *Pediatrician*, **15**, 183–90.

Southall, D. P. (1988b). Role of apnea in the sudden infant death syndrome: a personal view. *Pediatrics*, **80**, 73–84.

Southall, D. P. & Talbert, D. G. (1987). Sudden atelectasis apnea breaking syndrome. In *Current Topics in Pharmacology and Toxicology*, vol. 3, ed. M. A. Hollinger. New York: Elsevier, pp. 210–89.

Southall, D. P. & Talbert, D. G. (1988). Mechanisms for abnormal apnea of possible relevance to the sudden infant death syndrome. *Annals of New York Academy of Sciences*, **533**, 329–49.

Southall, D. P., Alexander, J. R., Stebbens, V. A., Taylor, V. G. & Janczynski, R. E. (1987a). Cardiorespiratory patterns in siblings of babies with sudden infant death syndrome. *Archives of Disease in Childhood*, **62**, 721–6.

Southall, D. P., Arrowsmith, W. A., Oakley, J. R., McEnery, G., Anderson, R. H. & Shinebourne, E. A. (1979). Prolonged QT interval and cardiac arrhythmias in two neonates: sudden infant death syndrome in one case. *Archives of Disease in Childhood*, **54**, 776–9.

Southall, D. P., Arrowsmith, W. A., Stebbins, V. & Alexander, J. R. (1986a). QT interval measurements before sudden infant death syndrome. *Archives of Disease in Childhood*, **61**, 327–33.

Southall, D. P., Lewis, G. M., Buchanan, R. & Weller, R. O. (1987b). Prolonged expiratory apnoea (cyanotic 'breath-holding') in association with a medullary tumour. *Developmental Medicine and Child Neurology*, **29**, 789–93.

Southall, D. P., Noyes, J. P., Poets, C. F. & Samuels, M. P. (1993). Mechanisms for hypoxaemic episodes in infancy and early childhood. *Acta Paediatrica*, **389** (Suppl), 60–62.

Southall, D. P., Richards, J. M., de Swiet, M., *et al.* (1983a). Identification of infants destined to die unexpectedly during infancy: evaluation of predictive importance of prolonged apnoea and disorders of cardiac rhythm or conduction. First report of a multicentred prospective study into the sudden infant death syndrome. *British Medical Journal*, **286**, 1092–6.

Southall, D. P., Richards, J. M., Shinebourne, E. A., Franks, C. I., Wilson, A. J. & Alexander, J. R. (1983b). Prospective population-based studies into heart rate and breathing patterns in newborn infants: prediction of infants at risk of SIDS? In *Sudden Infant Death Syndrome*, ed. J. A. Tildon, L. M. Roeder & A. Steinschneider. New York: Academic Press, pp. 621–52.

Southall, D. P., Richards, J. M., Stebbens, V., Wilson, A. J., Taylor, V. & Alexander J. R. (1986b). Cardiorespiratory function in 16 full-term infants with sudden infant death syndrome. *Pediatrics*, **78**, 787–96.

Southall, D. P., Samuels, M. P. & Stebbens, V. A. (1989). Suffocation and sudden infant death syndrome. *British Medical Journal*, **299**, 178.

Southall, D. P., Samuels, M. P. & Talbert, D. G. (1990). Recurrent cyanotic episodes with severe arterial hypoxaemia and intrapulmonary shunting: a mechanism for sudden death. *Archives of Disease in Childhood*, **65**, 953–61.

Southall, D. P., Stebbens, V., Abraham, N. & Abraham, L. (1987c). Prolonged apnoea with severe arterial hypoxaemia resulting from complex partial seizures. *Developmental Medicine and Child Neurology*, **29**, 784–9.

Southall, D. P., Stebbens, V. A., Alexander, J. R., Cardle, C. M. & Cogswell, J. J. (1986c). Cardiorespiratory patterns occurring in infants during and after recovery from respiratory tract infection. *Pediatrics*, **78**, 37–43.

Southall, D., Stebbens, V. & Samuels, M. (1990). Bedding and sleeping position in the sudden infant death syndrome. *British Medical Journal*, **301**, 492.

Southall, D. P., Talbert, D. G., Alexander, J. R., Stevens, A. V. & Wilson, A. J. (1988). Recordings of cardiorespiratory activity in relation to the problem of SIDS. In *Sudden Infant Death Syndrome. Risk Factors and Basic Mechanisms*, ed. R. M. Harper & H. J. Hoffman. New York: PMA Publishing, pp. 447–58.

Sparks, D. L. & Hunsaker, J. C., III (1988). The pineal gland in sudden infant death syndrome: preliminary observations. *Journal of Pineal Research*, **5**, 111–18.

Sparks, D. L. & Hunsaker, J. C., III (1991). Increased ALZ-50-reactive neurons in the brains of SIDS infants: an indicator of greater neuronal death? *Journal of Child Neurology*, **6**, 123–7.

Spiers, P. S. & Guntheroth, W. G. (1997). The seasonal distribution of infant deaths by age: a comparison of sudden infant death syndrome and other causes of death. *Journal of Paediatrics and Child Health*, **33**, 408–12.

Standfast, S. J., Jereb, S., Aliferis, D. & Janerich, D. T. (1983). Epidemiology of SIDS in upstate New York. In *Sudden Infant Death Syndrome*, ed. J. A. Tildon, L. M. Roeder & A. Steinschneider. New York: Academic Press, pp. 145–59.

Stanley, F. & Byard, R. W. (1991). The association between the prone sleeping position and sudden infant death syndrome (SIDS): an editorial overview. *Journal of Paediatrics and Child Health*, **27**, 325–8.

Stanton, A. N. (1984). Overheating and cot death. *Lancet*, **ii**, 1199–201.

Stanton, A. N., Scott, D. J. & Downham, M. A. P. S. (1980). Is overheating a factor in some unexpected infant deaths? *Lancet*, **i**, 1054–7.

Steinschneider, A. (1972). Prolonged apnea and the sudden infant death syndrome: clinical and laboratory observations. *Pediatrics*, **50**, 646–54.

Steinschneider, A. (1977). Nasopharyngitis and the sudden infant death syndrome. *Pediatrics*, **60**, 531–3.

Steinschneider, A. (1978). Sudden infant death syndrome and prolongation of the QT interval. *American Journal of Diseases of Children*, **132**, 688–91.

Steinschneider, A., Freed, G., Rhetta-Smith, A. & Santos, V. R. (1991). Effect of diphtheria-tetanus-pertussis immunization on prolonged apnea or bradycardia in siblings of sudden infant death syndrome victims. *Journal of Pediatrics*, **119**, 411–14.

Steinschneider, A., Weinstein, S. L. & Diamond, E. (1982). The sudden infant death syndrome and apnea/obstruction during neonatal sleep and feeding. *Pediatrics*, **70**, 858–63.

Sterman, M. B. & Hodgman, J. (1988). The role of sleep and arousal in SIDS. *Annals of New York Academy of Science*, **533**, 48–59.

Stewart, S., Fawcett, J. & Jacobson, W. (1985). Interstitial haemosiderin in the lungs of sudden infant death syndrome: a histological hallmark of 'near-miss' episodes? *Journal of Pathology*, **145**, 53–8.

Stoltenberg, L., Saugstad, O. D. & Rognum, T. O. (1992). Sudden infant death syndrome victims show local immunoglobulin M response in tracheal wall and immunoglobulin A response in duodenal mucosa. *Pediatric Research*, **31**, 372–5.

Storm, H., Rognum, T. O., Saugstad, O. D., Skullerud, K. & Reichelt, K. L. (1994). Beta-endorphin immunoreactivity in spinal fluid and hypoxanthine in vitreous humour related to brain stem gliosis in sudden infant death victims. *European Journal of Pediatrics*, **153**, 675–81.

Sturner, W. Q. (1995). Sudden infant death syndrome – the medical examiner's viewpoint. *Perspectives in Pediatric Pathology*, **19**, 76–86.

Sturner, W. Q. (1998). SIDS redux: is it or isn't it? *American Journal of Forensic Medicine and Pathology*, **190**, 107–8.

Sturner, W. Q. & Susa, J. B. (1980). Sudden infant death and liver phosphoenolpyruvate carboxykinase analysis. *Forensic Science International*, **16**, 19–28.

Sumbilla, C. M., Zielke, H. R., Krause, B. L. & Ozand, P. T. (1983). Gluconeogenic enzymes in fibroblasts from infants dying of the sudden infant death syndrome (SIDS). *European Journal of Pediatrics*, **140**, 276–7.

Summers, C. G. & Parker, J. C., Jr (1981). The brain stem in sudden infant death syndrome. A postmortem survey. *American Journal of Forensic Medicine and Pathology*, **2**, 121–7.

Summers, A. M., Summers, C. W., Drucker, D. B., Barson, A., Hajeer, A. H. & Hutchinson, I. V. (2000). Association of IL-10 genotype with sudden infant death syndrome. *Human Immunology*, **61**, 1270–73.

Sunderland, R. & Emery, J. L. (1981). Febrile convulsions and cot death. *Lancet*, **ii**, 176–8.

Suzuki, T., Kashimura, S. & Umetsu, K. (1980). Sudden infant death syndrome: histological studies on adrenal gland and kidney. *Forensic Science International*, **15**, 41–6.

Takashima, S. & Becker, L. E. (1985). Developmental abnormalities of medullary "respiratory centers" in sudden infant death syndrome. *Experimental Neurology*, **90**, 580–87.

Takashima, S. & Becker, L. E. (1991). Delayed dendritic development of catecholaminergic neurons in the ventrolateral medulla of children who died of sudden infant death syndrome. *Neuropediatrics*, **22**, 97–9.

Takashima, S., Armstrong, D., Becker, L. & Bryan, C. (1978a). Cerebral hypoperfusion in the sudden infant death syndrome? Brainstem gliosis and vasculature. *Annals of Neurology*, **4**, 257–62.

Takashima S., Armstrong, D., Becker, L. E. & Huber, J. (1978b). Cerebral white matter lesions in sudden infant death syndrome. *Pediatrics*, **62**, 155–9.

Takashima, S., Mito, T. & Becker, L. E. (1990). Dendritic development of motor neurons in the cervical anterior horn and hypoglossal nucleus of normal infants and victims of sudden infant death syndrome. *Neuropediatrics*, **21**, 24–6.

Takashima, S., Yamanouchi, H. & Becker, L. E. (1993). Development of catecholaminergic neurons and substance P-positive nerve fibres in the brain stem of victims of sudden infant death syndrome. In *Sleep Apnea and Rhonchopathy*, ed. K. Togawa, S. Katayama, Y. Hishikawa, Y. Ohta & T. Horie. Basel: Karger, pp. 13–18.

Talbert, D. G. (1990). SIDS, surfactant, and temperature. *Lancet*, **ii**, 690.

Talbert, D. G. & Southall, D. P. (1985). A bimodal form of alveolar behaviour induced by a defect in lung surfactant – a possible mechanism for sudden infant death syndrome. *Lancet*, **i**, 727–8.

Taylor, B. J. (1991). A review of epidemiological studies of sudden infant death syndrome in Southern New Zealand. *Journal of Paediatrics and Child Health*, **27**, 344–8.

Taylor, B. J., Williams, S. M., Mitchell, E. A. & Ford, R. P. K. (1996a). Symptoms, sweating and reactivity of infants who die of SIDS compared with community controls. *Journal of Paediatrics and Child Health*, **32**, 316–22.

Taylor, E. M. & Emery, J. L. (1982). Immunisation and cot deaths. *Lancet*, **ii**, 721.

Taylor, E. M., Sutton, D., Larson, C. R., Smith, O. A. & Lindeman, R. C. (1976). Sudden death in infant primates from induced laryngeal occlusion. *Archives of Otolaryngology*, **102**, 291–6.

Taylor, J. A. & Sanderson, M. (1995). A reexamination of the risk factors for the sudden infant death syndrome. *Journal of Pediatrics*, **126**, 887–91.

Taylor, J. A., Krieger, J. W., Reay, D. T., Davis, R. L., Harruff, R. & Cheney, L. K. (1996b). Prone sleep position and the sudden infant death syndrome in King County, Washington: a case–control study. *Journal of Pediatrics*, **128**: 626–30.

Templeman, C. (1892). Two hundred and fifty-eight cases of suffocation of infants. *Edinburgh Medical Journal*, **38**, 322–9.

Tennyson, S. A., Pereyra, P. M. & Becker, L. E. (1994). The development of the diaphragm in infants with sudden infant death syndrome. *Early Human Development*, **37**: 1–8.

Thach, B. T. (1983). The role of pharyngeal airway obstruction in prolonging infantile apneic spells. In *Sudden Infant Death Syndrome*, ed. J. A. Tildon, L. M. Roeder & A. Steinschneider. New York: Academic Press, pp. 279–92.

Thach, B. T. (1986). Sudden infant death syndrome. Old causes rediscovered? *New England Journal of Medicine*, **315**, 126–8.

Thach, B. T. (1989). The potential role of airway obstruction in sudden infant death syndrome. In *Sudden Infant Death Syndrome. Medical Aspects and Psychological Management*, ed. J. L. Culbertson, H. F. Krous & R. D. Bendell. London: Edward Arnold, pp. 62–93.

Thach, B. T. (2000). Sudden infant death syndrome: can gastroesophageal reflux cause sudden infant death? *American Journal of Medicine*, **108** (Suppl), 144–8S.

Thach, B. T., Davies, A. M. & Koenig, J. S. (1988). Pathophysiology of sudden upper airway obstruction in sleeping infants and its relevance for SIDS. *Annals of New York Academy of Sciences*, **533**, 314–28.

Thiene, G. (1988). Problems in the interpretation of cardiac pathology in reference to SIDS. *Annals of New York Academy of Sciences*, **533**, 191–9.

Thompson, J. A., Glasgow, L. A., Warpinski, J. R. & Olsen, C. (1980). Infant botulism: clinical spectrum and epidemiology. *Pediatrics*, **66**, 936–42.

Tildon J. T. & Roeder L. M. (1983). Metabolic and endocrine aspects of SIDS: an overview. In *Sudden Infant Death Syndrome*, ed. J. A. Tildon, L. M. Roeder & A. Steinschneider. New York: Academic Press, pp. 243–62.

Tildon, J. T., Chacon, M. A. & Blair, J. D. (1983). Changes in hypothalamic-endocrine function as possible factor(s) in SIDS. In *Sudden Infant Death Syndrome*, ed. J. A. Tildon, L. M. Roeder & A. Steinschneider. New York: Academic Press, pp. 211–19.

Tipene-Leach, D., Everard, C. & Haretuku, R. (2001). Taking a strategic approach to SIDS prevention in Maori communities – an indigenous perspective. In *Sudden Infant Death Syndrome. Problems, Progress and Possibilities*, ed. R. W. Byard & H. F. Krous. London: Arnold, pp. 275–82.

Tonkin, S. (1975). Sudden infant death syndrome: hypothesis of causation. *Pediatrics*, **55**, 650–61.

Tonkin, S. L. (1986). Epidemiology of cot deaths in Auckland. *New Zealand Medical Journal*, **99**, 324–6.

Tonkin, S. & Beach, D. (1988). The vulnerability of the infant upper airway. In *Sudden Infant Death Syndrome. Risk Factors and Basic Mechanisms*, ed. R. M. Harper & H. J. Hoffman. New York: PMA Publishing, pp. 417–22.

Tonkin, S. & Hassall, I. (1989). Infant sleeping position and cot death. *Australian Paediatric Journal*, **25**, 376–7.

Tonkin, S. L., Davis, S. L. & Gunn, T. R. (1994). Upper airway radiographs in infants with upper airway insufficiency. *Archives of Disease in Childhood*, **70**, 523–9.

Tonkin, S. L., Partridge, J., Beach, D. & Whiteney, S. (1979). The pharyngeal effect of partial nasal obstruction. *Pediatrics*, **63**, 261–71.

Tonkin, S. L., Stewart, J. H. & Withey, S. (1980). Obstruction of the upper airway as a mechanism of sudden infant death: evidence for a restricted nasal airway contributing to pharyngeal obstruction. *Sleep*, **3**, 375–82.

Towbin, J. A. & Friedman, R. A. (1998). Prolongation of the QT interval and the sudden infant death syndrome. *New England Journal of Medicine*, **338**, 1760–61.

Turner, K. J., Baldo, B. A. & Hilton, J. M. N. (1975). IgE antibodies to *Dermatophagoides pteronyssinus* (house-dust mite), *Aspergillus fumigatus*, and β-lactoglobulin in sudden infant death syndrome. *British Medical Journal*, **i**, 357–60.

Tyler, J. W. (1983). *Cot-death – the Ammonia Factor*. New Zealand: J. W. Tyler.

Valdes-Dapena, M. A. (1967). Sudden and unexpected death in infancy: a review of the world literature 1954–1966. *Pediatrics*, **39**, 123–38.

Valdes-Dapena, M. (1977). Sudden unexplained infant death, 1970 through 1975. An evolution in understanding. *Pathology Annual*, **12**, 117–45.

Valdes-Dapena, M. A. (1980). Sudden infant death syndrome: a review of the medical literature 1974–1979. *Pediatrics*, **66**, 597–614.

Valdes-Dapena, M. (1982). The pathologist and the sudden infant death syndrome. *American Journal of Pathology*, **106**, 118–31.

Valdes-Dapena, M. (1983). The morphology of the sudden infant death syndrome: an overview. In *Sudden Infant Death Syndrome*, ed. J. A. Tildon, L. M. Roeder & A. Steinschneider. New York: Academic Press, pp. 169–82.

Valdes-Dapena, M. (1985). Are some crib deaths sudden cardiac deaths? *Journal of American College of Cardiology*, **5**, 113–17B.

Valdes-Dapena, M. (1988a). A pathologist's perspective on possible mechanisms in SIDS. *Annals of New York Academy of Sciences*, **533**, 31–6.

Valdes-Dapena, M. (1988b). Sudden infant death syndrome: overview of recent research developments from a pediatric pathologist's perspective. *Pediatrician*, **15**, 222–30.

Valdes-Dapena, M. (1992a). A pathologist's perspective on the sudden infant death syndrome – 1991. *Pathology Annual*, **27** (part 1), 133–64.

Valdes-Dapena, M. (1992b). The sudden infant death syndrome: pathologic findings. *Clinics in Perinatology*, **19**, 701–16.

Valdes-Dapena, M. & Gilbert-Barness, E. (2002). Cardiovascular causes for sudden infant death. *Pediatric Pathology and Molecular Medicine*, **21**, 195–211.

Valdes-Dapena, M. A., Amazon, K., Gillane, M. M., Ross, D. & Catherman, R. (1980a). The question of right ventricular hypertrophy in sudden infant death syndrome. *Archives of Pathology and Laboratory Medicine*, **104**, 184–6.

Valdes-Dapena, M. A., Gillane, M. M., Cassady, J. C., Catherman, R. & Ross, D. (1980b). Wall thickness of small pulmonary arteries. Its measurement in victims of sudden infant death syndrome. *Archives of Pathology and Laboratory Medicine*, **104**, 621–4.

Valdes-Dapena, M. A., Gillane, M. M. & Catherman, R. (1976). Brown fat retention in sudden infant death syndrome. *Archives of Pathology and Laboratory Medicine*, **100**, 547–9.

Valdes-Dapena, M. A., Gillane, M. M., Ross, D. & Catherman, R. (1979). Extramedullary hematopoiesis in the liver in sudden infant death syndrome. *Archives of Pathology and Laboratory Medicine*, **103**, 513–15.

Valdes-Dapena, M., Hoffman, H. J., Froelich, C. & Requeira, O. (1990). Glomerulosclerosis in the sudden infant death syndrome. *Pediatric Pathology*, **10**, 273–9.

Van Belle, G., Hoffman, H. J. & Peterson, D. R. (1988). Intrauterine growth retardation and the sudden infant death syndrome. In *Sudden Infant Death Syndrome. Risk Factors and Basic Mechanisms*, ed. R. M. Harper & H. J. Hoffman. New York: PMA Publishing, pp. 203–19.

Variend, S. (1990). Infant mortality, microglial nodules and parotid CMV-type inclusions. *Early Human Development*, **21**, 31–40.

Variend, S. & Forrest, A. R. W. (1987). Carbon monoxide concentrations in infant deaths. *Archives of Disease in Childhood*, **62**, 417–18.

Variend, S. & Howat, A. J. (1986). Renal glomerular size in infants with congenital heart disease and in cases of sudden infant death syndrome. *European Journal of Pediatrics*, **145**, 90–93.

Variend, S. & Pearse, R. G. (1986). Sudden infant death and cytomegalovirus inclusion disease. *Journal of Clinical Pathology*, **39**, 383–6.

Vawter, G. F. & Kozakewich, H. P. W. (1983). Aspects of morphologic variation amongst SIDS victims. In *Sudden Infant Death Syndrome*, ed. J. A. Tildon, L. M. Roeder & A. Steinschneider. New York: Academic Press, pp. 133–44.

Vawter, G. F., McGraw, C. A., Hug, G., Kozakewich, H. P. W., McNaulty, J. & Mandell, F. (1986). An hepatic metabolic profile in sudden infant death (SIDS). *Forensic Science International*, **30**, 93–8.

Vege, Å. (1998). *Clues to Understanding the Death Mechanism in Sudden Infant Death Syndrome (SIDS)*. Oslo: University of Oslo Press.

Vege, Å., Rognum, T. O. & Opdal, S. H. (1998). SIDS – changes in the epidemiological pattern in Eastern Norway 1984–1996. *Forensic Science International*, **93**, 155–66.

Vege, Å., Rognum, T. O., Scott, H., Aasen, A. O. & Saugstad, O. D. (1995). SIDS cases have increased levels of interleukin-6 in cerebrospinal fluid. *Acta Paediatrica*, **84**, 193–6.

Verrier, R. L. & Kirby, D. A. (1988). Sleep and cardiac arrhythmias. *Annals of New York Academy of Sciences*, **533**, 238–51.

Verschoor, P. L., Wilschut, J. T., de Jonge, G. A. & Kostense, P. J. (1991). Frequent symptoms after DTPP vaccinations. *Archives of Disease in Childhood*, **66**, 1408–12.

Vesselinova-Jenkins, C. K. (1980). Model of persistent fetal circulation and sudden infant death syndrome (SIDS). *Lancet*, **ii**, 831–4.

Wagner, M., Samson-Dollfus, D. & Menard, J. (1984). Sudden unexpected infant death in a French county. *Archives of Disease in Childhood*, **59**, 1082–7.

Wailoo, M. P., Petersen, S. A., Whittaker, H. & Goodenough, P. (1989). The thermal environment in which 3–4 month old infants sleep at home. *Archives of Disease in Childhood*, **64**, 600–604.

Walker, A. M., Jick, H., Perera, D. R., Thompson, R. S. & Knauss, T. A. (1987). Diphtheria-tetanus-pertussis immunization and sudden infant death syndrome. *American Journal of Public Health*, **77**, 945–51.

Walker, A. M. & McMillen, C. (1993). *Second SIDS International Conference*. Ithaca, NY: Perinatology Press.

Walsh, J. K., Farrell, M. K., Keenan, W. J., Lucas, M. & Kramer, M. (1981). Gastroesophageal reflux in infants: relation to apnea. *Journal of Pediatrics*, **99**, 197–201.

Warnock, D. W., Delves, H. T., Campell, C. K., *et al.* (1995). Toxic gas generation from plastic mattresses and sudden infant death syndrome. *Lancet*, **346**, 1516–20.

Waters, K. A., Gonzalez, A., Jean, C., Morielli, A. & Brouillette, R. T. (1996). Face-straight-down and face-near-straight-down positions in healthy, prone-sleeping infants. *Journal of Pediatrics*, **128**, 616–25.

Weese-Mayer, D. E., Berry-Kravis, E. M., Maher, B. S., Silvestri, J. M., Curran, M. E. & Marazita, M. L. (2003). Sudden infant death syndrome: association with a promotor polymorphism of the serotonin transporter gene. *American Journal of Medical Genetics*, **117A**, 268–74.

Weese-Mayer, D. E., Morrow, A. S., Conway, L. P., Brouillette, R. T. & Silvestri, J. M. (1990). Assessing clinical significance of apnea exceeding fifteen seconds with event recording. *Journal of Pediatrics*, **117**, 568–74.

Weiler, G. & de Haardt, J. (1983). Morphometrical investigations into alterations of the wall thickness of small pulmonary arteries after birth and in cases of sudden infant death syndrome (SIDS). *Forensic Science International*, **21**, 33–42.

Weinstein, S. L. & Steinschneider, A. (1985). QTc and R-R intervals in victims of the sudden infant death syndrome. *American Journal of Diseases of Children*, **139**, 987–90.

Weinstein, S., Steinschneider, A. & Diamond, E. (1983). SIDS and prolonged apnea during sleep: are they only a matter of state? In *Sudden Infant Death Syndrome*, ed. J. A. Tildon, L. M. Roeder & A. Steinschneider. New York: Academic Press, pp. 413–21.

Weis, J., Weber, U., Schröder, J. M., Lemke, R. & Althoff, H. (1998). Phrenic nerves and diaphragms in sudden infant death syndrome. *Forensic Science International*, **91**, 133–46.

Wellby, M. L., Farror, C. J. & Pannall, P. R. (1987). Importance of postmortem changes in measurements of thyroid function in studies of sudden infant death syndrome. *Journal of Clinical Pathology*, **40**, 631–2.

Wennergren, G., Milerad, J., Lagercrantz, H., *et al.* (1987). The epidemiology of sudden infant death syndrome and attacks of lifelessness in Sweden. *Acta Paediatrica Scandinavica*, **76**, 898–906.

Werthammer, J., Brown, E. R., Neff, R. K. & Taeusch, H. W., Jr (1982). Sudden infant death syndrome in infants with bronchopulmonary dysplasia. *Pediatrics*, **69**, 301–4.

Whybourne, A., Zillman, M. A., Miliauskas, J. & Byard, R. W. (2001). Sudden and unexpected infant death due to occult lymphoblastic leukaemia. *Journal of Clinical Forensic Medicine*, **8**, 160–62.

Wigfield, R. E., Fleming, P. J., Berry, P. J., Rudd, P. T. & Golding, J. (1992). Can the fall in Avon's sudden infant death rate be explained by changes in sleeping position? *British Medical Journal*, **304**, 282–3.

Williams, A., Vawter, G. & Reid, L. (1979). Increased muscularity of the pulmonary circulation in victims of sudden infant death syndrome. *Pediatrics*, **63**, 18–23.

Williams, A. L. (1980). Tracheobronchitis and sudden infant death syndrome. *Pathology*, **12**, 73–8.

Williams, A. L. (1990). Sudden infant death syndrome. *Australian and New Zealand Journal of Obstetrics and Gynaecology*, **30**, 98–107.

Williams, A. L., Uren, E. C. & Bretherton, L. (1984). Respiratory viruses and sudden infant death. *British Medical Journal*, **288**, 1491–3.

Williams, S. M., Taylor, B. J. & Mitchell, E. A. (1996). Sudden infant death syndrome: insulation from bedding and clothing and its effect modifiers. The National Cot Death Study Group. *International Journal of Epidemiology*, **25**, 366–75.

Willinger, M., Hoffman, H. J., Wu, K. T., *et al.* (1998). Factors associated with the transition to nonprone sleep positions of infants in the United States: the National Infant Sleep Position Study. *Journal of the American Medical Association*, **280**, 329–35.

Willinger, M., James, L. S. & Catz, C. (1991). Defining the sudden infant death syndrome (SIDS): deliberations of an expert panel convened by the National Institute of Child Health and Human Development. *Pediatric Pathology*, **11**, 677–84.

Willinger, M., Ko, C. W., Hoffman, H. J., Kessler, R. C. & Corwin, M. J. (2000). Factors associated with caregivers' choice of infant sleep position, 1994–1998: the National Infant Sleep Position Study. *Journal of the American Medical Association*, **283**, 2135–42.

Winn, K. (1986). Similarities between lethal asphyxia in postneonatal rats and the terminal episode in SIDS. *Pediatric Pathology*, **5**, 325–35.

Wyatt, D. T., Erickson, M. M., Hillman, R. E. & Hillman, L. S. (1984). Elevated thiamine levels in SIDS, non-SIDS and adults: postmortem artifact. *Journal of Pediatrics*, **104**, 585–8.

Wynn, V. T. & Southall, D. P. (1992). Normal relation between heart rate and cardiac repolarisation in sudden infant death syndrome. *British Heart Journal*, **67**, 84–8.

Yeats, W. B. (1962). 'The Ballad of Moll Magee'. In *W. B. Yeats. Selected Poetry*, ed. A. N. Jeffares. London: Macmillan, pp. 7–9.

Yukawa, N. Carter, N., Rutty, G. & Green, M. A. (1999). Intraalveolar haemorrhage in sudden infant death syndrome: a cause for concern? *Journal of Clinical Pathology*, **52**, 581–7.

Zielke, H. R., Meny, R. G., O'Brien, *et al.* (1989). Normal fetal hemoglobin levels in the sudden infant death syndrome. *New England Journal of Medicine*, **321**, 1359–64.

Appendix I: Autopsy information pamphlet

Many of the deaths due to disorders in this text will be the subject of a medicolegal inquiry due to their sudden and unexpected nature, and so parental permission may not be required for the performance of an autopsy. However, where permission is required, the following information may be of use in explaining the process and purpose of an autopsy. It has been taken from a hospital information pamphlet prepared specifically for parents and guardians (Byard, 1992).

The autopsy: an explanation

The staff would like to extend their deepest sympathy to you and your family. The death of a child is one of the most terrible tragedies that can affect a family, and it is often hard to make decisions during this time of grief. A request for an autopsy examination may, therefore, seem intrusive and unnecessary.

Because of this, we have prepared this pamphlet to provide you with information about the autopsy and why we feel that it is so important. We hope it will provide answers to some of your questions and help you to make your decision.

Be assured that, with the exception of unexpected deaths from sudden infant death syndrome (SIDS) and those involving accidents such as drowning, etc., which come under the jurisdiction of the State Coroner, the right to decide what is to happen is entirely yours. The staff will always be guided by this and will be supportive of your decision.

What is an autopsy?

An autopsy is a systematic examination of the body of a person who has died, performed by a doctor who is a specialist in pathology in consultation with the doctors who were looking after the person during life. It begins with a full external examination followed by an examination of individual organs. The techniques are similar to those found in the operating theatre, except that every part of the body is examined. A number of special investigations are also performed, which include looking for infections, as well as looking at tissue under a microscope for the presence or absence of particular diseases.

Once the examination is completed, the pathologist prepares a detailed report of the findings and a summary of the person's medical history. A copy of this is then sent to the hospital doctor and, if requested, to the local doctor.

Why is it needed?

Sometimes parents feel that there was something extra that they could have done to prevent their child's death. This is a normal reaction to the loss of a person you love. In our experience, autopsies may help to alleviate these feelings of guilt by showing clearly the seriousness of the disease and the inability of anyone to prevent the final outcome.

Some people also feel that once a child has died, an autopsy can be of little or no help, but this is not true. Doctors are continually learning, not only about rare diseases but also about more common ones as well. An autopsy enables a full scientific study of all the different features of a particular illness, which then helps doctors to understand better the reasons for the outcome.

Greater understanding may then help children who present with the same or a similar illness in the future. In addition, performing an autopsy may be the only way that the cause of a particularly puzzling symptom can be explained. Sometimes, even the exact cause of death may not be obvious until after the autopsy.

New treatments and investigations are continually being developed and used in hospitals, and a complete autopsy examination may be the only way to assess fully the accuracy of new diagnostic procedures and the response of particular illnesses to new medicines or surgical techniques. By allowing an autopsy to be performed, the family enables direct feedback of this information to doctors, resulting in greater understanding of new technologies, procedures, and treatments. It is only by completely understanding new developments that progress in medicine can be made.

Other advantages of an autopsy include detection of abnormalities that were not obvious during life, as these may have relevance to other family members.

What is a "limited autopsy?"

Sometimes, a family may not want a complete autopsy performed. In this case, although it is less satisfactory, it may be sufficient for the pathologist to examine only one area of the body. For example, a limited autopsy may be restricted to the organs inside the chest in a patient who has heart or lung disease, or to the head in a patient who has a brain tumor. This is an option that you can discuss further with your doctor if you wish.

Will an autopsy be disfiguring?

With modern autopsies, there is almost no difference in the appearance of the body at the funeral, and a normal viewing can be held. Although incisions are made, they can usually be placed so that they will not be seen. They are also closed very carefully after the procedure, just as in operations. At all times, the body is treated with the utmost respect.

Will tissues be removed?

Tissues or organs such as the heart or brain may require very special examinations after the autopsy. This will depend on the disorder causing death and can be discussed with your doctors.

Will an autopsy interfere with funeral arrangements?

Autopsies are usually completed within a day of death, and so there should be no delay in making funeral preparations. Funeral directors are accustomed to working with pathologists and can arrange any service that the family may request. Embalming is still possible after an autopsy.

Will an autopsy be against religious beliefs?

Families are sometimes concerned that an autopsy may be against their religious beliefs. Autopsies have been performed on people from a wide range of religions, but if you are concerned it may be best to discuss the matter with someone from your church or religious group before deciding. Staff will be pleased to help you to contact the appropriate person.

We hope that this information has been of use to you in helping to show the value of the autopsy examination. If you have any further questions, your doctor or the pathologist will be most willing to answer them for you.

The following explanatory note to staff accompanies the autopsy pamphlet:

It is hoped that the attached pamphlet may be of assistance to you in discussing the possibility of an autopsy examination with parents. The pamphlet is intended to supplement discussions with the parents by providing information that they can take some time to read over. It is not intended in any way to interfere with, or replace, discussions between staff and parents, as these are an essential part of obtaining permission for an autopsy.

REFERENCE

Byard, R. W. (1992). *The Autopsy – An Explanation*. Adelaide: Women's and Children's Hospital.

Appendix II: Pediatric forensic autopsy guidelines

Introduction

Medicolegal inquiries into unexpected infant and early childhood death are characterized by marked variability, around the world, in the type and extent of the investigations that are performed. In response to a request from the South Australian State Coroner in 1999, a pediatric forensic pathology service was established at the Forensic Science Centre in Adelaide to coordinate the pathologic investigation and assessment of deaths in infants and children subject to coronial inquiry. The Forensic Science Centre provides autopsy services to the State Coroner for the state of South Australia, which has a population of approximately 1.5 million people. Over 90% of the state's adult coronial autopsies, and all pediatric coronial autopsies, are performed at the center.

While it is recognized that there cannot be a single approach to these deaths, the following protocol provides a summary of the way in which these cases are handled in one center, and provides a template for such a service. Investigations are based on modifications of:

1 the Sudden Unexplained Infant Death Investigation Report Form (SUIDIRF) (see Appendix III), and
2 the International Standardized Autopsy Protocol (see Appendix IV).

Further guidelines are available in other publications (Bove *et al.*, 1997).

A register of pediatric coronial cases is held at the Forensic Science Centre to enable peer review by Forensic Science Centre pathologists, with assistance from pediatric pathologists and pediatric forensic physicians when required. This provides a mechanism for examining specific issues regarding the implementation of protocols, public health and safety matters, and diagnostic problems with individual cases.

Unexpected infant and early childhood deaths

Overtly suspicious case

Following discussion by telephone of the case with attending police officers, scene attendance by the pathologist usually occurs, unless death has been in hospital. At the scene, the pathologist liaises with police officers, who will include Physical Evidence Section, Major Crime, Criminal Investigation Bureau, Family Violence Unit, and uniformed officers. The body is then examined, and preliminary assessments are made as to the presence and nature of injuries and the possible cause and time of death.

All other cases

Liaison with police officers, with examination of the body at the scene or in the mortuary at the earliest possible convenience. Discussion with attending officers also occurs, regarding the possible transfer of bedding, medication, feeding bottles, and scene videos to the mortuary for examination prior to performance of the autopsy.

All cases

In all cases, details are obtained of:
- the circumstances of death and events over the preceding 24 hours;
- the presenting and any hospital histories (particularly regarding methods of attempted resuscitation);
- prescribed medications, and any medications or drugs found at the scene;
- details of sleeping arrangements;
- the child's developmental level;
- any significant or recent illnesses;
- community health center records;
- any specific police concerns.

Contact

Contact is made with:
- the local child protection officer/physician for possible further background hospital and community health center information. The child protection officer/physician may also be invited to attend the autopsy for assistance in the evaluation of injuries;
- the local child abuse report line for further background information and notification of the case, particularly if there are concerns for the safety of other children in the family;
- the local Sudden Infant Death Syndrome Association for additional information if SIDS support workers have attended the family;
- ambulance officers if additional information from the scene is required;
- local medical officer/nursing staff if additional medical information is required;
- local children's hospital pathologists for case discussion with possible attendance at the autopsy.

External examination

The body is examined for external evidence of trauma and neglect. Limb deformities, swellings, bruises, lacerations, burns, abrasions, and skin and conjunctival petechiae are documented. The external auditory canals and nasal septum are exam-

ined by otoscope. Rectal/anogenital trauma is documented or excluded, and the core temperature is taken. The palms and soles of feet are examined for burns and injuries.

Radiology

A full skeletal survey is performed at the local pediatric hospital department of radiology prior to the autopsy. A verbal report is obtained from the reporting radiologist, and radiographs accompany the body back to the forensic science center mortuary if injuries have been found. (X-rays are routine for children under two years of age and discretionary after this, depending on history, circumstances, and external examination.)

Photography

Full external photographs are taken in addition to photographs during the autopsy (of positive or negative findings). Photographs include pictures of the front and back of the body, and close-ups of the face, the conjunctivae (using eyelid retractors if necessary), the inside of the lips and mouth, the dissected neck, chest, abdomen, back, and buttocks, and the pleural, peritoneal, and cranial cavities (with organs in situ and removed) (Figures AII. 1–AII.4).

Autopsy protocol

The autopsy examination of the three body cavities, soft tissues, and limbs is undertaken according to a modified international protocol (see Appendix IV).

Routine specimens

See Box AII. I.
- Peripheral blood from iliac vessels, if possible, for blood toxicology. This includes common prescription and illicit drugs and alcohol. Blood will usually have to be taken from the heart in infants.
- Urine, if available, for toxicology.
- Sample of liver for toxicology.

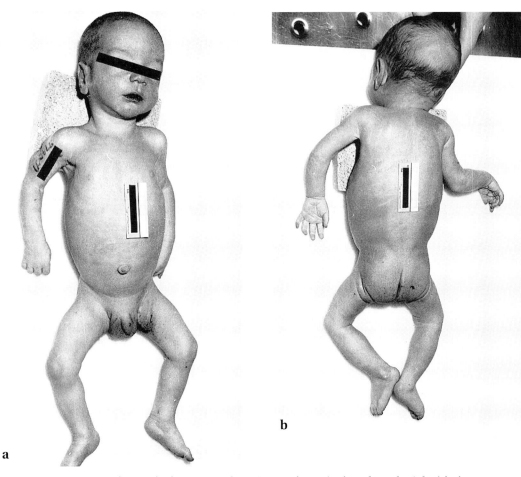

Figure AII.1 Routine autopsy photographs showing normal anterior (a) and posterior (b) surfaces of an infant's body.

- Heart blood, after searing the right atrium with a heated spatula or washing with isopropyl alcohol, for:
  - blood culture (anerobic and aerobic);
  - storage for DNA analysis if required.

Other specimens

- CSF, by anterior lower spinal approach prior to removal of the brain, for microbiology.
- Lung and spleen swabs for microbiology.
- Sample of heart for virology.
- Blood spots on paper for metabolic screening.

- Vitreous humor and liver for metabolic screening.
- Liver, any spare blood (centrifuged for serum), and possibly gastric contents are stored in the freezer. (Liver and serum to be stored indefinitely at $-20\,^{\circ}$C.)
- Hospital admission bloods and fluids are obtained by coronial warrant in suspicious cases for toxicologic analyses.

Additional steps to usual dissection and organ assessment

- Measurements include crown–heel length, crown–rump length, head circumference, chest

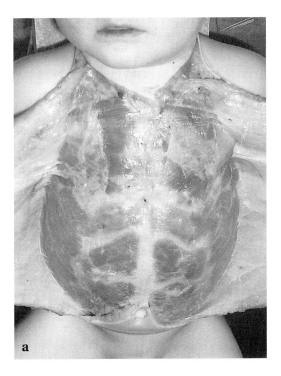

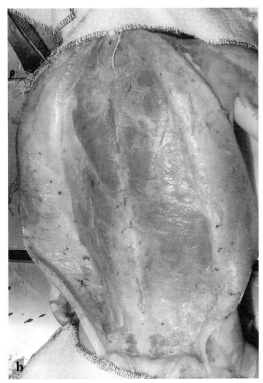

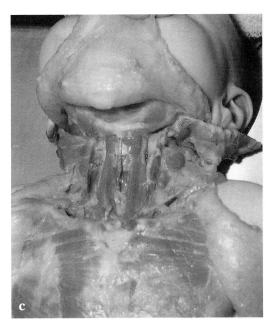

Figure AII.2 Careful layer dissection of skin and subcutaneous tissues of the anterior abdominal wall (a) and back (b), with exposure of neck strap muscles (c) prior to further dissection, performed either to assess the extent of soft tissue injury and hemorrhage or to check for possible occult bruising. In this case, no injuries were apparent.

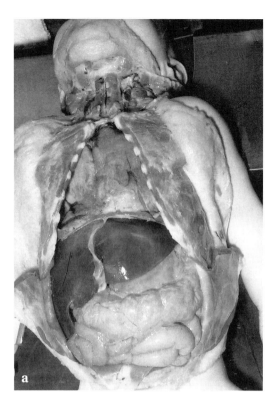

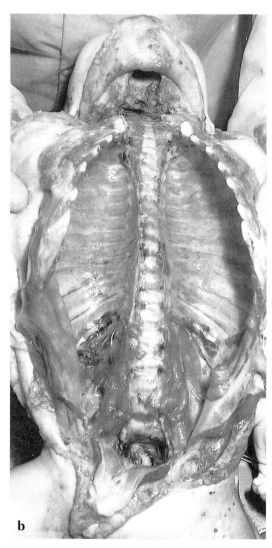

Figure AII.3 Internal organs in situ once the chest and abdominal cavities have been opened, showing normally formed and situated organs with no injuries or dehydration (a). After evisceration, no evidence of spinal, paraspinal, or rib injuries was seen (b).

circumference, thickness of fat at anterior abdominal wall, and maximum width of anterior fontanelle. (Normal values for age taken from standard charts are to be included in the autopsy report.)

- Skin and soft tissue layer dissections of neck, anterior chest wall, abdomen, and back are performed. Buttocks (and possibly backs of legs) are

incised for soft tissue bruising. (Dissections are photographed.)

- Organs, in particular the heart with its venous and arterial connections, are examined in situ prior to evisceration of the body by the pathologist. The calvarium may be removed by the mortuary attendant, but brain removal must be performed/supervised by the pathologist.

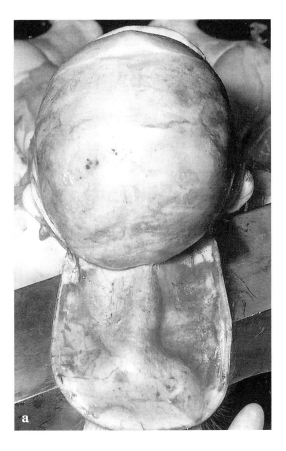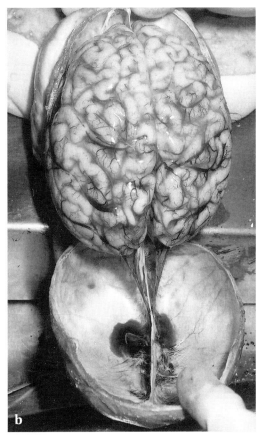

Figure AII.4 Reflection of the scalp, revealing no subgaleal hematomas or fractures (a). Normal brain after removal of the calvarium and dura, with no hemorrhages or edema. Pooling of blood in the calvarium is from artifactual seepage from dural sinuses, and not from trauma (b). Intact cranial cavity after removal of the brain, with no fractures or hemorrhages visible (c). Lifting of the vertebral column posteriorly to reveal the underlying spinal cord prior to removal (d).

- All organs are examined and weighed, including the thymus, adrenal glands, spleen, and pancreas. (Each lung and kidney is weighed separately.) (Normal weights for age taken from standard charts are to be included in the autopsy report.)
- In all cases of unexplained or suspicious infant and early childhood death, the brain is sent to the local department of neuropathology for formal examination and staining of sections for amyloid precursor protein. If there is any evidence of possible inflicted injury, or unusual features in the history or presentation, then the spinal cord is removed as

well. In such cases, the eyeballs are also removed and sections stained for hemosiderin.
- Samples taken for histology (in addition to any abnormal tissues) include the heart (two sections), lungs (five sections), kidneys (two sections), adrenal glands (two sections), pituitary gland, thymus gland, submandibular gland, tonsil, thyroid gland (including adjacent trachea and esophagus), rib (marrow and bone growth plate), liver, stomach, esophagus, small intestine, large intestine, appendix, spleen, pancreas, mesenteric fat and lymph nodes, bladder, gonad, and uterus. Brain sections

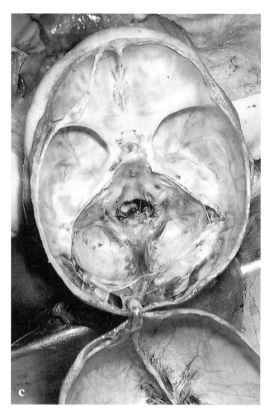

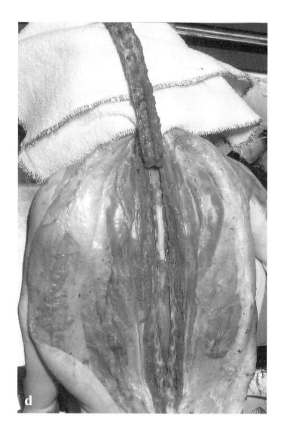

Figure AII.4 (cont.)

include the frontal lobe, centrum semiovale next to the angle of the lateral ventricle, corpus callosum and parasagittal white matter, basal ganglia, hippocampus, occipital lobe, midbrain, pons, cerebellum and dentate nucleus, and medulla. A representative lung section is also stained for hemosiderin.

• Samples taken for microbiological assessment (following searing of organ surfaces with a heated spatula, or washing with isopropyl alcohol) include a lung swab, spleen swab, blood culture from the right atrium, and heart tissue for virological study. The middle ears are examined and swabbed if moist.

Organ retention

Retention of whole organs, such as the brain, spinal cord, eyes, and heart, for further specialist examina-tion requires specific permission and formal authorization by the coroner.

Special circumstances

Inflicted injury

See also Appendix V.

• Bite marks are swabbed for DNA, photographed, and examined by a forensic odontologist.

• Finger or hand pressure marks are swabbed for DNA.

• Cases of possible/definite sexual assault are examined in conjunction with the local child protection officer, following the taking of radiographs. Colposcopic videos may be taken. Semen and microbiological swabs/smears of the anogenital region, mouth, and pharynx are performed.

<table>
<tr><td>

Box AII.1 Checklist for cases of unexplained infant death

Case number   Date

Attending personnel
1 Police   [ ]
2 Physical evidence officers   [ ]
3 Child protection physician   [ ]
4 Pediatric pathologist   [ ]
5 Others (specify)   [ ]

Samples
1 Blood/urine/liver for toxicology   [ ]
2 Blood/CSF for microbiological culture   [ ]
3 Lung/spleen swabs for microbiological culture   [ ]
4 Blood/vitreous/liver/skin for metabolic study   [ ]
5 Blood for DNA   [ ]
6 Heart tissue for virology   [ ]
7 Vitreous for electrolytes   [ ]
8 Liver/blood/gastric contents for   [ ]
  storage (−70 °C)
9 Filter paper storage:
  blood spot   [ ]
  urine spot (optional)   [ ]
  hair (optional)   [ ]

Specimens
1 Brain for neuropathology   [ ]
2 Spinal cord for neuropathology   [ ]
3 Eyeballs   [ ]
Photographs (see Figures AII.1–AII.4)
1 Front, back, face   [ ]
2 Eyes, mouth   [ ]
3 Soft tissue dissections   [ ]
4 Body cavities   [ ]
5 Other   [ ]

Phone numbers in cases of unexpected infant death
Forensic technician   _____
Police communications   _____
Child protection physician   _____
Child abuse report line/crisis care   _____
Pediatric pathologist   _____
SIDS Association   _____
Ambulance officers   _____

</td></tr>
</table>

- Representative fracture sites detected at autopsy, or shown radiographically, are removed for decalcification and histologic assessment.
- Bruises, burns, and skin lesions are sampled for microscopy (routine histology plus staining for hemosiderin).
- Fingernail cuttings and head-hair samples are taken for future DNA analysis if required.

Metabolic disease

See also Appendix VI.

The local pediatric hospital metabolic physician is contacted as soon as possible for case discussion and receiving samples. The autopsy may need to be performed immediately if a metabolic disorder is suspected. Specimens taken include:

- an alcohol-swabbed, sterile skin specimen for fibroblast culture (taken fresh and not frozen);
- fresh samples of liver, skeletal muscle, heart, and brain for snap-freezing;
- urine;
- blood;
- vitreous humour.

All specimens require immediate transfer to a metabolic laboratory for processing or optimal storage.

Gastroenteritis/heat deaths/dehydration

Specimens to be taken include:

- Fecal swabs for microbiology;
- Vitreous humor for electrolyte assessment.

Checklists for cases of possible sepsis or poisoning are found in Appendices VII and VIII.

REFERENCE

Bove, K. E. and the Autopsy Committee of the College of American Pathologists (1997). Practice guidelines for autopsy pathology. The perinatal and pediatric autopsy. *Archives of Pathology and Laboratory Medicine*, **121**, 368–76.

Appendix III: The Sudden Unexplained Infant Death Investigation Report Form

Reprinted from the Centers for Disease Control and Prevention (1996).
Morbidity and Mortality Weekly Report, **45**: 1, 7–19.

Guidelines for Death Scene Investigation of Sudden, Unexplained Infant Deaths: Recommendations of the Interagency Panel on Sudden Infant Death Syndrome

Summary

Because no uniform procedure has been developed for collecting and evaluating information on sudden, unexplained infant deaths (SUIDs) in the United States, the U.S. Senate and U.S. House of Representatives recommended in 1992 that the U.S. Department of Health and Human Services Interagency Panel on Sudden Infant Death Syndrome (SIDS) establish a standard scene investigation protocol for SUIDs. Two members of the panel, the Division of Reproductive Health of CDC and the National Institute for Child Health and Human Development of the National Institutes of Health, convened a workshop in July 1993 to gather information and ideas to use in developing such a protocol. Workshop participants, who included consultants having expertise in SIDS and representatives of public and private organizations concerned with SIDS, suggested that the Interagency Panel on SIDS develop both a short-form protocol and a longer, comprehensive protocol. The participants also recommended data items to include in the short-form protocol. This report includes the short form, which was developed to standardize the investigation of SUID scenes; ensure that information pertinent to determining the cause, manner, and circumstances of an infant death is considered in each investigation; and assist researchers in accurately determining the cause of and risk factors for SIDS. It can be used by medical examiners, coroners, death investigators, and police officers. Instructions for using the protocol are also included.

Instructions for Completing the Sudden Unexplained Infant Death Investigation Report Form (SUIDIRF)

Use

SUIDIRF may be used to assess the death of any infant for whom the cause of death is not apparent before autopsy. Applicable parts of the form may also be used to collect data about the death of any infant for whom the cause of death is known. The medical examiner or coroner (ME/C) or the death investigator acting on behalf of the former should complete the SUIDIRF. Police officers who report to the ME/C may also find the form useful.

Completion

The form may be completed by using blue or black ink or a #2 soft-lead pencil to facilitate electronic scanning, photocopying, and fax transmission. To ensure legibility of the forms, writing on the blank side (back) of the forms is discouraged. One blank page is provided for notes. If necessary, additional sheets of blank paper may be attached.

Design

The SUIDIRF pages are designed for use on a clipboard. The pages may be separated to allow other persons to complete, scan, photocopy, or fax the pages. Each page is printed on one side for legibility.

Compatibility with Other Forms

CDC's Medical Examiner and Coroner Information Sharing Program has published two generic death investigation report forms (DIRFs) – one for the investigator conducting the initial phases of the investigation (IDIRF) and another for the person who certifies the death or "closes" the investigation (CDIRF) (1, 2). The SUIDIRF is compatible with the DIRFs and has many data items in common. The CDIRF may be used in conjunction with the SUIDIRF. Although the generic IDIRF can be used for all death investigations irrespective of the age of the decedent, the SUIDIRF was designed specifically for infant deaths. On the SUIDIRF, the one-letter abbreviations in parentheses match the codes on the other DIRFs developed by CDC.

General Instructions

Use military time. Military time (midnight = 0000, noon = 1200) facilitates computer applications. Midnight (0000) corresponds to the same day as 0001 (one minute after midnight). The investigator may indicate a.m. and p.m. as long as the data entry personnel converts standard time to military time.

Month and day are sufficient for many fields. Birth date, death date, and the date the case was reported to the ME/C should each contain the month, day, and year, in that order, in numeric format (e.g. 01/05/97). For other events that occur in the same year as the report, indicating the month and day only is sufficient.

Indicate answers by an X. Multiple possible answers to an item are preceded by a line or followed by a box. Indicate the correct answer by writing an X on the appropriate line or in the appropriate box.

Use NA to indicate that a specific item is not applicable. If a given item is not applicable, write NA. If the respondent refuses to answer a question, write refused. Do not leave an item blank; the reviewer needs to know that an item has not been overlooked.

Correct errors by erasing or scratching through an incorrect response. If it is not possible to erase an answer, scratch out the incorrect response and indicate the correct one by using an X or by writing text as needed.

Glossary

Abbreviations used in the SUIDIRF

CPR Cardiopulmonary resuscitation
DC Death certificate
DOA Dead on arrival
DOB Date of birth
EMS Emergency medical services
IV Intravenous
ME/C Medical examiner or coroner
NA Not applicable
NOK Next of kin
OTC Over-the-counter medication
Rx Prescription medication
SIDS Sudden infant death syndrome
SS# Social security number
Unk Unknown

Terminology

EMS caller. The person who first called for emergency medical services, including an ambulance service, the police, or the fire department rescue team.

EMS responder. The person who first responded on behalf of the emergency medical service agency.

Father. The person serving as the father at the time of the incident. The relationship as natural (birth) father, stepfather, or other should be indicated.

Finder. The person who discovered the infant dead, unresponsive, or in distress.

First responder. The first person who attempted to render aid when the infant was found dead, unresponsive, or in distress.

Health-care provider. The physician, nurse, clinician, or other medical service provider who usually gave the infant medical care or well-baby checkups.

Last caregiver. The person who was last responsible for the care of the infant when he or she was discovered dead, unresponsive, or in distress (e.g. a baby-sitter, a child care custodian, or the mother).

Last witness. The person who last observed the infant alive or presumably alive in or near the area where he or she was discovered dead, unresponsive, or in distress.

Mother. The person serving as mother of the infant at the time of the incident. The relationship as natural (birth) mother, stepmother, or other should be indicated.

Placer. The person who last placed the infant in or near the area where he or she was found dead, unresponsive, or in distress.

Police. The law enforcement officer responsible for completing the police report on the death scene investigation.

Usual caregiver. The person responsible for providing the usual, ongoing care for the infant (e.g. changing diapers and feeding).

Page-by-Page Instructions

Many of the information items on SUIDIRF are self-explanatory. Instructions are provided here for items that require clarification.

Page 1

Use page 1 to document the date and time of critical events as well as to describe briefly circumstances of the infant's death. If the space on the blank page provided is not sufficient, additional pages for narrative descriptions may be attached.

Home address. The primary residence of the infant at the time of his or her death.

Age. The infant's age at death. Use MI for minutes (if less than 1 hour old), HR for hours (if less than 1 day old), DA for days (if less than 1 month old), and MO for months (until 23 months). Age at death can readily be calculated from the date of birth and date of death.

Race. The infant's race (based on the race of the birth mother). Use W for white, B for black, I for American Indian or Alaskan Native, A for Asian or Pacific Islander, and O for other.

Ethnicity. Whether the infant is of Hispanic descent. Additional information about the infant's national descent may be included here (e.g. Japan, China, Philippines, South Africa, Poland, or Germany).

Receipt by. The name of the ME/C or receptionist who first received notification of the infant's death.

NOK notified. The date and time the NOK not at the scene was notified of the infant's death, who was notified, and by whom. If the family was present at the scene and already knew of the infant's death at the time of its report, write NA in the date field.

Scene visit. The date and time the ME/C or the death investigator acting on behalf of the former visited the site where the injury or illness began or the death occurred. If ME/C staff visited the site, put an X by "ME/C staff" and name the person who went to the scene. If another agency and not ME/C staff went to the site, put an X by "Other agency" and name the agency or person. If no scene visit took place, place an X by "Not done"; however, use this form to collect information from telephone or in-person interviews of witnesses and from emergency medical service logs and reports.

Scene address. The address of the place where the injury or death occurred. Indicate if the scene address is the same as the home address. If the scene was not visited, give the presumed address.

Condition of infant when found. The condition of the infant at the time of his or her discovery. A dead infant is believed to be dead even after resuscitation is attempted. An unresponsive infant is unconscious but shows signs of life (e.g. has a pulse and is breathing). An infant in distress is in obvious trouble but retains some degree of responsiveness.

Sequence of events before death. A summary of the reported sequence of events leading to the infant's death. For example, "Infant found dead in crib at 3:00 a.m. No significant history." Use supplementary pages to detail the reported circumstances and sequence of events.

Injury. The date, time, and address of a known or suspected injury relevant to the infant's death.

Discovery. The date, time, and address of where the infant was found dead, unresponsive, or in distress.

Arrival. The date and time the infant arrived at a hospital (if such is the case).

Transport by. The mode of transport (e.g. ambulance or private motor vehicle) and the agency or person who transported the infant to the hospital.

Actual death. The specific date, time, and place where the death is believed or known to have occurred, not necessarily when or where death was pronounced. Options include where the infant was found (on scene), en route to a hospital, in a hospital emergency room, during surgery, and after being admitted to a hospital as an inpatient.

Infant placed. The date, time, and type of place where the infant was last placed as well as who placed the infant before he or she was found dead, unresponsive, or in distress. For example, a place might be listed as crib in bedroom, adult bed, sofa in living room, mattress on floor, or infant seat in vehicle.

Known alive. The date, time, and type of place where the infant was last seen or otherwise known (or assumed) to be alive as well as who believed the infant was alive.

First response. The date, time, and type of response (e.g. mouth-to-mouth resuscitation, chest compression, slapping, or shaking) rendered by the first person who attempted to aid or revive the infant as well as who rendered such aid.

EMS called. The date and time EMS was called, who called EMS, and the site from where the EMS caller called.

EMS response. The date and time EMS personnel arrived at the scene as well as the name of the EMS agency.

Police response. The date and time police arrived at the scene as well as the name of the police department.

Place of fatal event. For each choice, only one condition can apply. Indicate the correct choice with an X on the appropriate line.

Describe type of place. A concise but thorough description of the place where the events leading to death occurred. Examples include infant's bedroom at home, privately owned daycare center, child restraint in back seat of moving car, and infant seat in booth at a restaurant.

The name and relationship to the infant of all involved persons referenced on page 1 should be listed in the table at the top of page 4. On page 1 of the form, generic terms (e.g. mother, sister, uncle, or neighbor) can be used to indicate "By whom."

Page 2

Use page 2 to document the infant's usual healthcare provider, prenatal and birth history, medical history (e.g. recent symptoms, signs, and behavioral changes), and medication history as well as resuscitation attempts (including medical techniques and procedures) used in attempts to revive the infant. The letter codes can be used to identify the fields on supplementary pages and to facilitate data coding.

Medical source. The sources used to obtain medical information about the infant and the mother.

Use the section on specific infant medical history to describe relevant medical history. If further description or clarification is needed, use the space provided on the right of the form, use the blank supplement page, or attach additional pages.

Problems during labor or delivery. Includes problems with the placenta, membranes, or cord;

breech or malpresentation; cephalopelvic dispro-portion; prolonged labor; and fetal distress.

Maternal illness or complications during pregnancy. Includes eclampsia; incompetent cervix; maternal anemia; and pregnancy-induced hypertension, diabetes, cardiac conditions, and renal diseases.

Major birth defects. Includes central nervous system defects (e.g. spina bifida or meningocele, hydrocephalus, and microcephalus), cardiac malformations, gastrointestinal defects (e.g. rectal atresia or stenosis), Down's syndrome, and cleft lip or cleft palate.

Hospitalization of infant after initial discharge. Any overnight stay of the infant at a hospital after having been discharged from the hospital of delivery. Specify the date, reason, and outcome of each hospitalization.

Emergency room visits in past 2 weeks. The date, reason, and outcome of each visit.

Known allergies. Any allergies (e.g. to cow's milk, food, medication, or vaccine).

Growth and weight gain considered normal. If not normal, clarify.

Exposure to contagious diseases in past 2 weeks. Any contact with a person who had a communicable infectious disease (e.g. a cold, hepatitis, measles, pertussis, tuberculosis, or viral or diarrheal disease).

Illness in past 2 weeks. Any observed illness the infant experienced in the past 2 weeks. Specify the condition and its outcome.

Infant has ever stopped breathing or turned blue. Any episode of apnea before the infant died.

Infant was ever breast-fed. Breast-feeding was successfully initiated irrespective of whether the infant was still breast-feeding at the time of death.

Vaccinations in past 72 hours. Vaccinations against preventable childhood diseases. Specify which vaccinations were administered.

Deceased siblings. The cause and circumstances of death of the infant's deceased siblings.

Medication history. The type of medications given to the infant in the past. Place an X where it applies.

List the name of the medicines and doses taken. Indicate any home remedies given to infant, such as white clay or balms.

Emergency medical treatment. The types of medical treatment rendered to revive the infant. Explain further, if necessary, in the spaces provided below.

Page 3

When completing the questions on page 3, draw on personal observations. Use the section on household environment to indicate whether the household was visited and to document the presence or absence of selected environmental and social risk factors in the primary home of the infant (even if the events leading to death occurred somewhere else). Items for which the response is yes can be clarified in the space provided on the right. The letter codes can be used to identify the fields on supplementary pages and to facilitate data coding. Also use this section to document maternal sociodemographic information.

Type of dwelling. Concise description of the type of household (e.g. single family home, apartment, or trailer).

Water source. Source of drinking water (e.g. city water, well water, bottled water, or spring water).

Number of bedrooms. The number of rooms used as nighttime sleeping rooms, excluding living and dining rooms.

Estimated annual income. The estimated yearly income from all sources except public assistance.

On public assistance. Whether the householder receives public assistance (e.g. Aid for Families with Dependent Children [AFDC]).

Number of smokers in household. Includes both regular and occasional smokers in the household.

Use the section on infant and environment to document the immediate environment in which the events leading to death occurred. The immediate environment may or may not be the infant's primary home. If the infant was found in a crib or bed, put an X in the space provided. Indicate if the infant was sleeping alone or was sharing the crib or bed with others.

Temperature of area. A measured temperature where the infant was discovered. If a thermometer is not available, use subjective terms such as cold, cool, comfortable, warm, and hot.

The next items are included to help evaluate the possibility of asphyxia and external conditions as a cause of death. The questions evaluate the possibility of interference with breathing (e.g. covering of the nose and mouth) or hazards related to aspiration, choking, electrocution, excessive heat or cold, and other external factors. When possible, the manufacturer, brand, and lot or product number of relevant consumer products should be documented.

Sleeping or supporting surface. The characteristics of the crib, bed, floor, or other object that directly supported the infant when he or she was found dead, unresponsive, or in distress. Examples include sheepskin on cement floor, mesh seat of baby swing, sheeted mattress in crib, uncovered mattress on wood floor, and plastic-covered foam cushion on sofa. If the surface is easily compressed or deformed, that fact should be noted and the item should be obtained as evidence.

Clothing. A list and description of all articles of clothing worn by the infant, including diapers.

Other items in contact with infant. Any objects, other than the sleeping surface and articles of clothing, that were in contact with the infant (e.g. pacifier, dangling puppet on mobile, or plastic-covered, foam-filled bumper guard). These items should be secured as evidence.

Items in crib or immediate environment. Any other items in the immediate area to which the infant reasonably may have had access. Examples are pill on floor 16 inches from body, pacifier at opposite end of crib, and electric cord draping through crib. These items should be secured as evidence.

Devices operating in room. All electrical and mechanical devices in use in the room where the infant was found dead, unresponsive, or in distress. These devices include vaporizers, space heaters, fans, and infant electronic monitors (e.g. apnea monitor or heart rate monitor).

Cooling source in room and **Heat source in room**. The type of cooling and heat sources in the room where the infant was found. Examples of space devices include portable heaters, window air conditioners, and ceiling fans. Central devices include gas- or electricity-powered systems that heat or cool multiple rooms or an entire house.

Use the section on items collected to document material secured as evidence for presentation to the ME/C, crime laboratory, or other expert for further observation or analysis.

Page 4

Use page 4 to document interviews and procedures related to the investigation (e.g. review of medical records and referral of the case to a SIDS services agency), provide notes to the pathologist, indicate an overall assessment of whether findings suggest SIDS or another diagnosis or injury, indicate the family's interest in organ or tissue donation, and document disposition of the body. Use the section on interview and procedural tracking to record the names of informants, their relationship to the infant, phone number, and the date and time of interview.

Relationship to infant. Specific relationship to the infant (e.g. natural [or birth] mother, adoptive mother, foster mother, stepmother, maternal aunt, or neighbor).

Alternate contact person. If the mother cannot be located, the person who would be able to provide information about her.

Doll reenactment performed. Whether a doll was used to assist the witnesses in describing the body and face position of the infant when he or she was found dead, unresponsive, or in distress.

Detailed protocol completed. Whether the jurisdiction's detailed death investigation protocol was completed. Enter an X by "NA" if no such protocol exists for the jurisdiction.

Use the overall preliminary summary to provide notes to the pathologist (e.g. note and evaluate subtle mark on neck), indicate whether environmental hazards or consumer products may have contributed to the infant's death, and indicate whether the family is interested in organ or tissue donation. The last line is for the investigator to indicate whether, in his or her opinion, the investigation suggests SIDS, other causes of death, or trauma or injury.

In the section on case disposition, indicate whether the ME/C declined or accepted the reported case for investigation. A case can be declined because the cause and circumstances of death do not place the case within the ME/C's jurisdiction because of the topic (subject matter) or the location of death. A case is generally accepted so that an autopsy can be performed, an external examination can be conducted, and the cause and manner of death can be certified. Diagnosis of SIDS requires a complete autopsy, including histology, toxicology, and other tests as needed.

Transport agent. The person or transport service who brings the body to the morgue from its location at the time of the death report. Enter NA if the body is not brought to a morgue.

Funeral home. The funeral home authorized to handle the disposition of the body (regardless of whether the body has been brought to a morgue).

Page 5

Use page 5 to diagram the immediate area surrounding the infant when he or she was discovered dead, unresponsive, or in distress and to record selected observations about the area.

Page 6

Page 6 is an illustration of an infant's body that may be used to note marks, bruises, discolorations, drainage from orifices, and other observations.

REFERENCES

Centers for Disease Control and Prevention (CDC) (1996). Guidelines for Death Scene Investigation of Sudden Unexplained Infant Deaths. Recommendations of the Interagency Panel on Sudden Infant Death Syndrome. *Morbidity and Mortality Weekly*, **45**, 1, 7–19.

Hanzlick, R. & Parrish, R. G. (1994). Death investigation report forms (DIRFs): generic forms for investigators (IDIRFs) and certifiers (CDIRFs). *Journal of Forensic Sciences*, **39**, 629–36.

SUDDEN UNEXPLAINED INFANT DEATH INVESTIGATION FORM (SUIDIRF)   Case number

Infant's full name   Age   DOB
Home address   Race   Sex
City, state, zip   Ethnicity
County   SS#

Police complaint number   Police department

I. CIRCUMSTANCES OF DEATH

Action	Date	Time	By whom (person or agency)	Remarks
ME/C notified				Receipt by:
NOK notified				Person:
Scene visit				☐ME/C staff ☐Other agency ☐Not done
Scene address				

Condition of infant when found	☐Dead(D)	☐Unresponsive(U)	☐In distress(I)	☐NA(N)

Sequence of events before death:

Event	Date	Time	Location (street, city, state, county, zip code)
Injury			
Discovery			
Arrival			Hospital: Transported by:
Actual death			☐ On scene (S) ☐ Emergency room (E) ☐Inpatient(I)
			☐ En route or DOA (D) ☐ During surgery (O)
Pronounced			By whom:
dead			License#: Where:

Event	Date	Time	By whom (person)	Remarks
Infant placed				Place:
Known alive				Place:
Infant found				Place:
First response				Type:
EMS called				From where:
EMS response			Agency:	
Police response			Agency:	

Place of fatal event   **Describe type of place**
☐ Witness in room or area (W) or   ☐ Unwitnessed (U)
☐ At own home (H)   or   ☐ Away from home (A)
☐ Indoors (I)   or   ☐ Outdoors (O)
☐ In vehicle (V)   or   ☐ Not in vehicle (N)

II. BASIC MEDICAL INFORMATION

Health care provider for infant:	Phone:

Medical history   ☐ Not investigated (X)   ☐ Unk (U)   ☐ No past problems (N)   ☐ Medical problems (P)

Medical source   ☐ Physician (P)   ☐ Other health care provider (H)   ☐ Other (O)
☐ Medical records (M)   ☐ Family (F)   ☐ None (N)

Specific infant medical history	Yes	No	Unk	Remarks
A. Problems during labor or delivery Birth hospital: Birth city state:				
B. Maternal illness or complications during pregnancy Number of prenatal visits:				
C. Major birth defects				
D. Infant was one of multiple births (e.g. a twin) Birth weight: Gestational age at birth (weeks):				
E. Hospitalization of infant after initial discharge				
F. Emergency room visits in past 2 weeks				
G. Known allergies				
H. Growth and weight gain considered normal				
I. Exposure to contagious disease in past 2 weeks				
J. Illness in past 2 weeks				
K. Lethargy, crankiness, or excessive crying in the past 48 hours				
L. Appetite changes in past 48 hours				
M. Vomiting or choking in past 48 hours				
N. Fever or excessive sweating in past 48 hours				
O. Diarrhea or stool changes in past 48 hours				
P. Infant has ever stopped breathing or turned blue				
Q. Infant was ever breast-fed				
R. Vaccinations in past 72 hours				
S. Infant injury or other condition not mentioned above				
T. Deceased siblings				

Diet in past 2 weeks included: ☐ Breast milk   ☐ Formula   ☐ Cows milk   ☐ Solids
Date and time of last meal:
Content of last meal:

Medical history   ☐ Not investigated (X)   ☐ Unk (U)   ☐ Rx (P)   ☐ OTC (O)   ☐ Home remedies (H)   ☐ None (N)

Emergency medical treatment   ☐ None (N)   ☐ CPR (R)   ☐ Transfusion (T)   ☐ IV fluids (F)   ☐ Surgery (S)

Medicine names and doses; if prescription, include Rx number, Rx date, and name of pharmacy:	Describe nature and duration of resuscitation and treatments used to revive infant:	Describe any known injuries or marks on infant created or observed during resuscitation or treatment:

III. HOUSEHOLD AND ENVIRONMENT

Action	Yes	No	Unk	Remarks
A. House was visited				
B. Evidence of alcohol abuse				
C. Evidence of drug abuse				
D. Serious physical or mental illness in household				
E. Police have been called to home in past				
F. Prior contact with social services				
G. Documented history of child abuse				
H. Odors, fumes, or peeling paint in household				
I. Dampness, visible standing water, or mold growth				
J. Pets in household				

Type of dwelling   Water source   Number of bedrooms

Main language in home   Estimated annual income   On public assistance ☐Yes ☐ No

Number of adults (>18 years of age): ☐and children (<18 years of age):☐living in household. Total=☐people

Number of smokers in household: Does usual caregiver smoke? ☐Yes ☐No ☐Unk If yes,☐cigarettes/day

Maternal information ☐	Age: ☐	☐ Married (M) ☐ Single (S)	☐ Divorced (D) ☐ Widowed (W)	Cohabiting w/partner: ☐ Yes ☐No	☐Education (years)	☐Employed (E) ☐Not employed (N)

IV. INFANT AND ENVIRONMENT

☐In crib (C)   ☐In bed (B)   ☐Sleeping alone (A)   ☐NA (N)   Temperature of area:
☐Other (O)   ☐Sleeping with others (O)

Body position when placed	☐Unk	☐Back	☐Stomach	☐Side	☐Other
Body position when found	☐Unk	☐Back	☐Stomach	☐Side	☐Other
Face position when found	☐Unk	☐To left	☐To right	☐Facedown	☐Face up ☐To side
Nose or mouth was covered or obstructed	☐Unk	☐No	☐Yes		
Postmortem changes when found	☐Unk	☐None	☐Rigor	☐Lividity	☐Other

Number of cover or blanket layers on infant: ☐Covers on infant (C)   ☐Wrapped (W)   ☐No covers (N)

Sleeping or supporting surface: Clothing:

Other items in contact with infant: Items in crib or immediate environment:

Devices operating in room: Cooling source in room: Heat source in room:
                              ☐On (+) ☐Central (C) ☐None (N)   ☐On (+) ☐Central (C) ☐None (N)
                              ☐Off (-) ☐Space (S)   ☐Off (-) ☐Space (S)

Item collected	Yes	No	Item collected	Yes	No	Number of scene photos taken:
Baby bottle			Apnea monitor			Other items collected:
Formula			Medicines			
Diaper			Pacifier			
Clothing			Bedding			

V. INTERVIEW AND PROCEDURAL TRACKING

Contact	Name	Date	Time	Phone	Relationship to infant
Mother					
Father					
Usual caregiver					
Last caregiver					
Placer					
Last witness					
Finder					
First responder					
EMS caller					
EMS responder					
Police					
Alternate contact person:				Phone:	

Action	Date	Time	Action	
Medical record review for infant			Doll re-enactment performed	☐ Yes ☐ No
Medical record review for mother			Scene diagram completed	☐ Yes ☐ No
Physician or provider interview			Body diagram completed	☐ Yes ☐ No
Referral to social or SIDS services			Detailed protocol completed	☐ Yes ☐ No ☐ NA
Cause of death discussed with family			Other:	

VI. OVERALL PRELIMINARY SUMMARY

Notes to pathologist performing autopsy:

Indications that an environmental hazard, drug, poison, or consumer product contributed to death ☐ Yes ☐ No

Organ or tissue donation requested by family or agency ☐ Yes ☐ No ☐ Unk

Cause of death: ☐ Presumed SIDS ☐ Suspect trauma or injury ☐ Other

VII. CASE DISPOSITION

Case disposition	☐ Case declined (D) due to ☐ Topic (T) ☐ Locale (L)	☐ Case accepted (J) for ☐ Autopsy (A) ☐ Inspection (I) ☐ Certification (C)
Body disposition Who will sign DC?	☐ Brought in for exam (E) ☐ Brought in for holding or claim (C) ☐ Released from site (R)	
Transport agent:	Funeral home:	
Investigator and affiliation:	Date: Number of supplement pages attached:	

Appendix IV: International Standardized Autopsy Protocol

The International Standardized Autopsy Protocol for cases of unexpected infant death represents the first attempt to provide an international protocol aimed at standardizing autopsy practices and diagnoses. The protocol was developed by a working group set up by SIDS International and the NICHD in the 1990s (Krous, 1995; Krous & Byard, 2001). It aims to:

- standardize autopsy practices and improve diagnostic accuracy;
- provide additional information to supplement information obtained from the clinical history review and death scene examination;
- enhance opportunities to further reduce infant death rates and enable more meaningful comparisons of infant death rates to be made between populations;
- improve the quality of research into unexpected infant death.

The protocol has been endorsed by the National Association of Medical Examiners (NAME) and the Society for Pediatric Pathology (SPP) in the USA and has been implemented in a number of countries.

INTERNATIONAL STANDARDIZED AUTOPSY PROTOCOL
FOR SUDDEN UNEXPECTED INFANT DEATH

Decedent's Name		Local Accession Number
Age/Sex	Ethnicity	
Date Of Birth	Date/Time of Death	
Date/Time of Autopsy	Pathologist	
County/District	Country	

FINAL ANATOMIC DIAGNOSES

MICROBIOLOGY RESULTS:

TOXICOLOGY RESULTS:

CHEMISTRY RESULTS:

PATHOLOGIST---

DECEDENT'S NAME--.
ACCESSION NUMBER--
COUNTY & COUNTRY--
PATHOLOGIST--

	YES	NO	
MICROBIOLOGY Date/Time:,			
Done before autopsy,			
VIRUSES trachea stool,			
BACTERIA blood CSF fluids,			
FUNGI discretionary,			
MYCOBACTERIA discretionary,			
Done during autopsy,			
BACTERIA liver lung and myocardium,			
VIRUSES liver lung and myocardium,			
PHOTOGRAPHS include,			
Name Case number County Country Date,			
Measuring device Color reference,			
Consider front & back,			
Gross abnormalities,			
RADIOGRAPHIC STUDIES consider,			
Whole body,			
Thorax and specific lesions,			
EXTERNAL EXAMINATION,			
Date & Time of autopsy			
Date & Time of Autopsy,			
Sex (circle) Male Female,			
Observed race (circle),			
White Black			
Asian Arab			
Pacific Islander Gypsy,			
Hispanic, Other (specify),			
Rigor mortis: describe distribution,			
Livor mortis: describe distribution and if fixed,			
WEIGHTS AND MEASURES,			
Body Weight,			gm
Crown-Heel Length,			cm
Crown-Rump Length			cm
Occipitofrontal Circumference,			cm
Chest Circumference at Nipples,			cm
Abdominal Circumference at Umbilicus,			cm

DECEDENT'S NAME--
ACCESSION NUMBER--
COUNTY & COUNTRY--
PATHOLOGIST--

GENERAL APPEARANCE/DEVELOPMENT	YES	NO	NO EXAM
Development normal			
Nutritional status			
Normal			
Poor			
Obese			
Hydration			
Normal			
Dehydrated			
Edematous			
Pallor			
HEAD			
Configuration normal			
Scalp and hair normal			
Bone consistency normal			
Other			
TRAUMA EVIDENCE			
Bruises			
Lacerations			
Abrasions			
Burns			
Other			
PAST SURGICAL INTERVENTION			
Scars			
Other			
RESUSCITATION EVIDENCE			
Facial mask marks			
Lip abrasions			
Chest ecchymoses			
EKG monitor pads			
Defibrillator marks			
Venipunctures			
Other			
CONGENITAL ANOMALIES			
EXTERNAL			
INTEGUMENT			

DECEDENT'S NAME---
ACCESSION NUMBER---
COUNTY & COUNTRY--
PATHOLOGIST---

	YES	NO	NO EXAM
Jaundice			
Petechiae			
Rashes			
Birthmarks			
Other abnormalities			
EYES (remove when indicated and legal)			
Color circle Brown Blue Green Hazel			
Cataracts			
Position abnormal			
Jaundice			
Conjunctiva abnormal			
Petechiae			
Other abnormalities			
EARS			
Low set			
Rotation abnormal			
Other abnormalities			
NOSE			
Discharge (describe if present)			
Configuration abnormal			
Septal deviation			
Right choanal atresia			
Left choanal atresia			
Other abnormalities			
MOUTH			
Discharge (describe if present)			
Labial fenulum abnormal			
Teeth present			
Number of upper			
Number of lower			
TONGUE			
Abnormally large			
Frenulum abnormaL			
Other abnormalities			

DECEDENT'S NAME---

ACCESSION NUMBER---

COUNTY & COUNTRY--

PATHOLOGIST---

	YES	NO	NO EXAM
PALATE			
Cleft			
High arched			
Other abnormalities			
MANDIBLE			
Micrognathia			
Other abnormalities			
NECK			
abnormal			
CHEST			
abnormal			
ABDOMEN			
Distended			
Umbilicus abnormal			
Hernias			
Other abnormal			
EXTERNAL GENITALIA Abnormal			
ANUS abnormal			
EXTREMITIES abnormal			
INTERNAL EXAMINATION			
Subcutis Thickness Icm below umbilicus:			
Subcutaneous emphysema			
Situs inversus			
PLEURAL CAVITIES abnormal			
Fluid describe if present			
Right, ml			
Left, ml			
PERICARDIAL CAVITY abnormal			
Fluid, describe if present, ml			
Other abnormalities			
PERITONEAL CAVITY abnormal			
Fluid, describe if present, ml			
RETROPERITONEUM abnormal			

DECEDENT'S NAME--
ACCESSION NUMBER--
COUNTY & COUNTRY---
PATHOLOGIST--

	YES	NO	NO EXAM
PETECHIAE (indicate if dorsal and/or ventral)			
Parietal pleura			
Right			
Left			
Visceral pleura			
Right			
Left			
Pericardium			
Epicardium			
Thymus			
Parietal peritoneum			
Visceral peritoneum			
UPPER AIRWAY OBSTRUCTION			
Foreign body			
Mucus plug			
Other			
NECK SOFT TISSUE HEMORRHAGE			
HYOID BONE abnormal			
THYMUS			
Weight, gms			
Atrophy			
Other abnormalities			
EPIGLOTTIS abnormal			
LARYNX abnormal			
Narrowed lumen			
TRACHEA abnormal			
Stenosis			
Obstructive exudates			
Aspirated gastric contents			
ET tube tip location			
MAINSTEM BRONCHI abnormal			
Edema fluid			
Mucus plugs			
Gastric contents			
Inflammation			

DECEDENT'S NAME--

ACCESSION NUMBER---

COUNTY & COUNTRY--

PATHOLOGIST---

	YES	NO	NO EXAM
LUNGS			
Weight			
Right			gm
Left			gm
Abnormal			
Congestion, describe location, severity			
Hemorrhage, describe location, severity			
Edema, describe location			
Severity (circle)			
Consolidation, describe location, severity			
Anomalies			
Pulmonary artery			
Thromboembolization			
PLEURA abnormal			
RIBS abnormal			
Fractures			
with hemorrhages			
Callus formation			
Configuration abnormal			
DIAPHRAGM abnormal			
CARDIOVASCULAR SYSTEM			
Heart weight, gm			gm
Left ventricular thickness			cm
Right ventricular thickness			cm
Septal thickness maximum			cm
Mitral valve circumference			cm
Aortic valve circumference			cm
Tricuspid valve circumference			cm
Pulmonary valve circumference			cm
Myocardium abnormal			
Ventricular inflow/outflow tracts narrow			
Valvular vegetations/thromboses			
Aortic coarctation			
Patent ductus arteriosus			
Chamber blood (circle) fluid clotted			
Congenital heart disease			
Atrial septal defect			

DECEDENT'S NAME--

ACCESSION NUMBER---

COUNTY & COUNTRY---

PATHOLOGIST--

	YES	NO	NO EXAM
Ventricular septal defect			
Abnormal pulmonary venous connection			
Other			
Location of vascular cathether tips			
Occlusive vascular thrombosis locations			
Other abnormalities			
ESOPHAGUS abnormal			
STOMACH abnormal			
Describe contents and volume			
SMALL INTESTINE abnormal			
Hemorrhage			
Volvulus			
Describe contents			
COLON abnormal			
Congestion			
Hemorrhage			
Describe contents			
APPENDIX abnormal			
MESENTERY abnormal			
LIVER abnormal			
Weight			gm
GALLBLADDER abnormal			
PANCREAS abnormal			
SPLEEN abnormal			
Weight			
KIDNEYS abnormal			
Weight	███		
Right			gm
Left			gm
URETERS abnormal			
BLADDER abnormal			
Contents, volume			
PROSTATE abnormal			
UTERUS, F. TUBES, and OVARIES abnormal			

DECEDENT'S NAME--

ACCESSION NUMBER---

COUNTY & COUNTRY---

PATHOLOGIST--

	YES	NO	NO EXAM
THYROID abnormal			
ADRENALS abnormal			
Right			gm
Left			gm
Combined			gm
PITUITARY abnormal			
CONGENITAL ANOMALIES, INTERNAL			
CENTRAL NERVOUS SYSTEM			
Whole brain weight			
Fresh			gm
Fixed			gm
Combined cerebellum/brainstem weight			
Fresh			gm
Fixed			gm
Evidence of trauma			
Scalp abnormal			
Galea abnormal			
Fractures			
Anterior fontanelle abnormal			
Dimensions			
Calvarium abnormal			
Cranial sutures abnormal			
Closed (fused)			
Overriding			
Widened			
Base of skull abnormal			
Configuration abnormal			
Middle ears abnormal			
Foramen magnum abnormal			
Hemorrhage, estimate volumes (ml)			
Epidural			
Dural			
Subdural			
Subarachnoid			

DECEDENT'S NAME--
ACCESSION NUMBER--
COUNTY & COUNTRY--
PATHOLOGIST--

	YES	NO	NO EXAM
Intracerebral			
Cerebellum			
Brainstem			
Spinal cord			
Intraventricular			
Other			
Dural lacerations			
Dural sinus thrombosis			
BRAIN: IF EXTERNALLY ABNORMAL			
FIX BEFORE CUTTING			
Configuration abnormal			
Hydrocephalus			
Gyral pattern abnormal			
Cerebral edema			
Herniation			
Uncal			
Tonsillar			
Tonsillar necrosis			
Leptomeningeal exudates (culture)			
Cerebral contusions			
Malformations			
Cranial nerves abnormal			
Circle of Willis/basilar arteries abnormal			
Ventricular contours abnormal			
Cerebral infarction			
Contusional tears			
Other abnormalities			
SPINAL CORD			
Inflammation			
Contusion(s)			
Anomalies Other abnormalities			

DECEDENT'S NAME--

ACCESSION NUMBER--

COUNTY & COUNTRY--

PATHOLOGIST--

	YES	NO
MANDATORY SECTIONS TAKEN		
Skin, if lesions		
Thymus		
Lymph node		
Epiglottis, vertical		
Larynx, supraglottlc, transverse		
Larynx, true cords, transverse		
Trachea and thyroid, transverse		
Trachea at carina, transverse		
Lungs, all lobes		
Diaphragm		
Heart, septum and ventricles		
Esophagus, distal 3 cm		
Terminal ileum		
Rectum		
Liver		
Pancreas with duodenum		
Spleen		
Kidney with capsule		
Adrenal		
Rib with costochondral junction		
Submandibular gland		
Cervical spinal cord		
Rostral medulla junction		
Pons		
Midbrain		
Hippocampus		
Frontal lobe Cerebellum Choroid Plexus		

DECEDENT'S NAME--
ACCESSION NUMBER--
COUNTY & COUNTRY---
PATHOLOGIST--

	YES	NO
OIL RED O STAINED SECTIONS, IF INDICATED		
Heart		
Liver		
Muscle		
DISCRETIONARY MICROSCOPIC SECTIONS		
Supraglottic soft tissue		
Lung hilum		
Pancreatic tail		
Mesentery		
Stomach		
Colon		
Appendix		
Testes or ovaries		
Urinary bladder		
Psoas muscle		
Palatine tonsils		
Basal ganglia		
METABOLIC DISORDERS		
RETAIN ON FILTER PAPER IN ALL CASES		
Whole blood (I drop) Urine (I drop)		
Hair (taped down)		

DECEDENT'S NAME--
ACCESSION NUMBER--
COUNTY & COUNTRY--
PATHOLOGIST---

	YES	NO
TOXICOLOGY AND ELECTROLYTES		
FLUID AND TISSUES SAVED FOR 1 YEAR		
Whole blood and serum, save at -70°C and + 4°C		
Liver, save 100 gms at -700°C		
Frontal lobe, save at -70°C		
Urine, save at -700°C Bile		
Vitreous humor		
Serum		
Gastric contents		
Analyses performed, but not limited to:		
Cocaine and metabolites		
Morphine and metabolites		
Amphetamine and metabolites		
Volatiles (ethanol, acetone, etc.)		
Other indicated by history and exam		
FROZEN TISSUES, SAVE AT -70°C		
Lung		
Heart		
Liver		
Lymph node		

REFERENCES

Krous, H. (1995). An international standardised autopsy pro-
tocol for sudden unexpected infant death. In *Sudden Infant
Death Syndrome. New Trends in the Nineties*, ed. T. O. Rognum.
Oslo: Scandinavian University Press, pp. 81–95.

Krous, H. F. & Byard, R. W. (2001). International standardized
autopsy protocol for sudden unexpected infant death. In *Sudden Infant Death Syndrome. Problems, Progress and Possibilities*, ed. R. W. Byard & H. F. Krous. London: Arnold, pp.
319–33.

Appendix V: Autopsy checklist for possible non-accidental injury

Specific requirements:
- Complete body X-ray.
- Examination of mouth, eyes, palms, soles, genitalia, anus.
- Photography of all suspicious lesions.
- Shaving of hair and examination of underlying skin.
- Semen and microbiological swabs.
- Incision of livid areas.
- Representative sampling of wounds/bruises/fractures for histology.
- Excision of some wounds in toto.
- Removal of eyes in infants and young children.
- Toxicology.

Appendix VI: Autopsy checklist for possible metabolic disorders

Biochemical studies will be directed by histologic and electron-microscopic examinations. However, initially it is appropriate to collect as wide a range as possible of tissues and fluids. Many may not be needed, but those that are required must have been stored in a form that can be used (Bennett & Powell, 1994; Green & Hall, 1992; Moore *et al.*, 2000).

Specimens to be taken

- Urine
- Blood (10 ml):
  - with EDTA
  - with heparin
  - clotted
- Vitreous humour
- Skin or pericardium
- Other tissues – brain, heart, kidney, liver, skeletal muscle, adrenal gland

Minimum requirements

Urine, blood, skin, and liver.

Time interval

Although skin fibroblasts may still grow in tissue culture from specimens taken up to nine days after death (Vernon-Roberts, 1993), accurate tissue enzyme analysis requires specimens to be taken as soon after death as is practicable, i.e. within several hours of death. However, both MCAD and LCAD enzymes within liver tissue have been found to be stable for up to 100 hours if the body is refrigerated, and for at least five years if tissues are maintained at $-70\,°$C (Bennett *et al.*, 1990).

Method of taking and storing specimens

Urine

Withdrawn from the bladder by syringe after the abdominal cavity has been opened. If no urine can be obtained in this manner, the bladder can be opened, the renal pelvis can be aspirated, or urine may be squeezed from the diaper if this is otherwise clean. Storage is at $-70\,°$C in 1-ml aliquots for amino acid and organic acid analysis.

Blood

Blood with EDTA stored as whole blood. Heparinized blood centrifuged promptly to enable separate storage of packed cells and plasma in 1-ml aliquots. Stored at $-70\,°$C if possible, or at $-20\,°$C if not.

Vitreous humour

Withdrawn by syringe from the eye and sent for electrolyte and glucose analysis.

Skin or pericardium

Skin cleaned with alcohol and a 3.0×3.0-mm piece placed in sterile tissue transport media for fibroblast culture. Storage is possible at $-70\,^\circ$C if culture facilities are not available immediately.

Other tissues

- 1-mm cubes placed in 4% glutaraldehyde for electron microscopy.
- 10×1-cm^2 blocks snap frozen in liquid nitrogen and stored at $-70\,^\circ$C for biochemical assay/DNA analysis.
- 1-mm cubes quenched in liquid nitrogen and stored at $-70\,^\circ$C for enzyme histochemistry.
- 1-cm cubes of heart, liver, brain, muscle, adrenal gland, and kidney quenched in liquid nitrogen and stored at $-70\,^\circ$C for fat staining with Oil Red O.
- 5 g of spleen fresh or stored at $-70\,^\circ$C for DNA analysis.

REFERENCES

Bennett, M. J. & Powell, S. (1994). Metabolic disease and unexpected death. *Human Pathology*, **25**, 742–6.

Bennett, M. J., Allison, F., Pollitt, R. J. & Variend, S. (1990). Fatty acid oxidation defects as causes of unexpected death in infancy. *Progress in Clinical and Biological Research*, **321**, 349–64.

Green, A. & Hall, S. M. (1992). Investigation of metabolic disorders resembling Reye's syndrome. *Archives of Disease in Childhood*, **67**, 1313–17.

Moore, A., Debelle, G., Symonds, L. & Green, A. (2000). Investigation of sudden unexpected deaths in infancy. *Archives of Disease in Childhood*, **83**, 276.

Vernon-Roberts, E. (1993). Infant death due to congenital abnormalities presenting as homicide. *American Journal of Forensic Medicine and Pathology*, **14**, 208–11.

Appendix VII: Autopsy checklist for possible sepsis

Specimens that may be taken

- Blood: venous and arterial
- Cerebrospinal fluid
- Trachea swab/tissue
- Lung swab/tissue
- Liver swab/tissue
- Spleen swab/tissue
- Fecal swabs (multiple levels)
- Any other obviously infected/necrotic tissues
- In-dwelling catheters/devices

(Specimens taken for viral, bacterial, and fungal cultures.)

Autopsy sampling protocol for suspected fungal sepsis

See Figure AVII.1.

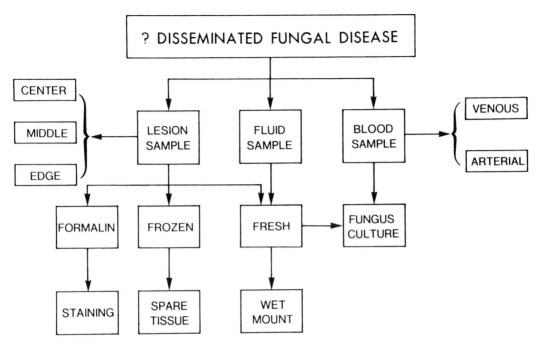

Figure AVII.1 Autopsy sampling protocol for suspected fungal sepsis.

Appendix VIII: Autopsy checklist for possible poisoning

Specimens to be taken
- Blood: cardiac and peripheral
- Gastric contents
- Fecal samples at multiple levels
- Urine
- Vitreous
- Gallbladder contents
- Liver
- Kidney
- Skeletal muscle
- Brain
- Liver
- Hair and nails

Index

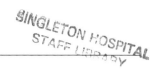

WITHDRAWN